I0030112

Boosting the Immune System

Natural Strategies to Supercharge Our Body's Immunity

By Case Adams, Naturopath

Boosting the Immune System: Natural Strategies to Supercharge Our Body's
    Immunity
Copyright © 2011, 2014, 2020, 2022 Case Adams
LOGICAL BOOKS
Wilmington, Delaware
http://www.logicalbooks.org
All rights reserved.
Printed in USA
Front cover image

The information provided in this book is for educational and scientific
research purposes only. The information is not medical advice and is not a
substitute for medical care or personal health advice. A medical practitioner or
other health expert should be consulted prior to any significant change in
lifestyle, diet, herbs or supplement usage. There shall neither be liability nor
responsibility should the information provided in this book be used in any
manner other than for the purposes of education and scientific research.

Publishers Cataloging in Publication Data
Adams, Case
        Boosting the Immune System: Natural Strategies to Supercharge Our
        Body's Immunity
First Edition
1. Medicine. 2. Health.
Bibliography and References; Index

ISBN-13: 978-1-936251-44-5

Other Books by the Author:

THE GLUTEN CURE: Scientifically Proven Natural Solutions to Celiac Disease and Gluten Sensitivities

THE HEALTHY BACK: Strategies for Low Back Pain (Course)

THE LIVING CLEANSE: Detoxification and Cleansing Using Living Foods and Safe Natural Strategies

THE MEANING OF DREAMS: The Science of Why We Dream, How to Interpret Them and How to Steer Them

THE SCIENCE OF LEAKY GUT SYNDROME: Intestinal Permeability and Digestive Health

TOTAL HARMONIC: The Healing Power of Nature's Elements

YOUR PLAN FOR LIFE: Personal Strategic Planning for Humans

Table of Contents

Introduction

Today our bodies are fighting a myriad of infections, outbreaks, autoimmune disorders, and other conditions. How will our bodies manage? With a strong immune system.

Yet immunosuppression is now at epidemic levels in modern society. What is causing this epidemic? What is causing all of the diseases that are borne from immunosuppression—many of which are fatal? And what can be done to turn the tide on this avalanche of inflammatory and immunity-related disorders?

Conventional medicine is utilizing an outmoded, out-dated perspective of the immune system. It's concept of immunity is a static system that assumes the immune system is solely run by legions of the body's immune cells, cytokines and immunoglobulins.

As we'll prove in this text, the immune system is more living than cellular. The immune system is not static. It is dynamic and alive with progressive probiotics that monitor and guard their territory with a vengeance.

That is, assuming our probiotic colonies are strong, and they are coordinated with the body's immune cells and processes.

This text advances this new vision of the immune system, together with those elements that depress it, and those elements that stimulate it. Here we will explore the science behind not only how the living immune system works, but how it can be damaged, how it can become immunosuppressed, and how it can be rejuvenated.

Towards this end we volunteer proven strategies that boost the living immune system. Most of these are supported by significant peer-reviewed research. This text is equipped to be scientifically substantial enough for the health professional to utilize, yet easy enough to understand for lay persons.

Nonetheless, the reader is advised to consult with their health professional before engaging any significant dietary, herbal or lifestyle changes: It is important to work with someone who understands our medical history and the relative risks of change.

With that's said, let's get right to it.

1

Chapter One

The Immune System

What weapons do our bodies have against the onslaught of bacteria, viruses, toxins and other invaders of the modern world? It seems that the combination of invasions into our body is practically insurmountable.

Yet nature has provided an answer. Nature has provided our bodies with not only an adaptive immune system, but a series of active combatants to swarm and overwhelm challenges to our body.

Why? Because these combatants want to protect their territory: Our bodies. These warriors, our antibodies, immune cells and probiotics, happen to be more prevalent in our bodies than our own tissue cells. We have between 30 and 40 trillion cells in the body but a healthy person will have as much as 70 trillion probiotic bacteria in and on the body. That means that our active body is comprised, two to one, of probiotics.

This also means that our body's immune system is more probiotic than cellular.

Yes, our probiotics also outnumber our immune cells. Our body contains some 25 billion immune cells. Many of these are in the bloodstream, but also billions of immune cells inhabit in our lymphatic system, organs, mucosal membranes and tissues.

In this chapter, we'll cover the body's immune system, including our own immune cells and our probiotic colonies.

When a toxin enters our body, our immune system immediately begins to reject it. This is because the living immune system recognizes the foreigner immediately. How does this happen? In this chapter, we'll show how the body's natural detoxification system works. This will help us understand how we can better utilize and even stimulate the immune system later.

The immune system is really located throughout the body. We find immune cells on the skin, in the blood, in the lungs, in the bones and in every organ system. We also find the immune system within trillions of probiotic bacteria scattered around the body.

The immune system has a number of intelligent abilities. The first is recognition. The immune system has the facility to recognize molecules that endanger the body's welfare. The immune system also maintains memory. The immune system can remember the identity of a toxin or pathogen by virtue of recognizing its antigens (byproducts or molecular structure). This is the rationale for vaccination. Vaccination exposes the body to a small amount of a particular pathogen so the immune system will develop the tools and the memory to recognize its antigens, so that the body can respond appropriately the next time it is exposed to the same pathogen.

The immune system is incredible in its ability to maintain specificity and diversity. These characteristics allow the immune system to respond to literally millions, if not billions of different antigens. Moreover, each particular antigen requires a completely different response.

The immune system is an intelligent scanning and review system intended to gauge whether a particular molecule, cell or organism belongs in the body. This is determined through a complex biochemical identification system. We might compare this system to an iris scan, often used as a password entry system. Utilizing a database of information, the immune system checks molecular structures against this database. If the molecular structure isn't recognized, or matches a structure considered foreign, the immune system launches an attack. This attack is referred to as an immune response or an inflammatory response.

Despite significant research in the areas of vaccination, antibiotics, and inflammation, modern medical science is still perplexed with the autoimmune syndrome. A massive list of degenerative diseases are now considered autoimmune, including irritable bowel syndrome, Crohn's, asthma, allergies, fibromyalgia, lupus, urinary tract disorders and many, many others. Physicians also classify most types of arthritis as autoimmune disorders. Why can't the immune system repair these disorders, as it does with most other types of injuries? What has gone wrong with the immune system in these cases? How about in a body that is overwhelmed with toxins?

Chemical toxins also invade the body via the digestive tract, the nose and sinuses, the genitals, the lungs, the skin, the ears and even the eyes. Microbial infections can also be caused by normal residents of the body, should they grow beyond their typical populations. These include *H. pylori*, *E. coli* and *Candida albicans*. These are also considered by the body as toxins, because these foreigners must be cleared from the body or otherwise controlled.

There are four processes the body uses to guard against and remove toxins:

Non-specific Immunity

The first is called the *non-specific* immune response. This utilizes a network of biochemical barriers that work synergistically to prevent infectious agents from getting into the body. The barrier structures include the ability of the body to shut down its orifices. We can close our eyes, mouths, noses and ears to prevent invaders or toxins from entering the body. Within these lie further defensive structures: Nose hairs, eyelashes, lips, tonsils, ear hair, pubic hair and hair in general are all designed to help screen out and filter invaders. Most of the body's passageways are also equipped with tiny cilia, which assist the body evacuate invaders by brushing them out. These cilia move rhythmically, sweeping back and forth, working caught pathogens outward with their undulations. The surfaces of most of the body's orifices are also covered with a mucous membrane. This thin liquid membrane film contains a combination of biochemicals and cells that prevent invaders from penetrating any further. These mucous membranes lining the passageways accomplish this with a combination of immune cells, immunoglobulins and colonies of probiotics.

The digestive tract is equipped with another type of sophisticated defense technology. Should any foreigners get through the lips, teeth, tongue, hairs, mucous membranes, cilia and sneak down the esophagus, they then must contend with the digestive fire of the stomach. The gastrin, peptic acid and hydrochloric acid within a healthy stomach keep a pH of around two. This is typically enough acidity to kill or significantly damage many bacteria. However, a person can mistakenly weaken this protective acid by taking antacids or acid-blockers. In this case, the stomach's ability to neutralize pathogens will be handicapped. In addition, a number of microorganisms are accustomed to acidic environments, and still others can tuck away into clumps of food—especially food that has not been chewed well enough.

Humoral Immunity

The second form of immune response involves a highly technical strategic attack that first identifies the invader's weaknesses, followed by a precise and immediate offensive attack to exploit those weaknesses. This is often called humoral immunity. More than a billion different types of antibodies, macrophages and other immune cells mobilize and execute specific attack plans. As an immune cell scans a particular invader, it may recognize a particular biomolecular or behavioral weakness within the toxin or pathogen. Upon recognizing this weakness, the immune system will devise a unique plan to exploit this weakness. It may launch a variety of possible attacks, using a combination of specialized B-cells (or *B-lymphocytes*) in conjunction with specialized antibodies.

Cruising through the blood and lymph systems, the antibodies and/or B-cells can quickly sense and size up invading microbes. Often this will mean the antibody will lock onto or bind to the invader to extract critical molecular information. This process will often draw upon databases held within certain helper B-cells that memorize vulnerabilities. The specific vulnerability is often revealed by molecular structures of pathogenic cell membranes. Each pathogen will be identified by these unique structures or antigens. The B-cell then reproduces a specific antibody designed to record and communicate that information to other B-cells through biochemical transception. This allows for a constant tracking of the location and development of pathogens, allowing B-cells to manage and constantly assess the response.

Cell-Mediated Immunity: Detoxing the Cells

The third process used by the immune system is the cell-mediated immune response. This also incorporates a collection of smart white blood cells, called T-cells. T-cells and their surrogates wander the body scanning the body's own cells. They are seeking cells that have become infected or otherwise damaged by microbes or toxic free radicals. Infected cells are typically identified by special marker molecules (antigens) that sit atop their cell membranes. These antigens have particular molecular arrangements that signal roving T-cells of the damage that has occurred within the cell. Once a damaged cell has been recognized, the cell-mediated immune system will launch an inflammatory response against the cell. This response will typically utilize a variety of cytotoxic (cell-killing) cells and helper T-cells. These types of immune cells will often directly kill the damaged cell by inserting toxic chemicals into it. Alternatively, the T-cell might send signals into the damaged cell, switching on a self-destruct mechanism within the cell.

Probiotics

The fourth and most powerful part of the immune system takes place among the body's probiotics. This is the backbone of the living immune system, because our probiotics drive many of our immune processes.

The human body can house more than 32 billion beneficial and harmful bacteria and fungi at any particular time. When beneficial bacteria are in the majority, they constitute up to 70-80% of the body's immune response. This takes place both in an isolated manner and in conjunction with the rest of the immune system.

Probiotic colonies work with the body's internal immune system to organize strategies that prevent toxins and pathogenic microorganisms from harming the body. Probiotics will communicate and cooperate with the immune system to organize cooperative strategies. They will stimulate the body's immune cells, activating the cell-mediated response, the humoral response, and indirectly, the body's exterior barrier mechanisms through immunoglobulin stimulation. As we will see in the research, they stimulate T-cells, B-cells, macrophages and NK-cells with smart messages that promote specific immune responses. They also activate cytokines and phagocytic cells directly to coordinate their intelligent immune response.

Probiotics can also quickly identify harmful bacteria or fungal overgrowths and work directly to eradicate them. This process may not directly involve the rest of the immune system. Even still, the immune system will be notified of any probiotic offensives. The immune system will support the process by breaking up and escorting dead pathogens out of the body.

Probiotics produce chemical substances that destroy invading microorganisms. Probiotics make up our body's own antibiotic system. Because probiotics are extremely intelligent and want to survive, they have developed various strategies to defend their homeland (our body). It is a territorial issue. Invading bacteria threaten their homes and families. Probiotics also learn how to fight newer bacteria species and new bacteria strategies. While static pharmaceutical antibiotics are counteracted by smart super-bugs, probiotics can alter their antibiotic strategies as needed. Our continued survival illustrates their intelligence.

Probiotics produce antimicrobial biochemicals that manage, damage or kill pathogenic microorganisms. In some cases, they will simply overcrowd the invaders with biochemistry and populations to limit their growth. In other cases, they will secrete chemicals into the fluid environment to eradicate large populations. In still other cases, they will insert specific chemicals into the invaders, which will directly kill them. Probiotic mechanisms are quite complex and variegated to say the least.

Dr. Mechnikov hypothesized that the beneficial effects of lactobacilli arise from the lactic acid they excrete. Indeed, the lactic acid produced by *Lactobacillus* and *Bifidobacteria* species sets up the ultimate pH control in the gut to repel antagonistic organisms. Lactic acids are not alike, however. There are different lactic acid molecular structures, and combinations with other chemicals. For example, some probiotics produce an L(+) form of lactic acid and other probiotics may produce the D(-) from. Many probiotic strains also produce a molecular combination with hydrogen peroxide called lactoperoxidase.

Probiotics also produce acetic acids, formic acids, special lipopolysaccharides, peptidoglycans, superantigens, heat shock proteins and bacterial DNA—all in precise portions to nourish each other, inhibit challengers and/or benefit the host.

Precision and proportion is the key. For example, some bifidobacteria secrete a 3:2 proportion of acetic acid to lactic acid in order to barricade certain pathogenic microbes.

Probiotics also secrete a number of key nutrients crucial to its host's (our body) immune system and metabolism, including B vitamins pantothenic acid, pyridoxine, niacin, folic acid, cobalamin and biotin, and crucial antioxidants such as vitamin K.

Probiotics also produce antimicrobial molecules called bacteriocins. *Lactobacillus plantarum* produces lactolin. *Lactobacillus bulgaricus* secretes bulgarican. *Lactobacillus acidophilus* can produce acidophilin, acidolin, bacterlocin and lactocidin. These and other antimicrobial substances equip probiotic species with territorial mechanisms to combat and reduce pathologies related to *Shigella, Coliform, Pseudomonas, Klebsiella, Staphylococcus, Clostridium, Escherichia* and other infective genera. Furthermore, antifungal biochemicals from the likes of *L. acidophilus, B. bifidum, E. faecium* and others also significantly reduce fungal outbreaks caused by *Candida albicans* (Shahani *et al.* 2005).

These types of antimicrobial tools give probiotics the ability to counter the mighty *H. pylori* bacterium—known to be at the root of a majority of ulcers. *H. pylori* inhibition has been observed in studies on *L. acidophilus* DDS-1, *L. rhamnosus* GG, *L. rhamnosus Lc705, Propionibacterium freudenreichii* and *Bifidobacterium breve Bb99,* as we will see later.

Furthermore, probiotics will specifically stimulate the body's own immune system to attack pathogens. For example, scientists from Finland's University of Turku (Pessi *et al.* 2000) gave nine atopic dermatitis children *Lactobacillus rhamnosus* GG for four weeks. They found that serum cytokine IL-10 levels specific to the infection increased following probiotic consumption.

Whatever the strategy, smart probiotic microorganisms work collectively and synergistically with the other three components of our immune system. Our probiotic system works within the non-specific immune system to help protect the body from invasions. Probiotics live within the oral cavity, the nasal cavity, the esophagus, around the gums, and in pockets of our pleural cavity (surrounding our lungs). They dwell within our stomach, within our intestines, within the vagina and around the rectum, and amongst other pockets of tissues. This means that for microbes to invade the bloodstream, they must first get through legions of probiotic bacteria that populate those entry channels—assuming a healthy body of course.

Probiotics participate deeply in immune activity. In one study, the probiotic organism *Bifidobacterium lactis* HN019 or a placebo was given to 30 healthy elderly volunteers (average age 69 years old) for nine weeks. The probiotic group had significant increases among total T-cells, helper T-cells (CD4+), activated (CD25+) T-cells, and natural killer T-cells. Cytotoxic capacity among mononuclear and polymorphonuclear phagocytes and tumor-cell killing activity among natural killer cells also increased among the probiotic group (Gill *et al.* 2001).

Probiotics modulate the inflammatory Th1/Th2 system. Illustrating this, yogurt with *Bifidobacterium longum* BB536 or plain yogurt was given to 40 patients with Japanese cedar pollinosis for 14 weeks. Peripheral blood mononuclear cells from the patients indicated that *B. fragilis* microorganisms induced significantly more helper TH cell type2 cytokines such as interleukin [IL]-6, and fewer Th1 cytokines such as IL-12 and interferon (Odamaki *et al.* 2007).

Probiotics utilize cytokine communications to transmit intelligent information to the body's network of white blood cells. Illustrating this, Scientists from the Slovak Institute of Cardiovascular Diseases (Hlivak *et al.* 2005) gave a placebo or probiotic *Enterococcus faecium* M-74 to human volunteers for 60 weeks. Peripheral blood analysis indicated significant decreases in cytokines sICAM-1, CD54 on monocytes, and CD11b on lymphocytes after one-year. These are related to anti-adhesion strategies following inflammatory responses to artery damage.

In order to better understand the relationship between probiotics and our immune system, let's discuss the other players among the body's immune system and their interaction with our probiotic populations.

Immune Cells

The immune system produces at least five different types of white blood cells. Each is designed to identify and target specific types of pathogens. After identification, they will either initiate an attack with other components, or directly begin their attack. The main types are lymphocytes, neutrophils, basophils, monocytes and macrophages. Each plays an important role in the pathogen-identification and inflammatory process. Lymphocytes are the body's self-specific immune response team.

The primary lymphocytes are the T-cells (thymus cells) or B-cells (bone marrow cells). These cells and their specialized proteins work together to strategically attack and remove invaders. Then they memorize the strategy in preparation for a future invasion.

All white blood cells are initially assembled by stem cells in the bone marrow. Following their release, T-cells undergo further differentiation and programming in the thymus gland. B-cells undergo a similar process of maturity before release from the spleen. Both T-cells and B-cells circulate via lymph nodes, the bloodstream and among tissue fluids. Both also have a number of special types, including memory cells and helper cells to identify and memorize invaders.

B-cells look for foreign or potentially harmful pathogens moving freely. These might include toxins or microbes. Once identified, B-cells will stimulate the production of a particular type of antibody protein, which is designed to destroy or break apart the foreigner. There are several different types of B-cells. Most are monoclonal, which means they will adjust to the specific type of invader. Some B-cells are investigative and surveillance oriented. They are focused on roaming pathogens. Once activated, they can then damage these invading pathogens using a variety of biochemical secretions or physical activities. B-cells that circulate and surveil the bloodstream are often called plasma B-cells. Others—like memory B-cells—record previous invasions for future attacks.

T-cells, on the other hand, are oriented toward the body's own cells. They are focused upon internal cellular problems, toxin absorption, or those pathogens that have invaded cells.

There are different types of T-cells. Each is programmed in the thymus to look for a different type of problem, and each has the capability of destroying different types of cells and infections. Many T-cells simply respond to a pathogen that has invaded the cell by destroying the cell itself—this is the *killer* T-cell. It does this by inserting special chemicals into the cell or submitting instructions for the cell to kill itself. Cell death is called apoptosis, and T-cells capable of killing our cells are called cytotoxic T-cells and natural killer T-cells.

T-cells work through a communication system of cytokines to relay instructions and information amongst the various T-cells. Prominent cytokine communications thus take place between helper T-cells, natural killer cells and cytotoxic T-cells.

The initial scanning of an infected cell by a helper T-cell utilizes electromagnetic scanning just as the B-cells do. The T-cell's support network also includes delta-gamma T-cells. Delta-gamma T-cells are stimulated by specific molecular receptors on cell membranes. In general, helper T-cells communicate previous immune responses, memorize current ones, and pass on strategic information on the progress of pending attack plans.

The helper T-cell scan surveys the cell's membrane for indications of either microbial infection or some sort of genetic mutation due to a virus or toxin. This antigen scan might reveal invasions of chemical toxins, protozoa, worms, fungi, bacteria and viruses that have intruded or deranged the cell. The scanning helper T-cell immediately communicates the information by releasing their tiny coded protein cytokines. These disseminate the information needed to coordinate macrophages, NK-cells and cytotoxic T-cells for attack.

Most cells contain tumor necrosis factor or TNF—a sort of self-destruct switch. When signaled from the outside by a T-cell, TNF will initiate a self-destruct and the cell will die.

Under some circumstances, entire groups of cells or tissue systems may be damaged. Macrophages may be signaled to cut off the blood supply to kill these deranged or infected cells.

The two primary helper T-cell types are the Th1 and the Th2. The Th1 T-cell focuses on the elimination of bacteria, fungi, parasites, viruses, and similar types of invaders. The Th2 cells, on the other hand, are focused upon allergic and antibody responses. The Th2 is thus explicitly involved in the responses of inflammation and allergic reaction. This is important to note, because research has revealed that stress, chemical toxins, poor dietary habits and lack of sleep tend to suppress Th1 levels and increase Th2 levels. With an abundance of Th2 cells in the system, the body is prone to respond more strongly to allergens and toxins, causing problems like hay fever and allergies. This is why we sometimes see people who are under physical or emotional stress overreacting with hives, psoriasis and other allergic-type responses.

Neutrophils are white blood cells that circulate within the blood stream, looking for abnormal behavior among various cells and tissues. Once they identify a problem, they will signal a mass assembly and begin the process of cleaning the area. This typically involves inflammation, as they work to break down and remove debris.

Neutrophils are also coordinated by probiotics. Researchers from the Liver Failure Group and The Institute of Hepatology at the University College London's Medical School (Stadlbauer *et al.* 2008) found in a study of 20 liver failure patients that neutrophil function and cytokines were significantly modulated by the probiotic *Lactobacillus casei* Shirota. Starting neutrophil phagocytic capacity was significantly lower than healthy controls (73% versus 98%) before probiotic treatment. Neutrophil phagocytic capacity after probiotic treatments were equal between the cirrhosis patients and the healthy volunteers at the end of the study— while the placebo group's neutrophil capacity did not change. In addition, endotoxin-stimulated TNF-receptors 1 and 2 and interleukin-10 (IL-10) levels were significantly lower among the probiotic group. The scientists concluded: "Our data provide a proof-of-concept that probiotics restore neutrophil phagocytic capacity in cirrhosis, possibly by changing IL10 secretion and TLR4 expression."

Monocytes are like the neolithic ancestors of the attack soldiers. After being produced in the marrow, monocytes differentiate into either macrophages or dendrite cells. The macrophages are particularly good at engulfing and breaking apart pathogens. Dendritic cells are interactive cells that stimulate certain responses. They may, for example, isolate and present a pathogen to the T-cells. Dendritic cells also stimulate the production of those special inter-white blood cell communication proteins called cytokines.

Coordinators

As mentioned, cytokines are communication devices that allow different immune cells to communicate. These typically come with complex names like interleukin (IL), transforming growth factor (TGF), leukemia inhibitory factor (LIF), and tumor necrosis factor (TNF). There are five basic types of cell communication: intracrine, autocrine, endocrine, juxtacrine and paracrine.

Autocrine communication takes place between two different types of cells. This message can be a biochemical exchange or an electromagnetic signal. The other cell in turn may respond automatically by producing a particular biochemical or electromagnetic message. We might compare this to leaving a voicemail on someone's message machine. Once we leave the message, the machine signals that the message has been received and will be delivered. Later the machine will replay the message. The immune system uses this type of autocrine message recording process to activate T-cells. Once the message is relayed, the T-cell will respond specifically with the instructed activity.

A paracrine communication takes place between neighboring cells of the same type, to pass on a message that comes from outside of the tissue system. Tiny protein antennas will sit on cell membranes, allowing one cell to communicate with another. This allows cells within the same tissue system to respond in a coordinated manner.

Juxtacrine communications take place via smart biomolecular structures. We might call these structures relay stations. They absorb messages and pass them on. An example of this is the passing of inflammatory messages via immune cell cytokines.

An intracrine communication takes place within the cell. First, an external message may be communicated into the cell through an antenna sitting on the cell's membrane. Once inside the cell, the message will be communicated around cell's organelles to initiate internal metabolic responses.

The endocrine message takes place between endocrine glands and individual cells. The endocrine glands include the pineal gland, the pituitary gland, the pancreas, adrenals, thyroid, ovary and testes. These glands produce endocrine biochemicals, which relay messages directly to cells. Their messages stimulate a variety of metabolic functions within the body. These include growth, temperature, sexual behavior, sleep, glucose utilization, stress response and so many others. One of the functions of the endocrine glands relevant to disease is the production of inflammatory co-factors such as cortisol, adrenaline and norepinephrine. These coordinate and initiate instructions that stimulate inflammatory processes.

Probiotics utilize these systems to communicate with the body's various cells. They utilize paracrine and juxtacrine communications to pass on messages about the location, type and weaknesses of invading organisms. These messages are then compared with the programmed history within helper T-cells and helper B-cells. This creates a coordinated response. For example, the immune system might launch phagocytic cells to help attack the pathogens a probiotic colony may be battling.

Scientists from the Nagoya University Graduate School of Medicine's Department of Surgery (Sugawara *et al.* 2006) found in a study of 101 patients that supplementation with probiotics increased NK activity and lymphocyte counts. Pro-inflammatory IL-6 cytokines decreased significantly among the probiotic group. Serum IL-6, white blood cell counts, and C-reactive protein also significantly decreased among the probiotic group.

Furthermore, probiotics have the ability to *uniquely modify* cytokines depending upon the condition and disease of the person. Illustrating this, a probiotic drink with either placebo or a probiotic combination of *Lactobacillus paracasei* Lpc-37, *Lactobacillus acidophilus* 74-2 and *Bifidobacterium animalis* subsp. *lactis* DGCC 420 (*B. lactis* 420) was given to 15 healthy adults and 15 adults with atopic dermatitis. After 8 weeks, CD57(+) cytokines levels increased significantly among the healthy group taking probiotics, while CD4(+)CD54(+) cytokines decreased significantly among the AD patients who were taking the probiotics, compared with the placebo group and compared to the levels at the beginning of the trial (Roessler *et al.* 2008).

Immunoglobulins

Immunoglobulins are proteins that are programmed for a particular type of response in the presence of particular pathogens in different areas and maturity. IgA immunoglobulins line the mouth and digestive tract, scanning for pathogens that might infect the body. IgDs sense infections and activate B-cells. IgEs attach to foreign substances and launch histamine responses—typically associated with allergic responses. IgGs cross through membranes, responding to growing pathogens that have already invaded the body. IgMs are focused on new intrusions that have yet to grow enough to garner the attention of the IgGs.

Each of these general immunoglobulin categories contain numerous sub-types geared to different types of pathogens and responses. Other immunoglobulin proteins also exist. Some of these aid macrophages and lymphocytes in identifying specific pathogens.

An element of immunoglobulins is the CD glycogen-protein complex. CD stands for cluster of differentiation. CDs are molecules that sit on top of immune cells to navigate and steer their behavior. They will sit atop T-cells, B-cells, NK-cells, granulocytes and monocytes, identifying pathogens and infected cells. They often negotiate and bind to pathogens. This allows the lymphocyte to proceed to attack the pathogen, often by inserting a toxic chemical that destroys the pathogen or the cell hosting it.

CDs are identified by their molecular structure: This is also referred to as a ligand. The specific molecular arrangement (or CD number) will also match a specific type of receptor at the membrane of the cell or pathogen. Each CD number will produce a bonding relationship with a certain receptor structure on the cell to allow the accompanying immunoglobulin or lymphocyte to have interactivity with the pathogen. This gives the immunoglobulin or lymphocyte an access point from which to attack the pathogen.

Immunoglobulins and CDs are also tools probiotics utilize to define or influence appropriate responses for the immune system. Probiotics stimulate IgAs through CDs, for example, when they discover a pathogen has invaded parts of the body's entry passageways.

CDs are also utilized by our body's probiotics to define the cells and tissue systems that have been damaged by toxins, bacteria, or viruses. Probiotics will respond appropriately, signalling back and forth with the immune system. This signalling often stimulates particular inflammatory and injury-healing responses.

Illustrating this, Finnish scientists (Ouwehand *et al.* 2009) gave healthy elderly volunteers lactitol (a milk sugar) with *Lactobacillus acidophilus* or a placebo. The group given the probiotics showed a significant modification of pro-inflammatory IgA and PGE2 levels. The researchers also noticed that levels of bifidobacteria in the stool of the elderly subjects were similar to those of a young person—as usually bifidobacteria colonies are reduced among the elderly. They also observed improved spermidine levels—an enzyme involved in DNA synthesis. These improvements suggested increased mucosal and intestinal immunity and probiotic content among the probiotic group.

In a study of 105 pregnant women, University of Western Australia scientists (Prescott *et al.* 2008) found that *Lactobacillus rhamnosus* and *Bifidobacterium lactis* stimulated higher levels of cytokine IFN-gamma, higher levels of TGF-beta1, and higher levels of breast milk IgA. Plasma of their babies had lower CD14 levels, and greater CB IFN-gamma levels. These indicated improvements in immune response stimulated by the probiotics.

In another example, researchers from the Turku University Central Hospital in Finland (Rinne *et al.* 2005) gave 96 mothers either a placebo or *Lactobacillus rhamnosus* GG before delivery and continued the supplementation in their infants after delivery. At three months of age, immunoglobulin IgG-secreting cells among breastfed infants supplemented with probiotics were significantly higher than the breastfed infants who received the placebo. In addition, IgM-, IgA-, and IgG-secreting cell counts at 12 months were significantly higher among the breastfed infants who supplemented with probiotics, compared to breastfed infants receiving the placebo.

In yet another example, researchers from the Teikyo University School of Medicine in Japan (Araki *et al.* 1999) gave *Bifidobacterium breve* YIT4064 or placebo to 19 infants for 28 days. Rotavirus shedding in the feces of the probiotic group was significantly reduced compared to the placebo group. IgA levels also significantly changed among the probiotic group.

The Thymus

One of the most important players in the body's purging of toxins is the thymus gland. The thymus gland is located in the center of the chest, behind the sternum. The thymus is one of the more critical organs of the lymphatic system. Some have compared the thymus gland of the lymphatic system to the heart of the circulatory system.

The thymus gland is not a pump, however. The thymus activates T-cells and various hormones that modulate and stimulate the immune and autoimmune processes. The thymus converts a type of lymphocyte called the thymocyte into T-cells or natural killer cells. These activated T-cells are released into the lymph and bloodstream ready to protect and serve. Within the thymus, the T-cells are infused with CD surface markers—which identify particular types of problematic cells or invading organisms. The CD markers define their mission.

In other words, the thymus codes the T-cells with receptors that will bind to particular toxins and the cells that have been invaded or damaged by toxins. The types of cells or toxins they bind to or identify are determined by the major histocompatibility complex, or MHC determinant. During the process of converting thymocytes to T-cells, their receptors are programmed with MHC combinations. This allows them to tolerate particular frailties within the body while attacking what the body considers to be true invaders (Kazansky 2008).

Therefore, it is the MHC that gives the T-cell the ability to identify the difference between *self* and *non-self* parts of the body. A non-self identification will produce an immunogen—a factor that stimulates an immune response. Once the immunogen is processed, it stimulates the inflammatory cascade.

The thymus gland develops and enlarges from birth. It is most productive and at its largest during puberty. From that point on, depending upon our diet, stress and lifestyle, our thymus gland will shrink over the years. By forty, an immunosuppressed person will often have a tiny thymus gland. In elderly persons, the thymus gland is often barely recognizable. For some, the thymus is practically non-functional.

Throughout its productive life, the thymus gland processes T-cells with the appropriate MHC programming. If the thymus gland is functioning, it will continue to produce T-cells with MHC programming that reflects the body's current status. The revised programming will accommodate the various genetic changes that can happen to different cells around the body as we age and adapt to our changing environment. With a shrunken and non-functioning thymus, however, its ability to re-program T-cells with a new MHC—enabling them to identify the body's cells that have adapted—is damaged. The T-cells will have to keep working off the old MHC programming. This means the T-cells will not be able to properly identify self versus non-self.

Herein we find at least part of the solution to the mystery of autoimmune disease.

Probiotics, on the other hand, stimulate a healthy thymus gland. Illustrating this, medical researchers from the University of Bari (Indrio *et al.* 2007) gave a placebo or a probiotic combination of *Bifidobacterium breve* C50 and *Streptococcus thermophilus* 065 to 60 newborns in a randomized, placebo-controlled study on thymus size. Thymus size was significantly larger in the probiotic group compared to the standard formula (placebo) group after the probiotic treatment period.

The Liver

The liver is the body's most important detoxifying organ. The liver is a blood filtering mechanism, where it screens out many toxins. The liver also produces numerous enzymes and proteins that break down and otherwise metabolize toxins.

The liver sits just below the lungs on the right side under the diaphragm. Partially protected by the ribs, it attaches to the abdominal wall with the falciform ligament. The ligamentum teres within the falciform is the remnant of the umbilical cord that once brought us blood from mama's placenta. As the body develops, the liver continues to filter, purify and enrich our blood. Should the liver shut down, the body would die within hours.

Into the liver drains nutrition-rich venous blood through the hepatic portal vein together with some oxygenated blood through the hepatic artery. A healthy liver will process almost a half-gallon of blood per minute. The blood is commingled within well cavities called sinusoids, where blood is staged through stacked sheets of the liver's primary cells— called hepatocytes. Here blood is also met by interspersed immune cells called kupffers. These kupffer cells attack and break apart bacteria and toxins. Nutrients coming in from the digestive tract are filtered and converted to molecules the body's cells can utilize. The liver also converts old red blood cells to bilirubin to be shipped out of the body. Filtered and purified blood is jettisoned through hepatic veins out the inferior vena cava and back into circulation.

The liver's filtration/purification mechanisms protect our body from various infectious diseases and chemical toxins. After hepatocytes and kuppfer cells break down toxins, the waste is disposed through the gall bladder and kidneys. The gall bladder channels bile from the liver to the intestines. Recycled bile acids combine with bilirubin, phospholipids, calcium and cholesterol to make bile. Bile is concentrated and pumped through the bile duct to the intestines. Here bile acids help digest fats, and broken down toxins are (hopefully) excreted through our feces. Assuming we have healthy probiotic colonies within the intestines.

The liver produces over a thousand biochemicals the body requires for healthy functioning. The liver maintains blood sugar balance by monitoring glucose levels and producing glucose metabolites. It manufactures albumin to maintain plasma pressure. It produces cholesterol, urea, inflammatory biochemicals, blood-clotting molecules, and many others.

Interspersed within the liver are functional fat factories called stellates. These cells store and process lipids, fat-soluble vitamins such as vitamin A, and secrete structural biomolecules like collagen, laminin and glycans. These are used to build some of the body's toughest tissue systems.

We know that our livers become burdened from the avalanche of toxins pelting our bodies. Today our diets, water and air are full of plasticizers, formaldehyde, heavy metals, hydrocarbons, DDT, dioxin, VOCs, asbestos, preservatives, artificial flavors, food dyes, propellants, synthetic fragrances and more. Every single chemical requires the liver to work harder.

Frankly, most livers are now overloaded and beyond their natural capacity. What happens then? Generally, two things. First, the hepatocytes collapse from overtoxification, causing genetic mutation, cell death, and liver exhaustion. Secondly, their weakened condition opens hepatocytes to diseases from infectious agents such as viral hepatitis.

Liver disease—where one or more lobes begin to malfunction—can result in a life-threatening emergency. Cirrhosis is a common diagnosis for liver disease, often caused by years of drinking alcohol or taking prescription medications. During its downfall into cirrhosis, the sub-functioning liver can also cause jaundice, high cholesterol, gallstones, encephalopathy, kidney disease, clotting problems, heart conditions, hormone imbalances and many others. As cirrhosis proceeds, it results in the liver cells' massive die-off and subsequent scarring, causing the liver to begin to shutdown.

While most of us have heard about the damage alcohol can have on the liver, many do not realize that pharmaceuticals and even some supplements can also be extremely toxic to the liver. The liver must find a way to break down these foreign chemicals. Many pharmaceuticals require a Herculean effort simply because the liver's various purification processes were not designed for these foreign molecules. As liver cells weaken and die their enzymes leak into the bloodstream. Blood tests for AST and ALT enzymes can reveal this weakening of the liver.

We must therefore closely monitor the quantity and types of chemicals we put into our body. Eliminating preservatives, food dyes and pesticides in our foods can be done easily by eating whole organic foods. We can eliminate exposures to many environmental toxins mentioned above by simply replacing them with natural alternatives.

A number of herbs help detoxify and strengthen the liver. These include goldenseal, dandelion, milk thistle and others.

Probiotics also play a large role in liver disease. When pathogenic bacteria get out of control in the intestines, they can overload the liver with endotoxins—their waste products. The bombardment of endotoxins onto the liver produces a result similar to alcohol or pharmaceuticals: When complex proteins (such as found in animal products) are putrefied by pathogenic bacteria, one of the metabolites is excessive ammonia. Ammonia is toxic to the liver.

In addition, urea is metabolized by pathogenic bacteria such as *Clostridium* spp., resulting in ammonia and carbon dioxide. Liver cells are damaged by this onslaught of endotoxins and metabolites produced by pathogenic bacteria.

In a study from scientists at the G.B. Pant Hospital in New Delhi (Sharma *et al.* 2008), 190 cirrhosis patients were given a combination of probiotics for one month. The probiotic group experienced a 51.6% improvement in symptoms, as measured by psychometric testing and blood ammonia levels.

Immune Respiration

Our lungs provide one of the body's most effective means of immunity, as well as an active filtering mechanism that screens out toxins.

With every breath, we purge the body of toxins. The epithelial cells of our airways house sub-mucosal ducts that push toxins out to the mucous membranes. As we breathe out and as our mucous is channeled out, we send these toxins out.

In addition, the lungs filter and prevent the body from inheriting more toxins. As air moves through the nostrils through to the *pharynx*, the *larynx* and the *trachea,* it passes over a mucous membrane lined with tiny hairs called *cilia.* These cilia capture foreign particles with a web of sticky mucous. After being stuck, the particles are gathered up within the mucous. The tiny cilia hairs will undulate the mucous and foreign particles towards exit points like the throat, nostrils and mouth. At these points, the particles can be sneezed or coughed out as phlegm, blown out through the nose, or swallowed down into the acidic abyss of the stomach.

More offensive particles like bacteria and viruses are attacked by the macrophages and probiotics that line the mucous membranes. They break down the foreigners and escort their parts out of the body. These may travel out with the mucous, or be absorbed into the lymph or blood and pushed out through urine, sweat or the colon.

About 97% of our incoming oxygen is delivered to the cells by hemoglobin molecules. After being escorted through the micro-capillaries to the cells, the oxygen disassociates from the hemoglobin. Only about 20% of oxygen disassociates from hemoglobin while we rest. More disassociates as needed. The rest stays in the bloodstream, on standby. This standby oxygen effectively alkalizes the blood, inhibiting oxidative radicals with the presence of O_2.

Cellular respiration proceeds in a process called *oxidative phosphorylation.* Here the two-phosphate ADP combines with oxygen and another phosphate atom to form a triple phosphate (ATP) structure. The resulting electromagnetic energy produced is held within the phosphate-oxygen bond. Once in ATP form, glucose interacts with one of the phosphates to release ADP, glucose 6-p along with heat and energy for metabolism. The process releases energy as the phosphoryl is transferred, producing a cyclic process of exchange between ADP (adenosine diphosphate) and ATP (adenosine triphosphate), which utilizes oxygen to feed the process.

The Krebs ATP/ADP cycle process releases kinetic energy and heat, along with carbon dioxide and other important byproducts such as cyclic AMP (which helps regulate the cell membrane). As carbon dioxide is released, the CO_2 combines with water to form carbonic acid. Carbonic acid releases hydrogen acid (H+) and blood bicarbonate (HCO_3) into the bloodstream. This creates an acidic environment, which means there are more H+ ions.

The freed H+ ions will then combine with dissociated hemoglobin. As this H+ rich hemoglobin and bicarbonate blood reach the alveoli capillaries, hemoglobin releases the H+, which reforms carbon dioxide (CO_2) as it reacts with the bicarbonate. Hemoglobin is then ready for another oxygen molecule and the CO_2 is ready to diffuse back through to the alveoli and out through the lungs to the atmosphere.

Should there not be enough oxygen available for the cell's energy needs; the cells will produce energy without the use of oxygen. This process has about 5% of the efficiency of aerobic respiration, however. This is called *anaerobic glycolysis,* and NAD+ and NADH become the vehicles for energy exchange instead of ATP and ADP.

During heavy exercise or breathing deficiencies, the blood will become laced with heavier doses of carbonic acid and carbonates, acidified with H+ hemoglobin. This acidic situation can become toxic to the tissue systems if it remains too long without clearance.

This lack of oxygen also increases anaerobic glycolysis. The problem with anaerobic glycolysis is that instead of easily-exchanged byproducts like carbon dioxide, glycolysis produces acidic lactates and other radicals that can buildup in the bloodstream. They are also difficult to clear. Muscle fatigue is often attributed to lactic acid buildup in the bloodstream and muscle tissues. But it is the significant acids (H+) produced by anaerobic glycolysis—creating acidosis—that produces muscle soreness. Thus, the faster we can alkalize the blood and tissues, the faster our muscle recovery will be.

Should exhalation not be able to deplete this acidic environment in the blood, one of the first locations of damage will be to the walls of the blood vessels and alveoli. The acidic radicals look for stability as they borrow atomic elements from the molecules making up these tissues. This leaves these tissues damaged and in need of repair.

This later process of energy production in the absence of oxygen (oxygen debt) produces many more acids than does the Krebs cycle. The result is a bloodstream subject to acidosis, which corresponds to overexertion.

The bottom line is that better and more complete breathing helps detoxify the bloodstream and keep the blood in more of a radical-free alkaline state.

The Respiratory Cilia

The bronchial epithelial cells of the airway passages are also equipped with microscopic hairs called cilia (see previous and next drawing). The cilia act like tiny brooms: They undulate towards the exits—the sinuses, mouth and pharynx. The little hairs "sweep" out the mucous, together with toxins and dead cell parts caught in the mucous membrane.

The ciliary hairs lining the airways beat rhythmically with the expansion and release of the lungs. This expansion and contraction increases the mucous surfactant as well.

Should toxin particles remain airborne, they will also likely be moved out through breathing and rhythmic ciliary hair undulations in healthy airways.

The membrane and ciliary hair move in slow waves—very similar to what we see among kelp beds as they move with undulating ocean waves. This wave-like action of the ciliary hairs acts as an effective transport system.

This transport mechanism—the clearing of toxins and cell parts out of the area by the cilia—is called the *mucociliary clearance apparatus*. This is a self-cleaning system of the airways: Should these 'automatic sweepers' become caught in the thick mucous of a toxin-rich and/or ionically imbalanced mucous membrane—they become ineffective.

The mucociliary clearance apparatus explains how we will gather an accumulation of phlegm within the throat and sinuses. Most of us clear our throats or blow our noses without a second thought. Little do we realize that much of that phlegm is the result of the cilias' self-cleaning undulations that sweep out toxins and mucous. This sweeping mechanism also helps prevent polluted air and particles from being absorbed into our blood. Those particles not tossed out with the breath or mucous get phagotized (broken down) and swept out. Or they may be transported to the blood or lymph and escorted out of the body through the colon, urinary tract or sweat glands.

However, should the mucosal fluid not be healthy and ionically balanced, thickened mucous will build up within the mucosal membrane. This will overwhelm and in effect *drown* the ciliary hairs—making them far less effective for removing toxins and toxin-rich mucous.

The cilia are stabilized by being seated in a thin pool of thicker mucous, with another layer of thinner mucous on top. The thinner mucous towards the surface of the mucous membrane allows the hairs to undulate faster near and at the surface of the mucous membrane.

It is essential that these cilia are healthy, vibrant, and free of toxin-debris. This is why, as we'll explain, that tar and soot from smoking and pollution can wreck such havoc on the lungs. The tops of the cilia—and mucous—become jammed up in this gummy residue.

Cilia must also have a warm temperature in a moist atmosphere. Should cold, dry air get into the passages where these sensitive airway cilia dwell, they may shut down or become uncoordinated. The ultimate temperature for productive cilia is about 98.6 degrees F with 100% relative humidity. This doesn't mean that outdoor temperatures must be that. A temperature of nearly 100 degrees F with 100% humidity would be practically unbearable.

Rather, the cilia are kept warm and moist by the combination of body heat, the warming of the air as it travels through the sinus turbinates, and the secretion of warm mucous in the airways.

Inflammation also involves reactive oxygen species. Indications of this during systemic inflammation include higher levels of superoxide anions and thiobarbituric acid-reactive products (TBARs), as well as hydrogen peroxide. This is because one of the main inflammatory byproducts of superoxide reactions is hydrogen peroxide (H_2O_2).

Research has illustrated that those with inflammatory conditions generate more hydrogen peroxide when they breathe out than normal people. In one study, asthmatics breathed out 26 times the levels of hydrogen peroxide as healthy subjects did. They also found that TBAR levels among asthmatics were 18 times the levels of healthy subjects (Antczak *et al.* 1997).

Inflammatory eosinophils—evidenced by higher eosinophil cationic protein (ECP) levels—are also significantly higher in inflammatory conditions. ECP can damage microorganisms such as viruses and bacteria, along with our body's cells. ECP damages cells by forming pores in the cell membranes, which produce a type of cell membrane damage called *permeability alteration.*

Research has indicated that ECP builds up in the airways and epithelial tissues in an inflammatory condition. While ECP is a defense measure in the case of infection, an overload of ECP damages the epithelial cells.

The build-up of ECP is simply part of an inflammatory process that occurs as part of an immune response: A deranged immune response that medical researchers call hyperreactivity.

The Mucosal Membranes

Mucous membranes cover just about every region of epithelial cells, including our skin, nose, throat, mouth, airways, digestive tract, urinary tract, vagina and other surfaces. Some surfaces, such as the skin, have very thin mucosal membranes. Other surfaces, such as the digestive tract and airways, have thick mucosal membranes.

The mucosal membrane is a thin layer of glycoproteins (mucin), mucopolysaccharides, special enzymes, probiotics, immune cells and ionic fluid. The ionic fluid provides a transporter medium, which escorts a host of elements back and forth between the epithelial cells and the surface of the mucosal membrane. These elements include chloride ions, sodium ions, oxygen, nitrogen, carbon dioxide, hydrogen carbonate and others.

Some of these—such as the sodium, bicarbonate and chloride ions— provide the transport mechanisms into the cells and tissues of the skin surfaces. These travel through openings or pores among the cells, attached to nutrients, oxygen and other elements—transporting them in, in other words.

Certainly, the body is choosy about what kinds of elements it will allow into the epithelial cells and tissues. There are countless toxins, microorganisms, debris allergens and other foreigners that the body wants kept out.

We might compare this to how oil lubricates and protects an engine from overheating and dirt. In a well-maintained car, good motor oil will be circulated through the rods and cylinders. The oil doesn't just allow the steel parts to move with minimal friction: The motor oil also helps keep the engine clean, and prevents dirt and other contaminants from clogging up the system. Imagine what would happen if a car were to run without oil for a few miles? The engine would surely seize up, and likely would break down completely. While this is a crude example, there are several elements that are consistent.

So just how does the body keep these invaders from penetrating the body's internal and external surfaces? The short answer is the mucosal membranes. This is why these membranes contain a host of immune cells. These include immunoglobulins such as IgA, B-cells, T-cells and others that are looking to trap foreigners before get any further. Once they find a foreigner, they will take it apart using a one of many immune system strategies.

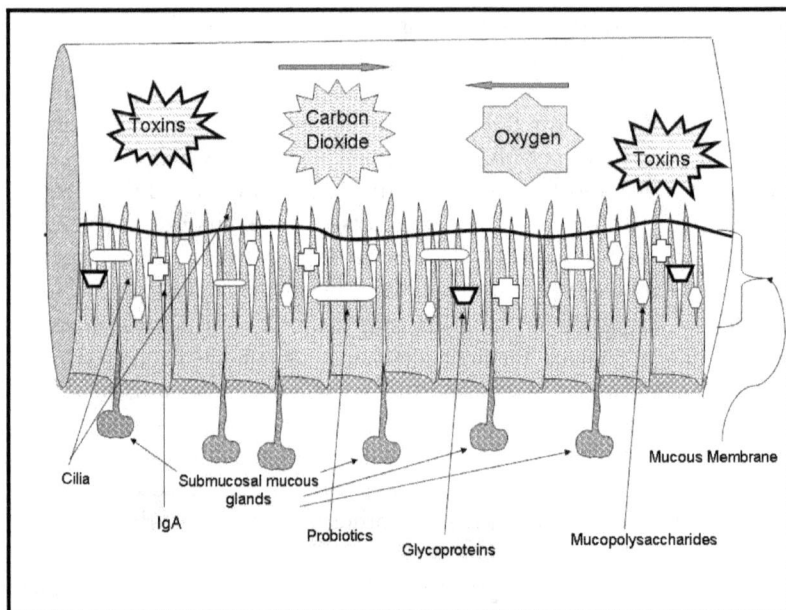

Airway Mucosal Membranes and Cilia

The mucous membranes are living structures. Probiotics populate our mucosal membranes, and are an important part of the "wall" of protection provided by these membranes. Tiny protective probiotic bacteria will inhabit all healthy mucosal membranes, including the skin. Like the immune system, these bacteria are trained to protect their territory. If an invading microorganism enters the mucosal membrane, the probiotics will lead an attack on them, with the immune cells in close pursuit.

The chemistry of the mucosal membrane also buffers and calms immune response. The mucosal membrane will help transport components such as corticosteroids from the adrenals to squelch inflammatory immune responses among our epithelial tissues. In other words, a healthy mucosal membrane is *calming* to our digestive tract, airways, skin and so on.

Other than our skin, which has been covered by placenta fluid, our mucosal membranes are raw and not well developed at birth. Gradually, as probiotics begin to colonize the sinuses, mouth and intestines—the mucosal membranes begin to mature. This maturity, as we'll discuss in detail, requires a host of nutrients as well as strong probiotic populations in order to populate the mucosal membranes. As this colonization occurs, the body's epithelial cells and mucous glands provide their balance of chemistry and protective attributes.

This is the basis for the hygiene theory, a product of many studies showing that infants and children that are allowed to roam the floors, parks, soils, and those among larger families have stronger immune systems. This is because all that roaming allows our bodies to collect a variety of probiotic species, which eventually colonize and territorialize our mucosal membranes.

Then there is the transporter mechanism. The mucous membranes utilizes this surfactant quality and ionic capabilities to transport nutrients among the epithelial cells, allowing them to function efficiently. It also transports toxins out of the area—assuming a healthy mucosal membrane.

Should this transport mechanism not be functioning properly, the region can become laden with a thickened, toxic mucous. Instead of the mucous membranes keeping these surfaces clean, the mucous itself becomes toxic.

This thickened mucous membrane is typical in hyperreactive airway responses among COPD, asthma, and hay fever conditions. In the intestines, the condition produces irritable bowel syndrome, colitis, Crohn's and other intestinal issues. In the lower esophagus and stomach, weakened mucosal membranes produces ulcers and acid reflux. And weakened skin mucosal membranes produce eczema, dermatitis, hives and other skin irritations.

Mucous is secreted by tiny mucous glands that lie within goblet cells scattered throughout these epithelia surfaces. They are called goblets because they are shaped like little goblet glasses, except their upper surface extends through the (internal) surfaces in tiny fingers. In the intestines and airways, they are called microvilli. On skin and other surfaces, they are become pores. They function almost identically with respect to their production of mucous.

The goblet cells and their end points both produce mucin through a process of contraction and glycosylation within the Golgi apparatus of the cells. This glycosylation of proteins produces the glycoproteins that are the mainstay in mucin.

The mucosal goblet cells of the respiratory tract are also similar to the gastric cells of the stomach and duodenum. The difference here is that these produce mucous fed by the pyloric glands in addition to the highly acidic gastrin. As we'll be discussing more at length throughout the remainder of the text, this similarity between the goblet cells, the villi and the gastric/pyloric cells facilitates an understanding of the mystery of GERD-related respiratory disorders.

The mucous membrane fluids can also become dehydrated if the ions that open the pores are blocked. Here the pores may be blocked due to an imbalance of ion chemistry in the sub-mucosal membrane. Tests have shown that chlorine and bicarbonate anions stimulate the opening of the pores that bring liquids into the mucous membrane. The mucin proteins produced by the submucosal membrane glands have to be diluted with these ion fluids to give the mucous membrane the right balance of stickiness and fluidity.

Among dehydrated mucosal membranes, the mucous is thickened and not fluid enough to provide its surfactant and transport functions.

In addition, exposure to toxins, pathogenic microorganisms, cold air and any number of other triggers can stimulate the production of mucous by the goblet cells. In a healthy body, this stimulates the quick removal of the toxin or invader, as the excess mucous is swept out by the cilia or other drainage facilities of the surface.

However, should the body be immunosuppressed or otherwise overwhelmed by the invasion, the goblet cells will over-produce mucous, which can swamp the epithelial surfaces with dead cell parts and toxins. When these surfaces are drowning in mucous, the removal process is deficient. The lack of mucous transport, combined with the need to remove toxins, produces inflammation as the immune system must engage to remove the toxins.

The Adrenals

The body's two adrenal glands are part of our endocrine system. The outer cortex is stimulated by master hormones from the hypothalamus and pituitary gland, while the inner medulla is stimulated directly with nerves. The adrenals produce an array of hormones, many of which are related to inflammation and/or stress.

For example, the medulla produces epinephrine and norepinephrine, and other catecholamines. Epinephrine (as well as norepinephrine) relaxes the smooth muscles of the airways and constricts the blood vessels, increases the heart rate, increases metabolism, dilates the pupils and halts digestive activity, all in an effort to reduce inflammation and respond to inflammation and stress.

This multi-organ adrenal response might seem beneficial, but it also comes with a double-edged sword: Epinephrine and norepinephrine also significantly slow the rate of mucous secretion by submucosal glands that feed the mucous membranes.

This effect can be quite dangerous to the highly-stressed individual, because the decreased mucous membranes also leave our lungs and digestive tracts open to irritation from toxins and environmental changes.

The adrenal glands also produce important steroids. Two of the most critical are cortisol and aldosterone.

Aldosterone is a mineralocorticoid. It and other mineralocorticoids are produced by the outer shell, or cortex, of the adrenal gland. Aldosterone and other mineralocorticoids adjust and balance the body's levels of sodium, potassium and other minerals; as well as alter sodium ion channels among various cells. These are critical to the acid/alkaline status of the blood and body fluids, and the body's ability to remove toxins through the kidneys, sweat glands and colon. Aldosterone is a critical player in maintaining blood pressure as well, and this affects the performance of respiration.

Aldosterone also balances the use and availability of cortisol and cortisone, because many aldosterone receptors also bind with cortisol. This means that a balanced production of these two steroids (cortisol is a glucocorticoid) by the adrenals is critical to the detoxification efforts of the body—along with the body's ability to balance inflammation with efforts to heal the body.

This means that adrenal glands stimulated by stress and inflammation repeatedly for long periods begin to wear down. As mentioned earlier, this is called adrenal exhaustion. When this happens, the adrenal glands produce inconsistently deficient levels of theses critical steroids and catecholamines.

This creates drastic imbalances within the body, affecting the body's ability to respond to toxins, inflammation and stress. Signs of adrenal exhaustion include being easily fatigued, overstressed and over-reactive to toxins and environmental changes. Adrenal exhaustion is typical in an immune system over-responding with hyper-inflammation.

Intestinal Immunity

What do the intestines have to do with cleansing and toxicity? Plenty.

This relates to the fact that the digestive tract protects against the penetration of toxins into our bloodstreams and tissues. When intestinal villi and their junctions are damaged, endotoxins (the poop and byproducts of pathogenic bacteria) and other toxins can get into the bloodstream—overloading the immune system and producing systemic inflammation.

The intestines utilize non-specific, humoral, cell-mediated and probiotic immunity to protect intestinal tissues from larger peptides, toxins and invading microorganisms.

This is all packaged nicely into what is referred to as the *intestinal brush barrier*. The intestinal brush barrier is a complex mucosal layer of mucin, enzymes, probiotics and ionic fluid—sealed by villi separated by tight junctions.

The intestinal mucosal membrane forms a protective surface medium over the intestinal epithelium. It also provides an active nutrient transport mechanism for nutrients and toxins. This mucosal layer is stabilized by the grooves of the intestinal microvilli. It contains glycoproteins, mucopolysaccharides and other ionic transporters, which attach to amino acids, minerals, vitamins, glucose and fatty acids—carrying them across intestinal membranes.

This mucosal layer is policed by billions of probiotic colonies, which help process and identify incoming food molecules; excrete various nutrients; and control toxins and pathogens.

The breakdown of the mucosal membrane causes it to thin. This depletes the protection rendered by the mucopolysaccharides and glycoproteins, probiotics, immune IgA cells, enzymes and bile. This thinning allows toxins and macromolecules that would have been screened out by the mucosal membrane to be presented to the intestinal cells.

In its entirety, the brush barrier is a triple-filter that screens for molecule size, ionic nature and nutrition quality. Much of this is performed via four screening mechanisms existing between the intestinal microvilli: tight junctions, adherens junctions, desmosomes, and colonies of probiotics. The tight functions form a bilayer interface between cells, controlling permeability. Desmosomes are points of interface between the tight junctions, and adherens junctions keep the cell membranes adhesive enough to stabilize the junctions. These junction mechanisms together regulate permeability at the intestinal wall.

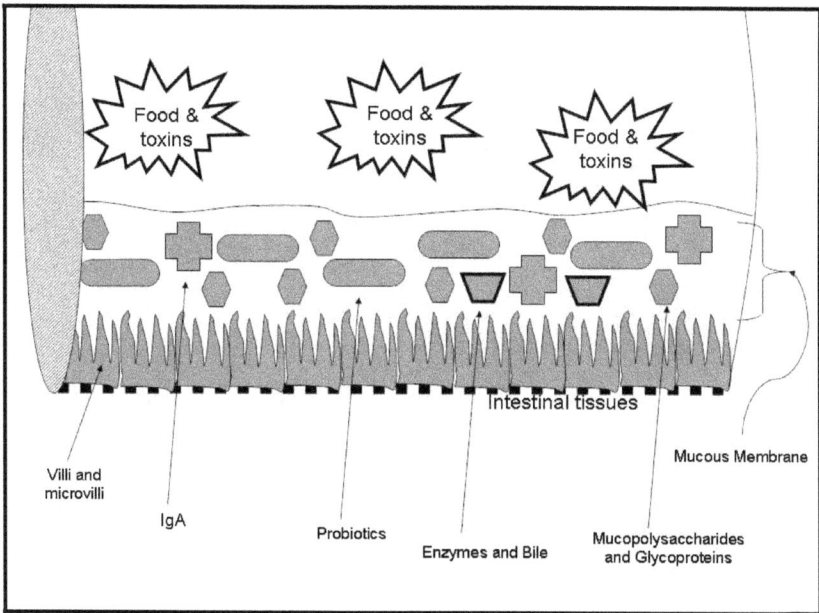

The Healthy Intestinal Wall

This mucosal brush barrier creates the boundary between intestinal contents and our bloodstream. Should the mucosal layer chemistry become altered, its protective and ionic transport mechanisms become weakened, allowing toxic or larger molecules to be presented to the microvilli junctions. This contact can irritate the microvilli, causing a subsequent inflammatory response. Research illustrates that this is a contributing cause of irritable bowel syndrome (IBS).

Should the mucous membrane thin, these mechanisms become irritated, producing an inflammatory immune response that causes the desmosomes and tight junctions to open. These gaps allow toxins and food macromolecules to enter the blood, where they can become allergens and contribute to systemic inflammation. Scientists call this condition *increased intestinal permeability.*

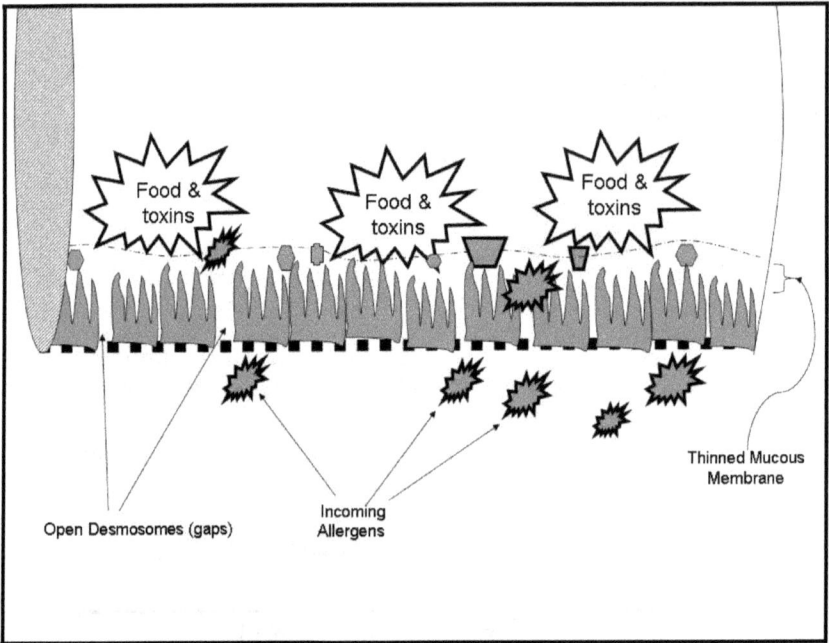

The Unhealthy Intestinal Wall

The Intestinal Permeability Index

How do scientists and physicians test for increased intestinal permeability? Intestinal permeability is typically measured by giving the patient indigestible substances with different molecular sizes. Urine samples then show relative levels of these, illustrating degrees of intestinal permeability. For example, alcohol-sugar combinations such as lactulose and mannitol are often used. These indicate intestinal permeability because of their different molecular sizes. A few (typically 5-6) hours after ingestion, the patient's urine is tested to measure the quantities of these two molecules in the urine.

Because lactulose is a larger molecule than mannitol, greater permeability will be indicated by high lactulose levels in the urine relative to mannitol levels. Intestines with normal permeability will have less lactulose absorption.

These relative levels create a ratio between lactulose and mannitol, which scientists call the L/M ratio. This L/M ratio is used to quantify intestinal permeability. When the lactulose-to-mannitol ratio is higher, more permeability exists. When it is lower, less (more normal) intestinal permeability exists. Higher levels are compared using what many researchers call the *Intestinal Permeability Index*.

Other molecule substances are also sometimes used to detect intestinal permeability using the same protocol of measuring recovery in the urine over a period of time. These other substances include polyethylene glycols of various molecular weights, horseradish peroxidase, EDTA (ethylenediaminetetraacetic acid), CrEDTA, rhamnose, lactulose, and cellobiose. Because these substances are not readily metabolized in the intestine or blood, and have varying molecular sizes, they can also give accurate readings on the relative intestinal permeability.

Chapter Two

Inflammation

Our immune system works utilizes a reactive process of protection called inflammation. You might say that inflammation is the visible side of immunity. When the immune system is fighting an invasion, the response will typically include inflammation.

Inflammation can come with a number of characteristics, including swelling, redness, pain, lack of motion and more.

This means that inflammation is both good and bad. Inflammation means the immune system is working. But inflammation also means there is a major threat to the body and the immune system must use this extreme mechanism to protect the body, as it routes healing forces to the site and seals off parts of the body against the invader.

At the same time, inflammation is used by the body to inform us of a problem. This can also mean we are dealing with pain. But without pain, we might continue doing something that continues the problem or makes the problem worse. So pain, like inflammation, might not feel good but they are important factors in our immune response.

Let's take a look at some of the mechanisms of inflammation, and some of the things that instigate inflammation in our bodies.

Most people think of inflammation as bad. Especially when they see that so many disease conditions involve inflammation. Rather, inflammation simply coordinates the various immune players into a frenzy of healing responses. Part of the response is to purge the area of toxins.

Our body's immune system launches inflammatory cells and factors that heal injury sites and prevent bleed-outs. This process is often stimulated by leukotrienes and prostaglandins.

Leukotrienes are molecules that identify problems and stimulate the immune system. They pinpoint and isolate areas of the body that require repair. Once they pinpoint the site of repair, one type of leukotriene will initiate inflammation, and others will assist in maintaining the process. Once the repair process proceeds to a point of maturity, another type of leukotriene will begin slowing down the process of inflammation.

This smart signalling process takes place through the biochemical bonding formations of these molecules. Leukotrienes are paracrines and autocrines. They are paracrine in that they initiate messages that travel from one cell to another. They are autocrine in that they initiate messages that encourage an automatic and immediate response—notably among T-cells, engaging them to remove bad cells. They also help transmit messages that initiate the process of repair through the clotting of blood and the patching of damaged tissues.

Leukotrienes are produced from the conversion of essential fatty acids (EFAs) by an enzyme produced by the body called arachidonate-5-lipoxygenase (sometimes called LOX). The central fatty acids of this process are arachidonic acid (AA), gamma-linolenic acid (GLA), and eicosapentaenoic acid (EPA). Lipoxygenase enzymes produce different types of leukotrienes, depending upon the initial fatty acid. The important point of this is that the leukotrienes produced by arachidonic acid stimulate inflammation, while the leukotrienes produced by EPA halt inflammation. The leukotrienes produced by GLA, on the other hand, block the conversion process of polyunsaturated fatty acids to arachidonic acid.

Prostaglandins are also produced through an enzyme conversion from fatty acids. Like leukotrienes, prostaglandins are messengers that transmit particular messages to immune cells. Their messaging is either paracrine or autocrine. Prostaglandins are critical parts of the process of injury repair. They also initiate a number of protective sequences in the body, including the transmission of pain and the clotting of blood.

Prostaglandins are produced by the oxidation of fatty acids by an enzyme produced in the body called cyclooxygenase—also called prostaglandin-endoperoxide synthase (PTGS) or COX. There are three types of COX, and each convert fatty acids to different types of prostaglandins. The central fatty acid that causes inflammation again is arachidonic acid. COX-1 converts AA to the PGE2 type of prostaglandin. COX-2, on the other hand, converts AA into the PGI2 type of prostaglandin.

The central messages that prostaglandins transmit depend upon the type of prostaglandin. Prostaglandin I2 (also PGI2) stimulates the widening of blood vessels and bronchial passages, and pain sensation within the nervous system. In other words, along with stimulating blood clotting, PGI2 signals a range of responses to assist the body's wound healing at the site of injury.

Prostaglandin E2, or PGE2, is altogether different from PGI2. PGE2 stimulates the secretion of mucus within the stomach, intestines, mouth and esophagus. It also decreases the production of gastric acid in the stomach. This combination of increasing mucus and lowering acid production keeps healthy stomach cells from being damaged by our gastric acids and the acidic content of our foods. This is one of the central reasons NSAID pharmaceuticals cause gastrointestinal problems: They interrupt the secretion of this protective mucus in the stomach.

This means that the COX-1 enzyme instigates the process of protecting the stomach, while the COX-2 enzyme instigates the process

34

of inflammation and repair within the body. In the case of autoimmune disease, the COX-2 process often lies at the root of pain and swelling.

Cyclooxygenase also converts ALA/DHA and GLA to prostaglandins. Just as lipoxygenase converts ALA/DHA and GLA to anti-inflammation leukotrienes, the conversion of ALA/DHA and GLA by cyclooxygenase produces prostaglandins that either block the inflammatory process or reverse it. This means that a healthy diet with plenty of GLA and ALA/DHA fats will balance inflammation response. ALA is found in walnuts, soybeans, flax, canola, pumpkin seeds and chia seeds. The purest form of DHA is found in certain algae, and the body produces EPA from DHA. Fish and krill also get their DHA up the food chain from algae. GLA is found in borage, primrose oil and spirulina.

Probiotics are often involved in the production of intermediary fatty acids used for these LOX and COX conversions, producing anti-inflammatory effects. To illustrate this, scientists from the University of Helsinki (Kekkonen *et al.* 2008) measured lipids and inflammation markers before and after giving probiotic *Lactobacillus rhamnosus* GG to 26 healthy adults. After three weeks of probiotic supplementation, the subjects had decreased levels of intermediary inflammatory fatty acids such as lysophosphatidylcholines, sphingomyelins, and several glycerophosphatidylcholines. Probiotics also reduced inflammatory markers TNF-alpha and CRP in this study.

The arachidonic acid conversion process that produces prostaglandins also produces thromboxanes. Thromboxanes stimulate platelets in the blood to aggregate. They work in concert with platelet-activating factor or PAF. Together, these biomolecules drive the process of clotting the blood and restricting blood flow. This is good during injury healing, but the inflammatory process must also be slowed down as the injury heals.

Probiotics help modulate that process. In the research from Poland's Pomeranian Academy of Medicine (Naruszewicz *et al.* 2002) mentioned earlier, scientists found that giving *Lactobacillus plantarum* 299v to 36 volunteers resulted in a 37% decrease in inflammatory F2-isoprostanes. Isoprostanes are similar to prostaglandins, formed outside of the COX process.

The probiotic and immunoglobulin immune system work together to deter and kill particular invaders—hopefully before they gain access to the body's tissues. Should these defenses fail, they can stimulate the humoral immune system in a strategic attack that includes identifying antigens and recognizing their weaknesses. B-cells and probiotics coordinate through the stimulation of immunoglobulins and clusters of differentiation (CDs).

This progression also stimulates an activation of neutrophils, phagocytes, immunoglobulins, leukotrienes and prostaglandins. Should cells become infected, they will signal the immune system using paracrines located on their cell membranes. Once the intrusion and strategy is determined, B-cells will surround the pathogens while T-cells attack any infected cells. Natural killer T-cells may secrete chemicals into infected cells, initiating the death of the cell.

Leukotrienes immediately gather in the region of toxicity or infection, and signal to T-cells to coordinate efforts in the process of repair. Prostaglandins initiate the widening of blood vessels to bring more T-cells and other repair factors (such as plasminogen and fibrin) to the site. Histamine opens the blood vessel walls to allow all these healing agents access to the injury site to clean it up.

Prostaglandins also stimulate substance P within the nerve cells, initiating the sensation of pain. At the same time, thromboxanes, along with fibrin, drive the process of clotting and coagulation in the blood, while constricting certain blood vessels to decrease the risk of bleeding.

Depending upon the toxin or invader, the inflammation response will also accompany an H1-histamine response. As mentioned earlier, histamine is primarily produced by the mast cells, basophils and neutrophils after being stimulated by IgE antibodies. This opens blood vessels to tissues, which stimulates the processes of sneezing, watering of the eyes and coughing.

These measures, though sometimes considered irritating, are all stimulated in an effort to remove the toxin and prevent its re-entry into the body. As histamine binds with receptors, one of the resulting physiological responses is alertness (also why antihistamines cause drowsiness). These are natural responses to help the body and mind remain vigilant in order to avoid further toxin intake.

At the height of the repair process, swelling, redness and pain are at their peak. The T-cells, macrophages, neutrophils, fibrin and plasmin all work together to purge the allergen from the body and repair the damage.

As macrophages continue the clean up, the other immune cells begin to retreat. Antioxidants like glutathione will attach to and transport the byproducts—broken down toxins and cell parts—out of the body. As this proceeds, prostaglandins, histamines and leukotrienes are signaled to reverse the inflammation and pain process.

One of the central features of the normalization process is the production of bradykinin. Bradykinin slows clotting and opens blood vessels, allowing the cleanup process to accelerate. A key signalling factor is the production of nitric oxide (NO). NO slows inflammation by promoting the detachment of lymphocytes to the site of infection or toxification, and reduces tissue swelling. NO also accelerates the clearing out of debris with its interaction with the superoxide anion. NO was originally described by researchers as endothelium-derived relaxing factor (or EDRF)—because of its role in relaxing blood vessel walls.

The body produces more nitric oxide in the presence of good nutrition and lower stress. Probiotics also play a big role in nitric oxide production in a healthy body. Lactobacilli such as *L. plantarum* have in fact been shown to remove the harmful nitrate molecule and use it to produce nitric oxide (Bengmark *et al.* 1998). This is beneficial to not only reducing inflammation: NO production also creates a balanced environment for increased tolerance.

Low nitric oxide levels also happen to be associated with a plethora of conditions, including diabetes, heart failure, high cholesterol, ulcerative colitis, premature aging, cancers and many others. Low or abnormal NO production is also seen among lifestyle factors such as smoking, obesity, and environmental air pollution.

In cases of toxicity from air pollutants, the cough reflex may be enlisted to help clear toxins. Irritated sites in the airways and lungs stimulate coughing, but this is also attenuated by a neural cough center located within the brainstem and within the cerebral cortex, where coughing is often initiated, suppressed or modified by consciousness. The cough reflex is, as put by Dr. John Christopher, *"a result of nature's effort to expectorate mucous from the lungs, after which breathing becomes easier."*

In other words, the stimulus for chronic coughing is the build-up of mucous in the airways. While incidental coughing might follow the inhalation of some smoke or other toxin, a chronic cough is stimulated by a build-up of thickened mucous in the airways.

And why is there this build up of mucous? Because the immune system is undergoing the inflammatory process by flushing out broken-down cells, broken down toxins, and even live infections. This thickened mucous is like the composition of flushed toilet water after a bowel movement: *it is full of crap.*

Allergic Response

An overload of toxins and subsequent systemic inflammation can stimulate a state of hypersensitivity within the body. In this state, the body is on high alert. This makes the body respond out of proportion to the actual threat. In other words, the body overwhelmed with toxins will over-react, just as an overworked person might blow up at an innocent remark by a co-worker.

Let's review the various hypersensitivity responses and see how they are connected to toxicity.

Atopic Hypersensitivity

This response occurs when IgE antibodies bind to an allergen. Antigens include air pollutants, pollen, dust mite allergens, and dander. An allergen can also be any food the immune system has become sensitized to. When this binding between an antigen and IgE takes place, the bound IgE will set off the release of inflammatory mediators from white blood cells called mast cells, basophils and/or neutrophils. The mediators released by these immune cells include histamine, prostaglandins and leukotrienes. Depending upon the location and type of mast/basophil/neutrophil cells, these mediators can spark an inflammatory response within the airways, and/or other tissues, including the sinuses, skin, joints, intestines and elsewhere.

This response can be further broken down into two stages: sensitization and elicitation.

Sensitization: The allergen sensitization process takes place when a potential antigen happens to come into contact with a type of immune cell called a progenitor B-cell. As part of their immune system responsibilities, these B-cells will break apart the allergen proteins into smaller parts— often called *epitopes*. These will become attached to hystocompatibility complex class II complex molecules.

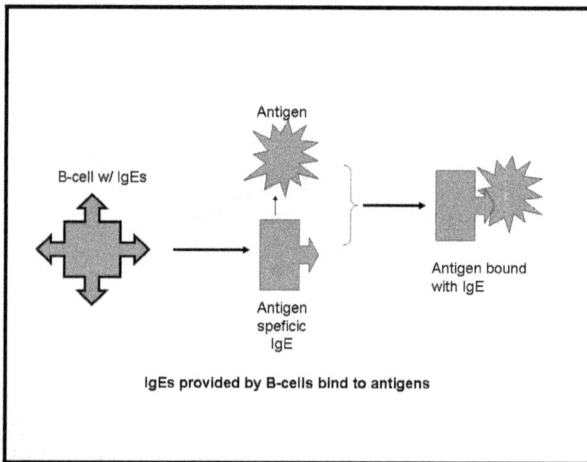

Antigen

B-cell w/ IgEs

Antigen bound with IgE

Antigen speficic IgE

IgEs provided by B-cells bind to antigens

The T-cell hystocompatibility complex is transferred onto the surface of the B-cell, which binds to a particular allergen. Once upon the B-cell surface, T-helper cells take notice of this foreign particle stuck to the B-cell. The T-helper cell cytokine CD4 receptors trigger a response, and this stimulates the production of the IgE immunoglobulins. These particular

IgE immunoglobulins are now sensitized to the particular epitope of the antigen in the future.

Elicitation: Once sensitized, the IgE associates with the specific IgE receptors that lie on the surface of the neutrophil, basophil or mast cells. Within these cells are packages called granules.

The granules are stock full of a variety of inflammatory mediators. The most notorious of these are the leukotrienes and histamines that are released into the bloodstream and lymph. These drive much of the symptoms of inflammation, including but not limited to hives, coughing, watery eyes, uritica, sinusitis and others.

The below diagram illustrates elicitation:

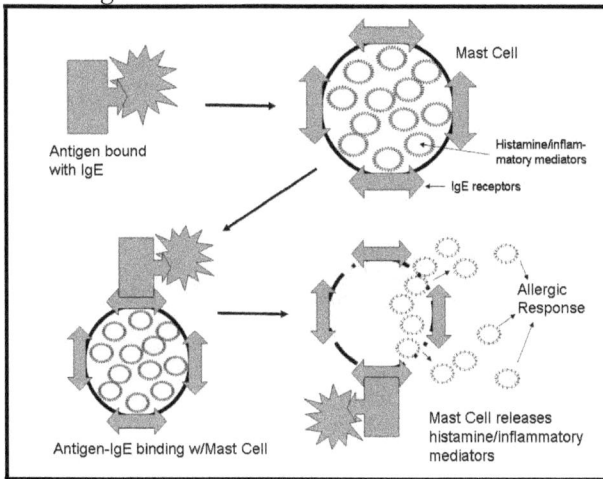

Cytotoxic Responses

In this type of immune response, antigens have penetrated the tissues, and the immune system is on a state of alert as it responds to kill these cells. This typically takes place through an antigen binding to IgG or IgM immunoglobulins in a delayed immune and inflammatory response. This response can happen concurrently to allergic responses; though it is most often a delayed response. This type of inflammatory response can last several days.

Should the red blood cells be involved in the antigen absorption, hemolysis (the destruction of red blood cells) and anemia (a lack of red blood cells) may result. These can in turn cause more inflammatory responses.

Immune Complex Responses

Here the allergen-bound antibody complex actually penetrates cell tissues and injures them. This can occur within the airway epithelial cells, intestinal cells, liver, or virtually anywhere around the body. Here the damage to the cells immediately stimulates the inflammatory response, regardless of whether there is an allergen trigger involved or not. Whatever is damaging the cells is considered a direct threat.

In some instances, these immune complexes can severely change alveoli permeability, vascular permeability and/or intestinal permeability, producing imbalances in respiration, circulation and digestion— sometimes even simultaneously.

This type of response is also often a delayed response, occurring hours or even a day or two after exposure to the toxin or allergen.

This alerted immune complex condition will also stimulate mast cells, basophils and/or neutrophils, resulting in continued degranulation of histamine, prostaglandins and leukotrienes, which in turn produce hypersensitivity to the foreigner.

Delayed T-Cell Responses

While the immune complex response may generate an immediate T-cell response once cells and tissues are damaged, a delayed T-cell response will occur over a period of time—as T-cells continue to destroy damaged airway cells. Here airway epithelial cells become damaged, and the T-cells are removing those damaged cells with an inflammatory response.

This type of response is the driving factor behind airway remodeling. In airway remodeling, the epithelial cell network that lines the airways become inflamed, damaged and chronically irritated. They are swollen and hyperreactive on an ongoing basis, in other words.

This same general condition can exist within the epithelial layers of many parts of the body. On the skin, this is seen as eczema. In the intestines, it is seen as colitis or Crohn's disease. In the sinuses, it is called sinusitis. In the urinary tract, it is called interstitial cystitis. In the stomach and lower esophagus, it is called GERD.

This response is also often attributed to autoimmunity, which is explained as the immune system attacking healthy cells. This notion is incorrect, however, because the immune system is not attacking healthy cells. The immune system is removing cells that have been damaged. Once these epithelial cells are damaged, T-cells stimulate the immune response to clear out the damaged cells. In other words, it is an inflammatory immune response to cellular and tissue toxicity.

Lipid Peroxidation

Considerable research has illustrated that a process called lipid peroxidation is implicated in those with inflammatory diseases, muscle fatigue, thyroid issues, reproductive issues, lung disorders, immune disorders and cognitive issues such as dementia and Alzheimer's. What is lipid peroxidation and how does it affect our bodies?

Researchers from the University of Alabama's School of Public Health (Stone *et al.* 2010) reviewed the association between low levels of selenium and higher rates of AIDS, HIV infections and other immune diseases. They found that HIV-infected persons who have low selenium levels have a faster progression of their disease to AIDS, and higher rates of mortality.

Selenium is a key ingredient in the liver's production of glutathione peroxidase. Glutathione peroxidase neutralizes toxins and free radicals, especially those relating to lipid peroxides.

In one of the early studies that established this link, researchers from Stockholm's Karolinska Institute (Hasselmark *et al.* 1993) gave 24 intrinsic asthma patients either placebo or 100 micrograms of sodium selenite per day for two weeks. The selenium group had higher glutathione levels and activity, and their asthma significantly improved as compared with the placebo group.

Researchers from Slovakia's Institute of Preventive and Clinical Medicine (Jahnova *et al.* 2002) also gave 20 asthmatic adults either a placebo or 200 micrograms of selenium per day for six months, in addition to inhaled corticosteroids and beta-agonists. They found that the selenium blocked IFN-gamma adhesion molecules, reducing inflammation.

Researchers from Britain's Imperial College (Shaheen *et al.* 2007) tested 197 patients with 100 micrograms of a selenium-yeast formula or a placebo for 24 weeks. Quality of life increased among the selenium patients but in this study, there was little difference between the selenium group and the placebo (yeast only) group. It should be noted, however, that the patients were all taking regular steroid medication and this study only used 100 micrograms of a blend of selenium and yeast. So the selenium dosage was substantially (less than half) the dosage of the studies that showed reductions in inflammation symptoms and improvement in lung function.

The recommended daily allowance for selenium is 55 micrograms. The studies above illustrated that those with inflammation require more like 200 micrograms for a therapeutic effect.

The critical component in this mystery is glutathione peroxidase—an enzyme produced in the liver. Glutathione peroxidase is the leading enzyme responsible for the breakdown and removal of lipid hydroperoxides. Lipid hydroperoxides are oxidized fats that damage cell membranes. As they do this, they create pores in the cell. The resulting damage eventually kills most cells. Lipid hydroperoxides are one of the most damaging molecules within the body. They are responsible for many deadly metabolic diseases, including heart disease, artery disease, Alzheimer's disease and many others.

When lipid hydroperoxides accumulate in the body, they can also damage the cells of the airways, causing irritation and inflammation. The damage from lipid hydroperoxides stimulates an inflammatory response. Researchers have called the initial signal from the cell that initiates this inflammatory response *lipid peroxidation/LOOH-mediated stress signaling*. In other words, the cells are stressed by lipid peroxidation, and this initiates a distress signal to the immune system.

This distress signal stimulates the contraction of the smooth bronchial muscles while stimulating leukotriene activity—which delivers cytotoxic (cell-destroying) T-cells and eosinophils into the region. This stimulates the production of more mucous, which drowns the cilia and restricts breathing.

The production of more mucous is intended to clear out the damaged cells. In other words, much of the increased mucous that drowns the cilia and produces wheezing is caused by the influx of dead cell matter from lipid hydroperoxide damage.

By virtue of removing lipid hydroperoxides, glutathione peroxidase—not to be confused with glutathione reductase—regulates pro-inflammatory arachidonic acid metabolism. In other words, glutathione regulates the release and populations of those pro-inflammatory mediators, the leukotrienes. Leukotriene activity is directly associated with the damage created by lipid hydroperoxides. Thus, when lipid hydroperoxide levels are reduced by glutathione peroxidase, leukotriene density is reduced.

Selenium is required for glutathione peroxidase production. Should the body be overloaded with lipid hydroperoxides, more glutathione is required to clear out the damage. As more glutathione is produced, more selenium is utilized, which runs selenium levels down.

This issue was illustrated by research from Britain's South Manchester University Hospital (Hassan 2008). The researchers studied 13 aspirin-induced asthmatics and a healthy matched control group. They found that the asthmatics maintained higher levels of selenium in the bloodstream—especially among blood platelets. This high selenium content in the bloodstream correlated with higher glutathione peroxidase activity. The research illustrated how selenium is used up faster in by those with inflammation through this glutathione peroxidase process.

Lipid peroxidation means that the lipids that make up the cell membrane are being robbed of electrons. This 'robbery' results in an unstable cell membrane. Let's take a closer look at the process of lipid peroxidation.

The first step takes place with the entry of a reactive oxygen species into the proximity of the cell. Reactive oxygen species are elements that require an electron—such as hydrogen (H+)—in order to become stable.

Fatty acids that make up the membranes of cells are the likely candidates for peroxidation. Remember, the name "lipid" refers to a fatty acid. Fatty acids include saturated fats, polyunsaturates, monounsaturates, and so on (see fatty acid discussions later on).

Several types of lipids make up the cell membrane. Fatty acids will combine with other molecules to make phospholipids, cholesterols and glycolipids. Saturates and polyunsaturates are typical, but there are several species of polyunsaturates. These range from long chain versions to short versions. They also include the cis- configuration and the trans-configuration. Cell membranes that utilize predominantly cis- versions with long chains are the most durable. Those cell membranes with trans-configurations can be highly unstable, and irregularly porous. This is one reason why trans fats are unhealthy. The other reason is that trans fats easily become peroxidized.

Cell membranes with more long chain fatty acids are more stable and are less subject to peroxidation. Shorter chains that provide more double bonds are less stable, because these are more easily broken. Also, monounsaturated fatty acids such as GLA are more stable.

Once the fatty acid is degraded by an oxygen species, it becomes a fatty acid radical. The fatty acid will usually become oxidized, making it a peroxyl-fatty acid radical. This radical will react with other fatty acids, forming a cyclic process involving radicals called cyclic peroxides.

This becomes a chain reaction that results in the cell membrane becoming completely destroyed and dysfunctional. This forces the cell to signal to the immune system that it is under attack and about to become malignant. The T-cell immune response will often initiate the cell's self-destruct switch: TNF—tumor necrosis factor. Alternatively, the cell may be directly destroyed by cytotoxic T-cells. The combined process stimulates inflammation. As these cells are killed or self-destruct, they are purged from the system—provoking increased mucous formation.

While this peroxidation and cell destruction is taking place, the immune system is not simply standing by. The body enters a state called *systemic inflammation*. As we discussed earlier, during systemic inflammation, the immune system launches an ongoing supply of eosinophils, neutrophils and mast cells, which release granulocytes that inflame the airways.

In other words, due to this ongoing peroxidation, the immune system is on a hair-trigger. Imagine a person at work who is stressed from being buried in work and a myriad of problems. You walk into their office and they immediately react: "And what do *you* want?" they ask.

If they were not overloaded with work, problems and deadlines, your coming into their office would probably be met without such a frantic response. But since they were overloaded, they reacted (hyper reacted is a better word) more defensively than needed, *because they thought you were going to add to their workload.*

In other words, inflammation is simply a defense measure by an immune system that is overwhelmed.

Typical associations with inflammation include artery damage and plaque build-up, obesity, diabetes, a sedentary lifestyle, and a diet high in saturated fats and/or fried foods. High blood pressure and fast or irregular heart rate, especially in persons over 40 years old, are also strong markers.

Along with these associations come higher levels of total cholesterol, low-density lipoprotein (LDL) and very low-density lipoprotein (VLDL) cholesterol, and total triglycerides are also key markers. The link between small LDL particle size and atherosclerosis is a key factor, and the oxidation of LDL particles is the match that lights the fuse. These involve hyperperoxides, as they readily form oxidative radicals. The cascade towards LDL oxidation also seems to be accelerated by lipooxygenases like 15-LOX-2 along with cyclooxygenases. The process as a whole is lipid peroxidation.

In addition to launching systemic inflammation due to widespread cell damage, the body also produces processes that attempt to halt the peroxidation cycle. One of these components is the glutathione peroxidase enzyme discussed earlier, formed by the body using selenium as a substrate. Depending upon the rate of lipid peroxidation, however, this could be like trying to blow out a forest fire. There is simply too much fire spreading too quickly.

Reactive Oxygen Species

Let's take a wider perspective on the problem. The initiation process of the lipid peroxidation is started by a reactive oxygen species. What is this?

This is also often called a free radical. A free radical is an unstable molecule or ion that forms during a chemical reaction. In other words, the molecule or ion needs another atom, ion or molecule to stabilize it. Once it is stable, it is not reactive.

While a free radical is unstable, it can damage any number of elements it meets. These include the cells, organs and tissues of the body.

Nature produces many, many free radicals. However, nature typically accompanies radicals with the molecules, atoms or ions that stabilize the radical. In the atmosphere, for example, radicals become stabilized by ozone and other elements. In plants, radicals become stabilized by antioxidants from nutrients derived from the sun, soil and oxygen. In the body, radicals are stabilized by antioxidizing enzymes, nutrients and other elements. These include glutathione peroxidase, as we discussed earlier.

Confirming this, the research from South Manchester University Hospital mentioned earlier concluded with a comment that the increased glutathione peroxidase activity related to radical oxidation: *"administration of aspirin to these patients increases the generation of immediate oxygen products…"*

Another anti-oxidation process within the body utilizes the *superoxide dismutase* (SOD) enzyme. The SOD enzyme is typically available within the cytoplasm of most cells. Here SOD is complexed by either copper and zinc, or manganese—similar to the way selenium is complexed with the glutathione peroxidase enzyme. Several types of SOD enzymes reside within the body—some in the mitochondria and some in the intercellular tissue fluids. SOD neutralizes superoxides before they can damage the inside and outside of the cell—assuming the body is healthy, with substantial amounts of SOD. The immune system produces superoxides as part of its strategy to attack microorganisms and toxins.

Superoxide dismutase secretion is extremely important to the nose and airways because it helps neutralize reactive oxygen species and reactive nitrogen species – both considered free radicals that will damage the body's cells if they are not neutralized. Many toxins and pollutants – especially air pollutants containing mercury, sulfur and other reactive elements from air pollution – will convert to radicals in the presence of oxygen, damaging lung and airway cells.

Phase 2 enzymes include glutathione transferases and quinone reductases. These are important enzymes for preventing genetic mutations – and those preventing cancerous cells from forming.

Another broad anti-oxidation process utilizes *catalase*. Here the body provides an enzyme bound by iron to neutralize peroxides to oxygen and water. It is a standard component of many metabolic reactions within the body.

Yet another enzyme utilized for radical reduction is *glutathione reductase*. This enzyme works with NADP in the cell to stabilize hydrogen peroxide oxidized radicals before they can damage the cell.

Notice that all of these antioxidizing enzymes require minerals. We have seen either selenium, copper, zinc, manganese or iron as necessary to keep these enzymes in good supply. Many other minerals and trace elements are used by other antioxidant and detoxifying enzyme processes.

These minerals, and many of the enzymes themselves, are supplied by various foods and supplements, as we'll discuss further.

Another tool that the healthy body utilizes to stabilize radicals are the antioxidants supplied by plant foods. Plants produce antioxidants to protect their own cells from radical damage. Thus, their plant material contains a host of these oxidation stabilizers, which our bodies use to neutralize radicals.

C-reactive Protein

A plethora of research has shown that higher C-reactive protein levels are indicative of systemic inflammation occurring somewhere in the body. The diagnostic measurement of CRP for cardiovascular disease is now standard care. This is because cardiovascular disease is typically the result of inflammation within the artery walls. This is usually companied by a body-wide inflammation condition called systemic inflammation.

CRP is now seen among many other inflammatory diseases. For expel, researchers from the Texas Tech University Health Sciences Center (Arif *et al.* 2007) studied the relationships between C-reactive protein (CRP) and asthma among 8,020 adults over the age of twenty. They found that those in the highest quarter of CRP levels had a 60% greater risk of current asthma than those with lower CRP levels. Those with the highest quartile of CRP levels had more than double the incidence of asthmatic wheezing, and more than triple the incidence of nighttime coughing. In other words, as we discussed in *Asthma Solved Naturally*, asthma is another sign of systemic inflammation.

So what causes systemic inflammation? As we'll discuss in the next chapter, localized inflammation is often caused by physical injuries like broken bones or tissue damage. Systemic inflammation, however, is typically caused by the bombardment and overload of toxins or pathological microorganisms.

Systemic inflammation indicates that the immune system is overburdened. The extent or combination of the elements mentioned simply overwhelms the immune system. Typically, the immune system can resolve most of these problems when it is presented with a small amount or a few of them at a time. But when an avalanche of them becomes too great, the immune system goes on alert, resulting in systemic inflammation.

Systemic inflammation is the immune system's version of all-out war. The immune system begins to launch the nukes. These can include fever, vomiting, diarrhea, swelling and pain.

The rest of this chapter will more specifically discuss lifestyle choices that produce or worsen systemic inflammation within the body. In other words, these are all *contributing causes.* This means that just one of these factors may not in itself cause systemic inflammation. But any one of these, in addition to others, can overwhelm the immune system—producing systemic inflammation.

Systemic Inflammation

Systemic and chronic inflammation creates hypersensitivity of the due to the immune system being stressed and on high alert status. In this situation, the immune system is overloaded by infection(s), chemical toxicity, or a diet that constantly exposes the body to toxins. One or a combination of these effects generally produces a whole-body diseased state. In such a state, the body will overreact to an exposure to stress in the airways. These triggers can be as simple as exercise, cold air, smoke or fragrance.

This type of systemic inflammatory status is evidenced by high C-reactive protein in the body. CRP levels are easily determined through blood analysis. We'll discuss some of the research that illustrates this later.

While toxin overload is the primary condition, the following list summarizes conditions that collectively contribute to systemic inflammation:

1) *Toxemia:* An overload of toxins that produce radicals.

2) *Infections:* Infection with microorganisms that produce mutagenicity, toxins and radicals: viruses, bacteria, yeasts and parasites.

3) *Antioxidant enzyme deficiencies:* An undersupply of anti-oxidizing enzymes that stabilize radicals, including glutathione peroxidase, glutathione reductase, catalase and superoxide dismutase.

4) *Dietary antioxidant deficiencies:* An undersupply of antioxidants from our foods to help stabilize radicals.

5) *Barriers to detoxification:* Lifestyle or physiological factors that block our body's ability to rid waste products and toxins. Detoxification requires exercise, fresh air, sweating, sunshine and so on.

6) *Poor dietary choices:* A poor diet burdens the body with toxins, unstable fatty acids, refined sugars and overly processed foods.

7) *Immunosuppression:* A burdened or defective immune system.

Example: Trans Fat

When palm and coconut oils are cooled, they become hardened. This makes them good thickening agents for cooking and good for frying. In an attempt to match nature, in 1902 German Wilhelm Normann patented the first hydrogenation process, which was eventually purchased by Proctor and Gamble, leading to Crisco® oil and eventually margarine. When nutritionists convinced us that *"all saturated fats are bad"* in the sixties and seventies, margarine sales took off. Processors also found that frying oil had a better shelf life and was cheaper if cottonseed oil and soybean oil were *partially hydrogenated*. Because these oils do not normally harden at room temperature as does palm, coconut and lard, hydrogenation allowed processors to use the less expensive oils for frying, spreading and cooking.

Hydrogenation means to *saturate* hydrogen onto all of the available bonds of the central molecule. Whereas a natural substance might have a double bond between carbon and other atoms, hydrogen gas can be bubbled through the substance—using a catalyst to spark the reaction—to attach more hydrogen to the molecule. To saturate carbon bonds with hydrogen, catalyst is added, and the oil undergoes the bubbling of hydrogen within a heated catalytic environment. This saturation synthetically changes the oil's melting point, giving it more versatility at a lower cost.

Let's review. Food scientists took real foods—oil extracted from soybeans or cottonseed—and synthetically converted it into what appeared to be the same molecular structure, but with a different melting point. Harmless, yes? Think again. After decades of use and millions of heart attacks and strokes later, health researchers began realizing that partially hydrogenated oils have damaging effects upon the cardiovascular system.

While the saturated or partially saturated molecule was the same formula, the synthetic process of hydrogenation created an unusual (transversed) molecular structure called a *trans-fat*. Trans-fat is now implicated in a various degenerative disorders, including atherosclerosis, dementia, liver disease, irritable bowel syndrome, and Alzheimer's disease among others. While the epidemic increase in cardiovascular disease has focused billions of dollars into research, the consumption of trans-fats was altogether overlooked. Why? Because researchers assumed that hydrogenated soybean oil was harmless because its molecularly-identical cousin—raw soybean oil—was harmless, and even healthy because it was a polyunsaturated oil.

The mechanism whereby trans-fats produce damage in the body—as we'll discuss later—is called lipid peroxidation. Because trans-fats are less stable than cis-fats, and because fats make up our cell membranes, trans-fats become more readily damaged, producing what is called lipid peroxides. Lipid peroxides damage blood vessel walls and other tissue systems, producing cardiovascular disease and other degenerative disorders.

So now researchers realize that the orientation—polarity and spin— of a molecule can have altogether different effects from the same molecule rotated in the orientation nature designed.

Nature normally orients healthy oil molecules—and many other nutrients—in *cis* formation: They are oriented so that the hydrogens are on the same side with the other molecular bonds. A *trans* configuration has hydrogens on the opposite side of the bonds.

Naturally occurring molecules are electromagnetically different than synthesized or disrupted molecules such as trans fats. The resulting quanta of spin and angular momentum produces an imbalance in the body that must be balanced. Natural lipids provide that balance by donation: They donate some of their electromagnetic character to balance the imbalanced trans fats.

What results is a lipid ripe for peroxidation. The reaction actually takes place almost simultaneously—the rebalancing of the trans fat opens the vulnerability to oxidation, and the peroxidation process proceeds, resulting in damaged cell membranes.

As the cell membranes become damaged, the body works to repair the damage. This is inflammation. As the inflammation process works to repair the cell damage, the tissue system is weakened. This is the case for arteriosclerosis. Once the cells of the artery walls are damaged by lipid peroxidation, they scab up and calcify. Some of these scabs can break off and clog blood vessels down the pipe.

The end result is, as the FDA has finally and appropriately identified, is that trans fats cause cardiovascular diseases.

This issue of peroxidation is not isolated to trans fats. Practically every toxin identified in the first chapter produces lipid peroxides and other types of oxidative radicals. These damage the body in the same—by damaging the cell membranes and thus damaging the tissue systems that the cell membranes make up.

While our bodies are built to handle moderate levels of free radicals, our synthetic world is overloading our body with synthetics, which produce these oxidized or oxidative radicals within the body. This oxidizing potency of toxins leads to an overload of acids (H+), causing excessive acidosis, and the subsequent degeneration of our tissue systems.

And among those synthetic chemicals that do not readily metabolize (break down) within the body, many will build up among the body's fat cells. This is because many synthetic toxins are *lipophilic:* fat-loving, or fat-soluble. This has the effect of the body storing up synthetic toxins within our fat cells, only to break down and pollute our bodies days, weeks or years later.

Chapter Three

Why Toxins are Bad

Just about every disease can now be attributed, at least in part, to toxins. And immune suppression—the weakening of our immune system, is often a direct result of toxin exposure.

The reality is that toxins burden our immune system because they require part of our immune system to remove them. As the immune system is breaking down and removing toxins it is less powerful against other invaders. Yes, a strong immune can fight many invaders at the same time. But when it is spread out it can also become depleted. This is called immunosuppression.

Even diseases primarily attributed to heredity have been traced to toxicity among previous generations. Before we further define why toxins are so bad, let's review the primary toxins that are currently bombarding modern humanity: chemical toxins, electromagnetic toxins, biological toxins and those environments that house those toxins.

Chemical Toxins

Over the past century, humankind has opened a Pandora's box of chemical manipulation. The brilliant marketing efforts of chemical manufacturers of the twentieth century convinced us that synthetic chemicals made life easier, more productive and healthier. Not only did they get this wrong, but we all bought in to it.

And now we are paying the price.

As this grand synthetic experiment has unfolded, we have discovered that many of these chemicals are not only toxic. They now risk humankind's future existence. After only a few decades of massive synthetic chemical manufacturing, we are beginning to suffer the horrific price synthetic chemicals come with: We are faced with increasing epidemics of cancer, asthma, nerve degenerative diseases and so many others.

Years ago scientists discovered that stress responses can be passed down over several generations within our genetic information – in a science termed epigenetics. New evidence is revealing that toxic exposures can also affect our grandchildren and their children.

Research from Washington State University, Case Western Reserve University School of Medicine, University of Toronto Medical School and the University of Texas (Guerrero-Bosagna *et al.* 2012) confirmed that our environment not only affects our genetic information (epigenetics): Exposure to toxins will produce metabolic changes, physiology changes, behavioral changes and cognitive changes two and three generations later.

University of Toronto and Case Western Reserve University researchers (Crews *et al.* 2012) determined that environmental stress will affect ones genes for several generations after the stressor. This precipitated from epidemiological research several decades ago showing that periods of starvation or famine caused metabolic affects in farming families two and three generations later. Now it appears that many other types of stressors, including environmental stress and toxic stress, can affect a family several generations later.

Another study from Washington State University (Matthews *et al.* 2012) found that dioxin, plastic compounds like bisphenol A and phthalates, and JP8 – a jet fuel – will produce DNA damage that affects metabolism in rats multiple generations after the initial exposure.

These results are consistent with epidemiology research that shows transgenerational effects caused by environmental and dietary factors can produce diseases such as cancer, heart disease and diabetes several generations later. Even asthma is linked to toxins such as hexavalent chromium.

The bottom line is that these epigenetic environmental stressors are toxins produced by our chemical industrial complex. Our choices are clear: Rethinking our (so far) irresponsible widespread use of synthetic chemicals, or face a widespread breakdown of health among our grandchildren, their children and successive generations – if humans survive that far.

Much of our drinking supplies are now laced with mercury, arsenic, DDT, PCB, nitrates, HTMs, plasticizers, pharmaceuticals and hundreds of other dangerous toxins. Much of the non-organic food we eat is now to full of various pesticide residues. We are gradually discovering that agribusiness' use of chemical fertilizers and pesticides is slowly poisoning our bodies. The toxins are building up in our cells—mutating DNA and suffocating our immune systems.

Most of the furnishings we purchase now are filled with formaldehydes, synthetic materials and preservatives. Most office buildings and many houses still contain hazards like asbestos and other components that cause toxicity. Our entire environment is laced with synthetic chemistry. If the human race stopped chemical production today, we still would have done so much damage over the past fifty years that it will take centuries for the earth's detoxification systems to purify herself.

Today we are building mountains of synthetic chemistry loading up our dumps, landfills, lakes, rivers, and oceans with toxic brews. These mountains are decomposing very slowly—outgassing and breaking down into potent poisons. *Time Magazine* reported on June 25, 2007 that

Americans generated 1,643 pounds of trash per person in 2005. A mere 32% of it was recycled.

Much of this waste is plastic. The problem with plastic is reflective of its benefit—it lasts far longer than do natural materials. While a plastic bag might not tear and rip as fast as a paper bag as we walk from the grocery store, a plastic bag will have as much as a 500-year half-life—depending upon its material. That is a long time. Whet happens to the bag while nature works to biodegrade it? It clogs our soils and waters. For this reason our lands, waters, and bodies are steadily becoming laced with polymers and plasticizers.

Plastics are made through reactions between monomers (small molecules) and plasticizers to create longer-chain molecules. Monomers are typically hydrocarbons such as petroleum. Combining ethane monomers and plasticizers forms polyethylene. Combining styrene monomers and plasticizers renders polystyrene. Combining vinyl chloride monomers and plasticizers results in polyvinyl chloride, or PVC. Combining propylene monomers and plasticizers gives us polypropylene. As these plastic combinations are broken down, guess what gets released into the environment?

Nature produces its own types of natural polymers such as rubber from rubber trees. But this isn't enough for our hungry appetite for luxury. In an attempt to improve upon nature, the 1855 lab of Alexander Parkes mixed pyroxylin from cellulose with alcohol and camphor to form the first type of plastic.

This clear, hard plastic was 'improved' by Dr. Leo Baekeland decades later with a polymer process using phenol and formaldehyde in early 1900s. "Bakelite" became a wildly successful product as it effectively replaced shellac and rubber as a general sheathing material. Because it was heat-resistant and moisture-proof, it quickly became the insulator of choice for engines, appliances, and electronics. Dr. Baekeland eventually sold his General Bakelite Company to Union Carbide in 1939 and retired a very wealthy man to Florida. His life was made easy through the 'miracle' of chemistry.

Nylon was an invention of DuPont researchers in the late 1930s. It was made initially with benzene from coal. The introduction of polypropylene as a synthetic rubber followed shortly thereafter. Polypropylene was an accidental discovery by a couple of researchers vying to convert natural gas for Phillips Petroleum.

The American industrial complex gearing up for World War II focused its attention on this synthetic version due to a shortage of natural rubber. Thanks to synthetic rubber, each soldier was able to wear 32 pounds of rubber in clothing and equipment. A tank needed about a ton.

America's military might was as likely due to its synthetic rubber as were its bombs. Again, chemistry was seemingly making our lives easier.

The synthetic polymer revolution surged after the Second World War. The plastic revolution raged, as both consumers and manufacturers bonded to replace anything natural with synthetic polymers.

A polychlorinated biphenyl is a grouping of chlorine atoms bonded together with biphenyl. Biphenyl is a molecule composed of two phenyl rings. It is an aromatic hydrocarbon occurring naturally in coal and petroleum. When synthetically combined with chlorine—another naturally occurring element—the result is highly toxic. PCB was banned in the early 1970s when biologists studied a population of dead seabirds and found they died of a toxic dose of PCBs. For more than forty years, PCBs have been used in paints, pesticides, paper, adhesives, flame-retardants, surgical implants, lubricating oil and electrical equipment.

Referred innocently as "phenols" for many years, the PCB ban followed suspicion of toxicity for over a decade. Massive PCB contamination in the Hudson River was found caused by local electrical manufacturing plants. Some two hundred miles of the river was eventually designated a toxic *superfund site*. This woke us up to PCB toxicity. PCBs break down slowly and bio-accumulate in living organisms.

When PCBs get into our waterways, they build up in the smallest organisms and work their way up the food chain, eventually reaching humans. Today the ban on PCBs does not include many applications considered "closed," such as capacitors and vacuum pump fluids. This means there are still considerable PCBs in our buildings and electrical equipment. PCB poisoning can cause immediate liver damage. Symptoms can include fever, rashes, nausea, and more.

One might argue that that combining earth-borne commodities like hydrocarbons cannot be so unnatural. After all, hydrocarbons are produced by the earth as part of her own recycling process. However, the process of converting nature's hydrocarbon monomers into polymers of our design requires various catalysts—*plasticizers*—to complete.

Plasticizers are used in plastic production to give the long polymer chain its flexibility. Without plasticizers inserted between the polymer chains, plastics would have no flexibility. Without plasticizers, polymers are clear, hard substances: rock-like. The gradations of flex added to polymer chains give the resulting plastic its particular usefulness. A plasticizer adds strength to this flexibility, making the new material difficult to tear or break.

Most plasticizers are *phthalates*. Phthalates are derived from phthalic acid, an aromatic ringed carbon molecule also referred to as dicarboxylic acid. Originally synthesized in 1836 through the oxidation of naphthalene tetrachloride, phthalic acid can also be synthesized from hydrocarbons and sulfuric acid with a mercury catalyst.

Common phthalates are di(2-ethylhexyl) phthalate (DEHP), dibutyl phthalate (DBP), and bisphenol A (BPA), among others.

Biphenyl A, for example, is used in many types of containers, including baby bottles. BPA can easily leach into food or formula when the bottle is exposed to heat or sunlight. A 2000 Centers of Disease Control study found 75% of those tested had phthalates in their urine, and subsequent studies have found some 95% of the U.S. population has detectable levels of biphenyl A within body fluids. Biphenyls are considered endocrine system disruptors. Long-term effects as their residues build up in our cells, organs and tissue systems are largely unknown.

More recently, researchers from the University of Michigan (Meeker and Ferguson 2011) confirmed that common phthalate plasticizers DEHP, DBP and BPA all disrupt human thyroid hormones—linked to increasing the incidence of thyroid diseases. The research compared and analyzed the metabolites from urine and serum thyroid levels of 1,346 adults and 329 adolescents.

Higher DEHP, DBP, and BPA levels were found to be associated with lower levels of the thyroid hormone metabolites of T4, free T3, total T3 and thyroglobin. Higher DEHP levels were associated with higher TSH levels, while higher BPA levels were associated with lower T3 and TSH levels. This means that the more plasticizers in the bloodstream, the more deranged the hormone levels. The researchers found that lower T4 metabolite levels has the strongest association with higher phthalates. High DEHP levels were associated strongly with lower TSH levels, while BPA was associated with lower T4 and TSH levels.

The study, published in the scientific journal, *Environmental Health Perspectives,* is the first national human study confirming that BPA and other common plasticizers definitely disrupt hormones. Over the past decade, the chemical industry has been disputing the link between BPA and hormone disruption as coincidental. This large study confirmed previous research that led to the suspicion that these plasticizers, common among food packaging, water bottles, can linings and other consumer goods, disrupt hormone levels.

University of Michigan assistant professor and lead researcher, Dr. John Meeker, commented that the highest 20% of DEHP exposures had as high as 10% decreased thyroid hormones.

Most aromatic carbon rings like the phenyl ring or the benzyl ring used for these polymers have otherwise proven to be hazardous to our environment and well-being. Note there are a number of aromatic carbon rings produced in nature. These, however, do not affect hormone levels, turning males to females, as has been found among fish.

Today there are hundreds of different plasticizers used to produce plastics. Most are variations of aromatic carbons or similarly hazardous compounds. When plasticizers from plastic polymers break down in the environment, these aromatic carbons are released. Our backyards, landfills and oceans—our entire environment for that matter—are silently being inundated by these insidious compounds.

Benzene, for example, is a popular phenyl plasticizer. Benzene has been classified as a volatile organic compound and a carcinogen by the Natural Institutes of Health's National Toxicology Program. Benzene is among the top twenty most used industrial chemicals. It is used to make adhesives, paint, pharmaceuticals, printed materials, photographic chemicals, synthetic rubber, dyes, detergents, paint and even food processing equipment. As a result, benzene is found throughout our environment—notably in our air and water—and has been implicated in numerous types of cancers.

The problems of synthetic chemicals are pervasive. About 80,000 chemicals have been approved for commercialization over the past fifty years. The *Toxic Substances Control Act of 1976* was set up to evaluate chemicals being introduced. Yet only about 65,000 have been reviewed. However only a small percentage of these chemicals have been carefully analyzed for their environmental and health effects.

Clinical research by Professor John G Ionescu, Ph.D. (2009) concluded that environmental pollution is clearly associated with the development of hypersensitivities. Dr. Ionescu's research indicated that environmental noxious agents, including many chemicals, contribute to the total immune burden, producing increased susceptibility for intolerances due to inflammation.

According to Dr. Ionescu, toxic inputs such as formaldehyde, smog, industrial waste, wood preservatives, microbial toxins, alcohol, pesticides, processed foods, nicotine, solvents and amalgam-heavy metals have been observed to be mediating toxins that produce the physical susceptibilities for toxin sensitization and subsequent inflammation.

This is also consistent with findings of other scientists—as discussed—that chemicals overload the immune system and cause inflammation.

Chemical toxins such as DDT, PBDEs, dioxin, formaldehyde, benzene, butane and chlorinated chemicals tend to accumulate within the body's tissues. This is because many of these are fat-soluble. Other compounds, such as phthalate plasticizers and parabens tend to clear the body faster because they are not fat soluble. Still, these can also cause toxicity issues if they are regularly presented to the body.

The compounding of these synthetics contributes to the body-wide status of systemic inflammation. As the immune system gears up to overdrive due to the overloading of multiple toxins, it becomes weaker and hypersensitive. This can cause a host of issues, including allergies, irritable bowel syndrome and many others.

Researchers from the U.S. Centers for Disease Control and Prevention (Ye *et al.* 2012) concluded that BPA and seven other toxins are building up within the bodies of U.S. children according to blood and urine studies.

The research comes from the CDC's National Center for Environmental Health. The researchers utilized data from Children's National Health and Nutrition Examination Survey results of children who were between three and eleven years old.

The research found that the blood of over 60% of these children contained significant levels of bisphenol A (BPA) and its metabolites, as well as seven other toxins referred to as phenols. These toxins include benzophenone-3, triclosan, 2,4-dichlorophenol, 2,5- dichlorophenol, and three parabens.

Benzophenone-3 is also referred to as oxybenzone, and it is a common ingredient in many sunscreens. This is because oxybenzone will absorb UV rays, preventing the skin from UV exposure (which, by the way, produces the all-important vitamin D).

Research from the Environmental Working Group has found that oxybenzone will also become absorbed into the skin, and may mutate DNA creating photosensitivity. Sunscreen producers argued against this notion, criticizing the EWG, but a 2008 study by the CDC confirmed that oxybenzone was found in 97% of urine samples in the 2003-2004 National Healthy and Nutrition Examination Survey.

Triclosan is a common ingredient in many antibacterial soaps, mouthwashes, underarm deodorants and toothpastes. Though banned in Europe in plastic, it is also a common ingredient in many food plastics. Triclosan is typically produced from 2,4-dichlorophenol (chlorinated phenol), so it is classified as a phenol. Byproducts of triclosan, as it is broken down in the body and on the skin, include dioxin and chlorophenols.

These toxins can harm us for generations according to other research.

A study from the University of Michigan (Clayton *et al.* 2011) found that triclosan is associated with reduced immunity and higher levels of allergies.

Besides its toxicity, triclosan has also been shown to produce superbugs, as bacteria can become resistant to it over time.

Dichlorophenols are used in many herbicides and pesticides, and are known toxins. Besides their toxicity, 2,5-DCP has been found to be associated with obesity among children, according to research by Georgia's Mercer University School of Medicine (Twum *et al.* 2011).

Parabens are ingredients in many skin lotions and they will readily become absorbed into the body. They are endocrine disruptors because they will attach to estrogen receptors. They have also been associated with breast cancer.

While one might assume only children using these chemicals are exposed, recent research has determined that many of these – including acyclovir, benzophenone-3, benzylparaben, carbamazepine, ethylparaben, fluconazole, fluoxetine, methylparaben, metronidazole, propylparaben, and ranitidine – are flowing into our waterways through municipal waste treatment facilities.

And because waste treatment plants cannot eliminate these in waste water streams, they are also flowing into our bathing and drinking water supplies as well. Other research has found that arsenic is common in many municipal drinking waters in the U.S. This means that arsenic toxicity is also present in many children.

This is a gigantic discussion, so here we will summarize the major categories and sources of toxic chemicals that add to our immune system burden:

Plasticizers and Parabens

Today, plasticizers and parabens are common amongst many of our medications, toys, foods packaged in plastic and other consumer items. Phthalates are also found in many household items. While phthalates have shorter half-lives than some toxins, they have been implicated in systemic inflammatory issues, hormone disruption, cancers and other conditions. Many cosmetics and antiperspirants contain parabens. They are thus readily absorbed into the skin where they can provoke inflammatory responses (Crinnion 2010).

Heavy Metals

Heavy metals are metal elements that exist naturally in trace quantities within our soils, waters and foods. However, extraordinary levels of heavy metals such as cadmium, lead and mercury are produced by humanity's industrial complex in the manufacturing of various consumer items.

We can cite many studies that have associated heavy metal exposure to immunosuppression. Mercury is one of these.

For example, in multicenter research from the Department of Medicine from the Lavoro Medical Center in Bari, Italy (Soleo *et al.* 2002), researchers studied the effects of low levels of inorganic mercury exposure on 117 workers. They compared these with 172 general population subjects. They found no difference in the white blood cell count between the two groups. However, the worker group exposed to mercury had increased levels of CD4+ and CD8+ cytokines, and CD4+ levels were particularly high. These indicated a state of systemic inflammation. In addition, significantly lower levels of interleukin (IL-8) occurred among the exposed workers—indicating immunosuppression.

This research concluded that even low levels of environmental exposure to mercury and other heavy metals (beyond the trace levels normally found in nature) suppresses the immune system and stimulates inflammation.

Cadmium is another heavy metal bombarding us. Among consumer products, cadmium is used in a number of metal coatings, batteries and colorings. Most cigarettes also contain cadmium.

Consumer Toxins

In conjunction with a mandate to lower toxin levels among the state's residents, in 2010 the Minnesota Department of Health compiled and released a list of the most toxic chemicals used in consumer products, building materials, pesticides, hair dyes, detergents, aerosols, cosmetics, furniture polish, herbicides, paints, cleaning solutions and many other common sources. The list also referenced research connecting the toxins to disease conditions.

The list contained 1,755 chemicals.

For each of these toxins, the liver and immune system must launch a variety of macrophages, T-cells and B-cells to break them apart and escort them out of the body. This means that each toxin represents an additional load the immune system must carry.

We might compare this to moving dirt. A small handful of dirt can be carried around easily, and dispersed without much effort. However, a truckload of dirt is another matter completely. What can we do with a truckload of dirt? If we dumped a truckload of dirt on our lawn, we'd have a hill of dirt that would bury the access to our front door and annihilate our lawn and/or garden.

This is a useful comparison because while our bodies can handle a small amount of toxins quite easily, modern society is increasingly dumping toxic 'dirt' into our atmosphere, water and foods, effectively inundating our bodies 'by the truckload.'

With this increased burden, the research shows that the body's defenses are lowered. The mucosal membrane is weakened. The immune system is on alert. Systemic inflammation becomes evident. In this immunosuppressed state, the body is more likely to succumb to a variety of disease conditions.

Water Pollutants

Our industrial society has been dumping massive amounts of synthetic chemistry into our waters for many decades, and we are paying the price. Water contamination comes from manufacturing, wastewater streams from houses, air pollution, ship and boat waste streams and pollutants, run-off from farms and the gutters and streets. All of these to one degree or another end up in our drinking water supplies.

While municipalities have extensive chlorination systems in place to clear microbiological content, removal systems for chemical pollutants are still in various stages of development. As a result, our drinking water supplies have numerous contaminants.

Even some of the cleaning agents used in some municipal water supplies are toxic. This includes trichloroethylene. Trichloroethylene is a chlorinated hydrocarbon used to separate oil from water. The solvent was popularized in the dry cleaning business, and is a common cleansing agent in many local water municipalities.

Pharmaceutical medicines in our water supplies make for a perfect example. In 2007, researchers from Finland's Abo Akademi University (Vieno *et al.*) released a study showing that pharmaceutical beta-blockers, antiepileptic drugs, lipid regulators, anti-inflammatory drugs and fluoroquinolone drugs were all found in river waters. The concentrations of these were well above drinking water limits. The researchers also found that water treatment only eliminated an average of 13% of the concentration of these pharmaceuticals. This means that 87% of these pharmaceutical medicines remained in the drinking water, ready to dose each and every person drinking that water with prescription medication.

Other pollutants that are commonly found in our drinking water supplies include PCBs, and other biphenol compounds, dioxin, chlorine metabolites, pesticides, herbicides, petroleum byproducts, nitrates, and many others.

Agricultural runoff is a huge source of drinking water contamination. In addition, nitrogen-rich fertilizers choke rivers and oceans with extra nitrogen, causing abnormal blooms of algae. These massive algal blooms cut off oxygen supplies and lead to the die-offs of many species of marine life. *Dead zones* have been reportedly growing in many of the world's waterways, as we will discuss shortly. The cause is the massive use of nitrogen-based synthetic fertilizers.

The use of pesticides on agricultural land, playgrounds, parks, home lawns, and gardens throughout the United States is staggering, and it is growing. In 1964, approximately 233 million pounds of pesticides were applied in the U.S. By 1982, this amount tripled to 612 million pounds. In 1999, the U.S. Environmental Protection Agency reported that some five *billion* pounds of these chemicals were applied per year throughout America's crops, forests, parks, and lawns.

One of the more increasingly popular pesticides is imidacloprid, a neonicotinoid. Introduced by Bayer in 1994, imidacloprid is used against aphids and similar insects on over 140 different crops. Touted as a chemical with a fairly short half-life of thirty days in water and twenty-seven days in anaerobic soil, imidacloprid's half-life is about 997 days in aerobic soil. While it has a lower immediate toxicity compared with hazards like DDT, imidacloprid's use is now widespread. It is rated by the EPA and WHO as *"moderately toxic"* in small doses. Larger doses can disrupt liver and thyroid function. While this pesticide does well at killing off increasingly resistant pests, it has also been shown to decimate bee populations.

Cleaning agents are used with or rinsed by water. They will thus immediately enter our greywater systems. According to the U.S. Poison Control Centers, about ten percent of all toxin exposure is caused by cleaning products, with almost two-thirds involving children under six years old. While we might be shocked to find a child toying with a bottle of drain cleaner containing sulfuric acid, hydrochloric acid and lye, we do not think twice about feeding this same product into our waterways. We wear gloves to protect our skin from the harmful affects of ammonia and bleach while we do our cleaning but assume they disappear once poured down the sink.

An example of this is 1,4-dioxane, a common ingredient in many shampoos and other cleaning products. The California EPA documented that 1,4-dioxane is a carcinogen that can also damage kidneys, nerves and lungs. It biodegrades very slowly and is becoming a threat to drinking water supplies. This is but one of many.

In a 2002 U.S. Geological Survey report on stream water contaminants, 69% of stream samples revealed non-biodegradable detergents, and 66% of the samples contained disinfectant chemicals. Phosphates—central ingredients in many commercial laundry soaps—have been banned for dumping in over eleven states in the U.S. because of their dangerous effects upon the environment. Yet many people still use these soaps without any consideration of their effects upon our waters.

Biphenyls are considered *xenoestrogens,* or endocrine system disruptors. Long-term effects as their residues build up in the tissues of aquatic species, and bio-accumulate up the ladder to our cells, organs and tissue systems. Research has found that biphenyls have produced sexual re-orientation of fish in some water supplies.

Our waters are filling up with plastic particles. As plastics break down into smaller particles, they are absorbed by filtering marine plants and aquatics and passed up the food chain. Research led by Captain Charles Moore of the *Algalita Marine Research Foundation* (2001; 2002; 2008) found an astounding six-to-one ratio of plastic particles-to-plankton in some areas. This means that for every pound of algae—the key nutrient for nearly all marine life—there are six pounds of plastic in the oceans. This also means that our marine life is eating plastic particles with their meals: and so are humans who eat fish.

Captain Moore was first alerted to the plastic problem in 1997 when he sailed through a region of the Pacific Ocean between Hawaii and California called the *North Pacific Gyre*. He came upon a large area of floating garbage, consisting primarily of plastic debris. The *Great Pacific Garbage Patch* is now documented from a number of studies, the earliest from a 1988 National Oceanic and Atmospheric Administration paper.

Requiring some 500 years to breakdown, plastics are known to disrupt hormones and accumulate hydrocarbons as mentioned earlier. It is estimated that about twenty percent of the plastic polluting our waters comes from discarded plastic pellets used to make plastic by manufacturers. These pellets are being swept or blown into the water from careless manufacturers and transport companies. The other eighty percent of the ocean's plastics is estimated to come from daily consumer use and the careless littering of waterways and runoffs.

These combined factors are increasingly problematic to a human population seeking to sustain life on the planet. Research by Slovenian researchers Tatjana Tisler and Jana Zagorc-Koncan (2003) has shown that we are drastically underestimating the effects of toxic industrial waste. Our typical method for toxicity research has been to study each individual chemical and its possible toxicity. What we are missing with this type of research is the combined effects of the thousands of chemicals we are putting into our waters. As these chemicals mix, they create a toxic soup of new chemical combinations. Some of these are combinations are exponentially more toxic than the individual chemicals.

Pesticides

By some accounts there are nearly nine hundred different pesticides being used in the United States. Of those, at least thirty-seven contain organophosphates—one of our more toxic chemical combinations. Organophosphates kill insects through nervous system disruption. These neurotoxins are also toxic to humans' nervous systems. The nerve gases Serin and VX are organophosphates, for example.

Organophosphates block cholinesterase—a key neuro-enzyme—from working properly within the body. With cholinesterase blocked, acetylcholine is not regulated. Unregulated acetylcholine causes an over-stimulation of nerve activity, resulting in nerve damage, paralysis, and muscle weakness.

Organophosphates are spreading through ground water, air and through dermal contact. They are exposing us through our breathing, skin contact, swimming, and consumption. Initial symptoms can include nausea, vomiting, shortness of breath, confusion, and muscle spasms. Some of the more common organophosphates include Malathion, Parathion, Diazinon, Phosmet, Clorpyrifos, Dursban and others.

The EPA actually banned Diazinon and Dursban in a phase-out beginning in March of 2001, to last through December 2003. Curiously, both Diazinon and Dursban are still in use today. Phased bans like this theoretically take several years to allow companies to run out their inventories. Also since these bans were aimed at consumer products, organophosphates are still used profusely in commercial agriculture—our food production.

In a 2003 study done by the Centers for Disease Control and Prevention, thousands of people were tested for 116 chemicals. Thirty-four of these were pesticides such as organophosphates, organochlorines, and carbamates. Nineteen of the thirty-four were found in either the blood or urine.

The use of pesticides on agricultural land, playgrounds, parks, home lawns, and gardens throughout the United States has growing by staggering proportions. In 1964, approximately 233 million pounds of pesticide active ingredients were used. By 1982, this amount tripled to 612 million pounds. In 1999, the U.S. Environmental Protection Agency reported that some five *billion* pounds of these chemicals were used per year throughout America's crops, forests, parks, and lawns.

One of the fastest growing of these pesticides has been imidacloprid, a neonicotinoid. Introduced by Bayer in 1994, imidacloprid is used against aphids and similar insects on over 140 different crops. Touted as a chemical with a fairly short half-life of thirty days in water and twenty-seven days in anaerobic soil, imidacloprid's half-life is about 997 days in aerobic soil. While it has a lower immediate toxicity compared with hazards like DDT, imidacloprid's use is now widespread. It is rated by the EPA and WHO as *"moderately toxic"* in small doses. Larger doses can disrupt liver and thyroid function. While this pesticide does well at killing off increasingly resistant pests, it also can decimate bee populations.

A world without bees, as described in Rachel Carson's classic *Silent Spring,* would insure a destiny of hunger and destitution in human society.

In France for example, some 500,000 registered hives were lost in the mid-1990s. Imidacloprid was implicated, and was subsequently banned for many crops in that country. Massive bee destruction has occurred in other regions of Europe also appear connected to imidacloprid use. A 2006-2007 loss of hives throughout Europe and the U.S.—referred to as *colony collapse disorder*—is now increasingly being connected to imidacloprid, although it also appears that other chemicals as well as possibly unnatural electromagnetic radiation work together to weaken the bees' immunity to viruses and other diseases. Imidacloprid and other chemicals can weaken the bee's immune system just as they weaken the human immune system—depending of course on the level of exposure.

Neonicotinoid pesticides have been banned from the European Union and for good reason. Not only are they harming bee populations because they are neurotoxic to bees. They are also neurotoxins in humans.

The European Food Safety Authority (EFSA) warns that the common pesticides categorized as neonicotinoids, which include acetamiprid and imidacloprid, will damage the human brain and nervous system.

The report, first released in 2013, suggested that permitted levels of exposure be reduced until more research is done to evaluate their neurotoxicity.

The report follows a new study from the Tokyo Metropolitan Institute of Medical Science. This studied the effects of acetamiprid and imidacloprid on developing nervous systems:

"This study is the first to show that of acetamiprid, imidacloprid and nicotine exert similar excitatory effects on mammalian nAChRs at concentrations greater than 1 μM. Therefore, the neonicotinoids may adversely affect human health, especially the developing brain."

The bottom line is that these neonicotinoids are neurotoxins not only to insects – including bees. They are neurotoxic to humans as well.

The EFSA stated in its release:

"The PPR Panel found that acetamiprid and imidacloprid may adversely affect the development of neurons and brain structures associated with functions such as learning and memory. It concluded that some current guidance levels for acceptable exposure to acetamiprid and imidacloprid may not be protective enough to safeguard against developmental neurotoxicity and should be reduced."

Chlorinated dioxins are also pervasive in today's environment. Significant sources include cigarettes, pesticides, coal-burning factories, diesel exhaust, and sewage sludge. Dioxins are also byproducts of the manufacturing of a number of products, including many resins, glues, plastics, and chlorine-treated products. Dioxins also bio-accumulate in fatty tissues and can take years to fully degrade. Dioxins are known endocrine disruptors. They have also been linked to liver toxicity and birth defects.

Thanks to the human industrial complex, there are now thousands of *volatile organic compounds* in our environment. A VOC is classified as such if it has a relatively high vapor pressure, allowing it to vaporize quickly and enter the atmosphere. Gasoline, paint thinners, cleaning solvents, ketones, and aldehydes are a few of the chemicals considered sources of VOCs. Methane-forming VOCs like benzene and toluene are also carcinogens. VOCs are often used as preservatives for pressed wood and other building materials. As a result, many buildings contain VOCs locked within its building materials. Once soaked in or inborn with the fabrication, VOCs are trapped within the material, causing them to outgas over time. This outgassing process is speeded up when the building is demolished or taken apart. As the building materials are broken up, VOCs can be released at toxic exposure levels.

VOCs will form ozone as they interact with sunlight and heat. VOC poisoning symptoms include nausea; headaches; eye irritation; inflammation of the nose and throat; liver damage; brain fog; and neurotoxic brain damage. Using cleaning or painting solvents indoors is a common cause of VOC poisoning.

In a study by Janssen *et al.* (2004) and *The Collaborative on Health and the Environment,* some two hundred diseases were found to be attributable to exposure to industrial chemicals. The diseases listed are some of the most prevalent diseases of our society—cancers, cardiovascular disease, autoimmune diseases and so on. The researchers found that over 120 diseases have been specifically linked by research to exposure to specific industrial chemicals. For another thirty-three diseases, the evidence for linking to specific chemicals was considered "good." For the rest of the diseases, research indicated a definite link but the evidence was considered "limited" (Lean 2004).

The Pandora's box of adverse effects of pesticides and herbicides is coming to roost in a multitude of ailments. Now we find pesticides and herbicides significantly increase the risk of thyroid disease such as hypothyroidism.

This may be obvious, but these chemicals are designed to kill life. There are a number of different types of pesticides, but most of them work as neurotoxins. This means they damage the nervous systems of insects, killing the insects in their tracks or flight paths.

Herbicides work in similar ways, but typically damage the metabolism of plants. This often means they ruin the plant's ability to protect itself. They also work to kill the circulatory system of the plant.

These killing chemicals often have similar effects upon humans, except at a more subtle basis. Neurotoxic pesticides will also hurt the human nervous system, without necessarily knocking it out completely. This is why, for example, pesticides have been linked to nervous system disorders such as Parkinson's disease.

But many pesticides and herbicides have an effect upon our body's hormonal systems as well. These are also an indirect result of neurotoxic chemicals, because our secretion of hormones are synchronized by our brain and nervous system.

These neurotoxic chemicals also bind to hormone receptors, as we'll discuss.

In particular, research is discovering that many pesticides and herbicides specifically reduce the secretion of thyroid hormones.

Many women today have a condition called hypothyroidism. This means the thyroid gland is not producing enough thyroid hormones. Hyperthyroidism, on the other hand, means the thyroid is overactive and producing too much thyroid hormones.

A 2019 study from the University of Nebraska (Shrestha *et al.* 2019) tested 35,150 men and women who had sprayed pesticides or herbicides. The researchers followed the men and women over a period of 20 years.

Pesticides tested included diazinon, malathion, dichlorvos, glyphosate, 2-4-D and others. They also included herbicides like RoundUp, which contains the glyphosate chemical.

The researchers found that the pesticides and herbicides increased their incidence of hypothyroidism by between 21 percent and 54 percent, depending upon the pesticide or herbicide used. Pesticides and herbicides tested included:
- Diazinon (organophosphate)
- Malathion (organophosphate)
- Dichlorvos (organophosphate)
- RoundUp (glyphosate)
- Dicamba
- Chlordane
- 2-4-D (phenoxyacetic acid) and others.
- Aldrin (organochlorine)
- Heptachlor (organochlorine)
- Lindane (organochlorine)

The most harmful chemical on the thyroid turned out to be lindane, at 54 percent. But the incidence of hypothyroidism was greatest among those who used chlordane the most.

The cases of hypothyroid also increased with age. Among those who were between 45 and 55 years old, the increased incidence among pesticide and herbicide applicators was 58 percent.

But among those between 56 and 65 years old, the incidence of hypothyroidism jumped to 97 percent higher (nearly twice the incidence compared to the general population). For those over 65 years old the incidence was 78 percent.

Another study (Shrestha. *et al.* 2018) on pesticides and thyroid conditions followed 24,092 wives of conventional farmers for over 20 years.

Again the researchers found links between certain types of pesticides and thyroid diseases. The study found that several fungicides (including benomyl, maneb/mancozeb, and metalaxyl), and the herbicide pendimethalin, as well as parathion and permethrin pesticides were all linked with increased incidence of hypothyroidism.

The average increased incidence among the farmer's wives ranged from 56 percent to nearly two-and-a-half times the general population.

Furthermore, some pesticides and herbicides increased the incidence of hyperthyroidism among the wives.

The use of these chemicals by their husbands increased the incidence of hyperthyroidism by between 35 percent higher and twice the incidence compared to the general population. These included diazinon (pesticide), maneb and mancozeb (fungicides), and metolachlor (herbicide).

Scientists from Brazil (Piccoli *et al.* 2016) studied 275 men and women who worked and/or lived on farms in Southern Brazil. The researchers collected blood samples during times when the farm workers were spraying, and also at other times when they weren't spraying.

They also compared the farm workers' levels of thyroid hormones in the blood with their longer-term exposure to pesticides on the farm.

The researchers found that during the spraying season, the working men's TSH levels significantly increased. Those with higher lifetime exposure to pesticides also had increased TSH levels.

The researchers also found that higher TSH levels were associated with higher concentrations of many pesticides in their bloodstream.

Higher TSH levels in the blood means the thyroid is underactive. It is not properly utilizing TSH to produce thyroid hormones.

A study from the University of North Carolina (Xiang *et al.* 2017) studied the interaction between a number of pesticides and thyroid receptors. Indeed, the researchers found 11 pesticides will bind with thyroid receptors, changing the way T3 was produced.

Pesticides are also linked to ADHD.

Pharmaceutical Toxins

There is no doubt that a number of pharmaceuticals have provided real life-saving benefits. Whether these same benefits could not have been provided by herbal medicines is debatable and we won't debate that here. We should mention, however, that more than half of pharmaceuticals are based upon the constituent agents provided by herbal medicines. However, this isolation and concentration of these constituents, along with the synthesized nature of pharmaceuticals provides toxicity and a wealth of side effects. We must therefore include pharmaceuticals and their excipients as toxins.

This was illustrated in a 1998 report published in the *Journal of the American Medical Association* (Lazarou *et al.* 1998). Approximately 2,300,000 people either end up being hospitalized, permanently disabled, or fatally injured as a result of pharmaceutical use in the United States alone every year. That is over 2.2 million people annually with *reported* injury from pharmaceuticals.

This study, done at the University of Toronto, also showed that approximately 106,000 people in the U.S. die each year from taking correctly prescribed pharmaceuticals approved by the FDA. This does not include the number of deaths resulting by overdose or by addiction to these same drugs. The U.S. FDA was sent 258,000 adverse drug events in 1999.

Harvard researcher and associate professor of medicine Dr. David Bates told the *Los Angeles Times* in 2001: *"...these numbers translate to 36 million adverse drug events per year"* (Rappoport 2006).

The plausibility of this number was confirmed in another study published in the *Journal of the American Medical Association* in 1995 (Bates *et al.*). This revealed that over a sixth month period, 12% of 4,031 adult hospital admissions had either a confirmed adverse drug event or a potentially adverse drug event. If we extrapolate this rate using the population of 300 million Americans, we would arrive at the same 36 million calculated in the study.

Practically any and every synthetic pharmaceutical can add to our body's total toxin burden. This is because the body must eventually break down any synthetic chemical in order to purge it from the body. The isolated or active chemical within the pharmaceutical may have its biological effect upon the body, but it must be broken down at some point. The body rarely if ever utilizes these chemicals as nutrients, in other words. They are foreigners to the body. Thus, enzymes such as glutathione must break down these chemical molecules into forms that can be excreted in urine, sweat, exhalation or stool.

This breakdown and disposal process requires work by the body's detoxification systems. This means that they further burden or stress a system that must remove many other toxins within the body, including other environmental toxins, microorganisms and their endotoxins, inflammatory mediators, broken-down cells and other toxins the body must get rid of. In other words, pharmaceuticals can contribute to, and even become another straw that breaks the camel's back.

Illustrating this, researchers from Britain's Imperial College (Shaheen *et al.* 2008) studied the association between acetaminophen use and asthma incidence among 1,028 asthmatics and healthy matched controls. They found that the weekly use of acetaminophen was significantly related to a diagnosis of asthma. The researchers concluded that: *"These data add to the increasing and consistent epidemiological evidence implicating frequent paracetamol [acetaminophen] use in asthma in diverse populations."*

Researchers from Norway's Oslo University Hospital (Bakkeheim *et al.* 2011) studied 1,016 mothers and their children from birth until six months old, and then followed up with the children at 10 years old. They found that acetaminophen use by the mother during the first trimester significantly increased incidence of allergic rhinitis at age ten. Furthermore, girls given acetaminophen had more than double the asthma incidence at age ten.

While these pharmaceuticals may be of concern specifically, we should look at any pharmaceutical as having the potential to increase the body's total toxic burden and raise the risk of systemic inflammation.

The Tryptophan Defect

As another example of the potential for pharmaceuticals to stimulate systemic inflammation is that some people have a defect in the availability of tryptophan, caused indirectly by the use of pharmaceuticals. Tryptophan is an amino acid critical for a number of processes in the body. If tryptophan is not properly metabolized, it can remain in the body at unhealthy high levels. This can be evidenced by extraordinary high levels of xanthurenic and knurenic acid in the urine.

One of the problems with high levels of tryptophan is that tryptophan is the precursor of serotonin. Thus, high tryptophan levels produce high levels of serotonin. And high serotonin levels can cause a variety of conditions, from fatigue and fibromyalgia to wheezing and lung disorders.

A link between tryptophan and inflammation is the indoleamine dioxygenase enzyme, or IDO. IDO regulates eosinophil inflammation, and tryptophan reduces IDO availability. This means that increased tryptophan presence in the blood has the effect of leaving eosinophils unregulated—which are directly involved in inflammation and pain, as we've discussed earlier.

There is reason to believe that oral steroids may increase the loss of vitamin B6 levels (Holt 1998). Vitamin B6 (pyridoxine) is required to metabolize and reduce tryptophan levels. Vitamin B6 also happens to diminish the effectiveness of steroid medications, because it inhibits steroid update into the nucleus and DNA (Gropper *et al.* 2008).

A number of pharmaceuticals have the effect of reducing levels of vitamin B6, which in turn increases tryptophan availability. This effectively produces continuous inflammation associated with high eosinophil levels by virtue of decreased levels of the IDO enzyme.

This effect was confirmed by researchers (Sur *et al.* 1993), who found that the medication theophylline significantly reduced pyridoxine (vitamin B6) levels within patients.

Another study (Collipp *et al.* 1975) found that asthmatic symptoms were significantly improved, together with a reduction of asthma medications, after B6 supplementation. This study followed 76 asthmatic children who were given 200 milligrams per day of pyridoxine (vitamin B6) for five months.

While this should not be interpreted as vitamin B6 as a panacea, its reduction is simply one sign that synthetic chemicals can interrupt the body's normal cleansing processes. Should we interrupt these processes, our body's ability to purify the body is blocked.

We can add to this discussion particular drugs and drug types that have been shown to be particularly toxic to particular organs, or toxic in general:

Drugs particularly hard on the liver:
- Acetaminophen
- Analgesics (pain-killers)
- Anesthetics (given during surgery)
- Antibiotics
- Anticoagulants
- Antihistamines
- Anti-inflammatory drugs
- Blood pressure drugs
- Chemotherapy drugs
- Cholesterol-lowering drugs
- Diabetes drugs
- Heart disease drugs
- Oral contraceptives
- Parkinson's drugs

> ➤ Tuberculosis drugs

Drugs that can stress or damage the kidneys:
> ➤ ACE inhibitors
> ➤ Acyoclovir
> ➤ Allopurinol
> ➤ Aminoglycosides
> ➤ Amphotericin
> ➤ Beta-blockers
> ➤ Captopril
> ➤ Cephalothin
> ➤ Chemotherapy drugs
> ➤ Chlorothiazide
> ➤ Chlopropamide
> ➤ Clofibrate
> ➤ Cyclosporine
> ➤ Diuretics
> ➤ Furosemide
> ➤ Isoproterenol
> ➤ Lithium
> ➤ Macanylamine
> ➤ Methotrexate
> ➤ Methysergide
> ➤ Morphine
> ➤ NSAIDs (acetaminophen, aspirin, ibuprofen)
> ➤ Penicillins
> ➤ Phenytoin
> ➤ Piperidine
> ➤ Probenecid
> ➤ Procaine
> ➤ Quinidine
> ➤ Sulfonamides
> ➤ Tolazoline

There are several conditions that will change the body's ability to metabolize drugs, and different factors that will increase or decrease the drug's effects. This can lead to serious outcomes. The factors include sex, age, race, weight, pregnancy, nursing, illness, alcohol consumption, food, multiple drugs, digestion variation, kidney damage, liver damage, nutritional deficiencies, supplements used, exposure to other toxins, exercise, stress and time of the day.

In particular, a number of drugs are metabolized differently in women than men. These include amitriptyline, benzodiazepines, beta-blockers, chlordiazepoxide, diflunisal, imipramine, methylprednisoline, oxazepam, piroxicam, prednisolone and trazodone.

Some drugs can lead to breast enlargement among men. These include AACE inhibitors, amitryptyline, cimetidine, digoxin, famotidine, ibuprofen, indomethacin, ketoconazole, ketoprofen, methyldopa, naproxen, spironolactone and terfenadine.

A number of drugs can cause intestinal issues and diarrhea. These include antibiotics, antidepressants, antihypertensive drugs, statins and heart drugs like digitalis, quinidine, hydralazine, beta-blockers, and ACE inhibitors.

The liver uses what is called the P-450 enzyme pathway to break down many drugs. However, the P-450 pathway can easily become overloaded by too many drugs, combined with other toxins. This can result in a few dire circumstances:

> The liver can be seriously damaged
> The drug's effects can be exaggerated, causing dangerous effects.
> The drugs can remain in the system longer, causing more side effects
> The unprocessed metabolites of these drugs can produce fatigue, chemical overload and immunosuppression.

Several drugs can block or overload the liver's P-450 pathway:

> Antirrhythmic drugs (disopyramide)
> Antihistamines (terfenadine, astemizole)
> Benzodiazepines
> Bromocriptine
> Caffeine
> Calcium channel blockers
> Statins
> Cimetidine
> Cisapride
> Macrolides
> Antifungals
> Phenytoin
> Tacrine
> Theophyllines
> Tricyclic antidepressants
> Warfarin

(Adapted from Mindell and Hopkins 1998)

Synthetic Food Additives

This is a large topic, because so many processed foods are chock full of many different artificial additives. These include hundreds of artificial food colors, preservatives, stabilizers, flavorings and a variety of food processing aids. A number of these additives have been found to cause sensitivities in some people.

Illustrating the effects that food additives can have, Australian researchers (Dengate and Ruben 2002) studied 27 children with irritability, restlessness, inattention and sleep difficulties. The researchers saw many of these symptoms subside after putting the children on the Royal Prince Alfred Hospital Diet, which is absent of food additives, natural salicylates, amines and glutamates.

Using preservative challenges, the researchers were also able to determine that the preservatives significantly affected the children's behavior and physiology adversely.

Researchers from Britain's University of Southampton (Bateman *et al.* 2004) screened 1,873 three-year old children for hyperactivity and the consumption of artificial food colors and preservatives. They gave the children 20 mg daily of artificial colors and 45 mg daily of sodium benzoate, or a placebo mixture. The additive group showed significantly higher levels of hyperactivity than the group that did not consume the artificial colors and preservative.

While these studies are not proof that these food additives are allergens, we can say that with confidence that they can cause food intolerances, as hyperactivity is considered a reaction to eating these "foods."

Once an additive has caused intolerance symptoms such as those from the research above, there is always the possibility that the immune system may begin to become sensitive to some of the foods these additives are associated with. This likelihood increases should the immune system become continually exposed to the foods together with the additives over a considerable period of time.

Sulfites

Sulfites provide a classic case. The sulfite ion will aggressively preserve a food. Sulfites can also produce wheezing, tightness of the throat and other symptoms almost immediately after eating foods preserved with them. However, the effects of sulfites may not be as significant as often portrayed. It may well be that many sulfite-sensitivities seen among wine drinkers are actually the product of the alcohol rather than the sulfites.

Illustrating this, researchers from Australia's Centre for Asthma (Vally *et al.* 2007) tested eight wine-sensitive subjects with sulfite wine and non-sulfite wine. The researchers found that the wine sensitivities were unlikely caused by the sulfites in the wine.

Today, sulfites are used to preserve many wines, dehydrated potatoes and numerous dried fruits. Sulfites include potassium bisulfite, sulfur dioxide, potassium matabisulfite and others. Often labels do not disclose the use of sulfites, because the preservative may have been used early in the processing of the raw ingredients instead of added into the finished product. In addition, under current U.S. labeling laws, if an ingredient such as sulfite is less than 10 parts per million, there is no requirement for putting the ingredient on the panel.

Sulfite sensitivity may be the result of B12 deficiency. In a study presented to the American Academy of Allergy and Immunology, 18 sulfite-sensitive persons were given sublingual B12. The B12 effectively blocked adverse reactions to sulfites in 17 of the 18 (Werbach 1996).

Monosodium Glutamate

Monosodium glutamate also gets a lot of attention for producing sensitivity symptoms. This has also been echoed among a number of studies.

To better understand this, Harvard researchers (Geha *et al.* 2000) set out to study the effects of MSG sensitivities in a multi-center study. They found that of 130 human volunteers who thought they were sensitive to MSG, 38% physically responded to MSG with allergic symptoms. However, 13% also responded to a placebo (they thought contained MSG). Subsequent retesting continued to show inconsistent responses among some of those who thought they were MSG-sensitive.

This led the researchers to conclude that people who believe they are sensitive tend to react more strongly to MSG, but their responses were not always consistent. This of course may be the result of differing levels of tolerance and periods of sensitivity—again depending upon immunity.

This research still confirms that MSG can cause sensitivity responses. Possibly MSG may be overhyped somewhat, but like so many other food additives, there is no doubt that it is not a natural part of our food supply.

Microparticles

Some researchers have suggested that substances with microparticles can lead to increased intestinal permeability and food sensitivities (Korzenik 2005).

Microparticles are particles smaller than 100 μm, but larger than 0.1 μm. (Smaller molecules, in the nanometer range, are called nanoparticles.) Products that are produced with microparticles include toothpaste and mouthwashes. Food products that contain microparticles include powdered sugars and some refined flours.

We might better classify microparticles in the same category as overly processed foods. The bottom line is that the body can become sensitive to unnaturally-processed constituents should they be exposed to intestinal tissues and bloodstream—and not be recognized by the immune system.

Artificial Sweeteners

A number of artificial sweeteners should be considered toxic. One is aspartame. Aspartame is a chemical combination of the amino acids phenylalanine and aspartic acid, bonded by methyl ester—a wood alcohol. Once inside the body, the wood alcohol and formaldehyde are released.

Another artificial sweetener sucralose. This is sweet yet not readily absorbed according to manufacturers. Yet studies have found that 11-27% is absorbed, and 20-30% of that absorbed quantity can be metabolized by the body. This requires the liver and kidneys to break it down and excrete it.

While this is a huge topic in itself, other questionable sweeteners that may provide toxicity once within the body include saccharin, acesulfame potassium and cyclamates. Stevia, mannitol and xylitol are plant-derived sweeteners that are considered by most to be relatively safe and non-toxic.

Air Pollutants

Clean air contains about 78% nitrogen, 21% oxygen, .9% argon, .03% carbon dioxide and a host of other trace elements. Depending upon the location and source, outdoor air pollution can contain carbon monoxide, nitrogen dioxide, sulphur dioxide, excess carbon dioxide, ammonia, various particulates, chlorofluorocarbons (CFCs), radon daughters, and a variety of toxic metals and volatile organic compounds (VOCs).

There are several types of air pollution, and most of them can overload the body with toxins. The first is *air particle* pollution—when particulate size ranges from .1 micron to 10 microns. This type of pollution is from soot, typical of automobile exhaust, industrial smoke stack exhaust, fireplace smoke, and smoke from forest fires, barbecues and other combustion. Soot is also called *black carbon* pollution, because the excess carbon burn off from burning fossil fuels is the primary component.

Noxious gases are another type of pollution category. These include gasses such as carbon monoxide, chlorine gas, nitrogen oxide, sulphur dioxide and various other chemical gases and vapors. CFCs are a type of noxious gas.

While these two pollution types are distinct, they are often tough to differentiate. Many pollutants are actually vaporized liquids. Molecules become suspended in vapor, appearing like gases or liquid vapors. They are airborne elements derived from synthetic solid and liquid compounds.

We should also specify a difference between *indoor* and *outdoor* air pollution. There are a number of pollutants specifically pervading building ventilation systems and indoor facilities. To this, we can add outdoor pollution entering the house. Examples of indoor pollutants include formaldehyde emitted by foam, treated wood plastics, and chlorine gas emitted in indoor swimming pools.

According to a 2007 *American Lung Association State of the Air* report, 46% or about 136 million Americans live within a county having *"unhealthful"* levels of either ozone or particle-based outdoor pollution. Over 38 million Americans live in a county with *"unhealthful"* levels of both ozone and particle pollution. A third of Americans live in *"unhealthful"* ozone level counties.

Interestingly, this is substantially better than a 2006 report indicating that almost half of Americans live in ozone-rich areas. It is unlikely that the source of ozone pollution—carbon emissions—went down this much in a year. Most likely—just as the ozone hole has been fluctuating with atmospheric rhythms—there are complicated relationships between weather systems, temperature, pressure and so on.

Meanwhile, more than ninety-three million Americans—about one in three—live in areas seasonally high in short-term particle pollution and about one in five Americans lives in an area of high year-round particle pollution. Unlike the fluctuating ozone levels, the number of high particle pollution areas has steadily increased over the past few years.

Smog

Research has illustrated that increased exposure to the particulates within smog, as well as the toxic burden presented by mercury, arsenic, sulfur dioxide, nitrogen dioxide and others, can contribute to systemic inflammation.

Illustrating this, researchers from Australia's University of Queensland (Barnett *et al.* 2005) studied respiratory hospital admissions among children of different ages in five Australian cities and two New Zealand cities. They found that increased rates of hospital admissions for asthma correlated with increased levels of particulate matter smaller than 2.5 micrometer and less than 10 micrometer (PM10-2.5), along with increased nitrogen and sulfur levels. A 6% hike in asthma admissions for children between five and fourteen years old related to a five parts per billion increase in nitrogen levels.

Ozone

Smog is primarily made up of ozone. There are two forms of ozone: The ozone that naturally makes up part of the stratosphere, often referred to as the ozone hole; and the ozone within the lower atmosphere, or troposphere. This latter ozone is called tropospheric ozone or ozone pollution. This form of O_3 gas is caused not by a nature's interaction between radiation and the atmosphere, but through the reaction between fuel vapors from automobiles and sunlight. For this reason, smog levels tend to peak during hot weather.

Smog levels are also higher in warmer regions like Southern California and urban areas in the southern U.S., such as Atlanta. Other cities also experience greater smog levels during the summer months. Wherever higher concentrations of vehicles combine with warm sunshine, smog levels go up. The 'perfect storm' of almost constant sunshine, warm weather, and vehicle concentration makes Southern California one of the worst smog and ozone regions in the United States.

Ozone will oxidize on a cellular and internal tissue level when taken into the body. These tissues will be damaged in almost the same way other oxidized radicals damage tissues. Ozone is readily absorbed through the alveoli as a gas. From there it can enter the bloodstream and damage artery walls and tissues. Ozone is also a major lung tissue irritant, causing inflammation and epithelial cell damage. This can result in decreased lung capacity and/or decreased lung growth development among children.

Ozone is directly linked to the incidence and worsening of respiratory conditions such as asthma, bronchitis, and COPD. Recent research indicates that this mechanism is the oxidation of lung surface lipids that line the cells of the lung. These oxidized lipids stimulate inflammation as the body seeks to mitigate ozone's damaging effects. The oxidation stimulates scavenger macrophages, which bind to the oxidized lipids in an effort to reverse the damage (Postlethwait 2007).

This means that ozone will release unpaired oxygen radicals, which can damage cell membranes and tissues, as we discussed earlier.

Ozone has some redeeming qualities as well. Ozone therapy is gaining recognition among the alternative medical community. Ozone is used in hot tubs as a purification measure. It is also used as an industrial cleaning and sanitizing substance. Ozone is part of our natural mix of gases in our air as well. Typical levels are between 25 and 75 parts per billion.

However, dangerous ozone levels occur with higher levels of carbon monoxide levels, sulphur dioxide, and other pollutants. Like the canary in the coalmine, high ozone levels provide a good indicator of unhealthy air. When combined with other pollutants, ozone has a worsening detrimental effect upon the body.

The EPA's Air quality index rates 85 parts per billion of ozone as unhealthy for sensitive people, and over 105 ppb as unhealthy for anyone. As ozone levels rise, it can irritate the lungs and throat, increasing the potential for inflammatory throat and lung infections. As a result, indoor ozone generating machines—which have become popular over the last decade—are discouraged by both the EPA and the FDA if they emit levels higher than 50 parts per billion.

Ironically, higher ozone levels in the air reflect its cleansing action upon other pollutants. Ozone is part of the atmosphere's normalizing systems. The very same cleaning and antibacterial effect we have begun to utilize are part of the earth's detoxification mechanisms to clean and break down particulate pollution. This doesn't mean it is healthy to breathe in ozone at these levels, however.

Particulates

Particulate pollution can produce severe toxicity. PM(10-2.5) refers to a particle size from 2.5 micron to 10 micron, and PM(2.5) refers to particle sizes below 2.5 micron. 2.5 micron or less is a *fine particulate,* while less than .1 micron is *ultra-fine.* Ultra-fine particles may also be considered noxious gas pollutants, because their molecular size is small enough to pass through the alveoli into the bloodstream.

Particles above 10 micron in size are usually trapped by the cilia and mucous membranes in the nose, throat, or mouth. As mentioned earlier, these are usually disposed through the movement of mucous or broken down by immune cells.

Fine particulates are small enough to escape this labyrinth and get into our lungs, but they are usually too large to get directly into the bloodstream. These particles can become lodged in the tissues of the lungs and bronchi and slowly break down. As they break down, their toxins become absorbed and dumped into the bloodstream. This accumulation of toxins can quickly overburden the liver and bloodstream, producing an inflammatory airway response. In other words, the pollution of the air quickly becomes the pollution of our bloodstream and liver—producing systemic inflammation.

The chemical makeup of these toxins depends upon the source of the pollution. Particle pollution caused by automobile exhaust will have various fluorocarbons and nitrate particles, while coal fired power plants will emit large numbers of sulphur dioxide molecules.

Course particulate pollutants are typically caused by mining, construction, or demolition. Building demolition can rain fumes of various dangerous substances a mile or more from the demolition site.

The most blatant illustration of the demolition effect is the World Trade Center bombing of 2001. The collapse of the towers caused such a toxic fume that there are still thousands of people suffering from a slow poisoning of the lungs. Dangerous chemicals like asbestos, formaldehyde and many others were breathed by thousands of people.

This effect was not limited to rescuers and those who escaped from the twin towers. Many others who happened to be in the vicinity are now suffering. One of the more prevalent diseases has been *sarcoidosis*—a life-threatening inflammation of the lungs. As toxin deposits build up and damage the airways, scar tissue forms—making mild asthma seem like a walk in the park.

This scar tissue affects the elasticity and efficiency of the lungs, causing life-threatening lung collapse. A recent study released by nine doctors (Izbicki *et al.* 2007) who researched the delayed health effects at Ground Zero reported that firefighters and rescue workers were diagnosed with sarcoidosis at a rate of five times the incidence rate prior to 9/11.

An epidemic of respiratory disorders and lung cancer was also an unfortunate result of the Trade Center bombing. While we know asbestos is toxic to the lungs, it is still a popular building material. Many structural components of new buildings use asbestos as an ingredient. Because it is a cheap fire retardant material, buildings still go up using it. Asbestos has been linked to thyroid cancer and lung cancer in many studies, which caused a number of high profile lawsuits and residential building restrictions.

Another toxin released when buildings collapse or are demolished is benzene. Benzene has been identified as a carcinogen, and certain types of leukemia are associated with benzene exposure. Other toxins thought to be released by building collapse include mercury, lead, cadmium, dioxin, polycyclic aromatic hydrocarbons (PAHs) and polychlorinated biphenyls (PCBs). Many of these components are still used to build buildings. All of them were used in buildings a few decades ago, when many of our current skyscrapers were built.

Besides the more publicized cases of cancer and sarcoidosis, ailments associated with the WTC bombing include reactive-airways syndrome, asthma, chronic throat irritation, gastroesophageal reflux disease (GERD—also referred to as heartburn) and persistent sinusitis. Other cases thought to be associated with the WTC have included miner's lung and thyroid cancer. While many thought these disorders were temporary, new diagnoses have continually increased. This is because toxins can build up and reside in lung tissue cells, affecting future lung capacity for many years to come. Studies on firefighters involved in the rescue report an average loss of 300 milliliters of lung capacity (Senior 2003).

It is thus safe to say that exposure to these sorts of particulates may not be symptomatic for years after the exposure. This was certainly the case with those exposed to Agent Orange in Vietnam. Cases of prostate cancer, skin cancer, and chronic lymphocytic leukemia did not appear in some veterans for decades later (Beaulieu and Fessele 2003).

Particulate pollution or soot is the most dangerous form of outdoor pollution. Auto exhaust, aerosols, and chemicals from power plants and wood burning are the major sources. While the particles themselves are too small to be seen by the naked eye, they can be seen as a whole in the form of a haze in the sunlight. While the body's cilia hair and mucous membranes in the nose and throat might filter and catch some of these particles, many will make it into the lungs where they can trigger inflammation.

Like any living organism, the earth and its atmosphere have means to cleanse toxins out of the system. The atmosphere conducts a number of self-cleaning currents, which move and break down pollutants. One such mechanism is the hydroxyl radical (OH) molecule. The immediate effect of the hydroxyl radical is to form photo-oxidants like nitric acid, which undergoes a photolysis reaction with nitrous acids. These can be highly toxic.

Humanity's intrusions into nature's course can produce other types of toxins. We might consider, for example, Owens Lake, California. For thousands of years, this beautiful lake offered respite from the heat and inhospitality of the California desert region known as Death Valley. The size of Owens lake was nearly 28,500 hectares—a huge body of water fed by the Sierra mountains. In 1900, the mountain rivers feeding the lake were diverted into the Los Angeles basin to feed a growing legion of humanity.

Within ten years, Owens Lake, which was often compared to the Aral Sea, turned into a dustbowl. Now the silt covering the water basin is coated with arsenic. Arsenic is a natural element, and in this case, it is providing resistance and restructuring for the soil at the lake bottom. This arsenic is also blowing around the region with the winds, increasing cancer rates among local residents (Raloff 2001).

Carbon Monoxide

Carbon monoxide is a substantial indoor air toxin. Carbon monoxide is released by burning gas, kerosene, or wood. It can thus arise from the use of wood stoves, fireplaces, gas stoves, generators, automobiles, kitchen stoves, and furnaces. Low concentrations of carbon monoxide in the indoor environment might cause fatigue and even chest pain.

Higher concentrations may result in headaches, confusion, dizziness, nausea, vision impairment and fever. This is due to carboxyhemoglobin formation in the bloodstream, which takes place when carbon monoxide attaches to hemoglobin instead of oxygen. This will in effect starve the body of oxygen, and higher concentrations can easily lead to death.

Acceptable carbon monoxide levels in households are about .5 to 5 parts per million. Levels near a gas stove might be 5 to 15 ppm. An improperly vented or leaking stove might cause 30 ppm or more near the stove, which becomes hazardous. The U.S. National Ambient Air Quality Standard for maximum carbon monoxide levels outside is 35 ppm for one hour and 9 ppm for eight hours. Standards for indoor carbon monoxide have not been determined.

Making sure that every appliance is vented properly is task number one in avoiding carbon monoxide poisoning. The appliance should also be checked for leaks, and those leaks should be sealed prior to use. Central heating systems should be inspected for leaks as well. Idling the car in the garage is a no-no. Open fireplaces should be avoided indoors, and wood stove doors should be kept closed. We shouldn't solely rely upon the draft up the fireplace chimney for the escape of carbon monoxide.

Nitrogen oxide

Nitrogen oxide is a gas byproduct of most engines and practically any gas-run appliance. Gas stoves, water heaters, wood stoves, gas heaters and cars are probably the biggest emitters in the home. Homes without these appliances will have very low levels of NO_2 compared to outside. Homes with these appliances may have double the levels. Nitrogen oxide can be a significant toxin if significant levels are taken in.

Researchers from Birmingham Heartlands Hospital (Tunnicliffe *et al.* 1994) tested one hour exposure to nitrogen dioxide on ten mild asthmatics with dust mite sensitivities. Forced expiratory volume (FEV1) levels were tested with non-NO_2 air, air with 100 parts per billion of NO_2, and air containing 400 ppb of nitrogen dioxide. FEV1 levels were 27% lower between the non-NO_2 air and the 400 ppb of NO_2 air. The average FEV1 among the asthmatics was nearly three times lower in the 400 ppb NO_2 air than in the clear air. The 100 ppb NO_2 air content did not seem to make a significant difference in FEV1, however. This gives us a yardstick for determining unhealthy NO_2 levels.

Cooking and Heating

Research from the University at Albany (Kaplan 2010) has revealed that about half of the people around the world utilize biomass such as wood, agricultural residues or coal to cook by and heat their homes with.

These fuels are not completely consumed by their ignition. They leave toxic residues in the form of carbon monoxide, arsenic and others that can significantly increase the body's burden of toxins when breathed in. This in turn increases the risk of systemic inflammation, as the body works to break down and remove these toxins.

Volatile Organic Compounds (VOCs)

Researchers from the Texas Tech University Health Sciences Center (Arif and Shah 2007) studied the effects of volatile organic compounds (VOCs). They collected data on ten VOCs and 550 adults. Aromatic compounds and chlorinated hydrocarbons were specifically categorized. Exposure to aromatic compounds increased the incidence of asthma by 63%. In addition, exposure to aromatic compounds increased wheezing incidence from the previous year by 68%, and chlorinated hydrocarbon exposure increased wheezing incidence from the previous year by 50%.

Exposures to VOCs ranged from 0.03 micrograms per cubic meter for trichloroethene up to 14 microg/m3 for toluene. In other words, the higher the level of toxic inhalation, the higher the incidence of respiratory disorders. This is because VOCs present toxins that are quickly absorbed into the bloodstream through the airways. Once in the bloodstream, the body launches an inflammatory response to remove them.

The researchers also found that as a group, Mexican-Americans experience the highest exposure levels to benzene—averaging 2.38 micrograms per cubic meter—compared with whites—who averaged 1.15 microg/m3—and blacks—who averaged 1.07 microg/m3. This relates to exposure levels that are relative to the type of work being done. In other words, this study indicates that Mexican-Americans are likely doing more work involving the use of VOCs, which in turn expose them to greater levels of benzene.

Benzene, like toluene and other VOCs, is highly disruptive to cells and tissues because of its highly reactive aromatic hydrocarbon structure. It can thus damage practically every cell and tissue system in the body, releasing numerous radicals. Not surprisingly, benzene is also known to be significantly carcinogenic.

Benzene and other VOCs can be found in many paints, glues, solvents, rubbers and many other workplace materials. Industries that use aromatic hydrocarbon solvents must provide significant ventilation and protection to avoid poisoning their workers.

First-, Second- and Third-Hand Smoke

Tobacco smoke is also an important source of indoor pollution. The American Cancer Society estimated in 2004 that 160,000 Americans die each year from lung cancer caused by smoking. Lung cancer maintains between an eleven and fifteen percent chance of survival beyond five years. It should be noted that the highest rates of global lung cancer occur for both men and women in North America and Europe (Field *et al.* 2006). Of course, these are also countries where indoor smoking rates are the highest.

Recent research has indicated that not only is second-hand smoke dangerous to non-smokers, but it has more than twice the amount of tar, nicotine and other toxins than the smoker inhales. While the smoker will inhale the smoke through the filtering mechanism provided by the packed tobacco inside the cigarette paper—and many cigarettes also have additional filters to screen out toxins—the second-hand smoker will breathe all the smoke. Second-hand smoke contains five times the amount of carbon monoxide—the lethal gas that de-oxygenates the blood—than the smoker inhales.

Second-hand smoke also contains higher levels of ammonia and cadmium. Its nitrogen dioxide levels are fifty times higher than levels considered harmful, and the concentration of hydrogen cyanide approaches toxic levels. Constant exposure to second-hand smoke increases the risk of lung disease by 25%, and increases the risk of heart disease by 10%. Second-hand smoke exposure has also been irrefutably linked to emphysema, chronic bronchitis, asthma and other ailments.

Despite significant educational programs, second-hand and third-hand smoke poisoning is still prevalent in the United States. The Centers for Disease Control's National Health and Nutrition Examination Survey from 1999-2008 (CDC 2010) revealed that between 2007 and 2008, about 88 million American nonsmokers over the age of three were consistently exposed to secondhand smoke. The good news is that the detectible blood nicotine levels among nonsmokers have declined from 52% between 1999 and 2000 to 40% between 2007 and 2008. Still, 40% is simply not acceptable. It should be noted that rates were the highest among children living in households below federal poverty levels.

Researchers from Britain's University of Southampton School of Medicine (Edgecombe et al. 2010) found in a study of 22 adolescents with severe asthma, that two-thirds lived with a smoker.

Researchers from the Respiratory Diseases Department of France's Hospital of Haut-Lévèque in Bordeaux (Raherison et al. 2008) studied 7,798 children among six cities in France. This focused on asthma and allergies among families who smoked. They found that about 20% of children were exposed to tobacco via their mother's smoking. Furthermore, they found that children born of mothers who smoked during pregnancy had significantly greater incidence of asthma.

There is now research that shows that anti-smoking laws decrease disease rates. Researchers from the Harvard School of Public Health (Dove et al. 2011) studied the National Health and Nutrition Examination Survey (NHANES) data—a research program run by the U.S. Centers for Disease Control and Prevention's National Center for Health Statistics (NCHS). NCHS's directive has been a continuous survey method focused on specific diseases among representative samples throughout the United States. About 5,000 persons each year are included in the data, from different counties across the nation.

The Harvard researchers used the 1999-2006 NHANES data to correlate locations that had some semblance of required smoke-free public places with asthma incidence. They found that smoke-free laws significantly reduced the odds of asthmatic symptoms among nonsmoking children and adolescents. Smoke-free laws were also linked to reduced asthma episodes ("attacks"), persistent wheeze, chronic night coughing and asthma medication use.

Fragrances

Various scents and fragrances used in deodorizers, decorations, soaps, and furniture can be downright toxic. While a fragrance might smell like flowers or delicious foods, the typical commercial fragrance contains at least ninety-five percent synthetic chemicals. A single perfume may contain more than 500 different chemicals. Benzene derivatives, aldehydes, toluene, and petroleum-derived chemicals are just a few synthetics used in commercial fragrances. Toluene alone, for example, has been linked to respiratory disorders among previously healthy people.

For this reason, we should carefully consider any product with an ingredient called "fragrances." This includes laundry detergents, dishwashing and other soaps, shampoos and other types of hair products, disinfectants, shaving creams, fabric softeners, fragrant candles, air fresheners, and of course perfumes and colognes. Discernment also should also be given to the word "unscented," as this still may have some of the same synthetics, used instead as fragrance masking elements.

In one study (Anderson and Anderson 1997), mice were submitted to breathing with a commercial air freshener for one hour at different concentrations. A number of concentrations, including levels typically used by humans in everyday use, caused sensory and pulmonary irritation, decreased breathing velocity, and functional behavior abnormalities.

Another study, performed by the same researchers (Anderson and Anderson 1998) and published a year later, revealed that mice who were subjected to five commercial colognes or toilet water for an hour suffered various combinations of negative effects, including sensory irritation, pulmonary irritation, decreased airflow expiration, and neurotoxicity.

Skin Lotions

Many of the chemical ingredients in many sunscreens have been identified as carcinogenic. These include benzophenone-3, homosalate, 4-methyl-benzylidene camphor, octylmethoxycinnamate, and octyl-dimethyl-PABA. These five, alone or in some combination thereof, are contained in about 90% of today's commercial sunscreens. All five have showed increased cancer cell proliferation both *in vitro* and *in vivo* in a study conducted at the Institute of Pharmacology and Toxicology at the University of Zurich (Schlumpf *et al.* 2001). This study also showed negative estrogenic and endocrine effects among mice from several of these chemicals.

A study done at the University of Manitoba in Winnipeg (Sarveiya *et al.* 2004) reported that all sunscreen ingredients tested—including octymethoxycinnamate and oxybenzone—significantly penetrate the skin. The penetration of common sunscreens was found to increase the penetration of even more dangerous herbicides—a concern for agricultural workers and non-organic gardeners (Pont *et al.* 2004). Furthermore, it has been established that some organic sunscreens can cause photo-contact allergies (Maier and Korting 2005). Research from Australia's Skin and Cancer Foundation (Cook and Freeman 2001) reported 21 cases of photo-allergic contact dermatitis caused by oxybenzone, butyl methoxy dibenzoylmethane, methoxycinnamate or benzophenone. The Cook and Freeman research has led to a conclusion that these sunscreen ingredients are the leading cause of photo-allergic contact dermatitis.

Contact dermatitis is actually quite rare amongst the general population. A study at the National Institute of Dermatology in Colombia conducted a study of eighty-two patients with clinical photo-allergic contact dermatitis. Their testing showed that twenty-six of those patients—31.7%—were shown to be positive for sensitivity to one or several of the sunscreen ingredients (Rodriguez *et al.* 2006).

The widespread proliferation of these harmful sunscreen ingredients—an occurrence increasing since the 1960s sunbathing era—is a significant factor in the skin cancer epidemic. Their addition to the epidermis layer create an environment of excessive oxidative radicals, as the sun in the presence of oxygen further oxidizes these synthetic molecules without nature's balancing biomolecules. At the bare minimum, these chemicals substantially increase the toxic burden within skin cells. This burden minimizes the body's ability to neutralize the oxidizing effects of the sun's radiation—intensifying the oxidizing factor. This intensification would essentially convert the sun's rays from therapeutic to dangerous.

Prior and concurrent to the prevalent use of sunscreen, sun-worshipers have ceremoniously applied various chemical- and oil-based sun lotions onto the skin. This is done to intensify the sun's tanning effects: to obtain that rich, brown tan to look more attractive. Many chemicals are/were in these products, including various hydrocarbons, which revert to oxidized radicals when exposed to the sun. In addition to sun lotion, sunbathers also apply various other chemical-based lotions onto the skin to condition, hydrate or treat sunburn. These various moisturizing lotions also contain a variety of synthetic chemicals that can become free radicals.

Furthermore, many sunscreens available today effectively absorb UV-B rays, but let UV-A rays through. Because UV-A rays are quite dangerous out of balance with UV-B to an unhealthy body, the risk of skin cancer using these sunscreens is even higher than without any sunscreen protection. In a 2007 study from the University of California at San Diego, researchers (Gorham *et al.* 2007) reviewed 17 studies of sunscreen use and melanoma. For those studies performed in latitudes over 40 degrees from the equator where skin types are fairer, there was a more significant correlation between sunscreen use and skin cancer.

Many other skin lotions should also be considered toxic. An example is DEET, or N,N-Diethyl-meta-toluamide. DEET is an effective mosquito repellent, yes. But it also poisons us as well. Research has shown that DEET exposure causes impairments to cognition, mood issues and insomnia. Whatever we put on our skin is absorbed into the epidermal and subdermal tissues, and eventually, into the bloodstream, and in the case of DEET, into our central nervous system.

Other toxic chemicals are used for lubricants, moisturizers, exfoliants and masks. Ingredients to steer clear of include methylisothiazalone, DMDM hydantoin, octenylsuccinate (a neurotoxin), methylchloroisothiazalone and triclosan—an antibacterial ingredient that is suspected to be an endocrine disruptor. Common among most soaps and cleansers are sodium laureth sulfate and ceteareth, which can bond to carcinogen chemicals used in manufacturing, such as ethylen oxide and 1,4-dioxane.

Toxic Household Materials

The same researchers (Anderson and Anderson 2000) found that pulmonary irritation and decreased lung capacity results from the use of synthetic mattress pads. They identified respiratory irritants such as styrene, isopropylbenzene and limonene among polyurethane mattresses. When subjecting organic cotton mattresses to the same test, the results were quite the opposite. Increased respiratory rates and tidal breathing volumes were observed with organic fiber mattresses.

Fabric softener emission is also a dangerous source of air toxicity. Several known irritants and toxins are typically found in fabric softeners, including styrene, isopropylbenzene, thymol, trimethylbenzene and phenols. In yet another study, Anderson and Anderson subjected mice to five commercial fabric softener emissions for 90 minutes using laundry dryers. The results clearly illustrated that fabric softeners significantly irritate airways. These negative health effects were also seen resulting from emissions of clothing driers containing fabric softener pads.

The researchers (Anderson and Anderson 1999) also found that pulmonary toxicity resulted from commercial diapers, adding that a number of chemicals found in diapers were known pulmonary and sensory irritants.

Another potential indoor trigger category is propellants. Propellants are used in sprays and pump bottles to disperse fluids. While chlorofluorocarbons (CFCs) have been practically eliminated from aerosols, today's aerosols and pump sprays often involves the use of volatile organic compounds (VOCs). Noxious propellants such as isobutane, butane and propane will typically linger in the air for several minutes after spraying. They can be quite toxic.

Asbestos

Asbestos exposure has become less likely since the *Environmental Protection Agency* passed the *Asbestos Ban and Phase Out Rule* as part of the *Toxic Substances Control Act* in 1989—which was for the most part overturned in 1991 by the U.S. *Fifth Circuit Court of Appeals*. What remain are various specific bans such as those from the *Clean Air Act* and remnants of *Toxic Substances Control Act*, including some continued restrictions supported by Congressional rulings.

The CAA has stimulated various bans since 1973. The bottom line is that although paper- and cardboard-based asbestos has been banned along with certain spray-on versions, many products still contain asbestos. These include cement sheets, clothing, pipe wrap, roofing felt, floor tiles, shingles, millboard, cement pipe, and various automotive parts.

Beyond the banned items, there is no ban preventing manufacturers from using asbestos. The important thing to remember is that the EPA does not monitor manufacturers for their ingredients. In general, asbestos inclusion into today's building materials should be considered a given.

Formaldehyde

Formaldehyde has been shown to be a significant and prevalent toxin. Today so many building materials and furniture are built using formaldehyde. These include pressed wood, draperies, glues, resins, shelving, flooring, and so many other materials. The greatest source of formaldehyde appears to be those materials made using *urea-formaldehyde* resins. These include particleboard, plywood paneling, and medium density fiberboard.

Among these, medium density fiberboard—used to make drawers, cabinets and furniture tops—appears to contain the highest resin-to-wood ratio. Another sort of resin called *phenol-formaldehyde* or PF resin. PF resin apparently emits substantially less formaldehyde than the UF resins. The PF resin is easily differentiated from UF resin by its darker, red or black color. The incidental *off-gassing* of formaldehyde into the indoor environment from these resins results from sun, heat, sanding and demolition. As the formaldehyde slowly off gasses, it becomes a chemical toxin once in the body.

Other Building Materials

There are many other toxins in our building materials—including many yet to be discovered. Certainly, we can safely say that any kind of building or decomposition of a modern building will likely impart various hazardous chemicals, including but not exclusively asbestos and formaldehyde.

Polybrominated diphenyl ethers or PBDEs provide one example. PBDEs is an organobromine used as a fire retardant. It is used to make automobiles, polyurethane foams, furniture, electronic goods, textiles, airplanes and of course, building materials.

This means that the air during any kind of sanding, crushing, fire or demolition should be treated with extreme caution. Using a particle or gas mask is more than a good idea under these circumstances, though it should be noted that most particle masks do not form a tight enough bond with the face to filter much at all. Best is to use a gas filter or a mask with a rubber barrier that fits tightly onto the face.

With regard to off-gassing, prior to bringing in any type of new furniture or wood into the house, it is best to off-gas the product by setting it in the sunshine for a couple of days or at least for a full day. As the sun's resonating waves connect with the material, many of its toxins are disassociated and released. Not such a good thing for the environment, but at least it will disburse outside of our immediate breathing environment. Off-gassing can help us avoid more than a potent toxin.

Fresh paint can also be toxic. This is because paint typically contains VOCs.

That New Car Smell

Many other indoor pollutants exist, depending upon the structure and condition of the environment. For example, automobiles, trains, planes, or buses can provide a whole range of triggers, from carbon monoxide to lead, formaldehyde and plasticizers—which can off-gas (also called *outgassing*), especially when the weather gets warmer.

This is especially the case for new cars. That 'new car smell' is the toxic off-gassing of a mixture of plasticizers, formaldehyde and other synthetics. In the case of older cars, air vents may be clogged with a number of molds, dust and bacteria, which may spray out whenever the "air" is turned on.

It might help to periodically clean out the filters of any car—especially older ones. In the case of a newer car, we might also consider leaving the windows cracked while parking in sunny locations between drives for a few weeks, to let the various materials outgas.

Electromagnetic Toxins

Ionizing or Non-ionizing?

Ionizing radiation is typically defined as electromagnetic radiation capable of disrupting atomic, molecular or biochemical bonds. This disruption takes place through an interference of waveforms between the ionizing radiation and the waveforms of atomic or molecular orbital bonds. As this interference is likely to cause the atom or molecule to lose electrons, ions are likely to develop as a result. These ions can often turn to oxidative species or otherwise imbalanced molecular species. Should ionizing radiation with enough intensity impact the physical body, it can result in cell injury or mutagenic damage. Various natural and synthetic radiation forms are considered ionizing. Natural ionizing radiation includes portions of ultraviolet radiation, x-rays, cosmic rays and gamma rays. Fire can also cause ionizing radiation at high temperatures if the radiation comes close enough. Synthetic versions of ionizing radiation include electrically produced x-rays, CAT-scans, mass accelerator emissions and a host of other electromagnetic radiation produced through alternating current.

Non-ionizing radiation also can be split into natural and synthetic versions. Natural versions include sound, light and radiowaves. Most natural non-ionizing radiation can also be synthetically produced. For example, sound may be digitally produced through the manipulation of alternating current by stereo receivers and speakers. This effect utilizes electrical semiconduction. Some scientists also categorize radiation from electrical power lines, electricity generating or transfer stations, appliances, cell phones, cell towers and other shielded electricity currents as non-ionizing radiation. Microwaves are also considered non-ionizing. Most assume that non-ionizing radiation is not harmful. This assumption, however, has undergone debate over the past few decades.

The 2005 National Academy of Sciences report, after a review of most of the available research regarding non-ionizing radiation, concluded that even low doses below 100 milliseiverts were potentially harmful to humans and could cause a number of disorders from solid cancer or leukemia. This jolted the scientific community, because for many years researchers thought that small doses of non-ionizing radiation were not that harmful.

A rem is one unit of radiation dose in roentgens. An mrem is one thousandth of a rem. One hundred rem equals one sievert. One sievert equals one thousand milliseiverts. Ten sieverts (10,000 mSv) will cause immediate illness and death within a few weeks. One to ten sieverts will cause severe radiation sickness, and the possibility of death. Above 100 mSv there is a probability of cancer, and 50 mSv is the lowest dose that has been established as cancer causing. Twenty mSv per year has been established as the limit for radiological workers. About one to three mSv per year is the typical background radiation received from natural sources, depending upon our location and surroundings. About .2 to .7 mSv per year comes from air. Soil sources are responsible for about .8 mSv. Cosmic rays give off about .22 mSv per year. Japanese holocaust victims received .1 Sv to 5 Sv from the bomb.

Our total radiation dose is a thus a combination of natural sources and those emitted by our artificial electromagnetic empire. A report from the Hiroshima International Council for Health Care of the Radiation-Exposed noted that the world's average radiation dose from natural radiation sources is 2.4 mSv. However, they also noted that Japan's natural radiation average is comparably low at 1.2 mSv. Japan's average radiation dose from medical radiation is higher than average, at 2.4 mSv. This gives Japan a significantly higher radiation average of 3.6 mSv.

UK's National Radiological Protection Board estimates that the national radiation exposure in Britain for the average person is 2.6 mSv, with an estimated 50% coming from radon gas, 11.5% coming from foods and drinks, 14% coming from gamma rays, 10% coming from cosmic rays and 14% originating from appliances—primarily medical equipment.

Recent research indicates that radiation from medical equipment is increasing. This is primarily driven by the growing use of CT scans, which generate a larger dose of radiation than the more traditional x-rays. About sixty-two million CT scans are now given a year in the U.S., as opposed to about three million per year in 1980. Brenner and Hall (2007) reported in the *New England Journal of Medicine* that a third of CT scans given today are unnecessary. The article also estimated that between one and two percent of all cancers are caused by CT scan radiation exposure.

In contrast, the maximum radiation a nuclear electricity generating plant will emit at the perimeter fence is about .05 mSv per year. A set of dental x-rays will render a dose of about .05-.1 mSv. A CT scan will can render a dose of about 10 mSv—*making a CT scan a hundred to a thousand times the dose of an x-ray.*

A grand electromagnetic human self-experiment is unfolding. Unsuspecting humans and animals are the subjects of this experiment. The findings will be available in a decade or two from now.

Most researchers are quick to say gamma rays—from radon and other natural sources—produce significantly more radiation than do appliances. This might be true for someone with a minimal amount of electrical appliances who rarely visits the hospital and dentist's office.

The question that persists is whether humankind's synthetic "non-ionizing radiation" is as innocuous as is currently assumed.

Power Lines

The American Physical Society, an association of 43,000 physicists, said in a 1995 National Policy (95.2) statement, *"....no consistent significant link between cancer and power line fields...."* This statement was reaffirmed by the APS council in April of 2005.

Power lines emit electromagnetic radiation at ELF or *extra low frequency* levels. Power lines typically release about 50 hertz of pulsed radiation. As an electric current moves through a wire or appliance, magnetic fields move perpendicular with electricity in a cross pattern. Thus, electricity fields form from the strength of the voltage while magnetic fields rise and break away from the electronic waveform's motion. While electricity voltage can shock us or burn the body, magnetic fields have more subtle yet lasting influences upon the body's natural biowave systems—such as brainwaves, neurotransmitter release, hormone production, and so on.

While magnetic influences are difficult to perceive directly, it is apparent they may substantially interrupt our immune systems. Between 1970 and 2000, about fourteen international studies analyzed the potential link between power lines and cancer among children. Eight of those studies showed a link between cancer rates and power line proximity, while four studies associated power lines with leukemia.

One of the U.S. studies to show a positive link in between cancer took place in 1979 in Denver, led by Dr. Nancy Wertheimer and Ed Leeper. This studied showed a more than double likelihood of cancer among children living within forty meters of a high-voltage line. Another Denver study published in 1988 (Savitz *et al.*) also found a 1.54x odds ratio (OR) positive link in all childhood cancers and high power lines. A Danish study (Olsen *et al.* 1993) also linked general cancer rates (1.5 OR) with power line proximity. A study done in Los Angeles (London *et al.* 1991) showed a 2.15 OR rate, a Swedish study (Feychting and Ahlbom 1992) showed a 3.8 OR risk and a Mexican (Fajardo-Gutierrez *et al.* 1993) study showed 2.63 OR increased rate of leukemia cancer rates among children with close proximity to high-voltage power lines. One Swedish study (Tomenius 1986) showed a 3.7 OR increased risk for central nervous system tumors among children living close to power lines. The Danish study mentioned above also showed a 5.6 OR increased potential of all cancers among children. The other positive link studies showed rates above 1 to 1.5 OR, which are not considered by mainstream science to be statistically significant.

Following the release of these studies, a number of governments took steps to warn housing developers of the potential risks of building close to high frequency power line hubs. In some municipalities across Europe and the U.S., building departments have even taken steps to dissuade or ban developments close to larger power lines.

Adult power line studies have yet to illustrate as large a correlation between power line proximity and cancer rates. Still a few have been significant enough to confirm the need for concern. Werthheimer and Leeper's (1982) studies showed increased rates of all cancers. Still, this 1.28 OR rate was not considered that significant. However a U.K. study (McDowall 1986) showed a SMR 215 increased rate of lung cancer and a SMR 143 increased risk (SMR 100 or less = no risk) of leukemia. Another study in the U.K (Youngson 1991) showed a statistically insignificant 1.29 OR rate for leukemia and lymphoma and Feychting and Ahlbom's (1992) Swedish study showed a 1.7 OR risk for leukemia subtypes. Another significant study (Schreiber *et al.* 1993) showed a SMR=469 rate for Hodgkin's disease.

It must be noted that these studies are epidemiological. They are population studies where groups living in close-proximity to high frequency power lines are compared with groups living further away. The problems that can occur with these studies focusing on cancer are several. In cancer pathology, there can be a two to twenty year delay between exposure and cancer diagnosis. While some of the populations involved in these studies might have been living in a particular house for many years, most may have only lived there for a year or two at the most.

In addition, some of the studies limited the disease group population, restricting the usefulness of the information. Cancer is seen primarily in the elderly and middle-aged, where there may be a host of various different types of exposures. These would include smoking, alcohol consumption, job-related exposures, chemical toxins, and so on. For this reason, these studies can be difficult to weigh against the costs of preventing exposure. The economic issues involving power lines are quite substantial. Relocating schools and families away from high-voltage lines or even relocating power lines comes with a substantial economic cost.

Nonetheless, this is increasingly becoming a problem for both homeowners and utility companies. For example, in the mid-nineties, the New Jersey Assembly enacted legislation requiring disclosure from homebuilders of vicinity transmission lines in excess of 240 kilovolts (kV). Other states have followed with real estate disclosure laws for power lines. Lawsuits have followed on power line proximity issues between schools, buyers, builders and utility companies.

One of the problems existing with some of the power line studies is the comparable limits of the distances between households and power lines. For example, is the effect of a transformer 40 meters away significantly different from one 50 meters away? Another difficulty with these epidemiological power line studies is that some of the studies measured utility wire codes (wire thickness) and distance, while other studies used spot physical measurements to determine exposure levels. In addition, there has been a variance of controls related to whether the child was born in the house or moved there recently.

With regard to the significance of the leukemia studies, we should consider the incidence of leukemia cancer among the childhood population—close to 1 in 10,000. A 2 or 3 OR among a group, unless the size of the groups are in the millions (most of the studies were significantly smaller—in the thousands), would relate to only a small handful of disease cases over the entire study population. If the study group size was five or ten million, then these numbers might be considered more reliable. As the increased rates have been smaller (rather than the 4 or 5 OR rate that appears in many study groups) then the size of the disease group is not considered to be a significant factor with which to judge the quality of the study. To this point, D'Arcy Holman, a professor at the University of Western Australia, calculated that the UK studies' worst projections might mean one extra childhood leukemia death in Western Australia every fifty years (Chapman 2001).

Occupational studies regarding exposure to EMR have shown unclear results with regard to leukemia and cancer (Kheifets *et al.* 2008). However, studies have pointed to the increased risk of amyotrophic lateral sclerosis (ALS) due to EMR exposure (Johansen 2004). Studies on electricians, electric utility line workers and other electrical workers have consistently showed higher rates of leukemia and central nervous system-related cancers. In a 2006 meta-study of fourteen studies by Garcia *et al.* (2008), Alzheimer's disease was associated with chronic occupational EMR exposure.

One of the difficulties with assessing the data on EMR effects is the sheer volume of studies of different types that has been published over the past twenty years. The breadth of variances between the studies of plants, animals, and human response to various degrees of radiation is substantial. Because of this huge base of studies, most researchers have been forced to rely upon various reviews by publications and government agencies to assess the implications of this large base of varying research. These groups have assessed and compared studies to figure out whether there is a correlation between study results, and whether they are significant. Government-sponsored reviews have included the United Kingdom's National Radiological Protection Board, the Associated Universities of Oak Ridge, the French National Institute of Health and Medical Research; councils in Denmark, Sweden, Australia and Canada together with U.S. agencies such as the Environmental Protection Agency and the Department of Transportation. In addition, the U.S. National Council on Radiation Protection and Measurements and the US National Academy of Sciences have also put together major reports on EMR research.

A number of respected journals have published reviews of EMR research as well. While some of these studies have found some epidemiological evidence notable, few found conclusive results, and some have presented skeptical views of any significant positive pathological correlation with non-ionizing EMR exposure. Multiple reviews were also presented (Savitz 1993) in *Environmental Health Perspectives*. No interaction mechanism between power line EMRs and biological organisms was determined.

An electrical field is substantially different a magnetic field. An electrical field is generated when there is a charge differential between two terminating points, regardless of whether current runs between them. An electric light bulb will still generate an electric field even when it is turned off. This electrical field allows alternating current to run between the two points when the switch is eventually turned on.

A magnetic field is created by a current flowing with electricity. The magnetic field will be emitted outward with perpendicular orientation to the electrical field. However, because magnetic fields have a particular polarity or direction, a current flowing in the opposite direction placed next to the current wire will cancel the magnetic field. Most power cords with double wires (hot and ground for a circuit loop) effectively cancel the magnetic field of the incoming current directly related to the distance between the wires. An increase in this separation increases the strength of the magnetic field. This occurs in power lines, where conductors are typically separated by poles and shields for fire protection.

For these reasons, excessive magnetic fields are considered to have the greatest potential for harm. The level of potential harm are thought to be related directly to the distance from the generating source, the distance between other conductors, the size of the coils on the transformer (if any) and of course the amount of current flowing through the system. It is generally accepted that the relative magnetic field strength halves with the amount of distance from the line. In other words, a line 100-foot away will have one-quarter of the magnetic field strength of a line 50-feet away.

Li *et al.* (1997), after testing 407 residences in northern Taiwan ranging from 50 meters to 150 meters from high-voltage power lines, found that the magnetic fields at the houses ranged from .93 mG for 50 meters to between .51 and .55 milliGauss for residences under 149 meters, and .29 mG for residences beyond 149 meters.

This data is somewhat contradicted by a 1993 cohort study from the Netherlands that revealed magnetic field intensities, ranging from 1 to 11 milliGauss from two kilovolt power lines connecting to one transformer substation (Schreiber 1993).

Higher voltage wires are typically thought to be an issue because the voltage and speed is boosted to travel longer distances. With a high-speed voltage line comes an increase in magnetic field. Magnetic fields have been connected with decreased melatonin secretion (Brainard *et al.* 1999). A number of studies have linked lower melatonin levels with higher incidence of a number of types of cancers. It would thus seem probable that since lower melatonin levels are associated with higher voltage, high-speed power lines could well be a mechanism for cancer (Ravindra 2006).

In comparison, a typical house or office will range from .8 to 1 mG in magnetic fields. The magnetic field strength from a kitchen appliance at close range for a person working in the kitchen is significantly greater than the strength coming from power lines 50-100 feet away. Stepping a few feet away from a microwave oven will dramatically reduce this field strength, while that same relative power line reduction will require a more significant change. A typical microwave oven might cause a field strength of 1,000 mG, which can be reduced to a minimal 1 mG by stepping a few feet away. Moving ones house further away from a power line obviously requires a significant commitment to the reduction of magnetic field strength, and a few feet will not make a significant difference.

Epidemiological studies involving electrical appliances have been limited. They are more difficult because of the control parameters. Nonetheless, a few appliances have undergone controlled studies over the years. Electric blankets have undergone several studies. Some of these illustrated significantly increased risk factors for postmenopausal cancer (Vena *et al.* 1991), testicular cancer (Verreault 1990), and congenital defects (Dlugosz 1992).

Radio Waves

Radiofrequency waves range from about 3 hertz to 300 gigahertz. This means their waves travel from speeds of 3 cycles per second up to 3,000,000 cycles per second. *Extremely low frequency* (ELF=3-30 Hz) and *super low frequency* (SLF=30-300 Hz) broadcasting has primarily been used for submarine communications, as these wavelengths transmit well through the water. This is also the frequency range that sound waves travel. *Ultra low frequency* (ULF=300-3000 Hz) has primarily been used in mines, where the waves can penetrate the depths. Above these levels, *very low frequency* and *low frequency* (VLF and LF = 3-300 kHz) have been used by beacons, heart rate monitors, navigation and time signaling. *Medium frequency* (300-3000 kHz) radiowaves are typically used for AM broadcasts, while *high frequency* (HF = 3-30 MHz) is used primarily for shortwave and amateur radio broadcasting. *Very high frequency* (VHF = 30-300 MHz) waves are used for FM radio, television and aircraft communications while *ultra high frequency* (UHF = 300-3000 MHz) waves are used for certain television ranges, but also cell phones, wireless LAN, GPS, Bluetooth and many two-way radios. While often considered outside the radio spectrum, *super high frequency* (SHF = 3-30 GHz) waves are used in microwave devices, some LAN wireless systems and radar. *Extremely high frequency* (EHF = 30-300 GHz) is used for long-range systems such as microwave radio and astronomy radio systems. The audio frequencies are primarily ELF through VLF brands, covering 20-20,000 Hz.

Note that EMR wavelengths inversely vary to their frequency. For naturally occurring EMR such as sunlight, the frequency will equal the speed of light divided by the wavelength. Thus, an ULF wave can range from 10,000 and 100,000 kilometers long. An UHF wave will range from one meter to ten millimeters in length, while an ELF wavelength will range from one millimeter and ten millimeters long.

Adulterated radiofrequencies have been utilized by humans for only about the last seventy-five years. Early use was primarily for radio transmission, while during the past few decades, various communication and signaling systems have been developed that utilize radiofrequencies. Radiofrequencies are generated with alternating current fed through an antenna at particular speeds and wavelengths.

Studies on radiofrequency radiation proximity at work have also studied possible reproductive and cardiovascular effects. While many of the reports are inconclusive, there have been positive correlations between radiofrequency exposure and delayed conception (Larsen *et al.* 1991), spontaneous abortion (Quellet-Hellstrom and Steward 1993; Taskinen *et al.* 1990), stillbirth (Larsen *et al.* 1991), preterm birth after father exposure (Larsen *et al.* 1991), and birth defects (Larson 1991). However, many of these results have either not been replicated or remain uncorroborated. Three studies examined male military personnel exposure to microwaves and radar (Hjollund *et al.* 1997; Lancranjan *et al.* 1975; Weyandt *et al.* 1996). All three found reductions in sperm density.

A number of animal studies have illustrated adverse health effects from radiowaves but doubt has been raised regarding the dose comparison with humans. In one study, GSM phone frequency radiowaves caused the cell death of about 2% of rat brains. Researchers hypothesized that the blood-brain barrier was being penetrated by the radiation (Salford 2003). This was correlated by three earlier studies that reported blood-brain barrier penetration with radiowave exposure (Shivers *et al.* 1987; Prato *et al.* 1990; Schirmacher *et al.* 2000). For several years following the release of this last study, other studies could not replicate the findings, nor could they establish a confirmation of the permeation of the blood-brain-barrier from radiofrequencies (Kuribayashi 2005; others). However, Shivers and colleagues, and Prato and associates had previously determined the effect of magnetic resonance imaging upon the rat brain. They showed that the exposure to radiofrequencies combined with pulsed and static magnetic fields gave rise to a significant pinocytotic transport of albumin from the capillaries into the brain.

Rates of breast cancer, endometrial cancer, testicular cancer and lung cancer have been studied with close range radiofrequency radiation, primarily in occupational settings. Slightly positive correlations with endometrial cancer (Cantor *et al.* 1995) and male breast cancer (Demers *et al.* 1991) were found. A potential link between testicular cancer and radiofrequency radiation from traffic radar guns, particularly among a small group of police officers (Davis and Mostofi 1993) was also established. Slightly increased ocular melanoma was established among occupational radiofrequency exposure (Holly *et al.* 1996) in another small group. French and Canadian utility workers were found to have an increased likelihood of lung cancer (Armstrong *et al.* 1994).

Cell phone tower radiofrequencies are popular concerns. The first cell phones communicated with analog frequencies of 450 or 900 megahertz, for example. By the 1990s, cell phones were using 1800 megahertz, and various modulation systems. Now the Universal Mobile Telecommunication System is adhered to, which uses 1900 to 2200 megahertz.

In 2000, over 80,000 cell tower base stations were in use in the United States. By 2006, this number was estimated at 175,000. CTIA, the International Association for Wireless Telecommunications Industry, estimates that by 2010 there will be about 260,000 towers. These base stations transmit radiowaves using around 100 watts of power. The range of GSM towers is about 40 kilometers, while the CDMA and iDEN technologies offer ranges of 50 to 70 kilometers. This obviously is relative to terrain. In a hilly area, the range can be a few kilometers.

In populated areas, cell base towers are placed from one to two miles apart, while in urban areas they can be as close together as a quarter of a mile. Some cell phone bases are mounted on primary towers, and some are built onto elevated structures such as buildings and hillsides.

A base cell tower antenna is comprised of a transmitter(s), a receiver(s)—often called transceivers—an electrical power source, and various digital signal processors. The circuits will utilize copper, fiber, or microwave connections. They may be connected to the network via T1, E1, T3 and/or Ethernet connections. They are typically strung together through base station controllers and radio network controllers, typically connected to a switched telephone network system. The radio network controller will connect to the SGSN network.

There has been scant research on the risks of radiofrequency waves from radio stations or television stations. The primary reason for this appears to be that most of these have been located outside of densely populated areas, on high towers enabling greater ranges. Cell towers have created more concern because of their close proximity and relatively lower heights.

Research has suggested that exposure from cell towers is reduced by a factor of one to one hundred times inside of a building, depending upon the building materials and style of the building. However, exposure also increases with height. Upper floors can have substantially greater exposure levels than lower floors (Schuz and Mann 2000). Whether this is a factor of pure height or whether the earth provides a buffering factor is not known.

Exposure levels in regions surrounding cell towers will range from .01 to .1% of ISNIRP (International Commission on Non-Ionizing Radiation Protection) permitted levels for general public exposure directly around the station, to .1 to 1% of ISNIRP permitted levels between 100 meters and 200 meters from the tower. Beyond the 200-meter level, the exposure returns to the .01 to .1% level and reduces as the range increases. It should be noted also that exposure levels from cell phone towers are not substantially greater than exposure levels of radiofrequencies (RF) emitted by radio broadcasting towers. In one Australian study, the greatest level found was .2% (Henderson 2006).

In a 2006 randomized double-blind study performed at the Institute of Pharmacology and Toxicology at the University of Zurich (Regel *et al.*) in Switzerland, UMTS signals approximating the strength of a cell phone tower emission were tested on 117 healthy human subjects, 33 of which reported themselves as sensitive to cell towers and 84 as non-sensitive. Physiological analyses included organ-specific tests, cognitive tests, and well-being questionnaires. Apparently, significant negative physiological or cognitive results were not found, although there appeared to be a marginal effect on one of the cognitive tests for each of the two groups. Because the difference was slight, and each group (sensitive versus control) had different results, this effect was considered insignificant.

In 2006, the British medical journal (Rubin *et al.*) reported a study done at the King's College in London, which tested 60 self-reported sensitive people and 60 control subjects with no reported sensitivities. Six different symptoms such as headaches were tracked, and subjects took questionnaires in an attempt to find whether the sensitive subjects could successfully judge whether a cell tower signal was on or off. While 60% of the sensitive subjects believed the tower signals were on when they were on, 63% believed the tower signals to be on when they were indeed off.

There have also been several international studies done on radiofrequency transmissions from masts. Tests in the United States, Britain, Australia and the Vatican City have shown no or low correlation between RF levels and health effects, rendering these studies for the most part, inconclusive. One study in the Netherlands using simulated mobile phone base station transmissions did conclude, however, that the UMTS-like spectrum of cell transmission might have an adverse affect upon the well-being of questionnaire respondents.

In July of 2007, an independent team of researchers (Eltiti *et al.*) from the University of Essex reported findings from a three-year double-blind study using a special laboratory to test potential cell phone tower effects. The study included 44 people who reported sensitivity to cell phone towers and 114 healthy people who had not. The study measured various physiological factors like skin conductance, blood pressure and heart rate while being exposed (or not) to 3G tower signals. During periods where the researcher and the subject knew the signals were on, sensitive people reported feeling worse, and their physiological factors were affected negatively. However when neither the subjects nor the researchers knew the cell tower signals were on during a series of tests, there was no difference between either the sensitive or non-sensitive subjects with regard to physiological factors. In fact, only two of the forty-four sensitive subjects were able to guess the cell tower signals being on correctly while five of the control subjects (non-sensitive) were able to guess correctly. Subjects who reported sensitivities to cell phone towers prior to the study reported negative symptoms more often, regardless of whether the cell tower transmitters were on or off.

Remote and Cell Phones

Typically, a digital cell phone operates at a power range of about .25 watts, while the newest digital phones might transmit as low as .09 watts. Analog phones were much higher power transmitters. The exposure level of a cell phone will depend greatly upon the way the phone is designed. The location of the antenna and the power supply/battery will typically govern the strength of the transmission to the dermal layers of the skin. The further away the antenna is from dermal contact (hand or ear), the less exposure.

The orientation of the power supply will also govern exposure. Some phones have shielding between the power supply and the antenna and earpiece. This is thought to reduce dermal exposure. In other words, the manner of carrying and holding the phone will vary the exposure.

There is another factor called *adaptive power*. When a cell phone is further away from a tower, or in a moving car, it will typically increase its internal transceiver power to send and receive signals. This increases the level of electromagnetic exposure as the phone is boosting power and transmissions. EMR cell phone exposure is thus typically less out of doors than indoors, because there is less interference from building materials out of doors. In addition, exposure to radiowaves is greatest on the side of the head the phone is most used and closest to where the antenna is located (Dimbylow and Mann 1994).

Radiofrequencies from handset use have been confirmed to heat the ear canal. In one controlled study of 30 individuals, 900 MHz and 1800 MHz phones against the ear for more than 35 minutes resulted in an increase of 1.2-1.3 degrees F (Tahvanainen *et al.* 2007). Other studies have confirmed this effect. For this reason there has been a great concern regarding the potential for tumor development either in the brain or in the areas surrounding the ears—referred to as an *acoustic neurinoma*.

Adverse effects of tissue temperature rise are not clear, but it is thought that the body's thermoregulation mechanisms may create an increased immune burden on the body. Lab studies have suggested a one-centigrade temperature rise at the tissue level will have immunosuppressive effects (Goldstein *et al.* 2003).

The International Agency for Research into Cancer has sponsored studies in thirteen countries to study the line between cell phone usage and cancer. So far, Australia, Canada, Denmark, Finland, France, Germany, Israel, Italy, Japan, New Zealand, Norway, Sweden and Britain have participated. Through 2005, the research tracked 6,000 glioma and menigioma cases (brain tumors), 1,000 acoustic neurinoma cases and 600 parotid gland cancers. Of these, the acoustic neurinoma results, primarily from Sweden, showed a significant link with handset use—from both cell phones and cordless phones. The German study also revealed a significant link between uveal melanoma and unspecified handset use. Other types of tumors had OR levels of around or just above 1 to 1.7 OR. The 2001

Swedish study on all brain tumors found a 2.4 OR link with ipsilateral cancer—more prevalent on the same side of primary handset use.

Again, we are faced with the fact that many of these associations are occurring at between 1 and 3 OR. A 2 or 3 level OR risk level creates questions in the minds of meta and review researchers. This should be combined with the fact that the rates of these tumors are so small among the general population (10-15 per 100,000 per year) for malignant brain tumors (Behin *et al.* 2003). Additionally, there is often a ten-year or more delay from exposure to diagnosis. This gives some researchers a myriad of reasons to question even the better correlations between cell phones and cancer.

Other researchers firmly disagree, stating that the weaker evidence is actually enhanced by the cancer diagnosis delay. Research from the Japanese nuclear victims of World War II has shown that many cancers arise ten to twenty years and more after the initial exposure. If we extrapolate this with cell phone use, we estimate that because cell phone use among the general population is still within this twenty-year period, especially for many younger adults (who were barely using cell phones five years ago). This means we should expect to see higher cancer rates among heavy cell phone users within the next five to ten years from now. Possibly this might be ameliorated somewhat by the improved cell phones being made now, with increased shielding (which begs the question; why did they increase the shielding if there was no danger?). Or not. We will see. The grand experiment with EMR rages on.

One of the more dramatic releases on cell phone use emerged in 2003 from a study conducted by Dr. Michael Klieeisen at Spain's Neuro Diagnostic Research Institute. This study revealed from a CATEEN scanner linked to a brainwave activity-imaging unit that radiowaves from cell phones could penetrate and interfere with the electrical activity of an eleven-year-old boy and a thirteen-year-old girl. Various hypotheses resulted from the release of this data. Among them, that radiowaves affect the moods, memory, and activities of children. Because brainwaves have been closely linked to moods, recollection, response time and other cognition skills, it is assumed that cell phone use has a disturbing effect upon cell phone users—particularly in children and adolescents.

In a 2004 study (Maier *et al.*), eleven volunteers' cognitive performance was tested with and without being exposed to electromagnetic fields similar to cell phones. Nine of the eleven (or 81.8%) showed reduced performance in cognition tests following exposure.

It should be noted that there is a tremendous market resistance to the information that cell phones and remote phones could be dangerous when used consistently. The cell phone industry is now a multi-billion dollar international business. The damage undeniable evidence of a health risk would have upon this industry is nothing short of monumental. It goes without saying that this would also have a significant impact upon the human lifestyle.

This effect may be effectively illustrated by the events reported by Dr. George Carlo and Martin Schram in their 2001 book *Cell Phones: Invisible Hazards in the Wireless Age*. Dr. Carlo was a well-respected epidemiologist/research scientist and pathologist. He was retained by the cell phone industry's chief lobbyist to study and comment on research regarding potential dangers of cell phone use. However, it was not expected that Dr. Carlo would speak out against cell phone use after examining the research data. In his book, Dr. Carlo describes the extraordinary efforts of the cell phone industry to discredit him. As Dr. Carlo began to announce negative cancer-related findings, his clients began to apply both political and financial pressure upon him.

We should however note that although U.S. brain cancer rates have increased substantially over the past three decades, brain cancer incidence increased until 1987, and has been slowly decreasing from that point (Deorah *et al.* 2006). This statistic does not concur with a model of increasing brain cancer rates with increasing cell phone usage. Quite possibly, some of the environmental etiologies involved in brain cancer prior to 1987 have been somewhat mitigated. Perhaps some of the toxin exposure levels—such as the rampant use of DDT and toxic waste dumping in waterways—have been curtailed due to some of the EPA actions of the 1960s and 1970s—decreasing brain cancer rates in the years following. We also cite further controls on nuclear leaks and a massive reduction in tobacco use. Epidemiologically, these could well be masking a slow rise in brain cancer levels due to cell phone use.

Cancer is not the only issue to consider with regard to cell phones, however. Researchers have examined other disorders with respect to radiofrequency exposure. Heavy cell users commonly report a wide variety of negative symptoms. In a study of 300 individuals at Alexandria University in Egypt (Salama and Naga 2004), cell phone usage was positively correlated with complaints of headaches, earaches, sense of fatigue, sleep disturbance, concentration difficulty and burning-face sensation. The results showed that 68% of the study population used cell phones. All of the above health complaints were significantly higher among the cell phone users, and 72.5% of the cell phone users had health complaints. The frequency duration of cell phone usage was also extrapolated together with health complaints, and it was discovered that the higher the cell phone use, the greater the incidence of health complaints. While the burning-face sensation complaint correlated positively with call frequency per day, complaints of fatigue also significantly correlated (positively) with both call duration and call frequency.

The warming of the ear, face and the scalp around our ear from cell phone use is logically taking place as a result of frequency and waveform interference between our body's natural waveforms and these synthetic waveforms. Our body's natural waveforms include the shorter waves of the brain and nerves, and the weaker biophoton waveforms of the cells, along with the molecular electromagnetic bonding waveforms within DNA. Should electronically driven waveforms interfere with these natural biowaves, the molecular bonding structures of our genetic information could gradually become deranged.

The effects of this interference should appear on a number of fronts. We should see lower cognition levels and brain fog, as unnatural waveforms interfere with our brainwave mapping system. We should see body temperature interference within the basal cell network. We should see damage to the blood-brain barrier and damage to nerve and brain cells. These effects should release greater levels of radical species from the imbalanced molecular structures—damaging cells and tissues. All of these effects have been documented in the research.

This waveform interference mechanism is illustrated by a recent study (Thaker et al. 2008) showing that a certain popular brand of MP3 player will interfere with the mechanisms of a pacemaker if held close to the chest for about five seconds. Appliance interference has been directly correlated with waveform interference. This is one reason why the U.S. Federal Communications Commission closely monitors and licenses bandwidths. When we consider that the body maintains various natural biowave "bandwidths" as it cycles hormones, thermoregulation, cortisol, melatonin and the Krebs energy cycle to name a few, it is not difficult to connect the waveform interference of cell phones and other appliances with the disruption of these natural cycles.

Video Display Terminals

VDTs and televisions emit about 60 hertz of electromagnetic fields. Although a number of early studies suggested the potential of a health risk, many studies over the past few years have suggested that VDTs pose little if any health risks. The National Academy of Sciences reviewed a number of studies in 1999 and stated, *"....the current body of evidence does not show that exposure to these fields presents a human health hazard..."* In 1994, the American Medical Association stated, *"no scientifically documented health risk has been associated with the usually occurring levels of electromagnetic fields..."* Their review included both epidemiological studies and various other direct studies of EMR effects from terminals.

Another report, published in *Lancet,* the British Medical Association's journal, documented the largest childhood study comparing childhood leukemia and cancer rates and exposure to 50-hertz non-ionizing magnetic fields. No link was found.

The National Radiological Protection Board in 1994 confirmed that while existing conditions might be aggravated, their review of the research showed no link between skin diseases or cataract formation and VDT use. However, the board's Chairman Sir Richard Doll, did confirm that VDT use might aggravate conditions that have already formed.

In addition, a bevy of clinical research regarding pregnancy outcome for those working around or on computers has failed to show any links between miscarriage or birth defects and VDT use. The National Radiological Protection Board from Oxford, U.K. confirmed this in a review of the research.

In 1998, the International Commission on Non-Ionizing Radiation Protection submitted low emission field guidelines. They suggested an upper limit of magnetic field exposure of 833 milliGauss (mG). The electric field limit was set at 4,167 volts per meter (V/m).

Both VDTs and televisions are far below these exposure levels when measured individually.

Regardless of these reports, problems associated with vision, fatigue and headaches have been reported from VDT use. These problems have been attributed to such ergonomic issues as the potential for glare on the screen, lighting location with the position of the screen, the distance from the screen, and whether there are regular breaks from looking at the screen.

Other issues reported have been associated with static electricity generated through the keyboard and screen, posture problems, and repetitive injuries such as keyboarding without rest, which can create a risk of carpal tunnel and other motor difficulties.

As for television, there have been numerous efforts to study the effects of television on children and adults. Most of these have leaned towards its behavioral effects, but a few have reported significant effects on physical health. In 2007, Crönlein *et al.* found a significant link between television viewing and adolescent children insomnia. Thakkar *et al.* (2006) and Paavonen *et al.* (2006) found that watching violence on television increased insomnia and sleep disturbances among young children. Bickham and Rich (2006) showed that increased television viewing—especially violent TV—was associated negatively with friendships. Hammermeister *et al.* (2005) showed that viewers who watched two hours or less television per day had a more positive psychosocial health profile. Viner and Cole (2005) determined that early childhood television viewing was associated with people who had a higher body mass index later in life. Other studies have also correlated increased television viewing with childhood obesity (Robinson 2001).

Meanwhile Zimmerman and Christakis (2005) found that children who watched a significant amount of television before the age of three years (2.2 hours/day) scored lower on Peabody reading comprehension, memory and intelligence testing at ages six and seven. Hancox *et al.* (2005) found in New Zealand that increased television viewing was associated with higher dropout rates and lower rates of university attendance. Collins *et al.* (2004) found that watching sex on television increases sex activity at a younger age in children. Huesmann *et al.* (2003) found that watching violence on television increased violent behavior during adulthood. Vallani (2001) illustrated that research since 1990 progressively showed that increased television viewing increases violent behavior, aggression, and high-risk behavior such as smoking, drinking, and promiscuousness.

However, Anderson *et al.* (2001) indicated that television content might have more to do with these associations. 570 adolescents were studied from preschool, and their programming was monitored. Educational program watching was linked to higher grades, increased reading, greater creativity and fewer violent activities.

Microwaves

Microwave ovens produce two different forms of radiation: High frequency radiowaves produce electromagnetic radiation in the range of 2450 megahertz and magnetic fields at 60 hertz. The central question is whether this is enough bombardment to cause harm to the food. While some claims have been made that microwave ovens cause the food particles to spin and rotate, this statement has not been confirmed by scientific investigation. What we know is that the microwaves increase the waveform energy states of the molecules using thin microwave beams in much the same way fire increases energy states. Whether this is accompanied by a spinning or rotation of the molecule appears to be speculative, though it appears likely—understanding the physics involved.

Indeed, microwaves do create unnatural molecular structure results. A well-cooked microwave dinner reveals dry and rubbery textures not seen in other forms of cooking. Is microwaved food healthy?

Dr. Robert Becker (1985) reported that various disorders such as cardiovascular difficulties, stress, headaches, dizziness, anxiety, irritability, insomnia, reproductive disorders, and cancer occurred in the Soviet Union among microwave-exposed workers when the Soviets were developing radar during the 1950s. In fairness, though technically correct, these were people working amongst microwave transmissions, not eating microwaved dinners.

Dr. Becker also reported that research from Russia indicated nutritional reductions of sixty to ninety percent in microwave oven tests. Decreases in bioavailable vitamin Bs, vitamin C, vitamin E, minerals, and oil nutrients were observed. Alkaloids, glucosides, galactosides and nitrilosides—all phytonutrients—were found damaged by microwaving. Some proteins were found to be denatured.

Research (Knize *et al.* 1999) at the University of California Lawrence Livermore Laboratory concluded that microwaves produced heterocyclic aromatic amines and polycyclic aromatic hydrocarbons. Both are suspected carcinogens. Frying meats also produces polycyclic aromatic hydrocarbons (Felton *et al.* 1994).

Dr. Lita Lee wrote in her 1989 book, *Microwaves and Microwave Ovens* that the Atlantis Rising Educational Center in Oregon reported that a number of carcinogens form during the microwaving of nearly all types of foods. Microwaving meats caused formation of the carcinogen d-nitrosodiethanolamine. Microwaving milk and grains converted amino acids into carcinogenic compounds. Thawing frozen fruit by microwave converted glucosides and galactosides into carcinogenic chemicals. Short-term microwaving converted alkaloids from plant foods into carcinogenic compounds. Carcinogenic free radicals formed during the microwaving of root vegetables, according to this report.

In December of 1989, the British Medical Association's *Lancet* reported that microwaves converted trans-amino acids to cis-isomers in baby formulas. Another amino acid, L-proline, converted to a d-isomer version. These isomers have been classified as neurotoxins (toxic to the nerves) and nephrotoxins (toxic to the kidneys).

Swiss food scientist Dr. Hans Ulrich Hertel and Dr. Bernard Blanc of the Swiss Federal Institute of Technology reported in a 1991 paper that microwave food created cancerous effects within the bloodstream. The small study had eight volunteers consume either raw milk; conventionally cooked milk, pasteurized milk; microwave-cooked milk; organic raw vegetables; conventionally-cooked vegetables; the same vegetables frozen and warmed in a microwave; or the same vegetables cooked in the microwave oven. Blood tests were taken before and after eating. Subjects who ate microwaved milk or vegetables had decreased hemoglobin levels, increased cholesterol levels and decreased lymphocyte levels. The increase in leucocytes concerned Dr. Hertel the most. Increased leukocyte levels in the bloodstream are generally connected with infection or tissue damage.

The controls in some of these studies may be in question, however. For example, in Dr. Hertel's study he was a participant, the group knew whether the food was microwaved or not, and the group members were predominantly macrobiotic. The Russian studies and the *Atlantis Rising* report statistics all come unconfirmed from secondary sources.

Various forms of cooking will also destroy nutrients and generate carcinogens—especially frying and barbequing. Overcooking in general destroys nutrients and can create a variety of free radicals that can be tumor forming if eaten in excess.

There are other dangers reported from microwaves. The leakage of various toxins from packaging during microwaving has been documented. A 1990 *Nutrition Action Newsletter* reported that various toxins will leach onto microwaved foods from food containers. Suspected carcinogens including benzene, toluene and xylene were among chemicals released into food. Also found was polyethylene terphtalate (PET). Various plasticizers are almost certainly to be included in this list, as they will quite easily outgas when heated.

In addition, microwaving—unless done for extended periods—rarely completely sterilizes a food. This should be a warning for all those who pack leftovers into storage containers and assume a few minutes in the microwave will produce a sterile, cooked food. This fact has been become obvious from the *Salmonella* outbreaks among those who took food home in doggie bags to microwave later.

Approaching this logically, it is apparent that nature did not design food to be cooked in microwaves.

This is evidenced by a simple experiment conducted in 2006. Marshall Dudley's granddaughter completed a Knoxville science fair project that compared plant water feeding between stove-boiled filtered water and the same filtered water source microwaved. She started with sets of plants of identical species, age, and health. One of each set was fed filtered water boiled in a pan and cooled. She fed another the same filtered water, but microwaved until boiling and cooled. This 'watering study' went on for a period of nine days, and pictures of the plant sets (which sat together in identical potted condition) were taken each day.

The simple assessment of each plant's health was clear by looking at the photographs. Each day the plant watered with microwaved-water looked worse. It became increasingly withered and slumped over in obvious stress. By the ninth day, the microwave-watered plant had lost most of its leaves. Meanwhile, the boiled-watered plant stood tall with crisp green leaves, growing healthier by the day.

Radon

As research in the nineties focused on power lines, research has illuminated the fact that electromagnetic fields can interact with various elements in the atmosphere, creating radon gas. A further potential danger has been proposed for households not properly wired with copper and insulation. A lack of shielding can also increase the potential interaction of household electricity with radon.

Radon 222 comes primarily from the nuclear decay of uranium. This natural process takes place within the earth. As this decay proceeds, radon gas is released, together with decay byproducts, called *radon daughters* or *radon progeny*. These particles are known carcinogens. Should we breathe these particles, they can be caught in the lungs. Breathing radon gas delivers the potential of it continuing to decay inside our bodies. This will effectively deposit the radioactive daughters inside our bodies.

The National Council on Radiation Protection and Measurement has developed a maximum safe dosage of radon to be 200 mrem per year.

The relationship between radon and outdoor power lines has not been clearly established, because in order to measure the interaction, an aerosol component (a pollutant of some sort) must accompany the electromagnetic field. Nonetheless, significant *radon daughters* have been measured (Henshaw *et al.* 1998) among power line fields.

The subsequent dose and tolerance of radon particles in the human body is also in question. In some research, heavy electromagnetic fields have been shown to penetrate with no more than about .0001 of the original field strength of radon emissions. Still this penetration effect alerted researchers to the fact that there might be a radon penetration into the lungs and basal tissues of the body (Fews *et al.* 1999).

The link between radon and lung cancer has become more evident in recent research. Lung cancer has been the most prevalent form of cancer worldwide since 1985, and has been responsible for more than one million deaths worldwide. The highest rates of lung cancer occurred in 2002 in North America and Northern or Eastern Europe. Although smoking is widely considered to be the primary etiology of lung cancer, uranium miners—who are exposed to increased levels of radon along with dust—experience higher rates of lung cancer (Tomasek *et al.* 2008). Epidemiological studies on radon-exposure and miners have also revealed that thousands of miners die per year of radon exposure (Field *et al.* 2006).

Research has illustrated that while living outdoors does not increase ones risk of lung cancer, unnatural living or working quarters without enough ventilation can lead to a drawing in and encapsulation of radon radiation. A household with poor ventilation poses a higher risk of radon exposure than a well-ventilated house. This is exasperated by other electromagnetic radiation in the local environment. Research has illustrated that ventilation around electromagnetic current exposure is an absolute requirement because of a release of radon daughters into the immediate atmosphere (Karpin 2005).

Darby *et al.* (2005) reported in the *British Medical Journal* on a collaborative analysis of thirteen case studies of 7,148 lung cancer cases together with 14,208 control subjects. This found that increased radon exposure is responsible for about 2% of European cancer deaths. Further research has revealed that most buildings, especially work environments that are full of various power lines and equipment, retain higher levels of radon. Radon levels are additionally increased with unventilated soils, higher air temperatures and higher atmospheric levels. Higher household radon levels are particularly associated with leaking and unventilated soils in the house. This research has caused legislation in many states in the U.S. requiring property sellers to disclose known radon issues.

The majority of our everyday radiation input comes from radon. Natural concentrations of radon are found in some granites, limestones and sandstones. Higher radon levels come from disturbed ground. Disturbing the normal landscape allows more permeability, allowing the release of the normally contained daughters. Once a house is built upon disturbed ground, the radon can come in through cracked foundations and spaces around piping and wiring. Because radon gas is pulled in through pressure changes within the house created by temperature gradients, it is important that our houses be well ventilated. This is particularly significant during the nighttime and during cold weather, as the warmer temperatures inside with colder temperatures outside cause the most pressure differential—the *Bernoulli effect*. Ventilation will not only allow the escape of indoor radon gas, but it will release some of this pressure, resulting in a lower draw of radon gas into the house.

Household radon levels tend to increase dramatically during the winter, and decrease substantially during the summer for these reasons. Radon levels also go up dramatically during the nighttime hours, as the outdoor temperature cools. This is when ventilation is most important. Disturbed landscaping ground can also leak increased radon daughters.

The U.S. Environmental Protection Agency has recommended safe levels of radon to be 4 *picocuries of radon per liter* (pCi/L). Levels any higher than this should be remedied by cementing over the exposed ground or sealing cracks in current cement foundations. Ventilation systems have also been known to help. Radon detection kits are quite inexpensive and easy to use.

Magnetic Fields

Nature's magnetic fields surround us, and pose little threat. Many species utilize nature's magnetic fields to navigate migration and nesting. In other words, our cells are tuned to the geomagnetic fields of the sun and the earth.

Synthetic magnetic fields, on the other hand, are dispersed with the distribution of unnatural alternating current. The proliferation of electricity and electrical appliances created by power-generating plants that convert nature's kinetic energy into alternating current has deluged our atmosphere with unnatural magnetism.

Most early research on the health effects of electrical appliances and wires focused on the electrical fields and ignored the magnetic fields given off by appliances. While most electrical fields are shielded by insulators within most appliances, magnetic fields can be more disruptive and insidious to the health of the body. This is because they can directly interfere with the body's internal biowaves. Normally, synchronic and harmonic biowaves—including brainwaves, nerve firings, and so on—travel with synchronicity throughout the body.

A magnetic field surrounding the body can induce an abnormal electrical current flow within the body. In a Swedish study (Wilen *et al.* 2004) of RF operators exposed to high levels of magnetic fields, currents were induced within the body at mean levels of 101 mA and maximum levels of one Amp. During this study, exposure levels correlated positively with the prevalence of fatigue, headaches, warm sensations in the hands, slower heart rates and more bradycardia episodes among the subjects.

In a study done by the Fred Hutchinson Cancer Research Center and the Epidemiology Division of Public Health Services in Seattle, Washington (Davis *et al.* 2001), 203 women aging from 20-74 years with no breast cancer history were studied between 1994 and 1996. Magnetic field and ambient light in the bedroom were measured for a 72-hour period during two seasons of the year. Urine samples were taken on three consecutive nights for each subject. After adjusting for hours of daylight, older age, higher body mass, alcohol use and medication use, those women with higher bedroom levels of magnetic fields had lower concentrations of 6-sulfatoxy-melatonin. It was thus concluded that increased levels of synthetic magnetic fields depress nocturnal melatonin.

While this illustrates how unnatural magnetism can significantly affect the body's biochemical rhythms, reduced melatonin also causes negative effects throughout the body. Over several decades since melatonin was discovered in 1958 by Dr. Aaron Lerner and his Yale colleagues, decreased melatonin levels have been linked to a variety of pathologies and immune function deficiencies.

A three milliGauss magnetic field at 60 Hertz will induce about one-billionth amp per square centimeter of the body. A magnetic field at 120 Hz frequency will have double the current effect the same field will have at 60 Hz. A typical American office building or home—filled with various electrical appliances—will contain magnetic fields at levels between .8 and

1 milliGauss. In a study done at a Canadian school by Akbar-Khanzadeh in 2000, workers, schoolteachers and administrative staff environments had magnetic field exposure levels ranging from .2 to 7.1 mG.

MilliGauss levels will be substantially higher in instrument-heavy environments. Hood *et al.* (2000) recorded the pilot's cockpits of a Boeing 767 with magnetic field levels of 6.7 milliGauss, while the Boeing 737 recorded at 12.7 mG of magnetic field strength. Nicholas *et al.* (1998) documented a mean magnetic field strength of 17 mG among the cockpits of B737, B757, DC9 and L1011 planes. Meanwhile, cabin measurements ranged from a high of 8 mG in the forward serving areas to 6 mG in the first class seats and 3 mG in the economy seats.

Rail maintenance workers experience magnetic field levels from 3 to 18 mG (Wenzl 1997). In a study published in the *Journal of the Canadian Dental Association* (Bohay *et al.* 1994), dental operating rooms with various ultrasonic scalars, amalgamators, and x-ray equipment revealed magnetic fields ranging from 1.2 to 2225 mG, with equipment distances from zero to thirty centimeters.

Most of these magnetic field readings were accompanied by lower level radiation frequencies ranging from 25 hertz to 100 hertz (though the airline cockpits research recorded up to 800 hertz).

In a population study of 969 women in San Francisco, miscarriage levels positively correlated with higher magnetic field exposure. Li *et al.* (2002) concluded that fields in the region of 16 mG or higher produced the greatest risk of miscarriage. While higher levels of magnetic fields have been shown not to significantly affect nervous system biowaves such as cardiac pacemakers (Graham *et al.* 2000), 12 milliGauss magnetic fields operating from radiation frequencies of 60 hertz were shown to block the inhibition of human breast cancer cells by both melatonin and tamoxifen *in vitro*. While melatonin and tamoxifen have different mechanisms of retarding cancer growth, it was confirmed by Harland and Liburdy (1997) that synthetic magnetic fields prevented their immunity effects. When we consider that the magnetic fields blocked the immune activities of *both* biochemicals—which work within different mechanisms—the affect of synthetic magnetic fields on the human body illustrates an *immune system magnetic interference* model.

This magnetic field interference model of electromagnetic exposure is further supported by research published in 2002 by Saunders and Jefferys. Brain tissue testing showed that even very low frequency electric and weak magnetic field exposure will induce electric fields and currents inside the body. These fields excited various nerve cells and retinal cells, inducing abnormal metabolic activity.

The immune system magnetic interference model mechanism is further confirmed by a study of magnetic and electric fields on neural cells by Blackman (1993). While magnetic fields stimulated abnormal neurite outgrowth between 22 and 40 mG, increased electric fields did not stimulate the same morphological change.

In contrast, the natural magnetic field strength of the earth ranges from about .2 gauss to .6 gauss (200-600 mG)—often also measured as .05 Tesla (1 Tesla=10,000 gauss). To give some reference with nature's levels, an MRI magnet will range from one to three Tesla, or 10,000 to 30,000 gauss. This is equivalent to 10,000,000-30,000,000 mG.

Appliance Magnetic Fields

Appliance	At 4 Inches	At 1 Foot	At 3 Feet
Blenders	50-220	5.2-1.7	.3-1.1
Can openers	1300-4000	31-280	.5-7.0
Clothes dryers	4.8-110	1.5-29	.1-1
Coffee makers	6-29	.9-1.2	<.1
Crock pots	8-23	.8-1.3	<.1
Electric drills	350-500	22-31	.8-2.0
Electric shavers	14-1600	.8-90	<.1-3.3
Faust blowers	3-120	.25-37	<.1-3.1
Fluorescent desk lamps	100-200	6-20	.2-2.1
Fluorescent fixtures	40-123	2-32	<.1-2.8
Hair dryers	3-1400	<.1-70	<.1-2.8
Irons	12-45	1.2-3.1	.1-.2
Microwave ovens*	39-75	2.7-6	.18-.75
Mixers	58-1400	5-100	.15-2.0
Portable heaters	11-280	1.5-40	.1-2.5
Saber and circular saws	200-2100	8-210	.2-10.0
Televisions	4.8-100	.4-20	<.1-1.5
Toasters	10-60	.6-7.0	<.1-.11
Vacuum cleaners	230-1300	20-180	1.2-18.0

Source: Gauger, 1985 *Gauger 1997 (at 3.6, 10.8 and 25.2 in)

Biological Toxins

Microorganisms and their endotoxins are collectively called *biological pollutants*. These microorganisms include bacteria, viruses, fungi and mold.

Bacteria can come from rotting food, plants, people and pets. Dander also can carry these creatures. Viruses can trigger inflammation initially, or once they infect the body's cells. Viruses damage DNA within the cells, and reproduce through the body via the DNA damage.

Microorganisms can grow on anything wet—especially mold. Almost any type of sitting water or dampness will grow mold, especially those in dark areas (as many fungi abhor sunlight).

Research has confirmed that infective microorganisms from viruses, bacteria and fungi can stimulate serious systemic inflammation. As we'll discuss later, microorganism infection requires a sharp living immune system—as we'll discuss in the next chapter. While a periodic super-cleanse might be helpful to clear microorganism toxins, a vibrant living immune system will consistently protect the body against infection. Let's talk about the possible microorganism infections we can face.

Bacteria were first discovered in 1673 by Dutch scientist Antony van Leeuwenhoek. Leeuwenhoek began writing letters to the Royal Society of London about the images he was seeing in his newly invented microscope. In 1674, Leeuwenhoek described his microscopic creatures as "wound serpent-wise and orderly arranged, after the manner of the copper or tin worms." He described "many very little living animalcules."

Today we are dealing with a multitude of infections from all of these types of microorganisms. Growing infectious diseases from this list include lyme disease (*Borrelia burgdorferi*), pneumonia, staphylococcus, streptococcus, salmonella, *E. coli*, cholera, listeria, salmonella, shigella, dengue fever, yellow fever, tuberculosis, cryptosporidiosis, hepatitis, rabies and others. Many of these microorganisms are growing despite our antibiotic and antiviral medications. Some are growing because of unsafe sex, unclean water or changes in land use. Many are growing because of new opportunities arising from our destruction of nature. Many are becoming resistant to our antibiotics. These are often referred to as *superbugs.*

One of the more dangerous of these superbugs is methicillin-resistant *Staphylococcus aureus* (MRSA). MRSA rates are on the rise, and nearly every hospital—the crown jewels of our antimicrobial kingdom—is infected with MRSA. In a 2007 survey of 1200 U.S. hospitals, 46 of every 1,000 hospital inpatients are colonized or infected with MRSA, with 75% of those being infected. Among the general population, the incidence of MRSA has skyrocketed from 24 cases per 100,000 people in 2000 to 164 cases per 100,000 people in 2005 (Hota *et al.* 2007). This means that MRSA is infecting nearly seven times the number of people it did in 2000.

The virulence of *Staphylococcus aureus* was first realized in 1929 by Alexander Fleming, a microbiologist who cultured a combination of *Staphylococcus aureus* in the vicinity of a growing mold. He noticed that the penicillin mold would kill some bacteria and not others. Fleming soon realized that *Staphylococcus aureus* adapted quickly to the penicillin. It became resistant. Even to this day, *Staphylococcus aureus* is still one of the most antibiotic-resistant bacteria.

Staphylococcus aureus is also one of the most lethal bacteria known to man. It secretes three cell-killing toxins: alpha toxin, beta toxin and leukocidin. Together these poisons bind to and dissolve cell membranes, allowing cytoplasm and cell contents to leak out. This, of course, immediately kills the cell. The immune system also has difficulty attacking and removing *Staphylococcus aureus* because it secretes enzymes that neutralize the immune system's attack strategies. *Staphylococcus aureus* adapts very quickly, so the more we throw at it, the stronger it becomes.

Infectious bacteria are not always suspected—or even detected—in many diseases. Increasingly, we are finding that many common diseases are caused or worsened by bacteria or fungal infections. We are also seeing an increase in many degenerative diseases connected to infection—including cardiovascular disease, arthritis, ulcer, irritable bowel syndrome, asthma, allergies and chronic fatigue syndrome.

A few diseases linked to microorganisms:

Disease	Some Suspected Microbes
Heart disease, stroke and cardiovascular disease	*Helicobacter. pylori* *Treponema pallidum* (syphilis) *Staphylococcus aureus* *Enterococci faecalis* *Streptococcus* spp. Herpes Simplex (I and II) *Pneumonococcal aerogenes* *Candida albicans* *Streptococcus mutans* *Escherichia coli* *Chlamydia pneumonia* *Porphyromonas gingivalis* *Tannerella forsynthensis* *Prevotella intermedia*
Gallstones	Eubacteria *Clostridium* spp.
Ulcers, ulcerative colitis and Crohn's	*Helicobacter pylori* *Clostridium* spp. *E. coli* *Mycobacterium pneumoniae*
Cancers	*Staphylococcus aureus* *Enterococci faecalis* *Streptococcus* spp. *Pneumonococcal aerogenes* *Streptococcus mutans* *E. coli* mammary tumor virus papilloma virus (HPV) *H. pylori* Heptitis B

Diabetes and metabolic disorders	*Bacteroides fragilis* *Borrelia burgdorferi* *Brucella melitensis* *Brucellae* spp. *Campylobacter jejuni* *Chlamydia trachomatis* Coxackle B virus Cytomegalovirus *Salmonella osteomyelitis* others suspected (see arthritis below)
Arthritis and other inflammatory diseases	*Bacteroides fragilis* *Borrelia burgdorferi* *Brucella melitensis* *Brucellae* spp. *Campylobacter jejuni* *Chlamydia trachomatis* *Clostridium difficile* *Corynebacterium striatum* *Cryptococcal pyarthrosis* *Gardnerella vaginalis* *Kingella kingae* *Listeria monocytogenes* *Moraxella canis* *Mycobacterium lepromatosis* *Mycobacterium marinum* *Mycobacterium terrae* *Mycoplasma arthritidis* *Mycoplasma hominis* *Mycoplasma leachii sp.* *Neisseria gonorrhoeae* *Ochrobactrum anthropi* *Pasteurella multocida* *Pneumocystis jiroveci* *Porphyromonas gingivalis* *Prevotella bivia* *Prevotella intermedia* *Prevotella loescheii* *Pseudomonas aeruginosa* *Pyoderma gangrenosum* *Roseomonas gilardii* *Salmonella entertidis* *Scedosporium prolificans* *Serratia fonticola* *Sphingomonas paucimobilis* *Staphylococcus aureus*

	Staphylococcus lugdunensis *Streptococcus agalactiae* *Streptococcus equisimilis* *Streptococcus pneumoniae* *Streptococcus pyogenes* *Streptococcus uberis* *Tannerella forsynthensis* *Treponema pallidum* *Vibrio vulnificus* *Yersinia enterocolitica*
Dementia	*Chlamydia pneumoniae* Borna virus *H. pylori* Spirochetes Herpes simplex I picornavirus

Overgrowths of yeasts like *Candida albicans* can also contribute to or be a primary cause for a number of diseases. Research has found that in some cases, *Candida albicans* can grow conjunctively with *Staphylococcus aureus*, resulting in the accelerated growth of both. This can result in a variety of diseases caused by combined yeast and bacteria infections. Viruses and bacteria can also grow in combination. We see this in many of the fatalities from the swine flu and other influenzas. Deaths often occur in immunosuppressed patients with concurrent bacteria infections.

Multiple toxic microorganisms will grow and prosper within the mouth, teeth and gums. These include *Streptococcus mutans*, *Streptococcus pyogenes*, *Porphyromonas gingivalis*, *Tannerella forsynthensis* and *Prevotella*. Additional microbes can grow within root canals. Root canals provide protected spaces for bacterial growth. Bacteria infecting root canals can include a variety of streptococci, staphylococci, and even dangerous spirochetes such as *Borrelia burgdorferi* among many others. Just about any bacteria that can infect the body internally can hibernate inside root canals. Because root canals are enclosed and the tissues around them die, the immune system cannot reach these areas to remove bacteria. As a result, a growing number of diseases are now being associated with root canal-harbored bacteria.

As these microbial populations grow, they not only can infect teeth and gums with gingivitis: They can also infect various other parts of the body. Infected gums have been implicated in a variety of fatal disorders, including heart disease, lung disease, liver disease, kidney disease, septic arthritis and others. A recent report from the Jos University Teaching Hospital in Nigeria (Adoga *et al.* 2009) reported that, "Most often the cause of cervical necrotizing fascitis is of dental origin." Necrotizing fascitis is a growing lethal infection of multiple bacteria that rapidly destroy tissues around the body, causing death very quickly.

Insect Endotoxins

Insect endotoxins—such as from dust mites—can be allergens as well as toxins. They can overload our immune system with toxicity and produce systemic inflammation. This overloaded immune system produces the allergy response.

Many other insects also produce endotoxins that one may become sensitized to. These include cockroaches, ladybugs, aphids and other household pests. We should be clear that insect endotoxins are practically everywhere. They are unavoidable. They are in our water, air, foods, carpets, seats, floors… literally everywhere.

Humans have been dealing with insect endotoxins since time immemorial. Furthermore, a strong immune system can easily tolerate these, simply because a natural immune system has the technology to break down and cleanse these toxins from the body.

However, an immune system that already is overloaded with toxins may have difficulty breaking these down and purging their metabolites from the body. In this case, there might be a need to reduce our exposure to dust mites and insect endotoxins.

While insects are ubiquitous, dust mites are especially insidious because they are so tiny and hardy. They live in beds, pillows, carpets, and other fabrics, and their favorite food is dead skin cells that slough off of our bodies and the bodies of our pets.

There are two prevalent household species: The American house dust mite (*Dermatophagoides farinae*) and the European house dust mite (*D. pteronyssinus*). Storage mite species include the *Acarus spp.* and *Tyrophagus spp.* Dust mites feed on organic matter—and they love dead skin. The primary allergens these mites create are the skin moltings they shed as they grow, and their feces. Because of their propensity for eating skin, mites are usually not found in vents or ducts.

Many health experts have advised that dust mites like warm and humid places, so they suggest placing a dehumidifier in the house. University of Cambridge researchers (Hyndman *et al.* 2000) tested this theory. They investigated 76 households given a dehumidifier, a behavior program, or nothing for one year. Other trap measures were also instituted to reduce dust mites. Every three months they tested each house for humidity, temperature, dust mite counts, dust mite allergens, and several other environmental elements. Not surprisingly, they found the relative humidity in houses with dehumidifiers were significantly lower than houses without dehumidifiers. However, the houses with dehumidifiers had no fewer dust mites than did the other houses.

Confirming this, researchers from New Zealand's Wellington School of Medicine (Crane *et al.* 1998) studied lowering humidity levels in heat-exchanger systems (MVHE) units. They tested ten buildings in Wellington, NZ. Again, lowering the humidity in these buildings did not reduce concentrations of the *Der p1* dust mite allergen.

German researchers (Kroidl *et al.* 2007) found, in a study of 132 patients with bronchial asthma, over half were sensitized to either storage mites or house mites. Only three patients were allergic to storage mites and not household dust mites. Farm workers, bakers and forestry and paper mill workers had the most risk of storage mite allergies.

Researchers from Italy's G. D'Annunzio University (Riccioni *et al.* 2001) studied the seasonal nature of mite and pollen sensitivity among 165 allergic patients. They found that pollen bronchial symptoms increased with pollen seasons as expected. However, asthmatic symptoms among patients allergic to dust mites increased in the fall—seemingly as mites or their endotoxin populations also increase.

Researchers from the UK's Imperial College (Atkinson *et al.* 1999) studied the relationship between allergen exposure and subsequent asthma among infants. They collected and analyzed dust samples from 643 homes. They coupled this with surveying each house and studying each infant. They found that higher dust mite allergen content was seen among houses that were carpeted, had double-glazed windows and less ventilation. Houses sampled in the winter had more dust mites than those sampled in other parts of the year. These conditions did not produce greater levels of cat allergens, however. Homes with more occupants had more dust mite and fewer cat allergens, regardless of cat ownership. Homes with smoking inhabitants had significantly fewer dust mites, but again had no difference in cat allergens.

Animal Dander

Animal dander is another toxin produced by the waste products of a living organism. A strong immune system should be well equipped to tolerate and manage these, but an overburdened immune system may not be.

Animal dander can come from any number of animals, including pets, farm animals, zoo animals and wild animals. This means that sources for animal dander include pet stores, zoos, vet clinics, farms, barns, and just about anywhere else that animals may occupy for extended periods.

The allergic or sensitive element of animal dander is not necessarily their hair, as one might think. It is typically the shedding of their skin as it flakes off their bodies. This can resemble dandruff, but may also be invisible to the naked eye. Dead skin or waste matter excreted by their skin is included in this. In other words, we are talking about the waste products of animals.

While we know now that greater levels of pet dander do not necessarily cause allergies, pet dander is one of the most prevalent allergy triggers. Illustrating this, researchers from Denmark's Roskilde County Hospital and Sweden's Sahlgrenska University Hospital (Plaschke *et al.* 1999) studied 1,859 adults to test atopic sensitization and asthma. They found that positive skin prick tests for allergens and allergen-specific IgEs included pets, grass pollens and mites. The greatest associations between allergies were made with cat and dog allergens.

Today, cat allergens (such as protein *Fel d1*) are found virtually everywhere. Scientists from New Zealand's Canterbury Respiratory Research Group and Christchurch Hospital (Martin *et al.* 1998) tested a variety of public places to understand exposure levels for the *Fel d1* cat allergen. They tested 203 floors, 64 beds and 24 seats in hotels, hospitals, rest homes, churches, schools, daycare centers, ski lodges, movie theaters, banks and airplanes. They found that 95% of the floors, 91% of the beds, and 100% of the seats maintained exposure levels of *Fel d1*. Furthermore, they found that theater seats and airplane seats contained the greatest levels, with more cat allergens than other public places, and most floors. Not surprisingly, cat allergen levels were greater on carpeted floors than on hard floors.

New Zealand has relatively high rates of asthma and allergies. About half of Kiwi households also have a cat, according to the research. To test the relationship between cat allergens and asthma, Wellington School of Medicine researchers (Patchett *et al.* 1997) tested the cat allergen (*Fel d1*) levels within schools and the clothing of children. They analyzed the clothing of 202 children and floors of 11 school classrooms. They found cat allergen practically everywhere, and highest on the clothing of children from homes that had cats. They also found a significant amount of cat allergen among the carpeted classes, significantly more than the floors without carpets.

While the researchers concluded that carpeting should be discouraged from schools and daycare centers, they could not correlate asthma frequency with increased cat allergens.

We are surrounded by microorganisms. Trillions upon trillions of bacteria, fungi, viruses, parasites, nanobacteria and extremophiles live within our clothes, cars, bathrooms, beds, floors, air, and all over our bodies. Just about everything we touch has millions of microbes living on it. Bacteria also live in and around just about every food. Our bodies are also densely populated with bacteria. There are more bacteria in our bodies than there are cells.

This situation has not changed for millions of years. Bacteria have been living amongst us and other creatures of our planet through the duration. Not only that, but for most of humankind's existence, we slept on earthen floors and straw beds. We farmed in our bare feet or in sandals made of rope. We crapped in holes in the ground and ate with our fingers. We drank out of the streams with our hands, and used twigs to brush our teeth.

How is it that over the past century we have become so fearful of bacteria? How is it that we now live in disinfectant-cleaned houses, and wash our hands with antibacterial soaps, and we still have a mortal fear of bacteria? How is it that despite these measures, we are still becoming infected?

Today, despite our various antibiotics, antivirals, disinfectants, mouthwashes and antiseptic cleaners, infectious diseases are on the rise. Rates of tuberculosis, influenza, shingles, mononucleosis, cytomegalovirus, malaria, HIV, AIDS and herpes are increasing worldwide. Estimates have calculated that 80% of the U.S. population may be infected with Herpes Simplex 1, while some 45 million are infected with the genital variety, HS2. More than half the world's population harbors *Helicobacter pylori* bacteria. About 1.5 million Americans are infected with sexually transmitted diseases gonorrhea, syphilis or chlamydia. Over 33 million people around the world were theoretically infected with HIV in 2005—a rise of 16% per year. In the U.S. alone, there are about 40,000 new cases of HIV documented every year. About one third of the world's population is infected with the tuberculosis bacterium. Every year about 6 million people die from TB according to the CDC. Millions more are infected with water-borne diseases throughout the world.

We end this section on biological toxins with a point that the immune system can readily adapt to many of these toxins. Assuming exposure at viable and reasonable levels, our immune system can become resistant to these types of toxins. We'll discuss how this happens and the difference between synthetic toxins and biological toxins later.

Sick Buildings

Over the last thirty years, researchers have become increasingly aware that certain buildings, especially older ones with older ventilation systems, can make people sick. This effect is often termed *sick building syndrome,* or SBS. The major symptoms reported in SBS include chronic fatigue, brain fog, headaches, allergies, nausea, chronic sore throat, bronchial congestion, and others.

Toxin overload becomes apparent in the case of toxins provided by older buildings, or buildings without sufficient ventilation or cleaning policies.

For example, research from the National Center for Healthy Housing (Jacobs *et al.* 2009) found that lower-income families tend to live in older homes, where there can be poor ventilation, more water leaks, more lead paint and greater moisture and mold levels. They found that these trends also relate to increased rates of respiratory illness, obesity and lead poisoning. They saw a clear association between respiratory disorders and home ventilation, home age, and the windows of homes. In other words, higher toxin exposure.

Researchers from the Vermont Department of Health's Division of Health Surveillance (Laney *et al.* 2009) studied a 2006 respiratory disorder cluster among workers who worked in a building that had water-damage. Physicians diagnosed increased incidence of sarcoidosis and asthma among the workers, and conducted pulmonary function tests.

As the researchers investigated the data, they found that adult respiratory disorders incidence in the office workers was 3.3/1,000 person-years prior to their working in the office, and 11.5/1,000 person-years after they began working in the building. Their respiratory disorders incidence tripled, in other words.

The workers were removed from the building while it was cleaned up.

In a study of school buildings (Sahakian *et al.* 2008), 309 school employees in two older elementary schools were tested. Excess dampness produced increased incidence of respiratory irritation, wheezing and rhinitis symptoms among the employees. The older, damper school of the two also produced more illness.

SBS is indicated when multiple workers or inhabitants of a building complain of one or more of these symptoms soon after beginning to work or live in the building. Sometimes, however, SBS can develop over time, or directly after or during an extreme change in the weather. A humid summer or heavy rainfall period, for example, may stimulate a growth in mold in the ventilation system. After a smoggy summer in a city or during a fire season, the ventilation system may become clogged with soot. Workers or occupants of the building need to speak up and request from management that filters and vents be periodically cleaned and flushed. The upholstery, walls and other parts of workplaces should also be cleaned periodically.

Occupational Toxicity

Scientists from the University of Texas School of Public Health (McHugh *et al.* 2010) analyzed the data from the National Health and

Nutrition Examination Survey (2001-2004) to determine the relative risks of toxicity in different occupations. They found that miners, health-care workers, and teachers have significantly higher rates of respiratory disorders than other occupations, including construction workers. Miners, for example had over four times the respiratory disorders incidence than construction workers. This of course relates to their exposure to indoor air pollutants at work.

Researchers from the National Institute for Occupational Safety and Health and the Centers for Disease Control (Greskevitch *et al.* 2007) investigated respiratory disease among agricultural workers using the 1988-1998 National Centers for Health Statistics' Multiple Cause of Death Data and the 1988-1994 Third National Health and Nutrition Examination Survey data (NHANES III). They studied mortality ratios for eleven respiratory illnesses in crop farm workers, livestock workers, farm managers, landscapers, horticultural workers, forestry workers, and fishery workers. Among the different occupations, the crop farm workers and livestock farm workers suffered significantly more deaths from respiratory conditions. Pneumonia with hypersensitivity was 10 to 50 times the normal levels. Landscapers and horticultural workers suffered more deaths from lung abscesses and COPD.

Wheeze and shortness of breath were also significantly elevated among the farm workers, especially among female farm workers. Respiratory disorders were heightened among agricultural workers, especially those who also smoked.

It is notable that these occupations each present particular toxins. In the case of miners, they are exposed to coal dust and soot, together with exhaust, with minimal ventilation. In the case of agricultural workers, landscapers and horticulture workers, they are exposed to chemical pesticides and herbicides. In the cases of teachers and healthcare workers, they are exposed to the contaminants that occupy their respective buildings and ventilation systems.

Exposure to specific toxins requires extensive ventilation and filtration systems. Whether these come in the form of protective breathing gear or building HVAC systems, the toxin exposures within a workplace must be minimized. Reducing exposure is, in fact, one of the driving purposes of the U.S. Occupational Safety and Health Administration (OSHA). Toxin exposure at the workplace has reached such significant levels that OSHA has put in place many regulations, such as Material Safety Data Sheets (MSDS), in efforts to protect workers from the effects of workplace toxins.

Why such an effort to protect workers from toxins? Today there are in the neighborhood of 100,000 different synthetic chemicals available in the marketplace. The chemical industry has produced many workplace chemicals for industrial uses over the past century, and many of these chemicals have been subsequently found to be carcinogenic or otherwise toxic. Keeping track of the effects and safeguards of each of these chemical toxins is a dizzying affair. Yet it is theoretically the responsibility of any business to make efforts to protect its workers from these toxins.

Here is a small list of occupations and their toxins:

Occupation	Exposures
Agricultural workers	Pesticides, herbicides
Plastics manufacturers	Plasticizers, VOCs, polymers
Painters	Paints/thinners (VOCs)
Drivers	Carbon, soot, formaldehyde, micro
Metal workers	Metallic dusts, heavy metals
Saw millers	Wood dust, preservatives
Janitorial and housekeepers	VOCs, cleaning chemicals
Bakers and food workers	Airborne food particles
Home builders	VOCs, formaldehyde, asbestos
Health workers	SBS, microorganisms, chemicals

Major Toxins and Their Sources

Source	Toxins
Air pollutants	Lead, mercury, carbon monoxide, sulfur, arsenic, nitrogen dioxide, ozone...
Animals	Dried skin, bacteria, waste excreted from animal (dander)
Carpets, rugs	Molds, dander, lice, PC-4, latex
Cigarette/Cigar/Pipe Smoke	Carbon monoxide, nicotine, aldehydes, ketones, soot, formaldehyde, others
Cosmetics	Aluminum, phosphates and chemicals
Spray cans	Propellants, other chemicals
Foods/Additives	Food colors, preservatives, trans fats, pesticides, arachidonic acids, acrylamide, phytanic acid, artificial flavors, refined sugars and much, much more
House	Radon, formaldehyde, pollen, dust, mold, dander, pesticides, cleaning products, asbestos, lead, paint, endotoxins

Household chemicals	Cleaners, pesticides, herbicides, paints
Insects	Endotoxins from dust mites, cockroaches and other insects
Laundry soaps	Fragrances, detergents, surfactants
Microorganisms	Mold, bacteria, viruses, parasites
Mattresses/pillows	Endotoxins, molds, formaldehyde
Paints	Lead, arsenic, VOCs, adhesives
Pets	Dander, up to 240 infectious diseases & parasites (65 from dogs/39 from cats)
Pharmaceuticals	Many-see short list on pages 112-113
Water	Chorine byproducts, pesticides, pharmaceuticals, many others
Pollinating plants	See pollen list on page 104
Pools and spas	Chlorine byproducts such as trihalomethanes (THMs), various carbonates
Soaps and Shampoos	Fragrances, detergents, surfactants
Stoves, Fireplaces	Carbon monoxide, NO_2, arsenic, soot
Work and school environments	SBS, practically all of the above

Chapter Four

Our Probiotic Defenses

In this chapter we'll introduce some of the hard-core evidence showing that probiotics, herbs and other natural elements stimulate the immune system and defend against infection, toxicity and disease in general.

Probiotics and Immunity

Immunosuppression is very simple: The immune system has been overburdened and compromised. This is the result of a myriad of combined effects, the primary being an overload of toxins and inadequate probiotic populations.

We might compare our toxin overload to a pile of dirt. A small handful of dirt can be carried around easily, and dispersed without much effort. However, a truckful of dirt is another matter completely. What do we do with a truckful of dirt? If we dumped it on our lawn, we'd have a hill of dirt blowing around and blocking us from getting in and out of the house.

This is a useful comparison because while our bodies can handle a small amount of toxins quite easily, modern society is increasingly dumping toxic 'dirt' into our atmosphere, water and foods, effectively inundating our bodies by the 'truckload.'

The modern world's toxin soup burdens an immune system trying to adapt and clean up each toxin and its damaging effects. Many of today's diseases, including arthritis, cancer, heart disease, Alzheimer's Disease and many others, are connected to immunosuppression due to the overload of toxins. Even a person's response to viruses or even the common cold may be related to the level of immunosuppression. An immunosuppressed person will likely get much sicker and can even die from an infection that a healthy body would throw off in a few days.

What does this have to do with probiotics? Lots. Probiotics are miniature workers that help carry our immune loads. They block many toxins and pathogens from getting into our bodies in the first place. Then they break down many toxins if they do get in. They will bind to and escort toxins out of the body by latching onto them like little bulldogs. More importantly, probiotics will stimulate the immune system. Let's look at the evidence:

Probiotics balance and temper our entire immune system. Probiotics increase IgA levels and reduce IgE allergic response. As we discussed earlier, IgA blocks toxins before they can enter the tissues and bloodstream.

Illustrating this, Finnish scientists (Ouwehand *et al.* 2009) gave healthy elderly volunteers *Lactobacillus acidophilus* or a placebo. The probiotics modulated IgA and PGE2 levels. The probiotics also improved spermidine levels—an enzyme involved in DNA synthesis. The researchers concluded that these improvements suggested increased mucosal and intestinal immunity among the probiotic group.

In a study of 105 pregnant women, University of Western Australia scientists (Prescott *et al.* 2008) found that *Lactobacillus rhamnosus* and *Bifidobacterium lactis* stimulated higher levels of cytokine IFN-gamma, higher levels of TGF-beta1, and higher levels of breast milk IgA. Plasma of their babies had lower CD14 levels, and greater CB IFN-gamma levels. These indicated that the probiotics strengthened immunity and moderated hypersensitivity.

Researchers from the Teikyo University School of Medicine in Japan (Araki *et al.* 1999) gave *Bifidobacterium breve* YIT4064 or placebo to 19 infants for 28 days. IgA levels significantly increased among the probiotic group.

Researchers from the Turku University Central Hospital in Finland (Rinne *et al.* 2005) gave 96 mothers either a placebo or *Lactobacillus rhamnosus* GG before delivery and continued the supplementation in their infants after delivery. At three months of age, immunoglobulin IgG-secreting cells among breastfed infants supplemented with probiotics were significantly higher than the breastfed infants who received the placebo. In addition, the non-hypersensitivity IgM-, IgA-, and IgG-secreting cell counts at 12 months were significantly higher among the breastfed infants who supplemented with probiotics, compared to the breastfed infants receiving the placebo.

Probiotics help modulate the inflammatory processes. In research from Poland's Pomeranian Academy of Medicine (Naruszewicz *et al.* 2002), scientists found that giving *Lactobacillus plantarum* 299v to 36 volunteers resulted in a 37% decrease in inflammatory F2-isoprostanes. Isoprostanes are similar to prostaglandins, formed outside of the COX process.

Probiotics also stimulate a healthy thymus gland. Illustrating this, medical researchers from the University of Bari (Indrio *et al.* 2007) gave a placebo or a probiotic combination of *Bifidobacterium breve* C50 and *Streptococcus thermophilus* 065 to 60 newborns. The thymus glands of the probiotic group were significantly larger compared to babies who consumed the standard (placebo) formula.

Scientists from the Nagoya University Graduate School of Medicine (Sugawara *et al.* 2006) found in a study of 101 patients that supplementation with probiotics increased NK activity and lymphocyte counts. Pro-inflammatory IL-6 cytokines also decreased significantly among the probiotic group. Serum IL-6, white blood cell counts, and C-reactive protein also significantly decreased among the probiotic group.

Furthermore, probiotics have the ability to *uniquely* modify cytokines—relative to the condition of the person. Illustrating this, a probiotic drink with either placebo or a probiotic combination of *Lactobacillus paracasei* Lpc-37, *Lactobacillus acidophilus* 74-2 and *Bifidobacterium animalis* subsp. *lactis* DGCC 420 (*B. lactis* 420) was given to 15 healthy adults and 15 adults with atopic dermatitis. After eight weeks, CD57(+) cytokines levels increased significantly among the healthy group taking probiotics, while CD4(+)CD54(+) cytokines decreased significantly among the atopic patients taking the probiotics (Roessler *et al.* 2008).

Researchers from Poland's Pomeranian Academy of Medicine (Naruszewicz *et al.* 2002) gave *Lactobacillus plantarum* 299v or placebo to 36 healthy volunteers for six weeks. Monocytes isolated from probiotic subjects had significantly reduced adhesion to endothelial cells, and the probiotic group had a 42% reduction in pro-inflammatory cytokine interleukin-6. No changes were observed among the placebo group.

Probiotics are often involved in the production of critical intermediary fatty acids used in LOX and COX enzyme conversions, producing anti-inflammatory effects. To illustrate this, scientists from the University of Helsinki (Kekkonen *et al.* 2008) measured lipids and inflammation markers before and after giving probiotic *Lactobacillus rhamnosus* GG to 26 healthy adults. After three weeks of probiotic supplementation, the subjects had decreased levels of intermediary inflammatory fatty acids such as lysophosphatidylcholines, sphingomyelins, and several glycerophosphatidylcholines. Probiotics also reduced hyper-inflammatory markers TNF-alpha and CRP in this study.

Researchers from the Osaka University Graduate School of Medicine (Morimoto *et al.* 2005) studied 99 addicted smokers for three weeks. They were given either a fermented milk containing *Lactobacillus casei* or a placebo. NK cell activity among peripheral blood mononuclear cells was measured before and after taking probiotics, and before and after smoking. NK cell activity reduced with the number of cigarettes smoked. However, NK cell activity was significantly higher after taking probiotics.

Ten healthy volunteers and nine volunteers with ileostomy underwent gastroscopy or ileoscopy along with *Lactobacillus reuteri* ATCC 55730 supplementation for 28 days (Valeur *et al.* 2004). After probiotic supplementation, gastric mucosal histiocyte numbers had reduced, and duodenal B-lymphocyte numbers had increased. *L. reuteri* supplementation also induced a significantly higher level of CD4-positive T-lymphocytes within the ileal epithelium. The scientists concluded that *L. reuteri* "is associated with significant alterations of the immune response in the gastrointestinal mucosa."

Researchers from Canada's Memorial University of Newfoundland (Arunachalam *et al.* 2000) gave *Bifidobacterium lactis* HN019 to 25 healthy elderly volunteers for 6 weeks. Interferon-alpha levels and polymorphonuclear cell phagocytic capacity increased substantially. The probiotic group also experienced enhanced phagocyte-mediated bactericidal activity. The researchers said that, "The results demonstrate that dietary consumption of *B. lactis* HN019 can enhance natural immunity in healthy elderly subjects, and that a relatively short-term dietary regime is sufficient to impart measurable improvements in immunity that may offer significant health benefits to consumers."

Researchers from the Teikyo University School of Medicine in Japan (Araki *et al.* 1999) gave *Bifidobacterium breve* YIT4064 or placebo to 19 infants for 28 days. After the treatment period, the probiotic group experienced significantly modulated levels of immunoglobulin IgA.

Scientists from The Netherlands (van Baarlen *et al.* 2009) gave living or heat-killed *Lactobacillus plantarum* to healthy adults. Biopsies were taken from the mucosa of their intestinal duodenums before and after the treatment period. These examinations indicated significantly different NF-kappaB-dependent pathways after the consumption of living *L. plantarum* bacteria in different growth phases. These mucosal gene expression patterns and cellular-immunity pathways correlated with increased immune tolerance among the subjects.

Pediatric medical researchers from the University of Bari (Indrio *et al.* 2007) gave a placebo or a combination of *Bifidobacterium breve* C50 and *Streptococcus thermophilus* 065 to 60 newborns. In addition, a control group of thirty newborns who were exclusively breastfed was included. Fecal pH of the breast-fed group and the probiotic formula group were similar—and significantly lower than the placebo group during the first few days of treatment. Meanwhile, thymus size was significantly larger in the probiotic group compared to the standard formula-placebo group. The probiotic group thymus sizes were similar to those of the breast-fed newborns.

Researchers from the Department of Immunology at Juntendo University's School of Medicine in Tokyo (Takeda and Okumura 2007) determined in a three-week study on 19 elderly volunteers that *Lactobacillus casei* strain Shirota significantly increased natural killer cell activity. This effect was particularly significant among those patients who began the study with low NK-activity levels.

Researchers at Belgium's University Hospital Leuven (De Preter *et al.* 2004) determined in a in a study of 19 healthy volunteers that *Lactobacillus casei* suppressed the production of toxic metabolites within the body.

Russian scientists (Bliakher *et al.* 2005) gave sickly children a *Lactobacillus* supplement, and assessed immune responses. They found the probiotics stimulated the immune system by modulating the activities of interferon, phagocytes, and cytokines among the children.

Researchers from the Department of Clinical Sciences at Spain's University of Las Palmas de Gran Canaria (Ortiz-Andrellucchi *et al.* 2008) studied the ability of *Lactobacillus casei* DN114001 to modulate immunity factors among lactating mothers and their babies. *L. casei* or a placebo was given to expecting mothers for six weeks. T helper-1 and T helper-2 (Th1/ Th2) levels were tested from breast-fed colostrum, early milk (10 days) and mature milk (45 days). Allergic episodes among the newborns were also observed throughout their first six months of life. Among the probiotic group, T and B lymphocyte levels were increased, and natural killer cells were significantly increased. Levels of the pro-inflammatory cytokine TNF-alpha was decreased in maternal milk. Significantly fewer gastrointestinal upsets occurred among the breast-fed children of the probiotic mother group as well.

Immune system suppression has been observed in students stressed during examinations. Spanish scientists (Marcos *et al.* 2004) gave 136 university students either a placebo or milk fermented with *Lactobacillus casei* for three weeks before examinations and during the three-week examination period. The probiotic group showed a significant increase in lymphocytes during the six weeks—which decreased among the placebo group. CD56+ cells decreased in the placebo group but stayed consistent in the probiotic group. The researchers concluded that *Lactobacillus casei* was "able to modulate the number of lymphocytes and CD56+ cells in subjects under academic examination stress."

Researchers from New Zealand's Massey University (Gill *et al.* 2001) investigated using probiotics to enhance risk of infectious and noninfectious disease and age-related lymphocyte activity. Twenty-seven elderly volunteers consumed low-fat and low-lactose milk supplemented with *Lactobacillus rhamnosus* HN001 or *Bifidobacterium lactis* HN019 for 3 weeks. The proportion of CD56+ lymphocytes among peripheral circulation was higher after probiotic supplementation. CD4+ and CD25+ activity increased among the probiotic group. PBMC tumor killing activity also increased. Subjects more than 70 years of age and those who were immune-suppressed experienced significantly greater improvements in immune system parameters than did the other subjects.

Researchers from the College of Medicine at National Taiwan University (Chiang *et al.* 2000) gave *Bifidobacterium lactis* HN019 to 50 persons aged from 41 to 81 years old. The probiotic group had significantly enhanced PMN cell phagocytosis and NK-cell tumor killing activity. The increases leveled off after *B. lactis* supplementation was discontinued, but still remained above the values at the beginning of the study.

Researchers from the Russia State Medical University in Moscow (Korschunov *et al.* 1996) studied five men who received accidental, uneven and high-dose, whole-body gamma-irradiation from exposure to an unshielded radiation source. Feces examinations 9-12 days after irradiation showed low numbers of anaerobes and high counts of enterobacteria and staphylococci in four of the five patients. All five were treated with ampicillin and gentamicin with oral nystatin starting 4-7 days after irradiation. Three were also given an antibiotic-resistant strain of *Bifidobacterium longum* for 30 days starting 10-12 days following irradiation while the other two received a placebo. After three weeks after irradiation, *B. longum* was observed in their feces, and this continued in the following weeks. In comparison, the two placebo patients' fecal flora was dominated by enterobacteria, including *Klebsiella, Staphylococcus* and *Serratia* spp. These showed resistance to multiple antibiotics. These pathogens were not found in the *B. longum*-treated group. One of the patients in the placebo group died. The other one continued to show high fecal counts of enterobacteria and staphylococci. The researchers concluded that, "Probiotic treatment with this antibiotic-resistant strain of *B. longum* may be of benefit in the treatment of radiation sickness, aiding normalization of the fecal flora and inhibiting colonization and overgrowth with opportunist pathogens."

Scientists from Bulgaria's National Oncological Centre (Krusteva *et al.* 1997) gave *Lactobacillus bulgaricus* to 78 patients who underwent combined chemotherapy and had subsequent moderate leukopenia (lack of white blood cells—a classic sign of immunosuppression). A recovery of WBC count (values above 3000) took place in all probiotic patients within three to five days. No infectious or febrile complications resulted from subsequent chemotherapy and probiotic treatment.

German scientists (Rayes *et al.* 2002) tested 172 patients who just had major abdominal surgery or liver transplantation with either conventional nutrition, *Lactobacillus plantarum* 299, or heat inactivated lactobacilli. Following treatment, bacteria infection after liver, gastric or pancreas resection was 31% in the conventional nutrition group, 13% in the heat-inactivated probiotic group and 4% in the probiotic group. Among the 95 liver transplant patients, 48% of the conventional nutrition group patients developed infections; while 34% of the inactive probiotic group and 13% of the live probiotic group developed infections (cholangitis and pneumonia were the most frequent). The use and duration of antibiotic therapy among the patients was also significantly shorter in the live probiotics group.

Within the intestines, probiotics attach to and dwell in between the villi and microvilli. This allows them to not only keep pathogenic bacteria from infecting those cells: It also allows them to monitor food molecule size of nutrients being presented to the intestinal wall for absorption. This helps prevent the body from absorbing molecules that are too large or not sufficiently broken down. As we will discuss further, large, atypical molecules that have entered the bloodstream will stimulate an inflammatory and allergic response. This is because these larger molecules are not recognized by the immune system.

Oral probiotics will vigorously defend the areas around the gums and teeth. The problem arises when our diets become overly sugary. As we will discuss later in more detail, probiotics require complex oligosaccharides like inulin, FOS (fructooligosaccharides) and GOS (galactooligosaccharides) for food sources. They do not thrive from simple sugars like glucose and sucrose. Pathogenic bacteria, on the other hand, typically thrive from these simple sugars. In fact, they can grow quite quickly, and may immediately begin to outnumber the probiotic populations, causing caries and gum infections.

These pathogenic bacteria, if unchallenged by oral probiotics, can also leak their endotoxins into the bloodstream, causing carotid artery damage.

The bottom line is that our body's probiotics head up the living immune system. At least 70% of the immune system *is* probiotic. Consider this carefully: If the intestine's probiotics were decimated by either a lethal bacteria infection or a course of antibiotics, *we would lose nearly three quarters of our gut's immune system.*

Probiotics aren't just the most important part of our immune systems. They also provide immunity in all parts of our ecosystem. An example is the role that soil bacteria play in providing nutrients and defending against disease among plants.

When an organism dies, *ammonifying bacteria* decompose the body and release ammonia into the soil. *Nitrosifying bacteria* oxidize the ammonia, converting it to nitrites, and *nitrifying bacteria* then oxidize the nitrites to soil nitrogen and ammonia ions. Plants utilize these to form amino acids and proteins. Nitrogen is also released into the air with *dentrifying* bacteria. As plant protein is eaten by animals and humans in plant food, these nitrogen amino acids become part of the proteins that make up our bodies. When our bodies die, the cycle begins again.

Throughout the nitrogen cycle, there is a precise balance of nitrogen in the atmosphere, the soils, and within each organism: Just enough to serve the combined purpose of all involved. Every species then gets a balanced dose of nitrogen, from the soil microbes and earthworms all the way up to humans.

This is of course, only one example of how bacteria are implicated in the life cycle. Now let's talk about some of the proof showing how probiotics provide immunity in the body.

Stimulating the Immune System

Probiotics are nature's smart army corps of engineers. They will help rebuild cellular functions and immune cell function, and help stimulate better immune system responses.

Many studies have illustrated these effects. Furthermore, some of the research has confirmed that somehow, probiotics are able to stimulate the effects of vaccines. How are they able to do that? Remember that probiotics are living organisms that can become aware of a pathogen entering the body. Then they can assist the immune system by stimulating specific immune responses. In the case of a vaccine, the vaccine is a small quantity of the pathogen itself, which stimulates the immune system to develop strategies to attack and rid the body of that pathogen should it invade the body later. Because probiotics help identify and stimulate immune responses, researchers have found that vaccination is often more productive when it is done concurrent to probiotic supplementation.

In a German study (de Vrese *et al.* 2005), 64 volunteers took either probiotics (*Lactobacillus rhamnosus* GG or *Lactobacillus acidophilus* CRL431) or placebo for five weeks. During the second week of treatment, the volunteers were given oral vaccinations against poliovirus 1, 2 and 4. As reported in other research, polio vaccination—even as documented by Dr. Salk—has caused on occasion the contraction of polio. Poliovirus factors—evident from poliovirus neutralizing antibody titers—increased significantly with probiotic treatment in this study. Increased vaccination response with probiotics ranged from two- to four-times higher. Furthermore, serum levels of *poliovirus-specific* IgA and IgG antibodies were significantly increased in the probiotic group. The researchers concluded that, "Probiotics induce an immunologic response that may provide enhanced systemic protection of cells from virus infections by increasing production of virus neutralizing antibodies."

Researchers from France's Université de Picardie (Mullié *et al.* 2004) gave 30 infants aged zero to four months poliovirus vaccinations along with a formula with *B. longum* and *B. infantis* or a placebo. In the probiotic group, antipoliovirus IgA responses significantly increased among the probiotic group versus the placebo group that received the vaccinations without probiotics. Antibody titers correlated with bifidobacteria levels,

132

especially with *B. longum/B. infantis* and *B. breve* supplementation doses. The researchers were puzzled by the mechanism, adding, "Whether this effect on the immune system is achieved through the bifidogenic effect of the formula (mainly through *B. longum/B. infantis* and *B. breve* stimulation) or directly linked to compounds (i.e. peptides) produced by milk fermentation remains to be investigated."

Scientists from Finland's University of Turku (Fang *et al.* 2000) gave *Lactobacillus* GG, *Lactococcus lactis* or placebo to 30 healthy volunteers for 7 days. On the first, third and fifth days, a *Salmonella typhi* Ty21 oral vaccine was given to each volunteer to mimic enteropathogenic infection. A greater increase in specific IgA was observed among the *Lactobacillus* GG group. Among the *L. lactis* group, significantly higher CR3 receptor expression on neutrophils was observed compared to the placebo or *Lactobacillus* GG groups. The researchers concluded that: "the immuno-modulatory effect of probiotics is strain-dependent."

Scientists from Finland's University of Tampere (Isolauri *et al.* 1995) studied the administration of *Lactobacillus* GG with oral rotavirus vaccines given to 2-5-month-old infants. Infants receiving the probiotic displayed an increased level of rotavirus-specific IgM secreting cells. The researchers concluded that, "these findings suggest that LGG has an immunostimulating effect on oral rotavirus vaccination."

Rebuilding the immune system with probiotics will return to the system the most vital part of preventing opportunistic infections: acquired immunity.

Illustrating this, Japanese scientists (Hirose *et al.* 2006) gave *Lactobacillus plantarum* strain L-137 or placebo to 60 healthy men and women, average age 56, for twelve weeks. Increased Con A-induced proliferation (acquired immunity), increases in IL-4 production by CD4+ T-cells, and a more balanced Th1:Th2 ratio was seen in the probiotic group. Quality of life criteria were also higher among the probiotic group.

Researchers from Britain's Scarborough Hospital (McNaught *et al.* 2005) gave a placebo or *Lactobacillus plantarum* 299v to 103 critically ill patients along with conventional therapy. On day 15, the probiotic group had significantly lower serum IL-6 levels compared to the control group.

Researchers from the Department of Immunology at Japan's Juntendo University School of Medicine (Takeda *et al.* 2006) gave a placebo or *Lactobacillus casei* Shirota to 9 healthy middle-aged adults and 10 elderly adults daily for three weeks. After three weeks of supplementation, *L. casei* significantly increased natural killer cell activity among the volunteers, especially among those who had low NK-cell activity before probiotic supplementation.

Researchers from the University of Vienna (Meyer *et al.* 2007) gave healthy women yogurt with starters *Lactobacillus bulgaricus* and *Streptococcus thermophilus*, with or without *Lactobacillus casei*. After two weeks, both yogurt groups had significantly increased blood levels of tumor necrosis factor-alpha (TNF-a): by 24% with the regular yogurt and by 63% with the *L. casei* yogurt. They also observed significantly higher levels of cytokines interleukin (IL)-1beta (by 40%) and interferon gamma (by 108%). In addition, IL-10 decreased during *L. casei*-enhanced yogurt treatment, but then significantly increased after the yogurt treatment was stopped (by 129%).

French scientists (Paineau *et al.* 2008) gave 83 healthy volunteers a placebo or seven probiotic strains, and tested their resulting antibody levels and immune response rates. IgG levels increased in the *Bifidobacterium lactis* Bl-04 and *Lactobacillus acidophilus* La-14 groups; and serum immunoglobulin levels increased significantly from six of the seven probiotic strains.

Researchers from the Department of Neurology and Geriatrics at Japan's Kagoshima University Graduate School of Medical and Dental Sciences (Matsuzaki *et al.* 2005) studied *Lactobacillus casei* Shirota as a treatment of HTLV-1 associated myelopathy/tropical spastic paraparesis. Ten HTLV-1 patients with myelopathy/tropical spastic paraparesis were given either a placebo or *Lactobacillus casei* Shirota fermented in milk for four weeks. NK-cell activity significantly increased. Spasticity—gauged by a modified Ashworth Scale—significantly decreased. Other urinary components indicating enhanced immunity were also seen following the probiotic treatment.

Researchers from Finland's University of Turku (Ouwehand *et al.* 2008) gave a placebo, *Bifidobacterium longum*, or *Bifidobacterium lactis* Bb-12 to 55 institutionalized elderly subjects for 6 months. The probiotic groups had modulated pro-inflammatory cytokine TNF-alpha and cytokine IL-10 levels compared with the placebo group.

Scientists from Spain's University of Navarra (Parra *et al.* 2004) investigated the effects of fermented milk with *Lactobacillus casei* DN114001 on 45 healthy volunteers, ages 51-58. The probiotic group showed increased oxidative burst capacity among monocytes, and increased NK-cell tumor suppression activity. The researchers concluded that *L. casei* can have "a positive effect in modulating the innate immune defense in healthy-middle-age people."

Probiotics and Early Immunity

Prematurity and Immunosuppression

When a baby is born premature, they are also likely to have a very low birth weight. Very low birth weights are considered one of the leading causes of death among premature infants. The problem is that with a low birth weight, the infant struggles to maintain metabolic and enzymatic activity. The key to stimulating weight among a low birth weight infant is thus proper digestion and assimilation of nutrients. The problem often with a premature infant is that they have yet to develop the mechanisms for the production of digestive aids such as bile, enzymes and gastrin that properly break down foods. This is where probiotics come into play. Probiotics help the body break down nutrients, and help stimulate the production of enzymes. Probiotics also help stimulate healthy mucosal membranes and intestinal barriers. Let's review some research that supports this:

Japanese scientists from the Osaka Medical Center (Kitajima *et al.* 1997) gave *Bifidobacterium breve* or placebo to 91 very low birthweight infants for eight weeks and followed up for three years. At two weeks of age, colonization rates of the administered bacteria were 73% versus 12% among the control group. The probiotic group showed significantly fewer abnormal abdominal signs and better weight gain than the control group.

Scientists from China's Medical University (Lin *et al.* 2005) gave 367 infants with very low birth weights either *Lactobacillus acidophilus* and *Bifidobacterium infantis* with their breast milk or breast milk alone. Those given the probiotics were five times less likely to contract necrotizing enterocolitis—a frequent disorder among very low birth weights—than did the control group. Furthermore, the probiotic group had no severe cases of necrotizing enterocolitis while the control group suffered six severe cases.

Another study—this time a multicenter study of 435 infants—from some of the same researchers (Lin *et al.* 2008) showed that death and necrotizing enterocolitis among low birth weight newborns significantly decreased for newborns who were supplemented with probiotics.

Researchers from Israel's Shaare Zedek Medical Center and the Faculty of Medicine from Hebrew University (Bin-Nun *et al.* 2005) gave a combination of *Bifidobacteria infantis*, *Streptococcus thermophilus* and *Bifidobacteria Bifidus* or a placebo to 145 low birth-weight infants. Necrotizing enterocolitis was significantly lower in the probiotic group than in the placebo group (4% versus 16%). Fewer severe cases also occurred in the probiotic infants. Three of the 15 babies who developed necrotizing enterocolitis died—with all the deaths sadly occurring among the placebo infants.

135

Researchers from the Neonatal Intensive Care Unit at Italy's Azienda Ospedaliera Regina Anna Hospital (Manzoni *et al.* 2006) studied 180 neonates with very low birth weight. They gave either a placebo or oral *Lactobacillus rhamnosus* beginning on the first three days of life through the earlier of six weeks or until discharge. The infants' health was tracked over a 12-month period. Incidence of *Candida* infections among the infants was significantly lower in the probiotic group (23.1% vs. 48.8%).

Researchers from India's Kolkata Medical College (Samanta *et al.* 2009) showed that death and necrotizing enterocolitis among low birth weight newborns significantly decreased for those newborns given probiotics.

Scientists from the University of Tartu's Department of Pediatrics in Estonia (Vendt *et al.* 2006) investigated *Lactobacillus rhamnosus* GG supplementation among normal healthy infants. One hundred and twenty healthy infants under two months old were given a probiotic-supplemented formula or a non-probiotic formula until the age of six months. Weight, length and head circumference were measured monthly. Combined, these measurements were all greater among the probiotic infants. In other words, infants given *Lactobacillus rhamnosus* GG with their feeding formula grew significantly faster than those not given probiotics!

Colic

Colic is the incessant crying of a baby, often resulting in radical oxygen reduction and further complications. Modern medicine does not understand colic very well. There are a number of theories as to its cause. Many believe that microbial infections are the main cause. Others feel that it has more to do with nutrition or perhaps their environment. Studies with probiotics give us another perspective on this mystery.

Researchers at Johns Hopkins University School of Medicine (Saavedra *et al.* 2004) gave a *Bifidobacterium lactis* and *Streptococcus thermophilus* combination or a placebo to 118 infants (average age 2.9 months) for 210 days. The probiotic group had a significantly lower frequency of colic and irritability, and a lower need (frequency) for antibiotics than did the placebo group.

Italian researchers from the University of Bari Policlinico (Indrio *et al.* 2008) gave 30 preterm newborns either a placebo or *Lactobacillus reuteri* ATCC 55730 for 30 days. Newborns fed with probiotics had a significant reduction in regurgitation and mean daily crying time. Probiotic newborns also had more stools compared with the placebo group. Gastric emptying rates significantly increased, and fasting antral area (inverse marker for digestive health) was significantly reduced among the newborns given *L. reuteri* and the breast-fed newborns, versus the placebo groups.

Researchers from Italy's Regina Margherita Children's Hospital (Savino *et al.* 2007) gave either simethicone (colic medication) or *Lactobacillus reuteri* to 90 children with infantile colic. After 28 days, 39 patients (95%) responded positively among the probiotic group, while only three patients (7%) responded positively among the simethicone group. Colicky symptoms among breastfed infants in the L. reuteri group improved within 1 week of treatment.

Probiotics and Infections

Intestinal infections leading to acute diarrhea are often caused by an overgrowth of certain bacteria or fungi within the intestines. This has been the most researched clinical use of probiotics, particularly among children, where diarrhea can easily cause death. Here is a sampling of the hundreds of clinical research on probiotics and intestinal infections:

Researchers from the Department of Pediatrics at Italy's University of Naples Federico II (Canani *et al.* 2007) investigated five different probiotics for the treatment of acute diarrhea among children. 571 children diagnosed with acute diarrhea received either 1) a placebo; 2) *Lactobacillus rhamnosus* strain GG; *Saccharomyces boulardii;* 3) *Bacillus clausii;* 4) *Enterococcus faecium* SF68; 5) or a combination of *L delbrueckii* var *bulgaricus, Streptococcus thermophilus, Lactobacillus acidophilus,* and *Bifidobacterium bifidum.* The average illness duration was significantly less for the probiotic group who took the combination of four strains (at 70 hours) and *L. rhamnosus* (at 78.5 hours), as compared with the placebo group (at 115.0 hours). The other probiotics given were not significantly better than the placebo.

Scientists from the University College of Medical Sciences and GTB Hospital in India (Agarwal and Bhasin 2002) studied 150 children with acute diarrhea. The children were given fermented milk with 1) a combination of *Lactobacillus casei* DN-114001, *Lactobacillus bulgaricus* and *Streptococcus thermophilus;* 2) Indian dahl supplemented with *Lactococcus lactis, Lactococcus lactis cremoris* and *Leuconostac mesenteroide;* 3) or a heat-treated yogurt with no live bacteria. Both live probiotic groups showed a significant reduction of illness compared to the heat-treated yogurt. The greatest reduction occurred with the *Lactobacillus casei* fermented milk.

Researchers from the Faculty of Medicine at London's Imperial College (Hickson *et al.* 2007) studied 135 elderly patients infected with *Clostridium difficile.* They were given a placebo or a combination of *Lactobacillus casei, Lactobacillus bulgaricus,* and *Streptococcus thermophilus* while taking antibiotics and then for one additional week after the antibiotic treatment was completed. Twelve percent of the probiotic group developed diarrhea (related to antibiotics) compared to 34% among the placebo group.

Italian scientists (Guarino *et al.* 1997) gave 100 children with rotavirus and non-rotavirus diarrhea a placebo or the probiotic *Lactobacillus rhamnosus* GG (also referred to as *Lactobacillus* GG). The duration of diarrhea was reduced from 6 to 3 days in all children (both rotavirus and non-rotavirus) receiving *Lactobacillus* GG.

Swedish researchers gave 26 adult volunteers with clostridia intestinal infections either a placebo or *Lactobacillus plantarum* DSM 9843. After 3 weeks, the probiotic group had significantly less sulfite-reducing clostridia (Johansson *et al.* 1998).

Scientists from the Liverpool School of Tropical Medicine (Raza *et al.* 1995) gave probiotics or placebo to 40 children hospitalized with acute diarrhea in Pakistan. Averaging 13 months of age, the children were given either *Lactobacillus* GG or the placebo for 2 days. The number of children with persistent watery diarrhea at 48 hours was 31% in the probiotic group versus 75% in the placebo group.

Researchers from the Universidad de Buenos Aires' Medical School (Gaón *et al.* 2003) tested 89 children aged 6-24 months with persistent diarrhea. They received a placebo, a combination of *Lactobacillus casei* and *Lactobacillus acidophilus,* or *Saccharomyces boulardii* for five days. Both probiotic treatments were effective in significantly improving those children compared to the placebo.

Scientists from Argentina's Universidad de Buenos Aires (Gaon *et al.* 2002) also studied 22 patients with chronic diarrhea. They were given either *Lactobacillus casei* and *Lactobacillus acidophilus* or placebo for three periods of seven days with untreated periods in between. The probiotic combination significantly reduced the diarrhea compared to the placebo group. In addition, probiotic effects were significantly reduced during the untreated periods, leading the researchers to suggest that continual use provides better efficacy.

Researchers from the Cathay General Hospital's Department of Pediatrics (Lee *et al.* 2001) studied one hundred hospitalized children with acute diarrhea. They were given either *Lactobacillus acidophilus* and *Bifidobacterium infantis* or a placebo for four days. The diarrhea frequency among the probiotic group improved on the first and second day of hospitalization significantly more than the placebo group.

In a multicenter study from France's Centre Hospitalier Universitaire de Grenoble (Chouraqui *et al.* 2004), *Bifidobacterium lactis* or placebo was given in formula to 90 healthy children for 8 months living in residential nurseries or foster care centers. The probiotic group had a 28.3% incidence of diarrhea compared to 38.7% among the placebo group. As for episode duration, the probiotic group had an average of 1.15 days of diarrhea compared to 2.3 days in the control group.

Scientists from Italy's University of degli Studi Pediatric Department (Michielutti *et al.* 1996) studied 63 children under 4 years old infected with intestinal bacteria. They were divided into three groups. One group was given *Lactobacillus acidophilus*. The other was given a placebo. The third group was given both antibiotic therapy and *L. acidophilus*. The first (probiotic-only) group showed significant clinical improvement over the second group. The third group illustrated that the probiotic therapy mitigated the adverse effects of dysbiosis following antibiotic treatment.

Finnish scientists from the University of Tampere (Kaila *et al.* 1995) tested the difference of effects between live and heat inactivated *Lactobacillus* GG on the immune system in patients with rotavirus infections. Their results in a rotavirus serum IgA enzyme immunoassay showed that antibody responses were significantly greater among infants treated with live *Lactobacillus* GG. While 10 of 12 infants receiving the live probiotics showed rotavirus-specific IgA secreting cells, only 2 of 13 infants receiving inactivated (dead) *Lactobacillus* GG showed the IgA secreting cells.

This is not to say that even dead probiotics do not lessen intestinal infections. Seventy-three children with diarrhea—50% of whom had rotavirus—were given either heat-killed *L. acidophilus* LB or a placebo. In 24 hours after treatment, the probiotic group had significantly less diarrhea. At the end of the study, the probiotics group had diarrhea for an average of 43 hours and the placebo group had diarrhea for an average of 57 hours (Simakachorn *et al.* 2000).

Scientists from Ramathibodi Hospital in Bangkok (Phuapradit *et al.* 1999) gave 175 children aged from 6 to 36 months old a placebo, *Bifidobacterium* Bb12 alone, or *Bifidobacterium* Bb12 combined with *Streptococcus thermophilus* in formula. During the 8-month study period, the non-probiotic group had a 4-fold increase in the IgA antibody titer for rotavirus, while both the *Bifidobacterium* Bb12 alone group and the group treated with Bb12 combined with *Streptococcus thermophilus* had no significant changes in their IgA antibody titer throughout the study period. This led the researchers to conclude that, "children receiving bifidobacteria-supplemented milk-based formula may be protected against symptomatic rotavirus infection."

Researchers from the Johns Hopkins University School of Medicine (Saavedra *et al.* 1994) gave *Bifidobacterium bifidum* and *Streptococcus thermophilus* or placebo to infants aged from 5 to 24 months old in a double-blind, placebo-controlled study. In all, 55 infants were assessed for 4,447 patient-days over a 17-month period. During the test period, 31% of the placebo infants developed diarrhea versus 7% of the probiotic group. In addition, 39% of the placebo group shed rotavirus during the study period versus 10% of the probiotic group.

Lactobacillus acidophilus and *Bifidobacterium infantis* probiotics were given to 1,237 newborns placed in intensive care at the Childrens University Hospital Lorencita Villegas in Bogotá, Colombia over one year (Hoyos 1999). The results were compared to (controls) 1,282 newborns not given probiotics while being hospitalized during the previous year. In the previous year, the controls experienced 85 cases of necrotizing enterocolitis, compared to 34 cases among the probiotic newborns. Furthermore, there were 35 NEC-associated deaths among the 1,282 newborns the previous year and only 14 fatalities among the 1,237 newborns given probiotics.

In research from two Finnish hospitals (Shornikova *et al.* 1997), 66 children between six months and three years of age with rotavirus infections and watery diarrhea were given a placebo or two dosages of *Lactobacillus reuteri* for up to 5 days. By the second day, watery diarrhea continued among 80% of the placebo group. In comparison, watery diarrhea continued among only 48% of the large dosage *L. reuteri* group.

Researchers at Spain's Hospital Materno-Infantil Vall d'Hebron (Tormo *et al.* 2006) treated 35 infants with gastrointestinal problems with either standard milk (placebo) or milk fermented milk *Lactobacillus casei* and *Streptococcus thermophilus*. The probiotic milk group was given the probiotic for six weeks and the placebo for six weeks. The placebo group drank the standard milk for twelve weeks. After the testing period, those receiving the probiotics showed a significant reduction of gastrointestinal gram-negative bacteria and an increase in secretory IgA levels (from 2.5 mg/dl to 3.4 mg/dl). Stool exams also confirmed the survival of *L. casei* through the gastrointestinal tract.

In a German (Mohan *et al.* 2006) study, 69 preterm infants were given placebo or *Bifidobacterium lactis* Bb12. The probiotic supplementation reduced cell counts of enterobacteria and clostridia while increasing counts of bifidobacteria.

Scientists from the Huddinge University Hospital in Sweden (Sullivan *et al.* 2003) compared the antibiotic clindamycin with probiotic yogurt containing *Bifidobacterium lactis* and *Lactobacillus* F19 on twenty-four people. One week of clindamycin treatment was compared to 14 days of probiotic treatment. Bacteria levels of *Bacteroides fragilis, Escherichia coli* and other gram-positive microorganisms were significantly lower in both treatment groups, but healthy probiotic levels were significantly higher among the probiotic group following the treatments.

Researchers from New Zealand's University of Otago (Dierksen *et al.* 2007) gave 219 children *Streptococcus salivarius*-supplemented milk for either

2 days or 9 days. At the beginning of the treatment, a significant number of the children had higher levels of infective *Streptococcus pyrogenes* (which can lead to strep throat and necrotizing fasciitis) populations on the tongue. Following probiotic supplementation, increased levels of salivaricin (produced by *Streptococcus salivarius*) was found among the probiotic group. This antibiotic substance produced by *Streptococcus salivarius* significantly inhibits *Streptococcus pyogenes*.

Scientists from Turkey's Celal Bayar University (Akil *et al.* 2006) gave *Saccharomyces boulardii* to 24 children aged 3-16 years old. *E. coli* colonies per gram in the children's feces declined from 384,625 to 6,283 following probiotic treatment.

The Gastroenterology Unit of the UK's Scarborough General Hospital (Jain *et al.* 2004) studied 90 patients admitted into its intensive care unit for sepsis (internal bacterial infection). Half were given a placebo and half were given a probiotic blend of *Lactobacillus acidophilus* La5, *Bifidobacterium lactis* Bb 12, *Streptococcus thermophilus* and *Lactobacillus bulgaricus* plus prebiotic oligofructose. After one week of treatment, nasogastric aspirate testing showed that the probiotic group had significantly lower incidence of pathogenic bacteria compared to the placebo group (43% versus 75%). The probiotic group also had fewer infections of pathogenic microorganisms (39% versus 75%).

Scientists from the Department of Nutrition at Spain's Universidad Completeness de Madrid (Jimenez *et al.* 2008) studied 20 women with staphylococcal mastitis in a randomized placebo-controlled study. The probiotic group was given *Lactobacillus salivarius* CECT5713 and *Lactobacillus gasseri* CECT5714 (both originally isolated from breast milk) for 4 weeks, and the control group was given a placebo. After 30 days, staphylococcal counts within the probiotic group were significantly lower than the control group (2.96 log(10) CFU/ml versus 4.79 log(10) CFU/ml). Furthermore, *L. salivarius* and *L. gasseri* were also isolated from the breast milk of 6 of the 10 women in the probiotic group. After 14 days of treatment, there were no clinical signs of mastitis observed within the probiotic group. Mastitis persisted among the placebo group.

Eighty burn patients from an Argentina hospital burn unit (Peral *et al.* 2009) had infected second- and third-degree burns, along with non-infected third-degree burns. They were given topical applications of probiotic *Lactobacillus plantarum* or silver sulphadiazine (SD-Ag). (SD-Ag is a typical antimicrobial paste used to prevent infection in burns, along with adverse side effects.) Among both infected and non-infected burns, *L. plantarum* prevented wound infection, and promoted wound granulation healing equal to or better than SD-Ag, without the side effects.

Researchers from the University of Paris (Schiffrin *et al.* 1997) gave 28 volunteers either *Lactobacillus acidophilus* or *Bifidobacterium bifidum* strain Bb12. Phagocytosis (killing) of *Escherichia coli* was enhanced in both probiotic groups.

Ukrainian scientists (Marushko 2000) examined 77 children with streptococcal tonsillitis. They found that the infections were symptomized by a reduction in "tonsil colony resistance." The study also found that *L. acidophilus* provided a "highly efficient means of treating tonsillitis of streptococcal etiology."

Candida Infections

Candida albicans is a normal inhabitant of the intestinal tract and several other locations throughout the body. Complications arise when *Candida* populations have been allowed to grow beyond their normal levels. Lower probiotic populations allow these fungi to easily grow beyond their healthy levels, infecting the intestines, vagina and many other parts of the body. The consumption of probiotics can help return *Candida* back to its normal population levels, as probiotics manage and control their colonies by secreting chemicals that limit their growth.

Researchers from Long Island Jewish Medical Center's Division of Infectious Diseases (Hilton, *et al.* 1992) studied thirty-three patients with vulvovaginal candida infections. Infection rates decreased by a third among patients consuming an eight-ounce yogurt (orally) with *Lactobacillus acidophilus* for six months. The infection rate was 2.54 per six months in the control group versus 0.38 in the yogurt group, while *Candida* spp. colonization rates were 3.23 in the control group versus only 0.84 in the yogurt group—through the six-month testing period.

Probiotics and Viral Infections

Scientists (Baron 2009) gave *Bacillus coagulans* GBI-30, 6086 to 10 healthy middle-aged men and women in a capsule for 30 days. After the treatment period, they had significantly increased T-cell production of TNF-alpha in response to adenovirus and influenza A (H3N2) exposure.

German scientists (de Vrese *et al.* 2005) gave a placebo or *Lactobacillus gasseri*, *Bifidobacterium longum* and *B. bifidum* to 479 healthy adult volunteers for three months. Total symptom score, duration of cold illness, and fever duration were significantly lower among the probiotic group—shortening common cold episodes by about 2 days—with a score of 79.3 versus 102.5 points. The probiotic group had significantly higher levels of cytotoxic T suppressor cells (CD8+) and higher activity among T helper cells (CD4+), along with reduced severity of symptoms.

Finnish medical researchers from the University of Turku (Rautava *et al.* 2009) conducted a clinical study to see if probiotics could reduce infection risk during infancy. Infants younger than two months of age were given formula supplemented with *Lactobacillus rhamnosus* GG and *Bifidobacterium lactis* Bb-12 or a placebo daily until they were 12 months of age. Incidence of infections was 22% among the probiotic infants and 50% among the placebo group. In addition, 28% of those receiving probiotics contracted recurrent respiratory infections, compared to 55% of the placebo group.

In research that began in the late 1950s, Dr. Don Weekes clinically administered a combination of *L. acidophilus* and *L. bulgaricus* to 180 patients with ulcers and/or herpes infections. After average treatment times of three days with four-times daily doses, 61 of 64 patients with herpes simplex labialis, 77 of 97 patients with mouth ulcers (aphthous stomatitis), 6 of 13 patients with dendrites ulcers, and 6 of 6 patients with genital herpes were either "cured" or "much improved" from the probiotic treatments (Trenev 1998; Weekes 1983; Weekes 1958).

Bulgarian researchers have also confirmed herpes simplex inhibition from species of lactobacilli (Dimitonova *et al.* 2007).

One hundred children from a slum of New Delhi between two and five years old were given either a probiotic curd with *Lactobacillus acidophilus* or a placebo for six months. The probiotic group had more growth, and had fewer incidences of colds, flu, diarrhea and fever than the placebo group (Saran *et al.* 2002).

Scientists from Finland's University of Tampere (Isolauri *et al.* 1995) studied the administration of *Lactobacillus casei* GG with oral rotavirus vaccines given to 2-5-month-old infants. Infants receiving the probiotic displayed an increased level of rotavirus-specific IgM secreting cells. The researchers concluded that, "these findings suggest that LGG has an immunostimulating effect on oral rotavirus vaccination."

Scientists from Taiwan's Buddhist Tzu Chi General Hospital (Lin *et al.* 2009) gave 1,062 children under the age of five a placebo or *L. rhamnosus*. The children given the probiotic had significantly lower rates of bacterial, viral and respiratory infections, along with increased T-cell activity.

Swedish researchers (Tubelius *et al.* 2005) gave 262 healthy employees at Sweden's TetraPak company either *L. reuteri* or placebo for 80 days. During the study, the placebo group's sick leave reporting was 26.4% compared to 10.6% among the *L. reuteri* group. The sick-day frequency was 0.9% among the placebo group and 0.4% among the *L. reuteri* group. Among 53 shift-workers, 33% in the placebo group reported being sick during the study period as compared to none in the *L. reuteri* group.

Lactobacillus casei DN-114001 was given to 360 elderly people for 3 weeks by Italian researchers (Turchet *et al.* 2003). The probiotic group suffered a 20% shorter duration of winter illnesses compared to the placebo group.

Scientists from Italy's University of Milan (Pregliasco *et al.* 2008) gave placebo or several combinations of *Lactobacillus plantarum, Lactobacillus rhamnosus,* and *Bifidobacterium lactis* together with prebiotics to healthy volunteers over three winter seasons (2003-2007). Acute respiratory infection episodes and upper respiratory tract infections were significantly lower among the probiotic groups. Severity of all illness episodes decreased significantly among probiotic groups, ranging from .73 days less to 1.12 days less in average duration compared to the placebo groups. The duration of upper respiratory infections ranged from 1.51 days less to 2.07 days less than the placebo groups. The probiotic groups also had an average of 1.25 to 1.4 days less flu illnesses than the placebo groups. There was also significantly less cold illnesses among the probiotics groups compared to the placebo groups.

Probiotics and Respiratory Infections

There is sufficient evidence that pathogenic bacteria such as *Staphylococcus aureus, Streptococcus pneumoniae* and *Heomonphilus influenzae* can infect the lungs. Little research seems to have been done to confirm whether or not the lungs also harbor probiotic bacteria, however. Research has confirmed that probiotic bacteria inhabit the nasal cavity, the mouth and the throat. Research has also confirmed that both ingested probiotics and probiotic sprays reduce lung infections. Probiotics in the lungs does not seem so radical: Certainly not as radical as the evidence showing probiotics from the intestinal tract can somehow inhibit bacteria in the lungs and nasal cavity.

In a study also mentioned earlier, scientists from the Swiss National Accident Insurance Institute (Glück and Gebbers 2003) gave 209 human volunteers either a conventional yogurt or a combination of *Lactobacillus* GG (ATCC 53103), *Bifidobacterium* sp. B420, *Lactobacillus acidophilus* 145, and *Streptococcus thermophilus* every day for 3 weeks. Nasal microbial flora was measured at the beginning, at day 21 and at day 28 (a week after). Significant pathogenic bacteria were found in most of the volunteers' nasal cavities at the beginning of the study. The consumption of the probiotic-enhanced milk led to a 19% reduction of pathogenic bacteria in the nasal cavity. The researchers concluded that, "The results indicate a [possible] linkage of the lymphoid tissue between the gut and the upper respiratory tract."

Scientists from Barcelona (Cobo Sanz *et al.* 2006) gave 251 children aged 3 to 12 years milk either with or without *Lactobacillus casei* for 20 weeks. The probiotic group of children experienced significantly less low respiratory tract infections, bronchitis and/or pneumonia (32% vs. 49%). The probiotic children also had a reduction in the duration of fatigue (3% vs. 13%). There was also a difference in the duration of sicknesses among the probiotic children compared to the placebo group.

French scientists (Forestier *et al.* 2008) assessed whether ventilator-associated pneumonia in intensive care units could be prevented or lessened by the use of probiotics. The 17-bed intensive care unit at the Clermont-Ferrand Teaching Hospital was used to test 208 patients with an intensive care unit stay of more than 48 hours. Patients were fed a placebo or *Lactobacillus rhamnosus* through a nasogastric feeding twice daily from their third day in the unit until discharge. Infective *Pseudomonas aeruginosa* cultures were measured at admission, once a week, and upon discharge. Bacteriological tests of the respiratory tract also were done to determine patient infections. The study results indicated that *P. aeruginosa* respiratory colonization and/or infection was significantly reduced among the probiotic group. Ventilator-associated pneumonia by *P. aeruginosa* in the probiotic group was reduced by more than 50% compared to the placebo group.

Researchers from the University of Arkansas' Medical School (Wheeler *et al.* 1997) studied 15 asthmatic adults in two 1-month crossover periods with placebo or yogurt containing *L. acidophilus*. The probiotic consumption increased immune system interferon gamma and decreased eosinophilia levels.

Greek scientists from the Faculty of Medicine of the University of Thessaloniki (Kotzampassi *et al.* 2006) gave a placebo or probiotic combination to 65 elderly critically ill, mechanically ventilated, multiple trauma patients for 15 days. The combination consisted of *Pediococcus pentosaceus* 5-33:3, *Leuconostoc mesenteroides* 32-77:1, *L. paracasei* subsp. *paracasei* 19; and *L. plantarum* 2,362; and inulin, oat bran, pectin and resistant starch as prebiotics. The probiotic patients had significantly lower levels of infection, sepsis and death than did the placebo group. Number of days in the ICU and number of days under ventilation were significantly reduced compared to the placebo group. The researchers concluded that: "The administration of this synbiotic formula in critically ill, mechanically ventilated, multiple trauma patients seems to exert beneficial effects in respect to infection and sepsis rates and to improve the patient's response, thus reducing the duration of ventilatory support and intensive care treatment."

Scientists from the University of Buenos Aires (Río *et al.* 2002) studied the incidence and severity of respiratory tract infections by giving 58 normal or undernourished children from 6 to 24 months old either a placebo or a combination of live *Lactobacillus acidophilus* and *Lactobacillus casei* probiotics. Their respiratory episodes were classified as pneumonia, bronchitis, recurrent obstructive bronchitis or upper respiratory tract infections. Total episodes in the probiotic group were 34; and 69 episodes occurred among the placebo group. The probiotic combination significantly suppressed pneumonia and bronchitis in both the normal and undernourished probiotic groups.

Probiotics and Cardiovascular Diseases

Atherosclerosis and Cholesterol

One of the most important indicators of heart or cardiovascular disease is atherosclerosis—the hardening and thickening of the arteries. Atherosclerosis occurs as artery walls are damaged from oxidized low-density lipoproteins, initiating an inflammatory response. Lipoproteins transport cholesterol and triglycerides through the bloodstream as either very-low density (VLDL), low-density (LDL), intermediate-density or high-density lipoproteins (HDL).

Cholesterol comes from our diet and from liver synthesis—which is sent with bile into the intestines. Here it is absorbed into the blood through the intestinal wall and transported via lipoproteins. Higher VLDL-c and LDL-c levels tend to oxidize more quickly, so these tend to cause more artery inflammation. HDL-cholesterol, on the other hand, does not oxidize as easily.

Probiotics will bind to and prevent LDL-cholesterol from being released back into the bloodstream. This effect reduces levels of cholesterol, and more importantly, levels of LDL-cholesterol in the blood. By reducing LDL-c and increasing HDL-c, less oxidation will take place and less artery damage will result.

Scientists from Denmark's The Royal Veterinary and Agricultural University (Agerholm-Larsen *et al.* 2000) gave 70 overweight and obese adult volunteers 1) placebo pills; 2) a placebo yogurt; 3) a yogurt with two strains of *Streptococcus thermophilus* and two strains of *Lactobacillus acidophilus*; 4) a yogurt with two strains of *Streptococcus thermophilus* and one strain of *Lactobacillus rhamnosus*; or 5) a yogurt with one strain of *Enterococcus faecium* and two strains of *Streptococcus thermophilus*. After eight weeks, LDL-cholesterol decreased by 8.4% (0.26) while fibrinogen increased (0.74) in the *Enterococcus faecium-Streptococcus thermophilus* group (#4). Groups #3 and #4 showed significant decreases in blood pressure as well.

Twenty healthy men were given either milk fermented with *Lactobacillus casei* or a placebo for eight weeks in a double-blind, placebo-controlled study from Japan (Kawase *et al.* 2000). Blood samples were taken before, after 4 weeks and after 8 weeks. After 4 and 8 weeks, the high-density lipoprotein cholesterol levels (HDL-c) were significantly higher for the probiotic group while the placebo group showed no change. The probiotic group also had lower triglycerides levels after 4 weeks while the placebo group showed no change.

Scientists from the University of Kentucky (Anderson and Gilliland 1999) conducted two studies: One a single-blind study, and the other a double-blind, placebo-controlled, crossover study. Volunteers completed three and four week trials with either placebo or two different strains of *L. acidophilus*. The combined analysis of both probiotic studies showed a 2.9% reduction in serum cholesterol. The authors commented that this converts to a potential 6 to 10% lowering of coronary heart disease.

Researchers from the Tehran University of Medical Sciences (Ataie-Jafari *et al.* 2009) gave 14 healthy subjects with serum total cholesterol levels of 200 to 300 mg/dL 300 grams of ordinary yogurt or yogurt fermented with *Lactobacillus acidophilus* and *Bifidobacterium lactis*. After the six-week period, the probiotic yogurt group showed a significant decrease in total cholesterol levels compared to the ordinary yogurt group.

Forty-three volunteers were given either a placebo or *Enterococcus faecium* M-74 plus 50 micrograms of organically bound selenium in a double-blind, placebo-controlled study (Hlivak *et al.* 2005). After 56 weeks, total cholesterol among the probiotic group reduced from 229 to 201 mg/dL. LDL cholesterol fell from 149 to 119 mg/dL. No significant changes were seen in the placebo group. The researchers concluded that *E. faecium* reduced serum cholesterol by 12% during the test period.

Researchers from Germany's Friedrich Schiller University (Kiessling *et al.* 2002) first gave 300 grams of control yogurt (with starter culture of *Streptococcus thermophilus* and *Lactobacillus lactis*) per day to 29 women for seven weeks. Then they had 18 women eat the same amount of yogurt enhanced with *Lactobacillus acidophilus* 145 and *Bifidobacterium longum* 913 per day while the others ate the control yogurt for the next seven weeks. During the third seven weeks, the two groups from the second period were reversed. After testing with all groups, the probiotic-enhanced groups had an average of 11.6 mg/dL increase in HDL cholesterol. Levels of LDL and total cholesterol were unchanged.

Scientists from The Netherlands' Nutrition and Food Research Institute in Zeist (Schaafsma *et al.* 1998) gave 32 healthy men either a placebo milk or milk fermented with yogurt starter, *Lactobacillus acidophilus* and fructooligosaccharides. After two treatment periods of three weeks separated by a week off, the probiotic group had 4.4% less total cholesterol and 5.4% lower LDL-cholesterol.

Japanese researchers (Xiao *et al.* 2003) gave yogurt with a combination of *Streptococcus thermophilus* and *Lactobacillus delbrueckii* subsp. bulgaricus

(SL), or the same combination with *Bifidobacterium longum* strain BL1 to 32 human subjects with total cholesterol from 220 to 280 mg/dL. After four weeks, the total cholesterol reduced by half in the *B. longum* group, while the cholesterol levels among the normal yogurt group remained nearly unchanged.

In research from Germany's Friedrich Schiller University (Klein *et al.* 2008), 26 healthy volunteers took a yogurt supplement with probiotic strains *L. acidophilus* 74-2 and *B. lactis* 420 or a placebo for five weeks. After the five weeks, they were tested and crossed over. Final test results revealed that the probiotic group's triglyceride levels decreased by 11.6%. Immune system granulocytes and monocytes with phagocytic activity significantly increased in the probiotic group as well.

High Blood Pressure

We might wonder how bacteria can lower blood pressure. Blood pressure is increased through an enzyme called ACE (angiotensin-converting enzyme). The ACE pathway, however, can be inhibited by two different tripeptides: isoleucyl-prolyl-proline (IPP) and valyl-prolyl-proline (VPP). These two tripeptides have been found in sour milks fermented with probiotic bacteria. Additional research (Narva *et al.* 2004) has indicated that probiotic-fermented dairy stimulate higher calcium levels than unfermented dairy. Higher serum calcium has also been associated with reduced blood pressure—and lower levels of osteoporosis.

Researchers from the University of Helsinki (Jauhiaimen *et al.* 2005) gave *Lactobacillus helveticus* LBK-16H fermented milk or placebo to 94 high blood pressure patients not receiving medications. After 10 weeks and a 4-week open period, the probiotic group had an average 4.1 mm Hg lower systolic and 1.8 mm Hg lower diastolic blood pressure.

Japanese scientists (Aihara *et al.* 2005) gave either *Lactobacillus helveticus* or a placebo to 40 high blood pressure patients for 4 weeks. During the treatment period, the probiotic group's blood pressure trended slightly higher than the placebo group, but at the end of the four weeks, the probiotic group had 5.0 mm Hg less diastolic blood pressure than the placebo group. No other changes, including pulse rate, was observed.

In the *L. casei* study mentioned earlier (Kawase *et al.* 2000), after 4 and 8 weeks, systolic blood pressure lowered significantly among the probiotic group, while there was no change in the placebo group.

This effect was also seen in the Agerholm-Larsen study mentioned earlier. *Enterococcus faecium* and *Streptococcus thermophilus* produced significant decreases in blood pressure in addition to their cholesterol-lowering effects.

Scientists from the Poland's Pomeranian Academy of Medicine (Naruszewicz *et al.* 2002) gave *Lactobacillus plantarum* 299v or placebo to 36 healthy smoker volunteers for six weeks, in a study we discussed earlier. The probiotic group had significant decreases in systolic blood pressure, leptin levels, and fibrinogen levels. No changes were observed among the placebo group.

Researchers from Finland's National Public Health Institute (Tuomilehto *et al.* 2004) gave 60 hypertensive volunteers not taking medication a placebo or *Lactobacillus helveticus* in fermented milk. During the first study period, the probiotic group had a 2 mmHg more reduction in systolic BP than the placebo group. During the second period, the crossover group experienced an average of 2.6 mmHg lower systolic blood pressure and 1.0 mmHg lower diastolic blood pressure.

Scientists from Tokyo's Kyorin University School of Medicine gave *Lactobacillus helveticus* and *Saccharomyces cerevisiae* fermented milk or placebo to 30 elderly high blood pressure patients—many taking antihypertensive medications. After 8 weeks, the probiotic group's systolic blood pressure decreased 14.1 mmHg. The probiotic group's diastolic blood pressure also decreased, by 6.9 mmHg. The placebo group, on the other hand, had no reduction in blood pressure.

Probiotics and Liver Disorders

The liver is one of the body's most important organs. It produces hundreds of thousands of enzymes, helps clear and detoxify the blood, and converts various nutrients into useable molecules. In liver disease such as cirrhosis, the cells of the liver become deranged or diseased. This decreases their effectiveness. Should enough of these hepatocytes become damaged, the liver can shut down. The American Liver Foundation estimates that more than 42,000 Americans die from liver disease every year. One in ten of us have some form of liver disease.

Probiotics interact significantly with the liver. Not only do probiotics help digest food: They also protect the liver and signal to the immune system when a threat to the liver exists. It is no coincidence that alcohol—which is tremendously damaging to the liver—also damages our body's probiotics.

Researchers from Russia's Northern State Medical University (Kirpich *et al.* 2008) studied 66 adult Russian males admitted to a psychiatric hospital with a diagnosis of alcoholic psychosis. They gave the patients standard therapy (abstinence plus vitamins) with *Bifidobacterium bifidum* and *Lactobacillus plantarum* 8PA3 or standard therapy alone without probiotics for five days. Stool cultures and liver enzymes were examined and compared with 24 healthy, matched non-drinker controls. The alcoholic patients had significantly fewer bifidobacteria, lactobacilli, and enterococci than did the healthy non-drinkers. The average starting levels of liver enzymes alanine aminotransferase (ALT), aspartate aminotransferase (AST), and gamma-glutamyl transpeptidase (GGT) were significantly greater in the alcoholic group compared to the healthy non-drinkers.

After 5 days of daily probiotics, alcoholic patients had significantly more bifidobacteria and lactobacilli populations compared to the control group. The probiotic group also had significantly lower AST and ALT levels at the end of treatment than the standard therapy control group. Of the 26 patients with mild alcoholic hepatitis, probiotic therapy significantly reduced liver enzymes ALT, AST, GGT, lactate dehydrogenase and total bilirubin. The researchers concluded that, "Short-term oral supplementation with *B. bifidum* and *L. plantarum* 8PA3 was associated with restoration of the bowel flora and greater improvement in alcohol-induced liver injury than standard therapy alone."

Scientists from Italy's University of Catania (Malaguarnera *et al.* 2007) gave 60 cirrhotic patients *Bifidobacterium longum* plus fructooligosaccharides (FOS) or placebo. After 90 days, fasting NH(4) serum levels significantly decreased among the probiotic patients. Other liver tests, including MMSE, Trail Making Test-A and Test-B also significantly improved among the probiotic group as compared with the placebo group.

Researchers from the Liver Failure Group and The Institute of Hepatology at the University College London's Medical School (Stadlbauer *et al.* 2008) studied neutrophil function and cytokine responses in alcoholic cirrhosis patients in an open-label study. Twenty patients with alcoholic cirrhosis were treated with a placebo or *Lactobacillus casei* Shirota for 4 weeks. The data were also compared to 13 healthy control subjects who did not receive probiotics. The cirrhosis patients' starting neutrophil phagocytic capacity was significantly lower than healthy controls (73% versus 98%) before probiotic treatment. Neutrophil phagocytic capacities after the probiotic treatments were equal among the cirrhosis patients and healthy volunteers at the end of the study—while the placebo group's neutrophil capacity did not change. In addition, endotoxin-stimulated TNF-receptor-1, TNFR-2 and interleukin IL10 levels were significantly lower among the probiotic group. The researchers concluded that, "Our data provide a proof-of-concept that probiotics restore neutrophil phagocytic capacity in cirrhosis, possibly by changing IL10 secretion and TLR4 expression."

China's Capital University of Medical Sciences and the Beijing Friendship Hospital (Zhao *et al.* 2004) studied fifty patients with liver cirrhosis. They tested and graded the entire group for intestinal probiotic content and severity of liver disease. The researchers found that the cirrhosis was directly associated with intestinal probiotic content. The more severe the cirrhosis, the more imbalanced the intestinal probiotic content was. The patients were randomized and given *Bifidobacterium, Lactobacillus acidophilus* and *Enterococcus faecium;* or *Bacillus subtilis* and *Enterococcus faecium* for 14 days. Fecal flora, pH and ammonia content, and plasma endotoxin levels were tested before and after. All levels improved after both probiotic treatments. In addition, those given *B. subtilis* and *E. faecium* showed a reduction in endotoxin levels among endotoxemia cirrhosis cases.

Researchers from the Department of Surgery at Japan's Nagoya University Graduate School of Medicine (Kanazawa *et al.* 2005) investigated the effects of *L. casei* with 54 patients following hepatectomy. Infection complications were 19% in the probiotic group and 52% in the placebo group.

Forty cirrhosis patients with hepatic encephalopathy were studied by researchers from the University of Naples (Loguercio, *et al.* 1987). They were given either *Enterococcus* probiotic strain SF68 or lactulose (standard treatment) for 10 days. The probiotics were as effective as lactulose in lowering blood ammonia and improving mental state. The beneficial effects of the probiotics persisted significantly longer after treatment was discontinued, however. In addition, reports of diarrhea and abdominal pain with lactulose treatment did not occur with probiotic treatment.

Gum Disease and Cavities

The gums and teeth are coated with legions of different bacteria—some probiotic and some pathogenic. Typical oral bacteria include *Streptococcus mutans, Streptococcus salivarius, Lactobacillus salivarius, E. coli, Streptococcus pyogenes, Porphyromonas gingivalis, Tannerella forsynthensis* and *Prevotella intermedia*. With a diet containing too many simple sugars and poor dental hygiene, the pathogenic bacteria can overwhelm the probiotics, causing infected gums and teeth. As pathogenic populations of *S. mutans, S. pyogenes, P. gingivalis, T. forsynthensis* and *P. intermedia* come into greater numbers, serious infections can occur. These conditions are often symptomized by gingivitis, teeth root infection, jawbone infections and general periodontal disease.

Streptococcus mutans was first isolated in 1924, but it was not linked to dental caries until the early 1960s. *S. mutans* and other cavity-forming bacteria consume sugars and carbohydrates from our foods, and produce destructive acids. These acids interact with the calcium in our tooth enamel, forming plaque. It is this interaction and plaque-formation that create cavities. There is now reason to believe that, like probiotics, *S. mutans* can be passed on from mother to infant.

This leads us to wonder whether *Streptococcus mutans* might actually be a eubiotic: a probiotic at controlled colony sizes. Like some other eubiotic yeasts and bacteria, perhaps it is a natural resident of the mouth that simply has grown beyond its healthy populations because of our eating and lifestyle imbalances.

All of the bacteria mentioned above and others can reside in both healthy and infected mouths. The strategy promoted by the modern medical and dental industries is to try to kill virtually all bacteria with various antiseptic mouthwashes and toothpastes. As we can see from continuing statistics on gingivitis and dental caries, these strategies are not working very well. A better strategy may be to use nature's probiotic populations to create a balance between the healthy bacteria and the disease-promoting bacteria. If probiotic populations are maximized, they will deplete and manage the pathogenic bacteria populations.

Let's see how this is supported by the research:

Researchers from the Istanbul's Yeditepe University Dental School (Caglar *et al.* 2008) gave oral lozenges of *Lactobacillus reuteri* or placebo to 20 healthy young women. After sucking on one lozenge a day for 10 days, salivary *Streptococcus mutans* levels were significantly reduced among the probiotic group, compared to the placebo group and before treatment.

Scientists from Yeditepe University (Caglar *et al.* 2007) gave placebo or *Lactobacillus reuteri* probiotic chewing gums to 80 healthy young adults for three weeks. The *L. reuteri* gums significantly reduced levels of salivary *Streptococcus mutans* compared to placebo and before treatment.

Scientists from Italy's University of L'Aquila, Department of Experimental Medicine (Riccia *et al.* 2007) gave 8 healthy volunteers and 21 chronic periodontitis patients *Lactobacillus brevis* lozenges. The probiotic treatment led to the total disappearance of all clinical symptoms among all patients. They also had a significant decrease in inflammatory markers nitrite/nitrate, PGE2, matrix metalloproteinase, and saliva IFN-gamma levels.

In another dental school study, *Lactobacillus reuteri* ATCC 55730 or placebo was given to 120 young adults through straw or lozenge daily for 3 weeks. *Streptococcus mutans* were significantly reduced in both probiotic groups as compared to the placebo group and before treatment (Caglar *et al.* 2006).

Researchers at Japan's Tohoku University Graduate School of Dentistry (Shimauchi *et al.* 2008) treated 66 human volunteers with freeze-dried *Lactobacillus salivarius* WB21 lozenge tablets or a placebo for 8 weeks. Periodontal testing confirmed that the probiotic group had significantly greater improvements in plaque index and probing pocket depth compared to the placebo group and before treatment.

Researchers from Turkey's Yeditepe University dental school (Caglar *et al.* 2008) gave 24 healthy young adult volunteers ice-cream containing *Bifidobacterium lactis* Bb-12 or a placebo ice cream for 40 days. Salivary *Streptococcus mutans* counts were significantly reduced in the probiotic ice cream group compared to the placebo group and before treatment.

Scientists from the University of Copenhagen (Twetman *et al.* 2009) gave three groups either chewing gum with placebo or two strains of *Lactobacillus reuteri* for 10 minutes a day for two weeks. Their gums were examined and given immunoassays for gingivitis inflammation. Bleeding on probing was significantly less among the probiotic subjects. TNF-alpha and IL-8 significantly decreased among the probiotic group. IL-1beta also decreased during the chewing period. The researchers concluded that, "The reduction of pro-inflammatory cytokines in GCF may be proof of principle for the probiotic approach combating inflammation in the oral cavity."

Researchers from the Institute of Dentistry at the University of Helsinki (Näse *et al.* 2001) investigated the effect of *Lactobacillus rhamnosus* GG on dental caries. Milk with or without *Lactobacillus rhamnosus* GG was given to 594 children ages 1 to 6 years old. The probiotic group had significantly less dental caries and significantly lower mutans streptococcus counts by the end of the study—especially among the 3- to 4-year-olds.

Scientists from the Universidad Nacional Autónoma de Mexico (Bayona *et al.* 1990) gave 245 seven-year-old children chewable tablets of either pyridoxine (vitamin B6) with heat-killed probiotics (streptococci and lactobacilli) or tablets with pyridoxine once a week for 16 weeks. Four evaluations were made over a two-year period from the beginning of the study. There was a 42% reduction of dental caries among the probiotic group compared to the placebo group.

Scientists from Sweden's Malmö University (Krasse *et al.* 2006) gave *Lactobacillus reuteri* or placebo to 59 patients with moderate to severe gingivitis. After 2 weeks of treatment, the gingival index and plaque index were established from measurements of two teeth surfaces and from saliva. The average gingival index and plaque index was significantly lower in the *L. reuteri* probiotic groups. The researchers concluded that, "*Lactobacillus reuteri* was efficacious in reducing both gingivitis and plaque in patients with moderate to severe gingivitis."

Finnish researchers from the University of Helsinki (Ahola *et al.* 2002) found that the long-term consumption of milk containing *Lactobacillus rhamnosus* GG significantly reduced dental caries. They found this same effect from probiotic cheese ingestion. To illustrate this later effect, the researchers gave 74 young adults a placebo or 60 grams of probiotic cheese per day for three weeks. There were significantly lower salivary *Streptococcus mutans* counts among the probiotic cheese group.

Italian scientists (Petti *et al.* 2001) gave healthy volunteers either yogurt with *Streptococcus thermophilus* and *Lactobacillus bulgaricus* or non-probiotic ice cream for 8 weeks. The probiotic group had lower levels of salivary *Streptococcus mutans* than the control group. However, *L. bulgaricus* was only transiently detected in the oral cavity, indicating that it did not colonize well within the mouth [in contrast with observations of other species such as *L. reuteri*].

Probiotics for Intestinal Disorders

Chronic digestive problems, which include bloating, indigestion, and cramping are often symptoms of IBS, Crohn's disease or colitis. These diseases (IBS, etc.) are also typically accompanied by chronic pain and intestinal inflammation, however. Occasional indigestion, bloating and cramping is often associated with a developing case of dysbiosis caused by antibiotic use, poor diet, or an overgrowth of specific pathogenic microorganisms. Enzyme deficiency can be caused by probiotic deficiencies. Probiotics produce a number of enzymes, including protease and lypase—necessary for the break down of proteins and fats. Poor digestion is often the result of a lack of these and other enzymes. Gastrointestinal difficulties in general are often caused by dysbiosis. This can include an overgrowth of yeasts, pathogenic bacteria or both. Here are a few of the many studies showing that digestion can improve with probiotic use:

IBS is one of those diseases that physicians like to qualify as an autoimmune disease. As we've discussed earlier, the concept that the body's immune system is attacking itself for no reason is not logical. There are reasons the immune system might target cells from within the body. These can range from the cells being damaged by environmental toxins, endotoxins, oxidative (free) radicals, viruses, to the immune system itself being damaged. How do probiotics intermix within these possibilities?

The research illustrates that probiotics directly attack foreign invaders like bacteria, viruses and fungi, often before they can damage the cells of the intestinal walls. Probiotics can also bind to oxidative radicals formed by many types of toxins. Probiotics will also line the intestinal cells, creating a barrier for toxins to enter the blood. They secrete lactic acid and other biochemicals that prevent endotoxic microorganisms from flourishing. Probiotics will also signal the immune system with the identities of pathogens, and then assist in their eradication.

Deficiencies of probiotics in the intestines usually result in overgrowths of pathogenic microorganisms like *Clostridia* spp., *E. coli, H. pylori* and *Candida* spp. These damage the cells of the intestinal wall and produce endotoxins that poison intestinal cells. In addition, a lack of probiotics means that food will not be properly broken down, as probiotics help break down many large food molecules into bioavailable nutrients. This means the intestinal cells will become under-nourished too.

Toxins from our foods will also more easily reach the intestinal wall cells without the protective agency that probiotics provide. For this reason, the intestinal cells have more exposure to various toxic chemicals from our foods and environment, including pesticides, herbicides and preservatives. These can damage intestinal cells to the point where they do not function normally. They can also mutate through adaptation to toxin exposure. Toxin exposure and subsequent genetic alteration can cause the immune system to launch an inflammatory attack on intestinal cells, in an effort to rid them from the body. This can result in the inflammation and pain associated with Crohn's and IBS.

Here is some research supporting these conclusions:

Researchers from the Medical University of Warsaw (Gawrońska *et al.* 2007) investigated 104 children who had functional dyspepsia, irritable bowel syndrome, or functional abdominal pain. They gave the children either placebo or *Lactobacillus rhamnosus* GG. for 4 weeks. The probiotic group had overall treatment success (25% versus 9.6%) compared to the placebo group. The IBS probiotic group had even more treatment success compared to the placebo IBS group (33% versus 5%). The probiotic group also had significantly reduced pain frequency.

French researchers (Drouault-Holowacz *et al.* 2008) gave probiotics or a placebo to 100 patients with irritable bowel syndrome. Between the first and fourth weeks of treatment, the probiotic group had significantly less abdominal pain (42% versus 24%) than the placebo group.

Researchers from Poland's Curie Regional Hospital (Niedzielin *et al.* 2001) gave *Lactobacillus plantarum* 299V or placebo to 40 IBS patients. IBS symptoms significantly improved for 95% of the probiotic patients versus just 15% of the placebo group.

Forty IBS patients took *Lactobacillus acidophilus* SDC 2012, 2013 or a placebo for four weeks in research at the Samsung Medical Center and Korea's Sungkyunkwan University School of Medicine (Sinn *et al.* 2008). The probiotic group had a 23% reduction in pain and discomfort while the placebo group showed no improvement.

Scientists from Italy's University of Parma (Fanigliulo *et al.* 2006) gave *Bifidobacterium longum* W11 or rifaximin (an IBS medication) to 70 IBS patients for two months. The probiotic patients reported a fewer symptoms and greater improvement than the rifaxmin patients. The researchers commented: "The abnormalities observed in the colonic flora of IBS suggest, in fact, that a probiotic approach will ultimately be justified."

Researchers from the University of Helsinki (Kajander *et al.* 2008) treated 86 patients with IBS with either a placebo or a combination of *Lactobacillus rhamnosus* GG, *L. rhamnosus* Lc705, *Propionibacterium freudenreichii* subsp. *Shermanii* JS and *Bifidobacterium animalis* subsp. *lactis.* After 5 months, the probiotic group had a significant reduction of IBS symptoms, especially with respect to distension and abdominal pain. The researchers concluded that, "this multispecies probiotic seems to be an effective and safe option to alleviate symptoms of irritable bowel syndrome, and to stabilize the intestinal microbiota."

Scientists from the Canadian Research and Development Centre for Probiotics and The Lawson Health Research Institute in Ontario (Lorea Baroja *et al.* 2007) studied 20 IBS patients, 15 Crohn's patients, 5 ulcerative colitis patients, and 20 healthy volunteers. All subjects were given a yogurt supplemented with *Lactobacillus rhamnosus* GR-1 and *L. reuteri* RC-14 for 30 days. IBS inflammatory markers were tested in the bloodstream. CD4(+) CD25(+) T-cells increased significantly among the probiotic IBS group. Tumor necrosis factor (TNF)-alpha(+)/interleukin (IL)-12(+) monocytes decreased for all the groups except the IBS probiotic group. Myeloid DC decreased among most probiotic groups, but was also stimulated in IBS patients. Serum IL-12, IL-2(+) and CD69(+) T-cells also decreased in probiotic IBS patients. The researchers also concluded that, "Probiotic yogurt intake was associated with significant anti-inflammatory effects..."

Researchers from the General Hospital of Celle (Plein and Hotz 1993) gave *Saccharomyces boulardii* or placebo to 20 Crohn's disease patients with diarrhea flare-ups. After ten weeks, the probiotic group had a significant reduction in bowel movement frequency compared with the control group. The control group's bowel movement frequency rose in the tenth week and subsided to initial frequency levels—consistent with flare-ups.

In another study from Finland (Kajander *et al.* 2005), a placebo or combination of *Lactobacillus rhamnosus* GG, *L. rhamnosus* LC705, *Bifidobacterium breve* Bb99 and *Propionibacterium freudenreichii* subsp. *shermanii* JS was given to of 103 patients with IBS. The total symptom score (abdominal pain + distension + flatulence + borborygmi) was 7.7 points lower among the probiotic group. This represented a 42% reduction in the symptoms of the probiotic group compared with a 6% reduction of symptoms among the placebo group.

In a study from Yonsei University College of Medicine in Korea (Kim *et al.* 2006), 40 irritable bowel syndrome patients were given either a placebo or a combination of *Bacillus subtilis* and *Streptococcus faecium* for four weeks. The severity and frequency of abdominal pain decreased significantly in the probiotic group.

Researchers from Sweden's Lund University Hospital (Nobaek *et al.* 2000) gave 60 patients with irritable bowel syndrome either a placebo or daily rose-hip drink with *Lactobacillus plantarum* for four weeks. Enterococci levels increased among the placebo group were unchanged in the test group. Flatulence was significantly reduced among the probiotic group compared with the placebo group. At a 12-month follow-up, the probiotic group maintained significantly better overall GI symptoms and function than the placebo group.

New York scientists (Hun 2009) gave 44 IBS patients either a placebo or *Bacillus coagulans* GBI-30 for 8 weeks. The probiotic group experienced significant improvements in abdominal pain and bloating symptoms versus the placebo group.

Scientists at Ireland's University College in Cork (O'Mahony *et al.* 2005) studied 77 irritable bowel syndrome patients with abnormal IL-10/IL-12 ratios—indicating a proinflammatory, Th1 status. The patients were given a placebo, *Lactobacillus salivarius* UCC4331 or *Bifidobacterium infantis* 35624 for eight weeks. IBS symptoms were logged daily and assessed weekly. Tests included quality of life, stool microbiology, and blood samples to test peripheral blood mononuclear cell release of inflammatory cytokines interleukin (IL)-10 and IL-12. Patients who took *B. infantis* 35624 had a significantly greater reduction in abdominal pain and discomfort, bloating and distention, and bowel movement difficulty, compared to the other groups. IL-10/IL-12 ratios—indicative of Th1 proinflammatory metabolism—were also normalized in the probiotic *B. infantis* group.

Researchers from the Umberto Hospital in Venice in Italy (Saggioro 2004) studied probiotics on seventy adults with irritable bowel syndrome. They were given 1) a placebo; 2) a combination of *Lactobacillus plantarum* and *Bifidobacterium breve*; or 3) a combination of *Lactobacillus plantarum* and *Lactobacillus acidophilus* for four weeks. After 28 days of treatment, pain scores measuring different abdominal regions decreased among the probiotic groups by 45% and 49% respectively, versus 29% for the placebo group. The IBS symptom severity scores decreased among the probiotic groups after 28 days by 56% and 55.6% respectively, versus 14% among the placebo group.

Sixty-eight patients with irritable bowel syndrome were treated at the TMC Hospital in Shizuoka, Japan (Tsuchiya *et al.* 2004) with either placebo or a combination of *Lactobacillus acidophilus*, *Lactobacillus helveticus* and *Bifidobacteria* for twelve weeks. The probiotic treatment was either "effective" or "very effective" in more than 80% of the IBS patients. In addition, less than 5% of the probiotic group reported the treatment as "not effective," while more than 40% of the placebo patients reported their placebo treatment as "not effective." The probiotic group also reported significant improvement of bowel habits.

Researchers from Britain's University of Manchester School of Medicine (Whorwell *et al.* 2007) gave a placebo or *Bifidobacterium infantis* 35624 to 362 primary care women with irritable bowel syndrome in a large-scale, multicenter study. After four weeks of treatment, *B. infantis* was significantly more effective than the placebo in reducing bloating, bowel dysfunction, incomplete evacuation, straining, and the passing of gas.

Scientists from Denmark's Hvidovre Hospital and the University Hospital of Copenhagen (Wildt *et al.* 2006) gave 29 colitis-IBS patients either *Lactobacillus acidophilus* LA-5 and *Bifidobacterium animalis* subsp. *lactis* BB-12, or a placebo for twelve weeks. The probiotic treatment group had a decrease in bowel frequency from 32 per week to 23 per week. Furthermore, the probiotic group had an average reduction in the frequency of liquid stools from 6 days per week to 1 day per week.

Scientists at Poland's Jagiellonian University Medical College (Zwolińska-Wcisło *et al.* 2006) tested 293 ulcer patients, 60 patients with ulcerative colitis, 12 patients with irritable bowel syndrome and 72 patients with other gastrointestinal issues. Compared to placebo, *Lactobacillus acidophilus* supplementation resulted in a lessening of symptoms, a reduction of fungal colonization, and increased levels of immune system cytokines TNF-alpha and IL-1 beta.

Medical researchers from Finland's University of Helsinki (Kajander *et al.* 2007) sought to understand the mechanism of probiotics' proven ability to reduce IBS symptoms. They gave either a placebo or a combination of *Lactobacillus rhamnosus* GG, *Lactobacillus rhamnosus* Lc705, *Propionibacterium freudenreichii* subsp. *shermanii* JS and *Bifidobacterium breve* Bb99 to 55 irritable bowel syndrome patients. After six months of treatment, feces and intestinal microorganism content illustrated a significant drop in glucuronidase levels in the probiotic group compared to the placebo group. The researchers concluded that there was a complexity of different factors, and so far unknown mechanisms explaining "the alleviation of irritable bowel syndrome symptoms by the multispecies probiotic."

French researchers (Guyonnet *et al.* 2009) gave *Bifidobacterium lactis* DN-173010 with yogurt strains to 371 adults reporting digestive discomfort for 2 weeks. 82.5% of the probiotic group reported improved digestive symptoms compared to 2.9% of the control group.

Another group of French scientists (Diop *et al.* 2008) gave 64 volunteers with high levels of stress and incidental gastrointestinal symptoms either a placebo or *Lactobacillus acidophilus* Rosell-52 and *Bifidobacterium longum* for three weeks. At the end of the three weeks, the stress-related gastrointestinal symptoms of abdominal pain, nausea and vomiting decreased by 49% among the probiotic group.

Probiotics and Allergies

Allergies have been increasing over the past few decades. Modern medical research is puzzled with this progression. Why are suddenly more people becoming allergic to the plants and pollens that have surrounded humans for thousands of years? This is a huge topic, but we do know from the research that the lack of healthy probiotic colonies is at least a contributing factor.

Probiotics mechanisms have been increasingly connected to inflammatory and allergic responses. They play a critical role in maintaining the epithelial barrier function of the intestinal tract. Allergies appear to increase with intestinal permeability. Without an adequate intestinal barrier, larger food molecules, endotoxins and microorganisms can enter the bloodstream more easily. These increase the body's total toxin burden, making it more sensitive to environmental inputs such as pollen.

Research from Sweden's Linköping University (Böttcher *et al.* 2008) gave *Lactobacillus reuteri* or a placebo to 99 pregnant women from gestational week 36 until infant delivery. The babies were followed for two years after birth, and analyzed for eczema and allergen sensitization and immunity markers. Probiotic supplementation lowered TGF-beta2 levels in mother's milk and babies' feces and slightly increased IL-10 levels in mothers' colostrum. Lower levels of TGF-beta2 are associated with lower sensitization and lower risk of IgE-associated eczema.

German researchers (Grönlund *et al.* 2007) tested 61 infants and mother pairs for allergic status and bifidobacteria levels from 30-35 weeks of gestation and from one-month old. Every mother's breast milk contained some type of bifidobacteria, with *Bifidobacterium longum* found most frequently. However, only the infants of allergic, atopic mothers had colonization with *B. adolescentis*. Allergic mothers also had significantly less bifidobacteria in their breast-milk versus non-allergic mothers. Infants of allergic mothers also had less bifidobacteria in the feces than did infants from non-allergic mothers.

Japanese scientists (Xiao *et al.* 2006) gave 44 patients with Japanese cedar pollen allergies *Bifidobacterium longum* BB536 for 13 weeks. The probiotic group had significantly decreased symptoms of rhinorrhea (runny nose) and nasal blockage versus the placebo group. The probiotic group also had decreased activity among plasma T-helper type 2 (Th2) cells and increased activity among Japanese cedar pollen-specific IgE. The researchers concluded that the results, "suggest the efficacy of BB536 in relieving JCPsis symptoms, probably through the modulation of Th2-skewed immune response."

Researchers from the Wellington School of Medicine and Health Sciences at New Zealand's University of Otago (Wickens *et al.* 2008) studied the association between probiotics and eczema in 474 children. Pregnant women took either a placebo, *Lactobacillus rhamnosus* HN001, or *Bifidobacterium animalis* subsp *lactis* strain HN019 starting from 35 weeks gestation, and their babies received the same treatment from birth to 2 years old. The probiotic infants given *L. rhamnosus* had significantly lower incidence of eczema compared with infants taking the placebo. There was no significant difference between the *B. animalis* group and the placebo group, however.

Researchers from Japan's Kansai Medical University Kouri Hospital (Hattori *et al.* 2003) gave 15 children with atopic dermatitis either *Bifidobacterium breve* M-16V or a placebo. After one month, the probiotic group had a significant improvement of allergic symptoms.

Japanese scientists (Ishida *et al.* 2003) gave a drink with *Lactobacillus acidophilus* strain L-92 or a placebo to 49 patients with perennial allergic rhinitis for eight weeks. The probiotic group showed significant improvement in runny nose and watery eyes symptoms, along with decreased nasal mucosa swelling and redness compared to the placebo group. These results were also duplicated in a follow-up study (2005) of 23 allergy sufferers by some of the same researchers.

Researchers from Tokyo's Juntendo University School of Medicine (Fujii *et al.* 2006) gave 19 preterm infants placebo or *Bifidobacterium breve* supplementation for three weeks after birth. Anti-inflammatory serum TGF-beta1 levels in the probiotic group were elevated on day 14 and remained elevated through day 28. Messenger RNA expression was enhanced for the probiotic group on day 28 compared with the placebo group. The researchers concluded that, "These results demonstrated that the administration of *B. breve* to preterm infants can up-regulate TGF-beta1 signaling and may possibly be beneficial in attenuating inflammatory and allergic reactions in these infants."

Scientists from Britain's Institute of Food Research (Ivory *et al.* 2008) gave *Lactobacillus casei* Shirota (LcS) to 10 patients with seasonal allergic rhinitis. The researchers compared immune status with daily ingestion of a milk drink with or without live *Lactobacillus casei* over a period of 5 months. Blood samples were tested for plasma IgE and grass pollen-specific IgG by an enzyme immunoassay. Patients treated with *Lactobacillus casei* milk showed significantly reduced levels of antigen-induced IL-5, IL-6 and IFN-gamma production compared with the placebo group. Levels of specific IgG also increased and IgE decreased in the probiotic group. The researchers concluded that, "These data show that probiotic supplementation modulates immune responses in allergic rhinitis and may have the potential to alleviate the severity of symptoms."

Researchers from the Skin and Allergy Hospital at the University of Helsinki (Kukkonen *et al.* 2007) studied the role of probiotics and allergies with 1,223 pregnant women carrying children with a high-risk of allergies. A placebo or lactobacilli and bifidobacteria combination with GOS was given to the pregnant women for 2 to 4 weeks before delivery, and their babies continued the treatment after birth. At two years of age, the infants in the probiotic group had 25% less chance of eczema and 34% less chance of contracting atopic eczema.

The same researchers from the Skin and Allergy Hospital and Helsinki University Central Hospital (Kukkonen *et al.* 2009) studied the immune effects of feeding probiotics to pregnant mothers. 925 pregnant mothers were given a placebo or a combination of *Lactobacillus rhamnosus* GG and LC705, *Bifidobacterium breve* Bb99, and *Propionibacterium freudenreichii* ssp. *shermanii* for four weeks prior to delivery. Their infants were given the same formula together with prebiotics, or a placebo for 6 months after birth. During the infants' six-month treatment period, antibiotics were prescribed less often among the probiotic group by 23%. In addition, respiratory infections occurred less frequently among the probiotic group through the two-year follow-up period (even after treatment had stopped) compared to the placebo group (an average of 3.7 infections versus 4.2 infections).

Finnish scientists (Kirjavainen *et al.* 2002) gave 21 infants with early onset atopic eczema a placebo or *Bifidobacterium lactis* Bb-12. Serum IgE concentration correlated directly to *Escherichia coli* and bacteroides counts, indicating the association between these bacteria with atopic sensitization. The probiotic group had a decrease in the numbers of *Escherichia coli* and bacteroides.

Sonicated *Streptococcus thermophilus* cream was applied to the forearms of 11 patients with atopic dermatitis for two weeks. This led to a significant increase of skin ceramide levels, and a significant improvement of their clinical signs and symptoms—including erythema, scaling and pruritus (Di Marzio *et al.* 2003).

Japanese researchers (Odamaki *et al.* 2007) gave yogurt with *Bifidobacterium longum* BB536 or plain yogurt to 40 patients with Japanese cedar pollinosis for 14 weeks. *Bacteroides fragilis* significantly changed with pollen dispersion. The ratio of *B. fragilis* to bifidobacteria also increased significantly during pollen season among the placebo group but not in the *B. longum* group. Peripheral blood mononuclear cells from the patients indicated that *B. fragilis* microorganisms induced significantly more Th2 cell cytokines such as interleukin-6, and fewer Th1 cell cytokines such as IL-12 and interferon. The researchers concluded that, "These results suggest a relationship between fluctuation in intestinal microbiota and pollinosis allergy. Furthermore, intake of BB536 yogurt appears to exert positive influences on the formation of anti-allergic microbiota."

Scientists from the Department of Oral Microbiology at Japan's Asahi University School of Dentistry (Ogawa *et al.* 2006) studied skin allergic symptoms and blood chemistry of healthy human volunteers during the cedar pollen season in Japan. After supplementation with *Lactobacillus casei*, activity of cedar pollen-specific IgE, thymus, chemokines, eosinophils, and interferon-gamma levels all decreased among the probiotic group.

Researchers from the School of Medicine and Health Sciences in Wellington, New Zealand (Sistek *et al.* 2006) determined in a study of *Lactobacillus rhamnosus* and *Bifidobacteria lactis* on 59 children with established atopic dermatitis that food-sensitized children responded significantly better to probiotics than did other atopic dermatitis children.

French scientists (Passeron *et al.* 2006) found that atopic dermatitis children improved significantly after three months of *Lactobacillus rhamnosus* treatment, based on SCORAD levels of 39.1 before and 20.7 afterward.

Scientists from Finland's National Public Health Institute (Piirainen *et al.* 2008) gave a placebo or *Lactobacillus rhamnosus* GG to 38 patients with atopic eczema for 5.5 months—starting 2.5 months before birch pollen season. Saliva and serum samples taken before and after indicated that allergen-specific IgA levels increased significantly among the probiotic group versus the placebo group (using the enzyme-linked immunosorbent assay (ELISA)). Allergen-specific IgE levels correlated positively with stimulated IgA and IgG in saliva, while they correlated negatively in the placebo group. The researchers concluded that the research showed that *L. rhamnosus* GG displayed "immunostimulating effects on oral mucosa seen as increased allergen specific IgA levels in saliva."

Children with cow's milk allergy and IgE-associated dermatitis were given a placebo or *Lactobacillus rhamnosus* GG and a combination of four other probiotic bacteria (Pohjavuori *et al.* 2004). The IFN-gamma by PBMCs at the beginning of supplementation was significantly lower among cow's milk allergy infants. However, cow's milk allergy infants receiving *L. rhamnosus* GG had significantly increased levels of IFN-gamma, showing increased tolerance.

The British medical publication *Lancet* published a study (Kalliomäki *et al.* 2003) where 107 children with a high risk of atopic eczema were given either a placebo or *Lactobacillus rhamnosus* GG during their first two years of life. Fourteen of 53 children receiving the probiotic developed atopic eczema, while 25 of 54 of the children receiving the placebo contracted atopic eczema by the end of the study.

In a study from the University of Western Australia School of Pediatrics (Taylor *et al.* 2006), 178 children born of mothers with allergies were given either *Lactobacillus acidophilus* or a placebo for the first six months of life. Those given the probiotics showed reduced levels of IL-5 and TGF-beta in response to polyclonal stimulation (typical for allergic responses), and significantly lower IL-10 responses to vaccines as compared with the placebo group. These results illustrated that the probiotics had increased allergen resistance among the probiotic group of children.

Researchers from the Department of Otolaryngology and Sensory Organ Surgery at Osaka University School of Medicine in Japan (Tamura *et al.* 2007) studied allergic response in chronic rhinitis patients. For eight weeks, patients were given either a placebo or *Lactobacillus casei* strain Shirota. Those with moderate-to-severe nasal symptom scores at the beginning of the study given probiotics experienced significantly reduced nasal symptoms compared to the placebo group and before treatment.

Probiotics and Pancreatitis

A variety of studies has shown that the pancreas can be damaged by either pathogenic bacteria endotoxins that leak in from the intestines or pathogenic bacteria themselves (called pancreatic sepsis). Because the pancreas is critical to the production of insulin and other key biochemicals that assist in energy metabolism, an infected pancreas can mean the shut down or slow down of energy production, strength and vitality.

Medical researchers from Hungary's Petz Aladár Teaching Hospital (Oláh *et al.* 2003; Kecskés *et al.* 2003) gave *Lactobacillus plantarum* 299 or placebo to 45 patients with acute pancreatitis who had arrived at the hospital within 48 hours after the onset of symptoms. Twenty-two of the pancreatitis patients received treatment with live *L. plantarum,* and 23 received heat-killed *L. plantarum* 299. Infected pancreatic necrosis and abscesses were found in only 1 of the 22 patients in the live probiotic group, versus 7 of the 23 among the inactivated probiotic group. The mean hospital stay was 13.7 days in the live probiotic group versus 21.4

days among the inactivated probiotic group. The researchers concluded that, "Supplementing *Lactobacillus plantarum* 299 is an effective tool to prevent pancreatic sepsis, to reduce the number of operations and length of stay. The only patient who developed sepsis in the treatment group did so eight days after the treatment had been discontinued."

In terms of the mechanisms of pancreatitis mechanisms, the researchers also confirmed that, "Colonization of the lower gastrointestinal tract and oropharynx, mostly with gram-negative but sometimes also gram-positive bacteria is known to precede the contamination of the pancreatic tissue by a few days."

Probiotics and Kidney Disorders

Kidney stones and kidney disease is rampant within the western world because of a combination of poor diet, high levels of chemical toxins in our foods and water, and dysbiosis. Our kidneys must push out many toxins and this puts a strain on the glomeruli within the kidneys. Especially tough on the kidneys is increased levels of uric acid, which is often caused by high dietary protein content. Yes, the western world eats too much protein. While our bodies only require 30-50 grams of a mixture of essential amino acids per day, the western diet often contains 75-150 grams of protein per day. This overabundance of protein in the form of amino acids and polypeptides produces excess uric acid, which can build up in cells throughout the body. Gout, for example, is the build up of uric acid crystals within the joints.

Excess uric acid can overload the kidneys. Combined with fatty acids and minerals, several different types of kidney stones can form as a result of uric acid overload. This combined with an overload of chemical toxins from our foods and water, and endotoxins from an overgrowth of pathogenic bacteria, can be dangerous to the kidneys.

Probiotics can be helpful for excess uric acid and kidney problems because they help reduce levels of endotoxins produced by pathogenic bacteria. These endotoxins increase the acidity of the blood, and thus increase the rate of uric acid crystals (oxalate) formation. Endotoxins also produce an additional toxic load the kidneys must filter and deal with.

Researchers from the S. Orsola University Hospital's Department of Nephrology in Bologna, Italy (Campieri *et al.* 2001) gave a combination of *L. acidophilus*, *L. plantarum*, *L. brevis*, *S. thermophilus*, and *B. infantis* to six patients with idiopathic calcium-oxalate urolithiasis and mild hyperoxaluria (oxalate kidney stones) for four weeks. They were tested for urine oxalate levels before and during treatment. Probiotic treatment resulted in a significant reduction in urine oxalate (from SD levels of 55.5 to 28.3 in thirty days) and a significant reduction in fecal oxalate excretion.

Researchers from the Mayo Clinic (Lieske *et al.* 2005) gave 10 patients with chronic fat malabsorption, calcium oxalate kidney stones, and hyperoxaluria *Lactobacillus* probiotics or placebo for three months. Patients treated with probiotics had a 20% drop in urinary oxalate excretion after the three months. The study authors also noted that other research concluded that people with inflammatory bowel disease have a 10 to 100 times increased risk of nephrolithiasis (kidney disease) related to hyperoxaluria (high uric acid). The researchers concluded that, "Manipulation of gastrointestinal (GI) flora can influence urinary oxalate excretion to reduce urinary supersaturation levels. These changes could have a salutary effect on stone formation rates."

Researchers from the Jefferson Medical College (Simenhoff *et al.* 1996) gave 8 kidney hemodialysis patients *Lactobacillus acidophilus* in an attempt to curtail the progression of small bowel bacteria overgrowth—a typical occurrence in end-stage kidney failure. Probiotic treatment lowered serum dimethylamine (a marker for kidney disease) levels from 224 to 154 micrograms/dl and nitrosodimethylamine (another kidney disease marker) from 178 to 83 ng/kg. Serum albumin, body weight, appetite and muscle mass also improved.

Researchers (Schulman 2006) at Vanderbilt University School of Medicine found in a preliminary clinical study that *Bifidobacterium longum* slowed progression of chronic kidney disease.

Probiotics and Vaginosis and Vaginitis

The vagina is lined with probiotic bacteria just as the mouth is. These bacteria protect the woman's internal tissues and organs from being overwhelmed by pathogenic bacteria, yeasts and other pathogens. Without a balance of probiotic bacteria, overgrowths can take place easily. Normal colonies within a healthy vagina include lactobacilli, *Gardenella vaginalis, Candida albicans* and other microorganisms—all existing in balance.

Vaginosis is the alteration of the normal microbiological ecology. Vaginitis is an overgrowth of pathogenic bacteria, and their resulting infection. Two common infective microorganisms within the vagina are *Candida albicans* and *Trichomonas vaginalis.* The use of antibiotics, antiseptics and chemical toxins can stress probiotic populations, allowing overgrowths to take place.

Vaginitis can easily lead to urinary tract infections as pathogenic bacteria colonies expand. Vagina microbial infection is often symptomized by stinging sensations and a fishy odor from the vagina. As we'll discuss later and as indicated in the research, internal supplementation (through the mouth) and external application (into the vagina) both have been shown to help replenish the probiotic populations within the vagina.

Estrogen production can also be a factor. Researchers from Israel's HaEmek Medical Center (Colodner *et al.* 2003) determined from research that, "The lack of lactobacilli in the vagina of postmenopausal women due to estrogen deficiency plays an important role in the development of bacteriuria."

Researchers from the School of Medicine at Italy's Università degli Studi di Siena (Delia *et al.* 2006) treated 60 healthy women with vaginosis with either a vaginal suppository containing *Lactobacillus acidophilus* or a suppository containing *Lactobacillus acidophilus* and *Lactobacillus paracasei* F19. At the end of three months of treatment—and again three months afterward—both groups showed significant improvement in vaginosis, a significant reduction in vaginal pH, and significant decrease in vagina odor.

In a study from the University of Milan (Drago *et al.* 2007), forty women with vaginosis took a douche with *Lactobacillus acidophilus* for six days. After treatment, only 7.5% of the women still had the vaginosis. The odor typical in vaginosis discontinued in all the women, and the pH went to normal levels of 4.5 in 34 of the 40 women.

Scientists from the University of Western Ontario (Reid *et al.* 2001) gave 42 women oral encapsulated *Lactobacillus rhamnosus* GR-1 plus *Lactobacillus fermentum* RC-14 probiotics, or *L. rhamnosus* GG orally for 28 days. Vaginal flora—normal in only 40% of the cases—resolved to healthy flora in 90% of the women in the GR-1 group, and the 7 of 11 women with microbial vaginosis at the beginning of the study were resolved within a month. *L. rhamnosus* GG did not have an effect.

In a similar study (Reid *et al.* 2003), 64 women were given placebo or *Lactobacillus rhamnosus* GR-1 and *Lactobacillus fermentum* RC-14 daily for 60 days. The treatment resulted in the restoration from microbial vaginosis microflora to normal lactobacilli-colonized microflora in 37% of the women treated with the probiotic, versus only 13% among the placebo group.

Researchers from Israel's Central Emek Hospital (Shalev *et al.* 1996) gave 46 microbial vaginosis patients either yogurt with live *L. acidophilus* or a placebo for several months. The probiotic group had significantly less vaginosis than the control group.

Researchers from Sweden's Uppsala University Hospital (Hallén *et al.* 1992) gave 60 women infected with microbial vaginosis either a placebo or *Lactobacillus acidophilus*. At the end of the study, 16 of the 28 women treated with lactobacilli had normal vaginal wet smear results while no improvement occurred among the 29 women treated with the placebo.

Infective vagina bacteroides were eliminated from 12 of 16 women in the probiotic group.

Italian scientists (Cianci *et al.* 2008) investigated the use of *Lactobacillus rhamnosus* GR-1 and *Lactobacillus reuteri* for the treatment and prevention of vaginosis and microbial vaginitis. Fifty women with diagnosed microbial vaginosis and vaginitis took either a placebo or an oral combination of *Lactobacillus rhamnosus* GR-1 and *Lactobacillus reuteri* RC-14 following antibiotic therapy. The researchers found that 92% of the patients significantly benefited from the probiotic treatment.

Scientists from Brazil's Universidade de Sao Paulo (Martinez *et al.* 2009) gave 64 women with microbial vaginosis tinidazole with placebo or with a combination of oral *Lactobacillus rhamnosus* GR-1 and *Lactobacillus reuteri* RC-14 daily for four weeks. The probiotic group experienced a cure rate of 87%, while the placebo group experienced a 50% cure rate. Normal vagina flora resumed in 75% of the probiotic group and in only 34% of the placebo group. This research team (2009) found similar results in another study on 55 women with vulvovaginal candidiasis.

Researchers from the Department of Obstetrics and Fetomaternal Medicine at Austria's Medical University of Vienna (Petricevic and Witt 2008) tested 190 women with microbial vaginosis. They were given either placebo or topical plus oral *Lactobacillus rhamnosus* after antibiotic treatment for 7 days. Sixty-nine of 83 (or 83%) in the probiotic group significantly improved, versus 31 of the 88 women (35%) in the placebo group.

Another study done by researchers from the Medical University of Vienna (Petricevic *et al.* 2008) gave *Lactobacillus rhamnosus* GR-1 and *Lactobacillus reuteri* RC-14 or placebo to 72 postmenopausal women with vaginosis for seven days. Both the placebo group and the probiotic group had received antibiotic treatment for seven days prior. Four weeks after treatment concluded, 60% (21 of 35) of the probiotic group demonstrated a significant improvement, while only 6 of the 37 non-probiotic subjects (16%) showed the same level of improvement.

Probiotics and Ear Infections

Most of us would laugh at the prospect that probiotics would help or prevent ear infections. Think again.

Scientists from Sweden's University of Gothenburg (Skovbjerg *et al.* 2009) studied the effect of probiotic treatment on secretory otitis media— an ear infection with fluid in the middle ear cavity. Sixty children suffering from chronic secretory otitis media who were scheduled for tympanostomy tube insertion were given a nasal spray of placebo, *Streptococcus sanguinis* or *Lactobacillus rhamnosus* for 10 days prior to surgery.

"Complete or significant clinical recovery" occurred in 7 of 19 patients treated with *S. sanguinis;* in 3 of 18 patients treated with *L. rhamnosus;* and in 1 of 17 of the placebo patients.

Probiotics and Cancer

At first glance, it might seem outlandish to propose that probiotics can prevent or even cure cancer. However, a number of studies—*in vitro, in vivo* and clinical research on humans—have confirmed that probiotics inhibit tumor cells through possibly several mechanisms. These include the inhibition of the enzymes beta-glucosidase, beta-glucuronidase, and urease. These enzymes have been conclusively associated with increased tumor cell growth in hundreds of other studies. Beta-glucuronidase, for example, seems to convert certain molecules into procarcinogens. In addition to blocking these enzymes, probiotics also stimulate natural killer cells and cytotoxic T-cells that eliminate tumor cells. Let's examine some of the clinical research:

Researchers from the Gastrointestinal Research Department of the University Hospital Gasthuisberg in Belgium (De Preter *et al.* 2008) determined, in study of 53 healthy volunteers, that probiotic combinations such as *Lactobacillus casei* Shirota, *Bifidobacterium breve* and *Saccharomyces boulardii* were able to significantly reduce beta-glucuronidase activity in the colon. Beta-glucuronidase activity, as mentioned above, has been associated with reducing carcinogenic metabolites within the colon.

Thirty-eight healthy volunteers were given either a placebo or a combination of *Lactobacillus rhamnosus* and *Propionibacterium freudenreichii* subsp. *shermanii* JS for four weeks (Hatakka *et al.* 2008). The probiotic group had significantly lower levels of beta-glucosidase activity and urease activity compared to the placebo group.

Researchers from the Department of Urology and the Faculty of Medicine from the University of Tokyo (Aso *et al.* 1995) conducted a study of 138 patients with superficial transitional cell carcinoma of the bladder following transurethral resection surgery. They gave patients either *Lactobacillus casei* or a placebo. The probiotic groups showed significantly better results than the placebo group in all cases except for those with recurrent multiple tumors—where there was no significant difference between the probiotic and placebo group. The researchers concluded that *L. casei* "was thus safe and effective for preventing recurrence of superficial bladder cancer."

In an earlier study by some of the same medical researchers from the University of Tokyo (Aso and Akazan 1992), *Lactobacillus casei* or placebo was given to 48 patients with bladder cancer following transurethral resection. The recurrence-free interval was significantly prolonged by the probiotic treatment, to 350 days, compared to the 195 days in the control (non-probiotic) group.

Scientists from Japan's Osaka University Medical School (Masuno *et al.* 1991) tested *L. casei* on 76 patients with malignant pleural effusions secondary to lung cancer. Response rates for treatment with intrapleural doxorubicin plus the probiotic was 73.7%, while the response rate without the probiotic was 39.5% in the control group treated with doxorubicin alone. The probiotic group also had a significantly longer survival rates than the control group. The probiotic group also had significantly greater improvement in symptoms such as chest pain, chest discomfort, and anorexia than the control group.

Researchers from the Graduate School of Medical Sciences at Japan's Kyushu University (Naito *et al.* 2008) studied 207 patients diagnosed with superficial bladder cancer who underwent transurethral resection, followed by treatment with the pharmaceutical epirubicin. One hundred of the patients were randomized to receive *Lactobacillus casei* every day for one year in addition to the epirubicin treatment. The lack of recurrence in three years was significantly higher among the probiotic group (74.6% versus 59.9%).

Japanese researchers (Matsumoto and Benno 2004) gave yogurt with *Bifidobacterium lactis* LKM512 or placebo to seven healthy adults for two weeks. The yogurt group showed increased anticarcinogenic fecal spermidine levels and significantly reduced mutagenicity (the likelihood of mutations) levels (48% versus 79%) compared to the placebo group.

Scientists from the Taipei Medical College Hospital and the College of Medicine at Taiwan's National University of Taiwan (Sheih *et al.* 2001) gave *Lactobacillus rhamnosus* HN001 in low-fat milk or lactose-hydrolyzed low-fat milk for 3 weeks to elderly adults with an average age of 64. PMN phagocytic activity increased among the two probiotic groups by 19% and 15%, respectively. NK cell tumor-killing activity increased by 71% and 147%. These declined after the supplement periods, but remained higher than before treatment.

Researchers from the School of Health Sciences and Nursing at the University of Tokyo (Ohashi *et al.* 2002) studied 180 cases of bladder cancer and 445 control subjects in a multi-center (7) study. Subjects given fermented milk products with *Lactobacillus casei* had a significantly reduced risk of bladder cancer, depending upon the frequency and dosage.

This Japanese study (Okamura *et al.* 1989) tested *L. casei* with and without mitomycin on patients with stomach cancer. The probiotic was given either alone or with the mitomycin C with 29 patients enrolled. The positive response rate was 60% for the probiotic group and 70% for those given both the probiotic and mitomycin. The researchers concluded that this probiotic strain "might be a useful therapeutic agent against carcinomatous peritonitis of gastric cancer whether used alone or in combination with mitomycin."

Japanese researchers (Okawa *et al.* 1993) investigated a combined therapy of radiation with heat-killed *Lactobacillus casei* on 228 patients with Stage IIIB cervical cancer. They found that probiotic combination therapy significantly increased tumor regression, and prolonged survival rates. It also increased the relapse-free intervals of patients. In addition, they found that radiation-induced leukopenia was significantly less among the probiotic group.

Researchers from the Japan's Hyogo College of Medicine (Ishikawa *et al.* 2005) studied the association between fiber, probiotics and colorectal tumors. They gave 398 volunteers who were currently free from tumors but who had at least two colorectal tumors removed in the past either wheat bran, *L. casei*, a combination of both or neither. The *L. casei* groups showed a significantly lower risk of atypia—cell abnormality—compared with the non-probiotic groups.

Researchers from the University of Wuerzburg's medical college (Bartram *et al.* 1994) concluded from several clinical studies that, "diet-induced changes in the colonic microflora seem to play a role in colon carcinogenesis."

Scientists from Sweden's Karolinska Institute (Rafter *et al.* 2007) examined probiotics' ability to inhibit colon cancer in a twelve-week study mentioned earlier. Thirty-seven colon cancer patients were given either a placebo or a combination of *Lactobacillus rhamnosus* GG and *Bifidobacterium lactis* Bb12 with FOS. The probiotic group had significant changes in fecal flora. Fecal *Bifidobacterium* and *Lactobacillus* levels increased, while *Clostridium perfringens* levels decreased. The probiotic group also had significantly reduced colorectal proliferation; and fecal water from this group could better induce necrosis (killing) of tumor cells. The probiotic group also had increased interleukin-2 production from peripheral blood mononuclear cells, and increased interferon gamma production among the cancer patients—all anticarcinogenic mechanisms.

German scientists (Roller *et al.* 2007) tested a combination of probiotics and prebiotics in colon cancer patients. Thirty-four colon cancer patients who underwent colon resection were given either a placebo or capsules with *Lactobacillus rhamnosus* GG and *Bifidobacterium lactis* Bb12 with inulin/FOS. At six weeks and twelve weeks, researchers found that IL-2 cytokines from activated PBMCs increased significantly, IFN-gamma production capacity increased—both anticarcinogenic mechanisms.

Researchers from Japan's Nagoya University Graduate School of Medicine's Department of Surgery (Sugawara *et al.* 2006) studied 101 patients with liver/biliary cancer following liver surgery. NK-cell activity and lymphocyte counts were significantly higher following surgery, and pro-inflammatory cytokine IL-6 decreased significantly in the probiotic group. C-reactive protein (another pro-inflammatory marker) also significantly decreased among the probiotic group. Postoperative infectious complications occurred in 30.0% of the placebo group and 12.1% of the probiotic group.

Medical researchers from the Institute of Immunology and Faculty of Medicine of Bratislava's Comenius University (Ferenčík *et al.* 1999) summarized the benefits of lactic acid bacteria: "These include: 1. Lactose digestion, improvement of diarrheal disorders (including traveler's diarrhea), prophylaxis of intestinal and urogenital infections—as a result of formation or reconstruction of a balanced indigenous microflora. 2. Inhibition of the mutagenicity of the intestinal contents and reduction of the incidence of intestinal tumors. 3. Immunomodulatory effects resulting in the improved host resistance. 4. Depression of the serum cholesterol level." These effects were seen during the researchers' nine-week clinical study. Lyophilized *Enterococcus faecium* M-74 in the form of waffles were used. Among the probiotic subjects, beta-D-glucuronidase in stool samples was reduced compared to those of the placebo group. The probiotic group also showed higher production of reactive oxygen species-neutralizing superoxide and peripheral neutrophils. This also accompanied an increase in IgG from peripheral blood mononuclear cells, increased activity from myeloperoxidase and elastase in peripheral neutrophils. The researchers concluded that, "intake of *E. faecium* M-74 in the form of waffles may have a significant immunostimulatory effect on both phagocytosis performed by neutrophils and antibody production."

Probiotics for HIV and AIDS

Aren't we taking the benefits of probiotics a bit too far now? Actually, no. HIV stands for *Human Immunodeficiency Virus*. AIDS stands for *Acquired Immune Deficiency Syndrome*. What are these, then? Once again, we find the immune system has become compromised—this time after being overburdened by viral infection on top of the other toxic burdens our modern society throws at our bodies.

To clarify, we must ask why there is a great disparity between survival rates of HIV-infected persons. One HIV sufferer may live for decades, while another may be diagnosed with AIDS and die within a year. The difference lies in the efficiency and strength of the immune system. The big questions include: How capable is the immune system at suppressing the virus? How well does the immune system interact with its various components to keep its defenses up?

In a study from Italy's University of Milan, researchers (Clerici *et al.* 1996) examined 26 long-term HIV-positive patients who were not progressing into AIDS, and compared them to 28 HIV-positive patients who were progressing rapidly and 24 HIV-seronegative controls (who tend to live longer). They found that cytokine levels, cytokine production rates and the surface marker expression of peripheral blood mononuclear cells (PBMCs) related directly to whether the patient had a longer survival rate. Let's review the research more analytically:

HIV Patient Type	Cytokine levels
Nonprogressing (long term survival, not progressing into AIDS)	Reduced IL-2 Reduced IFN-gamma Increased IL-4 Increased IL-10 Decrease in CD57, CD4, CD7 lymphocytes
Rapidly progressing	Increased IL-2 Increased IFN-gamma Decreased IL-4 Decreased IL-10 Increase in CD57, CD4, CD7 lymphocytes
Seronegative (long term survival)	same as Nonprogressing

We can see here that the ability to fight off the virus is directly related to the immune system's effectiveness and efficiency. Cytokines—the immune system's targeted signaling devices—are produced by the immune system. When it is healthy and not overburdened, it has greater capacity to produce effective cytokines. Lymphocytes with CD programming are specifically programmed to attack certain types of invaders. The production of certain CD lymphocytes indicate an overwhelmed and weakened immune response.

What does this have to do with probiotics? Everything. Probiotics stimulate the production of cytokines, often specific to the type of infection a person might have. This may seem surprising. How would a tiny probiotic know what is attacking the body, and how can it relay that information to the immune system?

Probiotics are conscious living organisms. They want to survive. Like any living being, when their survival is threatened, they get serious. They begin to devise strategies to increase their colonies' chance of survival.

Probiotics are also smart organisms. They utilize several means of communication, including biochemical ligands, biophoton signaling, and a colony communication process called quorum sensing. The orchestrated illumination of tiny algae that appears on the ocean at night is an example of quorum sensing. Even yeasts have these facilities (Chwirot and Popp 1991).

As we have seen from the research covered previously, probiotics often stimulate the production of cytokines specific to the particular ailment. Because the same species of probiotics are stimulating different immune responses for different ailments, this can only mean that the probiotics are responding in an intelligent manner to specific threats to their host.

This ability of probiotics to stimulate specific immune responses in specific disease pathologies has been illustrated in the probiotic research with HIV/AIDS sufferers:

Brazilian scientists (Trois *et al.* 2008) gave a placebo or a formula containing *Bifidobacterium bifidum* and *Streptococcus thermophilus* to 77 HIV-infected children. The average CD4 count in the probiotics group increased by +118 cells mm(-3), while CD4 decreased in the placebo group by -42 CD4 cells mm(-3). Stool consistency also increased among the probiotics group. The researchers concluded: "Our study showed that probiotics have immunostimulatory properties and might be helpful in the treatment of HIV-infected children."

Researchers from the University of Benin in Nigeria (Anukam *et al.* 2008) investigated probiotics in the treatment of HIV/AIDS in women. Yogurt with *Lactobacillus delbruekii* subsp. *bulgaricus*, *Streptococcus thermophilus*, *Lactobacillus rhamnosus* GR-1 and *L. reuteri* RC-14 was given to 24 HIV/AIDS adult female patients. Prior to treatment, they exhibited moderate diarrhea and CD4 counts over 200. They were not receiving antiretrovirals or other dietary supplements for 15 days prior to treatment. A placebo of conventional (unsupplemented) yogurt was used.

The probiotic yogurt group was measured in the beginning, at 15 days and at 30 days. Average CD4 cell counts remained the same or increased in 11 of 12 supplemented probiotic subjects, compared with only 3 of 12 among the placebo group. Diarrhea, flatulence, and nausea were resolved in 12 of 12 probiotic patients within 2 days, versus 2 of 12 in the placebo group. The researchers concluded that this study, "suggests that perhaps a simple fermented food can provide some relief in the management of the AIDS epidemic in Africa."

Researchers from Yale University's School of Nursing (Williams *et al.* 2001) studied 164 HIV women with vaginal candidiasis. They were given either weekly vaginal applications of placebo, *Lactobacillus acidophilus* or clotrimazole for 21 months. Those using the probiotics experienced a significant reduction of episodes—similar to the results of the antifungal ointment clotrimazole.

Research from the Institute of Nutritional Sciences at Germany's University of Giessen (Juszkiewicz *et al.* 2018) studied 73 women who were infected with HIV. The women were all from Cameroon, a sub-Sahara African country.

The researchers divided the patients into two groups. For three months, one group was given five grams per day of Arthrospira platensis – also known as spirulina or Spirulina platensis. The other group was given a placebo supplement. To eliminate possible effects of the nutrients within spirulina, the placebo supplement had a comparable nutritional makeup as spirulina – an equal amount of protein and so forth.

Before and after the 90 days, the patients were tested for CD4 T-cell counts. They also measured "viral load" – the level of viral infection in the body – and another type of T-cell, the CD8 T-cell, which expresses the cytokine CD38. This T-cell is best when it is decreased.

The researchers also measured antioxidant activity within the blood of the patients, and kidney function. The later was measured with creatinine, urea and kidney filtration rates.

After the 90 days treatment, both groups showed weight increase due to the extra protein intake, but the spirulina group showed more weight gain – a good thing for an infection that tends to waste the body.

The spirulina group also experienced no accompanying infections, while the placebo group experienced three infections during the test period.

During the treatment, the spirulina group also experienced nearly half of the associated events of HIV infection – such as liver and kidney conditions. Of the placebo group, 70 percent (21 of 30) experienced events related to HIV and among the spirulina group only 43 percent of the patients – 12 of 28 experienced associated HIV events.

In addition, in the two weeks following the three-month treatment, 10 of the placebo group patients' conditions had worsened to a point where they had to start antiretroviral treatment (ART). Meanwhile only three of the spirulina group was determined to require antiretroviral treatment during the two weeks after the study.

In addition, more of the placebo group had to start antiretroviral treatment during the study. This was only three total patients, but it is useful to consider.

A clinical study (Azabji-Kenfack *et al.* 2011) treated 52 HIV-positive patients who were undernourished in Sub-Sahara Africa. Half (26) of the patients were treated with spirulina and half were given a placebo of soybeans that matched the protein content of the spirulina. Again, the treatment period lasted three months.

Instead of a mere 5 grams of spirulina per day regardless of the patient's weight, this study considered the weight of each patient. The dose of spirulina was 0.37 grams per kilogram of the patient's body weight for the first month and 0.20 grams per kilo for the next two months. This was calculated to be approximately a quarter of the patients' total protein intake.

The average body weight of the patients was 53 kilograms at the beginning of the study. This means the patients were given about 19 grams of spirulina per day during the first month and about 12 grams of spirulina during the last two months, give or take the patient's average weight during that period.

Once again, this study showed the spirulina group gained considerable body mass and fat-free mass – critical for keeping ones health up. The difference in body mass was slightly higher in the soybean group (about 14 pounds to nearly 11 lbs). But the spirulina group had a significantly higher fat-free mass increase than the soybean group – by 92 pounds to 86 pounds.

In this study, the CD4 counts significantly increased among the spirulina group compared to the soybean group. And the viral load levels were significantly decreased in the spirulina group compared to the beginning of the study. The viral load levels for the spirulina group went down significantly more than the soybean group.

One of the main differences between the two studies is that the second study from Africa tested patients that were given antiretroviral drugs from the beginning of the study. Both the placebo group and the spirulina group took the antiretroviral drugs. As mentioned above, most of the patients were not on antiretroviral drugs, and slightly more of the placebo group started the ART therapy during the treatment period.

Yet another difference – one that should be considered carefully – is the dosage. The second trial utilized 2.5 to nearly four times the dose – and related the dose to weight rather than a flat five gram dose as in the first study. The second study used from 12 to 19 grams depending upon the patient's weight.

A clinical study from researchers from Cameroon's University of Yaoundé along with Germany's University of Giessen (Winter *et al.* 2014) studied 73 women infected with HIV. The researchers found that five grams a day significantly boosted the antioxidant capacity and those taking the spirulina had 27 percent fewer associated HIV symptoms.

Should spirulina HIV treatment include ART therapy?

Given the unblemished safety record of spirulina, the inclusion of spirulina supplementation for HIV conditions appears obvious from these studies. But what about antiretroviral therapy?

As the two studies above are examined side by side, the treatment that combined spirulina with antiretroviral drugs did produce more CD4 T-cells. But it should also be noted that given the fact when the trial began, none of the first study's patients needed antiretroviral drugs in the opinion of their doctors, while all of those in the second trial did. This means the patients in the first study were experiencing a different progression of the infection.

This of course means antiretroviral drugs should be determined by ones physician who is privy to the specific symptoms and diagnostic testing that would determine the progression of the infection.

Probiotics and Autoimmunity

In some ways, this section overlaps with some of the other topics because many diseases are described as autoimmune. Nevertheless, probiotics interact with the immune system in ways that help identify rouge cells more accurately. They do this by stimulating the immune factors appropriate to a particular type of problem. They also help to eliminate the possibility that these cells come under attack in the first place.

Researchers from China's Westchina Hospital and Sichuan University (Bai *et al.* 2006) took colonic biopsies from active ulcerative colitis patients. They were co-cultured for 24 hours with *Bifidobacterium longum*. Tumor necrosis factor (TNF)-alpha and interleukin (IL)-8 were lower than colitis patient samples cultured without *B. longum*. The number of lamina propria mononuclear cells (LPMC) with nuclear factor-kappa B (NF-kappaB) P65 positive among co-cultured tissues was also significantly less in the *B. longum* group. The researchers concluded that, "probiotics could inhibit NF-kappaB activation in LPMC and down-regulate inflammatory cytokine secretion from inflamed tissues of active ulcerative colitis."

Medical researchers at the Università dell'Aquila in Italy (De Simone *et al.* 1992) gave *Bifidobacterium bifidum* and *Lactobacillus acidophilus* or placebo to 25 elderly persons for 28 days. After treatment, inflammatory factors among the subjects showed a significant reduction in colonic inflammation, without any altering of T-cells, B-cells and leu7 cells within the digestive system. B-cell activity within the intestinal peripheral bloodstream increased in the probiotic group. The researchers concluded that, "the overall results suggest that the regular administration of *B. bifidum* and *L. acidophilus* leads to a modulation of the immunological and inflammatory response in elderly subjects."

Healthy elderly volunteers were given either lactitol with a placebo or lactitol (a milk sugar-alcohol) plus *Lactobacillus acidophilus*. The group given the probiotics showed a modification of inflammatory markers (prostaglandin-1 and IgA); and produced levels of *Bifidobacterium* in the stool typical for younger persons with stronger immune systems (Ouwehand *et al.* 2009).

Scientists from the University of Helsinki (Kekkonen *et al.* 2008) measured lipids and inflammation markers before and after three weeks of treatment of *Lactobacillus rhamnosus* GG on 26 healthy adults. After three weeks, the probiotic decreased levels of inflammatory fatty acids lysophosphatidylcholines, sphingomyelins, and several glycerophosphatidylcholines. Meanwhile pro-inflammatory triglycerides decreased, and inflammatory markers TNF-alpha and CRP also decreased after the probiotic treatment.

Japanese scientists (Matsumoto and Benno 2006) found that acute inflammation was inhibited by the consumption of *Bifidobacterium lactis* LKM512 yogurt. Tumor necrosis factor (TNF)-alpha production was modulated, and inflammatory cytokines produced by macrophages were modulated—consistent with a reduction of inflammation.

Researchers from Japan's Osaka University Graduate School of Medicine (Shimizu *et al.* 2009) studied 58 patients with severe systemic inflammatory response syndrome (SIRS), and C-reactive protein (CRP) levels greater than 10 mg/dl. The patients received a placebo or a combination of *Bifidobacterium breve*, *Lactobacillus casei*, and GOS (prebiotic). Instances of enteritis, pneumonia, and bacteremia were significantly lower among the probiotic group compared to the placebo group. The probiotics significantly reduced complications in the SIRS patients.

University of Helsinki scientists (Kekkonen *et al.* 2008) also studied the possible anti-inflammatory effects of probiotics with 62 volunteers who received either a placebo or a milk-drink with either *Lactobacillus rhamnosus* GG, *Bifidobacterium animalis* subsp. *lactis,* or *Propionibacterium freudenreichii* subsp. *shermanii* JS. Fecal, venous blood and saliva samples were taken before, during and at the end of the trial period. Serum hsCRP levels were reduced in the all the probiotic groups. TNF-alpha from peripheral blood mononuclear cells was significantly lower in the *L. rhamnosus* LGG compared to the placebo group. IL-2 from peripheral blood mononuclear cells (PBMCs) was significantly lower in the *B.*

animalis group compared to the placebo group. The researchers concluded that, "probiotic bacteria have strain-specific anti-inflammatory effects…"

Summary of Probiotic Mechanisms

We have seen a lot of research on the effects of probiotics. Let's summarize some of the basic functions, mechanisms and effects probiotics have shown among human clinical studies:

Allergies	reduce Th1/ Th2 ratio; decrease Th2 levels; lower TGF-beta2; increase IgE
Anorexia nervosa	increase appetite; increase assimilation; increase lymphocytes
Antibiotics	produce antibiotic and antifungal substances (such as acidophillin and bifidin) that repel or kill pathogenic bacteria, adjusting to pathogen and resistance
B-cells	modulate and redirect B-cell activity
Bile	break down bile acids
Biochemicals	secrete lactic acids, lactoperoxidases, formic acids, lipopolysaccharides, peptidoglycans, superantigens and others to manage pH and repel pathogens.
Bladder cancer	reduce recurrent bladder cancer incidence and inhibit new tumors
Blood pressure	reduce hypertension; inhibit ACE
Calcium	increase serum calcium; decrease parathyroid hormone
Cancer (general)	reduce mutagenicity; increase natural killer tumoricidal activity; increase survival rates
Candida overgrowth	control populations; reduce overgrowths
CD cell orientation	modulate and direct particular CD cells depending upon condition, including CD56, CD8, CD4, CD25, CD69, CD2, others
Cell degeneration	slow cellular degeneration and associated diseases among elderly persons
Colds and Influenza	reduce infection frequency; reduce infection duration; reduce symptoms; prevent complications; decrease worker sick days
Colic	reduce crying time; decrease infection; increase stool frequency; decrease bloating and indigestion
Colon cancer	reduce recurrence; increase survival rates; reduce beta-glucosidase; inhibit cell abnormality and mutation; increase IL-2
Constipation	increase bowel movement frequency; ease colon and impacted feces

Control pathogens	compete with pathogenic organisms for nutrients, thus checking their growth
C-reactive protein	reduce levels in blood
Cytokines	stimulate the body's production of various cytokines, including IL-6, IL-3, IL-5, TNF alpha, and interferon
Dental caries	reduce and control cavity-causing bacteria
Digestion	reduce gas, nausea and stress-related gastrointestinal digestive difficulty
Digestive difficulty	secrete digestive enzymes; help break down nutrients from fats; proteins and other foods
Diverticulosis	reduce polyps and strengthen intestinal wall mucosa
Ear infections	hasten otitis media healing response; prevent infections
EFAs	manufacture essential fatty acids, including important short-chained FAs, and help body assimilate EFAs
Fiber digestion	aid in soluble fiber fermentation, yielding fatty acids and energy
Food poisoning	increase resistance to food poisoning; battle and remove pathogenic organisms; reduce diarrhea and other symptoms
Glucose metabolism	improve glucose control
Gum disease	reduce gum infections; deplete gingivitis
H. pylori	reduce *H. pylori* infections; reduce ulcers
HIV/AIDS	stimulate immune system; reduce symptoms; reduce co-infections; increase survival rates
Hormones	balance and stimulate hormone production
Hydrogen peroxide	manufacture H2O2 - oxygenating/antiseptic
IBS	decrease bloating, pain, cramping
Immunoglobulins	modulate IgA, IgG, IgE, IgM to weakness
Inflammation	modify prostaglandins (E1, E2), IFN-gamma, reduce CRP; modulate TNF-alpha; increase IgA; slow inflammatory response as needed
Intestinal Permeability	protect against IIPS; block penetration of toxins; work cooperatively with villi and microvilli; attach to mucosa; improve barrier function
Intestine walls	protect walls of intestines against toxin exposure and colonization of pathogens
Iron absorption	increase iron assimilation; increase hemoglobin count
Keratoconjunctivitis	decrease burning, itching and dry eyes
Kidney stones	reduce urine oxalates; reduce blood oxalates
Lipids/Cholesterol	reduce LDL, triglycerides and total cholesterol; increase HDL

Liver	stimulate liver cells (hepatocytes); stimulate liver function; reduce cirrhosis symptoms; reduce liver enzymes
Liver cancer	stimulate immune response; decrease infection and complications after surgery
Lung cancer	increase survival rates; reduce chest pain and other symptoms
Mental state	improve mood; stimulate positive mood hormones like serotonin and tryptophan
Milk digestion	aid dairy digestion for lactose-intolerant people; produce lactase
Monocytes	increase oxidative burst capacity
Mucosa	coat intestines, stomach, oral, nasal and vagina mucosa, providing protective barrier
NF-kappaB	modulate activity to condition
NK-cells	stimulate natural killer cell activity
Nutrition	manufacture biotin, thiamin (B1), riboflavin (B2), niacin (B3), pantothenic acid (B5), pyridoxine (B6), cobalamine (B12), folic acid, vitamin A and/or vitamin K; aid in assimilation of proteins, fats and minerals
Pancreatitis	reduce pancreas infection (sepsis); reduce necrosis; speed healing
pH control	produce a number of other acids and biochemicals, modulating pH (see biochemicals)
Phagocytes	increase phagocytic activity as needed
Phytonutrients	convert to bioavailable nutrient forms
Premature births and Low birth weights	speed growth; reduce infection; improve immune response; increase nutrition
Protein assimilation	break down amino acid content; inhibit assimilation of allergic polypeptides
Respiratory infections	inhibit pneumonia; reduce duration of infection; inhibit bronchitis; inhibit tonsillitis
Rotavirus infections	speed healing times; prevent infection; ease abdominal pain; eradicate infective agents
Spleen	stimulate spleen activity
Stomach cancer	inhibit tumors; reduce *H. pylori* overgrowths
T-cells	modulate T-cell activity to condition
Th1 - Th2	decrease Th2 activity; increase Th1 (increases healing and decreases allergic response)
Thymus	increase thymus size and activity
Toxins	break down toxins; inhibit assimilation of heavy metals, chemicals, and endotoxins
Ulcers	control *H. pylori*; speed healing; improve mucosa; moderate acids; reduce pain

Vaccination	increase vaccine effectiveness
Vaginosis/Vaginitis	reduce infection; re-establish healthy pH; reduce odor

This summary of primarily randomized, double-blinded, and placebo-controlled human clinical research is by no means a complete list of all the probiotic effects that have been found by researchers. Furthermore, medical scientists have only chosen a small portion of probiotics' possible health benefits for controlled human research. The effects shown in these studies illustrate a variety of other possible benefits for specific infections and diseases. As we can see from probiotics' ability to specifically stimulate the immune system, there are many other possible applications for probiotics in medicine. The research has only begun.

Probiotic Supplementation

After reviewing hundreds of human clinical studies—some quoted in this book and many more discussed and referenced in the author's two books, *Probiotics–Protection Against Infection* and *Oral Probiotics*—we have selected the probiotic species shown in research to be useful for reducing systemic inflammation.

Below is a brief discussion of each organism. The references for these benefits can be found in the author's books on probiotics mentioned above.

Lactobacillus acidophilus is by far the most familiar probiotic to most of us, and is also by far the most-studied probiotic species to date. They are key residents in the human gut, although supplemented strains may still be transient. In addition to helping digest lactose, probably the most important benefit of *L. acidophilus* is their ability to inhibit the growth of pathogenic intestinal microorganisms such as *Candida albicans, Escherichia coli, Helicobacter pylori, Salmonella, Shigella* and *Staphylococcus* species.

<u>Research illustrates that *L. acidophilus* can:</u>

➤ Help digest milk
➤ Reduce stress-induced GI problems
➤ Inhibit *E. coli*
➤ Reduce infection from rotavirus
➤ Reduce necrotizing enterocolitis
➤ Reduce intestinal permeability
➤ Control *H. pylori*
➤ Modulate PGE2, IgA and IgG
➤ Reduce dyspepsia
➤ Relieve and inhibit IBS and colitis
➤ Inhibit and control *Clostridium* spp.

➢ Inhibit *Bacteroides* spp.
➢ Inhibit *Candida* spp. Overgrowths
➢ Reduce allergic response
➢ Decrease allergic symptoms
➢ Inhibit upper respiratory infections

Lactobacillus helveticus was made popular by cheese-makers from Switzerland. The Latin word *Helvetia* refers to Switzerland. *L. helveticus* is used to make Swiss cheese and other varietals, as it produces lactic acid but not other probiotic metabolites that can often make cheese taste bitter or sour.

Research illustrates that *L. helveticus* can:

➢ Normalize blood pressure by producing natural ACE inhibitors
➢ Stimulate intestinal mucosal immunity
➢ Promote healthy sleep

Lactobacillus salivarius are residents of most humans. They are found in the mouth, sinuses, larynx, pharynx, airways and small intestines, colon, and vagina. They are hardy bacteria that can live in both oxygen and oxygen-free environments. *L. salivarius* is one of the few bacteria species that can also thrive in salty environments. *L. salivarius* produce prolific amounts of lactic acid, which makes them hardy defenders of the teeth and gums. They also produce a number of antibiotics, and are speedy colonizers.

Research illustrates that *L. salivarius* can:

➢ Inhibit mutans streptococci in the mouth
➢ Reduce dental carries
➢ Reduce gingivitis and periodontal disease
➢ Reduce mastitis
➢ Reduce risk of strep throat caused by *S. pyogenes*
➢ Reduce ulcerative colitis and IBS
➢ Inhibit *E. coli*
➢ Inhibit *Salmonella* spp.
➢ Inhibit *Candida albicans*

Lactobacillus casei are transient bacteria within the human body, but are typical residents of cow intestines. They are readily found in natural raw milk and colostrum. *L. casei* have been reported to reduce allergy symptoms and increase immune response. This is accomplished by their regulating the immune system's CHS, CD8 and T-cell responsiveness—an effect seen among immunosuppressed patients. *L. casei* are also competitive bacteria that will overtake other probiotics in a combined supplement. Hence, it is best to supplement *L. casei* individually.

Research illustrates that *L. casei* can:

➤ Inhibit pathogenic microbial infections
➤ Reduce occurrence, risk and symptoms of IBS
➤ Inhibit severe systemic inflammatory response syndrome
➤ Inhibit respiratory tract infections
➤ Inhibit bronchitis
➤ Maintain remission of diverticular disease
➤ Inhibit *H. pylori* (and ulcers)
➤ Reduce allergy symptoms
➤ Inhibit *Pseudomonas aeruginosa*
➤ Decrease milk intolerance
➤ Increase CD3+ and CD4+
➤ Increase phagocytic activity
➤ Support liver function
➤ Decrease proinflammatory cytokine TNF-alpha
➤ Strengthen the immune system
➤ Inhibit and reduce diarrhea episodes
➤ Stimulate cytokine interleukin-1beta (IL-1b)
➤ Stimulate interferon-gamma
➤ Inhibit *Clostridium difficile*
➤ Reduce inflammation
➤ Reduce constipation
➤ Decrease beta-glucuronidase
➤ Stimulate natural killer cell activity (NK-cells)
➤ Increase IgA levels
➤ Increase lymphocytes
➤ Decrease IL-6 (pro-inflammatory)
➤ Increase IL-12 (stimulates NK-cells)
➤ Reduce lower respiratory infections
➤ Inhibit *Candida* overgrowth
➤ Inhibit vaginosis
➤ Prevent colorectal tumor growth
➤ Restore NK-cell activity in smokers
➤ Stimulate the immune system among the elderly
➤ Increase CD56 lymphocytes
➤ Decrease rotavirus infections
➤ Decrease colds and influenza
➤ Reduce risk of bladder cancer
➤ Increase (good) HDL-cholesterol
➤ Decrease triglycerides
➤ Decrease blood pressure
➤ Inhibit viral infections
➤ Inhibit malignant pleural effusions secondary to lung cancer
➤ Reduce cervix tumors when used in combination radiation therapy
➤ Inhibit tumor growth of carcinomatous peritonitis/stomach cancer

> Break down nutrients for bioavailability

Lactobacillus rhamnosus: These bacteria can colonize in the intestines and airways. Much of the research on this species has been done on a particular strain, *L. rhamnosus* GG. *L. rhamnosus* GG have been shown in numerous studies to significantly stimulate the immune system and inhibit allergic inflammatory responses. This is not to say, however, that non-GG strains will not perform similarly. In fact, studies with *L. rhamnosus* GR-1, *L. rhamnosus* 573/L, and *L. rhamnosus* LC705 strains have also showed positive results. The GG strain is trademarked by the Valio Ltd. Company in Finland and patented in 1985 by two scientists, Dr. Sherwood Gorbach and Dr. Barry Goldin, who also led most of the exhaustive research on this strain.

Research illustrates that *L. rhamnosus* can:

> Inhibit a number of pathogenic microbial infections

> Improve glucose control

> Reduce risk of respiratory infections

> Decrease beta-glucosidase

> Reduce eczema

> Reduce colds and flu

> Strengthen the immune system

> Increase IgA levels in mucosal membrane

> Increase IgA levels in mothers breast milk

> Inhibit *Pseudomonas aeruginosa* infections in respiratory tract

> Inhibit *Clostridium difficile*

> Inhibit enterobacteria

> Reduce IBS symptoms

> Decrease IL-12, IL-2+ and CD69+ T-cells in IBS

> Reduce constipation

> Reduce the risk of colon cancer

> Modulate skin IgE sensitization

> Inhibit *H. pylori* (ulcer-causing)

> Reduce atopic dermatitis in children

> Increase Hib IgG levels in allergy-prone infants

> Reduce colic

> Stimulate IgM, IgA and IgG levels (modulates IgE)

> Stabilize intestinal barrier function (decreased permeability)

> Increase INF-gamma

> Modulate IL-4

> Help prevent atopic eczema

> Reduce *Streptococcus mutans*

> Stimulate tumor killing activity among NK-cells

> Stimulate IL-10 (anti-inflammatory)

> Reduce inflammation

Lactobacillus reuteri is a species found residing permanently in humans. As a result, most supplemented strains attach fairly well, though temporarily, and stimulate colony growth for resident *L. reuteri* strains. *L. reuteri* will colonize in the mouth, airways, stomach, duodenum and ileum regions. *L. reuteri* will also significantly modulate the immune response of the gastrointestinal mucosal membranes. This means that *L. reuteri* are useful for many of the same digestive ailments that *L. acidophilus* are also effective for. *L. reuteri* have several other effects, including the restoration of our oral cavity bacteria. They also produce a significant amount of antibiotics.

Research illustrates that *L. reuteri* can:

➢ Inhibit gingivitis
➢ Reduce pro-inflammatory cytokines
➢ Stimulate growth and feeding among preterm infants
➢ Inhibit and suppress *H. pylori*
➢ Decrease dyspepsia
➢ Reduce nausea
➢ Reduce flatulence
➢ Reduce diarrhea (rotavirus and non-rotavirus)
➢ Reduce TGF-beta2 in breastfeeding mothers (reducing eczema)
➢ Reduce salivary *mutans streptococcus*
➢ Strengthen the immune system
➢ Reduce plaque on teeth
➢ Decrease symptoms of IBS
➢ Increase (inflammatory) CD4+ and CD25 T-cells (in IBS)
➢ Decrease (inflammatory) TNF-alpha (in IBS)
➢ Decrease (inflammatory) IL-12 (in IBS)
➢ Reduce eczema-specific IgEs in infants
➢ Reduce infant colic
➢ Reduce colds and influenza
➢ Stabilize intestinal barrier function (intestinal permeability)
➢ Decrease atopic dermatitis

Lactobacillus plantarum has been part of the human diet for thousands of years. They are used in numerous fermented foods, including Sauerkraut, Gherkins, Olive brines, Sourdough bread, Nigerian Ogi and Fufu, Kocha from Ethiopia, Sour Mifen noodles from China, Korean Kimchi and other traditional foods. *L. plantarum* are also found in dairy and cow dung.

L. plantarum is a hardy strain. They will colonize the oral cavity, airways, stomach and intestines. Temperature for optimal growth is 86-95 degrees F. *L. plantarum* are not permanent residents, however. When supplemented, they vigorously attack pathogenic bacteria, and create an environment hospitable for incubated resident strains to expand before departing. *L. plantarum* also produce lysine, and a number of antibiotics, including lactolin. They also strengthen mucosal membranes and reduce intestinal permeability.

Research illustrates that *L. plantarum* can:

➢ Strengthen the immune system
➢ Help restore healthy liver enzymes (and alcohol-induced liver injury)
➢ Reduce frequency and severity of respiratory diseases
➢ Reduce intestinal permeability
➢ Inhibit various intestinal pathobiotics (incl. *Clostridium difficile*)
➢ Reduce Th2 (inflammatory) levels and increase Th1/Th2 ratio
➢ Reduce inflammatory responses
➢ Reduce symptoms of multiple traumas among injured patients
➢ Reduce fungal infections
➢ Reduce IBS symptoms
➢ Reduce pancreatic sepsis (infection)
➢ Reduce (inflammatory) interleukin-6 (IL-6) levels
➢ Decrease flatulence

Lactobacillus bulgaricus: We owe the *bulgaricus* name to Ilya Mechnikov, who named it after the Bulgarians—who used the bacteria to make the fermented milks that produced the original kefirs apparently related to their extreme longevity. In the 1960s and 1970s, Russian researchers, notably Dr. Ivan Bogdanov and others, began focused research on *L. bulgaricus*. Early studies indicated antitumor effects. As the research progressed into Russian clinical research and commercialization, it became obvious that even heat-killed *L. bulgaricus* cell fragments have immune system-stimulating benefits.

L. bulgaricus bacteria are transients that assist in *bifidobacteria* colony growth. They significantly stimulate the immune system and have antitumor effects as mentioned. They also produce antibiotic and antiviral substances such as bulgarican and others. *L. bulgaricus* bacteria have also been reported to reduce IBS symptoms. *L. bulgaricus* require more heat to colonize than many probiotics—at 104-109 degrees F.

Research illustrates that *L. bulgaricus* can:

➢ Reduce intestinal permeability
➢ Decrease IBS symptoms
➢ Help manage HIV symptoms
➢ Stimulate TNF-alpha
➢ Stimulate IL-1beta
➢ Decrease diarrhea (rotavirus and non-rotavirus)
➢ Decrease nausea
➢ Increase phagocytic activity
➢ Increase leukocyte levels
➢ Increase immune response

➤ Increase CD8+ levels
➤ Lower CD4+/CD8+ ratio (reducing inflammation)
➤ Increase IFN-gamma
➤ Lower total cholesterol
➤ Lower LDL levels
➤ Lower triglycerides
➤ Inhibit viruses
➤ Reduce salivary mutans in the mouth
➤ Increase absorption of dairy (lactose)
➤ Increase white blood cell counts after chemotherapy
➤ Increase IgA (immunity) to rotavirus
➤ Reduce intestinal bacteria

Bifidobacterium bifidum are normal residents in the human intestines, and by far the largest residents in terms of colonies. Their greatest populations occur in the colon, but also inhabit the lower small intestines. Breast milk typically contains large populations of *B. bifidum* along with other bifidobacteria. *B. bifidum* are highly competitive with yeasts such as *Candida albicans*. As a result, their populations may be decimated by large yeast overgrowths. This will also result in a number of endotoxins, including ammonia, being leached out of the colon into the bloodstream. As a result, *B. bifidum* populations are extremely important to the health of the liver, as has been illustrated in the research. They produce an array of antibiotics such as bifidin and various antimicrobial biochemicals such as formic acid. *B. bifidus* populations can also be severely damaged by the use of pharmaceutical antibiotics.

Research illustrates that *B. bifidum* can:

➤ Increase cell regeneration in alcohol-induced liver injury
➤ Stimulate immunity in very low birth weight infants
➤ Increase TGF-beta (anti-inflammatory) levels
➤ Reduce allergies
➤ Reduce *H. pylori* colonization
➤ Increase CD8+ T-cells as needed
➤ Establish infant microflora
➤ Inhibit *E. coli*
➤ Reduce intestinal bacteria infections
➤ Reduce acute diarrhea (rotavirus and non-rotavirus)

Bifidobacterium infantis are also normal residents of the human intestines—particularly among children. As implicated in the name, infants colonize a significant number of *B. infantis* in their early years. They will also colonize in the vagina, leading to the newborn's first exposure to protective probiotic bacteria. For this reason, it is important that pregnant mothers consider probiotic supplementation with *B. infantis*.

B. infantis are largely anaerobic, and thrive within the darkest regions, where they can produce profuse quantities of acetic acid, lactic acid and formic acid to acidify the mucosal membranes and intestinal tract.

Research illustrates that *B. infantis* can:

➢ Reduce acute diarrhea (rotavirus and non-rotavirus)
➢ Reduce or eliminate symptoms of IBS
➢ Reduce death among very low birth weight infants
➢ Increase immunity among very low birth weight infants
➢ Establish infant microflora
➢ Normalize Th1/Th2 ratio
➢ Reduce inflammatory allergic responses
➢ Normalize IL-10/IL-12 ratio
➢ Improve immune system efficiency

Bifidobacterium longum are also normal inhabitants of the human digestive tract. They dominate the colon but also live in the small intestines. They are one of our top four bifidobacteria inhabitants. Like *B. infantis,* they produce acetic, lactic and formic acid. Like other bifidobacteria, they resist the growth of pathogenic bacteria, and thus reduce the production of harmful nitrites and ammonia. *B. longum* also produce B vitamins. Healthy breast milk contains significant *B. longum* counts.

Research illustrates that *B. longum* can:

➢ Reduce death among very low birth weight infants
➢ Reduce sickness among very low birth weight infants
➢ Reduce acute diarrhea (rotavirus and non-rotavirus)
➢ Reduce vomiting
➢ Reduce nausea
➢ Reduce ulcerative colitis
➢ Reduce or alleviate symptoms of IBS
➢ Stabilize intestinal barrier function (decreased permeability)
➢ Inhibit *H. pylori*
➢ Increase TGF-beta1 (anti-inflammatory) levels
➢ Decrease (inflammatory) TNF-alpha
➢ Decrease (inflammatory) IL-10 cytokines
➢ Reduce lactose-intolerance symptoms
➢ Reduce diarrhea
➢ Increase helper T-cells type2 (Th2)
➢ Increase (anti-inflammatory) IL-6
➢ Reduce (inflammatory) Th1
➢ Reduce pro-inflammatory IL-12 and interferon
➢ Stimulate healing of liver in cirrhosis
➢ Reduce constipation
➢ Reduce hypersensitivity
➢ Reduce IBS symptoms

➤ Inhibit intestinal pathogenic bacteria
➤ Decrease prostate cancer risk
➤ Decrease itching, nasal blockage and rhinitis in allergies
➤ Reduce (inflammatory) NF-kappaB
➤ Reduce (inflammatory) IL-8 levels
➤ Reduce progression of chronic liver disease
➤ Increase absorption of dairy nutrients

Bifidobacterium animalis/B. lactis was previously thought to be distinct from *B. lactis,* but today they are considered the same species with *B. lactis* being a subspecies of *B. animalis. B. lactis* has also been described as *Streptococcus lactis.* They are transient bacteria typically present in raw milk. They are used as starters for traditional cheeses, cottage cheeses and buttermilks. They are also found among certain plants.

Research illustrates that *B. animalis* can:

➤ Reduce constipation
➤ Improve digestive comfort
➤ Decrease total cholesterol
➤ Increase blood glucose control
➤ Reduce respiratory diseases (severity and frequency)
➤ Strengthen the immune system
➤ Reduce salivary mutans in mouth
➤ Increase body weight among preterm infants
➤ Reduce (inflammatory) CRP levels
➤ Reduce (inflammatory) TNF-alpha levels
➤ Reduce acute diarrhea (rotavirus and non-rotavirus)
➤ Reduce (inflammatory) IL-10 levels
➤ Reduce (inflammatory) TGF-beta1 levels
➤ Reduce (inflammatory) CDE4+CD54(+) cytokines
➤ Stimulate improvement in atopic dermatitis patients
➤ Reduce IBS symptoms
➤ Reduce diarrhea
➤ Normalize bowel movements
➤ Decrease intestinal permeability
➤ Reduce blood levels of interferon-gamma
➤ Stimulate IgA among milk-allergy infants
➤ Improve atopic dermatitis symptoms and sensitivity
➤ Inhibit *H. pylori*
➤ Reduce allergic inflammation
➤ Increase T-cell activity as needed
➤ Increase immunity among the elderly
➤ Increase absorption of dairy

Bifidobacterium breve are also normal inhabitants of the human digestive tract—living mostly within the colon. They produce prolific acids, and also B vitamins. Like the other bifidobacteria, they reduce ammonia-producing bacteria in the colon, aiding the health of the liver. They have been shown to reduce allergies and respiratory condition severity. They also inhibit and control populations of *H. pylori*. Remember that *H. pylori* overgrowths are seen in conditions of GERD and ulcers. Latin *brevis* means short.

Research illustrates that *B. breve* can:

➢ Reduce severe systemic inflammatory response syndrome
➢ Increase resistance to respiratory infection
➢ Reduce (inflammatory) TNF-alpha
➢ Reduce (inflammatory) IL-10
➢ Reduce (inflammatory) TGF-beta1
➢ Reduce IBS symptoms
➢ Decrease (pro-colon cancer) beta-glucoronidase
➢ Inhibit *H. pylori*
➢ Increase antipoliovirus vaccination effectiveness
➢ Reduce acute diarrhea (rotavirus and non-rotavirus)
➢ Reduce allergy symptoms
➢ Increase growth weights among very low birth weight infants

Streptococcus thermophilus are common participants in yogurt making. They are also used in cheese making, and are even sometimes found in pasteurized milk. They will colonize at higher temperatures, from 104-113 degrees F. This is significant because this bacterium readily produces lactase, which breaks down lactose. (This is the only streptococci known to do this.) Like many other supplemented probiotics, *S. thermophilus* are temporary microorganisms in the human body. Their colonies will typically inhabit the system for a week or two before exiting (unless consistently consumed). During that time, however, they will help set up a healthy environment to support resident colony growth. Like other probiotics, *S. thermophilus* also produce a number of different antibiotic substances, including acids that deter the growth of pathogenic bacteria.

Research illustrates that *S. thermophilus* can:

➢ Reduce acute diarrhea (rotavirus and non-rotavirus)
➢ Reduce intestinal permeability
➢ Inhibit *H. pylori*
➢ Help manage AIDS symptoms
➢ Increase lymphocytes among low-WBC patients
➢ Increase (anti-inflammatory) IL-1beta
➢ Decrease (inflammatory) IL-10
➢ Increase tumor necrosis factor-alpha (TNF-a)
➢ Increase absorption of dairy
➢ Decrease symptoms of IBS
➢ Inhibit *Clostridium difficile*

➤ Increase immune function among the elderly
➤ Restore infant microflora similar to breastfed infants
➤ Increase (anti-inflammatory) CD8+
➤ Increase (anti-inflammatory) IFN-gamma
➤ Reduce acute gastroenteritis (diarrhea)
➤ Reduce baby colic
➤ Reduce symptoms of atopic dermatitis
➤ Reduce nasal cavity infections
➤ Increase HDL-cholesterol
➤ Increase growth in preterm infants
➤ Reduce intestinal bacteria
➤ Reduce upper respiratory tract infections from *Staphylococcus aureus*, *Streptococcus pneumoniae*, beta-hemolytic streptococci, and *Haemophilus influenzae*
➤ Reduce salivary mutans streptococci in the mouth
➤ Reduce flare-ups of chronic pouchitis
➤ Reduce LDL-cholesterol in overweight subjects
➤ Reduce ulcerative colitis

Streptococcus salivarius are vigorous probiotic bacteria that station themselves throughout the upper respiratory tract, but primarily inhabit the oral cavity and pharynx. *S. salivarius* are the primary and most aggressive of our oral cavity probiotic bacteria. They are extremely territorial, and produce a number of antibiotics, including salivaricin A and salivaricin B, along with a host of other antibiotic substances.

They are also permanent residents in the human body, being primarily inherited from mom. *Streptococcus salivarius* are organizers. They produce a number of enzymes and acids that manage the growth of other bacteria. One might conclude that *Streptococcus salivarius* are one of the most important bacteria to maintaining the health of the airways, because they are the principal gatekeepers when it comes to preventing the entry and survival of infective microorganisms.

Research illustrates that *S. salivarius* can:

➤ Reduce dental plaque
➤ Reduce dental caries
➤ Inhibit gingivitis
➤ Inhibit *Streptococcus pyogenes* (strep throat)
➤ Prevent mastitis among breast-feeding mothers
➤ Reduce ulcerative colitis

Saccharomyces boulardii are yeasts (fungi). They render a variety of preventative and therapeutic benefits to the body. Yet should this or another yeast colony grow too large, they can quickly become a burden to the body due to their dietary needs (primarily refined sugars) and waste products. *S. boulardii* are known to enhance IgA—which, as we've discussed, will typically reduce IgE atopic sensitivities. This is likely why this probiotic helps clear skin disorders. *S. boulardii* also help control diarrhea, and have been shown to be helpful in Crohn's disease and irritable bowel issues. *S. boulardii* have also been shown to be useful in combating cholera bacteria (*Vibrio cholerae*).

Research illustrates that *S. boulardii* can:

➤ Decrease infectious *Entameba histolytica* (intestinal)
➤ Inhibit *H. pylori*
➤ Decrease intestinal permeability
➤ Decrease diarrhea infections
➤ Stimulate T-cells as needed
➤ Decrease C-reactive protein
➤ Decrease beta-glucoronidase enzyme (associated with colon cancer)
➤ Inhibit *E. coli*
➤ Reduce ulcerative colitis
➤ Reduce symptoms of Crohn's disease
➤ Reduce *Clostridium difficile*

Supplementing with Probiotics

The main consideration in probiotic supplementation is consuming *live* organisms. These are typically described as "CFU" which stands for *colony forming units.* In other words, live probiotics will produce new colonies once inside the intestines. Heat-killed ones are not as beneficial, although they can also stimulate the immune system. So the key is keeping the probiotics alive while in the capsule and supplement bottle, until we are ready to consume them. Here are a few considerations about probiotic supplements:

Capsules: Vegetable capsules contain less moisture than gelatin or enteric-coated capsules. Even a little moisture in the capsule can increase the possibility of waking up the probiotics while in the bottle. Once woken up, they can starve and die. Enteric coating can minimally protect the probiotics within the stomach, assuming they have survived in the bottle. Some manufactures use oils to help protect the probiotics in the stomach. In all cases, encapsulated freeze-dried probiotics should be refrigerated (no matter what the label says) at all times during shipping, at the store, and at home. Dark containers also better protect the probiotics from light exposure, which can kill them.

A newer development in probiotic encapsulation is microbeads. Microbeads are tiny beads of probiotic colonies. The beads give the probiotics much more protection against the elements, significantly increasing their longevity, even outside of refrigeration.

Powders of freeze-dried probiotics are subject to deterioration due to increased exposure to oxygen and light. Powders should be refrigerated in dark containers and sealed tightly to be kept viable. They should also be consumed with liquids or food, preferably dairy or fermented dairy. Powders can also be used as starters for homemade yogurt and kefir.

Caplets/Tablets: Some tablet/caplets have special coatings that provide viability through to the intestines without refrigeration. If not, those tablets would likely be in the same category as encapsulated products, requiring refrigeration.

Shells or Beads: These can provide longer shelf viability without refrigeration and better survive the stomach. However, because of the size of the shell, these typically come with less CFU quantity, increasing the cost per therapeutic dose. Another drawback may be that the intestines must dissolve this thick shell. An easy test is to examine the stool to be sure that the beads or shells aren't coming out the other end whole.

Lozenges: These are the newest way to supplement with probiotics, and should be a consideration for sinus infections and respiratory disorders. A correctly formulated chewable or lozenge can inoculate the mouth, nose and throat with beneficial bacteria to compete with and fight off pathogenic bacteria as they enter or reside in our mouth, nose, throat and airways of the lungs.

Probiotic supplements that survive well among the mucous membranes of the airways, sinuses and oral cavity include *L. reuteri, L. rhamnosus, L. plantarum, L. paracasei, and Streptococcus salivarius.* As we discussed in the research, several of these, notably *L. reuteri,* have been shown to increase airway health and decrease lung infections.

However, most of the probiotics in a lozenge will not likely survive the stomach acids and penetrate the intestines. (Therefore, intestinal probiotics in one of the forms above are recommended in addition to probiotic lozenges.)

As the research showed in the last chapter (see topic on oral probiotics), lozenges are an excellent way to help prevent new infections and sore throats during increased exposures. The bacteria in a good lozenge or chewable will allow the probiotics to colonize around our gums and throat, fending off microorganisms that threaten their welfare.

This type of supplement should still be kept sealed, airtight and cool. Refer to the author's book *Oral Probiotics* for detailed information regarding species, strategies and additional research on these probiotics.

Liquid Supplements: There are several probiotic supplements in small liquid form. One brand of *L. reuteri* has a long tradition and a hardy, well-researched strain. A liquid probiotic should be in a light-sealed, refrigerated container. It should also contain some dairy or other probiotic-friendly substrate, giving the probiotics some food while awaiting delivery to the intestines.

Probiotic Hydrotherapy: This method of supplementation is a great way to implant live colonies of probiotics into the lower colon. Colon hydrotherapy (or colonic) is one of the healthiest things we can do for preventative and therapeutic health in general. Colon hydrotherapy is performed by a certified colon hydrotherapist who uses specialized (and sanitary) equipment to flush out the colon with water. This colon flushing usually takes about 30 minutes. Once the process is complete, the hydrotherapist can "insert" a blend of probiotics into the tube and "pump" the probiotics directly into our colon. Colon hydrotherapy is a wonderful treatment recommended for most anyone, especially those with disorders related to systemic inflammation.

Colonic treatments are relatively inexpensive, compared with their benefit. Two to three colonics a year are often recommended for ultimate colon health. Those with sensitive or irritable bowels should consult with their health professional before submitting to a colonic, however.

Probiotic Dosage: A good dosage for intestinal probiotics for prevention and maintenance can be ten to fifteen billion CFU (*colony forming units*) per day. Total intake during an illness or therapeutic period, however, will often double or triple that dosage. Much of the research shown in this text utilized 20 billion to 60 billion CFU per day, about a third of that dose for children and a quarter of that dose for infants. (*B. infantis* is often the supplement of choice for babies.)

Supplemental oral probiotic dosages can be far less (100 million to two billion), especially when the formula contains the hardy *L. reuteri*.

People who must take antibiotics for life-threatening reasons can alternate doses of probiotics between their antibiotic dosing. The probiotic dose can be at least two hours before or after the antibiotic dose. (Always consult with the prescribing doctor.)

Remember that these dosages depend upon delivery to the intestines. Therefore, a product that passes into the stomach with little protection would likely not deliver many colonies to the intestines. Such a supplement would likely require higher dosage to achieve the desired effects.

Chapter Five

Immunity Boosting Herbs

Herbal Medicines that Boost Immunity

There are numerous herbs that have been utilized in traditional medicine to modulate the immune system and stimulate the body's purification processes. Some of these were in response to serious disease conditions.

In addition, a number of modern companies have developed cleansing formulations that stimulate the body's immunity processes in a dramatic way. Some of these formulations pile up upwards of 10-15 different herbs, some of which are laxatives, purgatories and emetics.

Some of the herbs within these are quite harsh upon the body, and can result in stressing the body to the point of producing full body toxemia. Examples of these include black walnut hulls, wormwood, cat's claw and others.

Now for diseased conditions of parasites, Lyme disease and other infective situations, some of these intense herbs could be called for. But these would require a careful evaluation by a medical professional, and clear guidelines on dosage, strength and duration.

This text does not advocate the use of such intense medicinal herbs to stimulate the body's own immune systems, without a specific prescription by a medical professional and herbalist.

What this text advocates is that incorporation of common culinary spices and herbs that have a gradual and gentle effect upon the body. These effects will be seen by the stimulation of the strength of those organs and tissue systems that drive our body's purification programs. They will:

➢ Strengthen the immune system
➢ Increase tolerance
➢ Stimulate detoxification processes
➢ Donate key nutrients
➢ Balance and strengthen the adrenal glands
➢ Subdue anxious nervous response
➢ Strengthen mucous membranes
➢ Feed probiotics
➢ Reverse systemic inflammation
➢ Alkalize the bloodstream
➢ Rebuild the airways
➢ Relax smooth muscles
➢ Neutralize free radicals

> Strengthen the adrenal glands

Our discussion is far from exhausting. One of the reasons is because just about every medicinal herb can affect and stimulate the body's purification systems in one way or another. We will focus, instead, upon those common herbs that are easily accessible in western society to the public: In other words, they can easily be grown in our gardens, purchased and blended into our food recipes, or mixed and steeped into herbal teas.

These uses are by far the most sustainable means to use these herbs, and they are also the safest. This is because nature provides a full spectrum of nutrients among an herb's active ingredients among the natural parts of the plant. The roots, stems, leaves and flowers of one of these herbal plants typically provide a safe means of consumption—assuming we are selecting one of these herbs and not some poisonous plant we have never seen.

On the contrary, an herbal formulation that has undergone extraction or refining can eliminate some of these natural buffers—such as fibers, polysaccharides and mucilages. Cooking these away can result in side effects and pronounced effects that might not be expected.

This presentation of the science and traditional use of medical herbs is not simply the personal opinion of the author. Rather, this discussion utilizes the medical science and research of numerous researchers, scientists and physicians trained in herbal medicines. Here traditional clinical uses of herbal medicine have been derived from a number of *Materia Medica* texts from various traditions, as well as from documented histories of using these herbs upon significant populations over centuries—some even over thousands of years. Unless otherwise noted in the text, this information utilizes the following reference materials (see reference section for complete citation):

Bensky *et al.* 1986; Bisset 1994; Blumenthal 1998; Blumenthal and Brinckmann 2000; Bruneton 1995; Chevallier 1996; Chopra *et al.* 1956; Christopher 1976; Clement *et al.* 2005; Duke 1989; Ellingwood 1983; Fecka 2009; Foster and Hobbs 2002; Frawley and Lad 1988; Gray-Davidson 2002; Griffith 2000; Gundermann and Müller 2007; Halpern and Miller 2002; Hobbs 2003; 1997; Hoffmann 2002; Hope *et al.* 1993; Jensen 2001; Kokwaro 1976; Lad 1984; LaValle 2001; Lininger *et al.* 1999; Mabey 1988; Mehra 1969; Mindell and Hopkins 1998; Murray and Pizzorno 1998; Nadkarni and Nadkarni 1908/1975; Newall *et al.* 1996; Newmark and Schulick 1997; O'Connor and Bensky 1981; Potterton 1983; Schulick 1996; Schauenberg and Paris 1977; Schulz *et al.* 1998; Shi *et al.* 2008; Shishodia *et al.* 2008; Tierra 1992; Tierra 1990; Tiwari 1995; Tisserand 1979; Tonkal and Morsy 2008; Weiner 1969; Weiss 1988;

Williard 1992; Williard and Jones 1990; White and Foster 2000; Wood 1997.

Bupleurum

Bupleurum (*Bupleurum chinense* or *Bupleurum falcatum*) has also been called Hare's Ear, Saiko and Thorowax. Bupleurum belongs in the Umbelliferae family, and thus is related to fennel, dill, cumin, coriander and others—and exerts similar medicinal effects.

The root is typically used, and its constituents include triterpenoid saponins called saikosides, flavonoids such as rutin, and sterols such as bupleurumol, furfurol and stigmasterol. The saikosides in Bupleurum have been known to boost liver function and reduce liver toxicity. In general, Bupleurum appears to also stimulate immunity.

Bupleurum is used to stimulate the spleen, purify the blood and rejuvenate the liver—and has been used to treat hepatitis. Bupleurum was studied by researchers at the Beijing University of Traditional Chinese Medicine (Chen *et al.* 2005) on 58 patients with spleen deficiency. After one month of treatment, tests showed that levels of epinephrine and dopamine were decreased and beta-endorphin levels had increased substantially among the Bupleurum-treated group. They concluded that Bupleurum significantly *"regulates nervous and endocrine systems."*

Szechwan Pepper

This is the fruit from *Zanthoxylum simulans* which is also sometimes referred to as *Fructus Zanthoxyli Bungeani* or *Pericarpium zanthoxyli bungeani* in traditional Chinese medicine. More precisely, this herb is also referred to as Sichuan pepper. The tree is also called Prickly ash, and is grown around the world. The small peppers that come from the Prickly ash tree can be dried and ground or used fresh.

Chuan Jiao is also referred to as Fagara, Sansho, Nepal pepper or Szechwan pepper.

Because it is very spicy and hot, it is often used in Sichuan dishes—known for their spiciness. Chuan Jiao contains limonene, geraniol and cumic alcohol, among with a number of other medicinal constituents.

In traditional Chinese medicine, Chuan Jiao is known to remove abdominal pain, vomiting, nausea and parasites—especially roundworm. It is also used as a skin wash for eczema, and has a mild diuretic effect.

Dong Quai

This is *Angelica sinensis,* also referred to as *Corpus radix angelicae sinensis* in traditional Chinese medicine. The roots and rhizomes are used. In Western herbology, it is sometimes referred to simply as Angelica. It is also called Dong quai.

This herb contains courmarins and a number of volatile oils. Thus it is known to lower blood pressure, relax tense muscles and improve circulation, as it inhibits platelet aggregation. It is also known as a potent anti-inflammatory, and is known to rejuvenate the adrenal glands.

Dong quai is also considered antispasmodic, which means it reduces hypersensitivity. It stimulates tolerance. It is a very popular herb for balancing the female reproductive system and irregular menstruation. It is considered a tonic in general, and has been used in traditional medicine for colds, fevers, inflammation, arthritis, rheumatic issues and anemia.

Licorice and Gan Cao (Chinese Licorice)

Glycyrrhiza uralensis is also called Chinese Licorice. It is not the common Licorice (*Glycyrrhiza glabra*) known in Western and Ayurvedic herbalism. However, the two plants have nearly identical uses and constituents. So this discussion also serves *Glycyrrhiza glabra*.

Chinese licorice is known in Chinese medicine as giving moisture and balancing heat to the lungs. It has thus been extensively used to stop coughs and wheezing. It is also known to clear fevers. Taken either internally or topically, it is known to ease carbuncles and skin lesions. It is also soothing to the throat and eases muscle spasms. The root is thus described as antispasmodic.

Researchers from New York's Mount Sinai School of Medicine (Jayaprakasam *et al.* 2009) extensively investigated *Glycyrrhiza uralensis*. They found that *G. uralensis* had five major flavonoids: liquiritin, liquiritigenin, isoliquiritigenin, dihydroxyflavone, and isoononin. Liquiritigenin, isoliquiritigenin, and dihydroxyflavone were found to suppress inflammation via inhibiting eotaxin. Eotaxin stimulates the release of eosinophils during inflammation.

Licorice also contains glactomannan, triterpene saponins, glycerol, glycyrrhisoflavone, glycybenzofuran, cyclolicocoumarone, glycybenzofuran, cyclolicocoumarone, licocoumarone, glisoflavone, cycloglycyrrhisoflavone, licoflavone, apigenin, isokaempferide, glycycoumarin, isoglycycoumarin, glycyrrhizin and glycyrrhetinic acid (Li *et al.* 2010; Huang *et al.* 2010).

One of its main active constituents, isoliquiritigenin, has been shown to be a H2 histamine antagonist (Stahl 2008). Chinese Licorice has been shown to prevent the IgE binding that signals the release of histamine. This essentially disrupts the histamine inflammatory process while modulating immune system responses (Kim *et al.* 2006).

Another important constituent, glycyrrhizin, is a potent anti-inflammatory biochemical. It has also been shown to halt the breakdown of cortisol produced by the body. Let's consider this carefully. Like cortisone, cortisol inhibits the inflammatory process by interrupting interleukin cytokine transmission. If cortisol is prevented from breaking down, more remains available in the bloodstream to keep a lid on inflammation.

This combination of constituents gives Licorice aldosterone-like effects. This means that the root stimulates the production and maintenance of steroidal corticoids. Animal research has confirmed that Licorice is anti-allergic, and decreases anaphylactic response. It also balances electrolytes and inflammatory edema (Lee *et al.* 2010; Gao *et al.* 2009).

Echinacea

The roots of Echinacea (E. purpura or E. angustifolia) are often used to boost immunity. Conventional medicine offers no preventative agent for the common cold. This is not the case for echinacia. Echinacia is a natural therapy that can help prevent and reduce the duration of a cold.

Researchers from the UK's Cardiff University (Jawad *et al.* 2012) conducted a gold-standard double-blind, randomized, placebo-controlled study of 755 healthy adults. They were given either an Echinacea extract or a placebo for four months.

The subjects completed diaries and were interviewed and analyzed once a month. The researchers also collected nasal mucous during cold or viral episodes. Blood samples were also collected and analyzed.

Those who took the echinacea had significantly fewer colds and virus infections during the treatment period. In addition, duration of illnesses were significantly reduced among the Echinacea group compared to the placebo group.

The subjects in the placebo group had 188 colds, compared to 149 among the Echinacea group. The placebo group's collective duration of illness was 850 episode-days, compared to 672 episode-days for the echinacea group.

Recurrent colds were significantly reduced. The researchers also found that only 65 infections recurred in 28 subjects among the Echinacea group compared 100 recurrent infections among 43 people in the placebo group, a difference of 59%.

The study also found that the placebo group took 52% more pain medication to help relieve infection symptoms than did the Echinacea group.

Ginger

This is *Zingiberis officinalis,* also called *Rhizoma zingiberis officinalis* in traditional Chinese medicine. It is quite simply common Ginger root.

Ginger is extensively used in both Chinese and Ayurvedic medicine. It is also commonly used in Western herbalism and a number of other traditional medicines around the world.

Ginger is one of the most versatile food-spice-herbs known to humanity. In Ayurveda—the oldest medical practice still in use—Ginger is the most recommended botanical medicine. Ginger is referred to as *vishwabhesaj*—meaning "universal medicine"—by Ayurvedic physicians.

An accumulation of studies and chemical analyses has determined that Ginger has at least 477 active constituents. As in all botanicals, each constituent will stimulate a slightly different mechanism—often moderating the mechanisms of other constituents. Many of Ginger's active constituents have anti-inflammatory and/or pain-reducing effects. These include a number of gingerols and shogaols.

Clinical evaluation has documented that Ginger blocks inflammation by inhibiting lipoxygenase and prostaglandins in a balanced manner. This allows for a gradual reduction of inflammation and pain without the negative GI side effects that accompany NSAIDs. Ginger also stimulates circulation, inhibits various infections, and strengthens the liver.

Properties of Ginger supported by traditional clinical use include being analgesic, anthelmintic, anticathartic, antiemetic, antifungal, antihepatotoxic, antipyretic, antitussive, antiulcer, cardiotonic, gastrointestinal motility, hypotensive, thermoregulatory, analgesic, tonic, expectorant, carminative, antiemetic, stimulant, anti-inflammatory, antimicrobial and more.

Ginger has therefore been used as a traditional treatment for bronchitis, rheumatism, asthma, colic, nervous disorders, colds, coughs, migraines, pneumonia, indigestion, respiratory ailments, fevers, nausea, colds, flu, ulcers, hepatitis, liver disease, colitis, tuberculosis and many digestive ailments to name a few.

Myrrh/Guggulu

Myrrh is from the gum oleoresin taken from the *Commiphora mukul* tree. This tree grows abundantly in India and Asia. In fact, many trees of the genus *Commiphora*—more than 200 species—have been called myrrh and used to treat pain, skin afflictions, inflammatory disorders, diarrhea, and periodontal diseases The frankincense and myrrh trade, along with gold and other spices, was an important commerce between the east, middle east and Africa thousands of years ago. Ayurvedic physicians consider it the most important medicinal resin used. "Guggul" is actually a general term meaning tree resins, but the widespread use of *Commiphora* has taken over the term. Myrrh has been widely used in India and the Middle East for thousands of years for a variety of ailments, including arthritis, rheumatism, gout, gastrointestinal problems, lumbago, nervousness, urinary tract issues, bronchitis, diabetes, asthma, obesity, phthisis, hemorrhoids, skin diseases, ulcers, infected gums, sore throat, intestinal worms, boils, liver disorders, vitiligo, edema, menstrual dysfunction, paralytic seizures and other ailments. It is applied both externally and taken internally. It is calming, considered an all-around tonic for the body, and slightly laxative. More recently, it has been recognized as significantly reducing serum triglycerides and cholesterol. It is considered stimulant, aromatic, expectorant, emmenagogue (stimulates menstruation flow), astringent (externally), antiseptic, antiparasitic, antineoplastic (preventing neoplasms), anesthetic (produces anesthesia), and anticarcinogenic.

A number of studies over the years have confirmed myrrh's immune-stimulating, antimicrobial and antitumor effects (Tonkal and Morsy 2008).

Research done by Banarus Hindu University researchers (Devaraj 1985) showed guggul resin had significant anti-inflammatory and anti-arthritic effects.

In 2008, laboratory testing (Raut *et al.* 2008) confirmed that myrrh oleoresin was effective at breaking down microcrystals that build up in the joints, kidneys and gallbladder.

Researchers from the University of Kansas (Ding and Staudinger 2005), determined that the plant sterol pregnane X receptor inhibits the expression of the gene cytochrome Cyp2b10. Cyp2b10 apparently plays a role in liver metabolism. This illustrates not only one mechanism of myrrh in terms of its ability to protect the liver. It also shows the capability of botanicals to modulate human gene expression—for the better.

In an *in vivo* study from Glasgow's University of Strathclyde (Duwiejua *et al.* 1993), myrrh significantly reduced joint swelling. The researchers concluded myrrh was an anti-inflammatory agent.

Juniper

Juniper is a round evergreen bush that grows to about ten feet tall. It has short, pointed leaves, small yellow flowers, and produces small green or blue-black berries (actually small cones). Juniper grows throughout Europe, Asia, and the United States—among both plains and alpine regions. Traditional uses have included a variety of inflammatory diseases and infectious diseases including chronic and rheumatic arthritis, edema, gout, bronchitis, colds, fungal infections, hemorrhoids, wounds, gynecological diseases and general inflammation. It is known to purify and balance blood chemistry. It stimulates appetite and digestion. American Indians used juniper for tuberculosis, fevers, colds, coughs, sore throats, liver and kidney infections, and intestinal disorders.

Tinctures from its berries and branches have been used for skin irritations and alopecia (baldness). It has also been used to combat urinary tract infections. In the Middle Ages, herbalists used juniper to prevent the contraction of various contagious diseases. When treating a person during the Black Death epidemic, many herbalists would keep a few juniper berries in the mouth to stave off infection—forming an antiseptic barrier of sorts. North American Indians used juniper berries as a liniment and an infusion for colds, sore throats and tuberculosis. Juniper is considered to be expectorant (detoxifying), analgesic, diuretic, stomach tonic, carminative, rubefacient (irritant when rubbed on), and disinfectant (antimicrobial).

Juniper is also part of the Ayurvedic Indian Materia Medica, as it is quite commonly found in the Himalayan mountains and valleys of India. In Ayurveda, juniper is suggested for urinary issues, digestive ailments, rheumatism, and as an antiseptic. Today herbalists frequently use juniper for cystitis, gout, and rheumatic joints. The German Commission E monograph recommends the dried fruit on a daily basis for rheumatic disorders.

In a study from the Karl-Franzens-University's School of Pharmacognosy, juniper extract inhibited LOX activity—the enzyme conversion process involved in the production of pro-inflammatory leucotrienes (Schneider *et al.* 2004).

Researchers from the University of Zagreb tested juniper essential oil against sixteen different bacterial species, seven different yeast-like fungi, three different yeast species, and four dermatophytes. Juniper illustrated antibacterial properties against both gram-positive and gram-negative bacteria; showed fungicidal activity; and significantly inhibited dermatophytes (Petlevski *et al.* 2008).

The berry extract showed significant antimicrobial ability against gram-positive bacteria. Studies show significant prostaglandin-2 inhibition, producing an anti-inflammatory effect and the blocking of pain (Akkol *et al.* 2009).

A study from Italy's University of Cagliari (Angioni *et al.* 2003) determined that juniper inhibited *Staphylococcus aureus*. Tests have shown juniper's essential oils produce a number of different antifungal effects (Pepeljnjak *et al.* 2005).

Juniper extract exhibited significant antimicrobial effects upon *Candida albicans, Aspergillus niger,* and others (El-Ghorab *et al.* 2008).

In a study from Turkey's Gebze Institute of Technology (Karaman *et al.* 2003), juniper inhibited 57 different strains of bacteria, including those of *Xanthomonas, Staphylococcus, Enterobacter, Cinetobacter, Bacillus, Brevundimonas, Brucella, Escherichia, Micrococcus* and *Pseudomonas.* Eleven *Candida albicans* species were also shown to be inhibited by juniper.

Juniper was shown effective against tumor cells (Moujir *et al.* 2008). This chemoprotective quality seems to relate to the lignans.

In tests against a variety of viruses, juniper essential oils were found to inhibit replication of the SARS-CoV and HSV-1 (herpes simplex) viruses (Loizzo *et al.* 2008; Sassi *et al.* 2008).

Juniper leaves and berries also contain a significant amount of antioxidant potency and free radical scavenging abilities. (Al-Mustafa 2008; Lim *et al.* 2002).

Juniper's safety has been established in a number of reports (Petlevski *et al.* 2008; Wang *et al.* 2002; Schilcher and Leuschner 1997).

Juniper extract also appears to increase the level of phosphorylation in adipose tissue with increased AMP-activated protein kinase—in mice studies this reduced obesity and increased the efficiency of insulin and leptin (Kim *et al.* 2008).

The polysaccharides in juniper stimulated macrophage and mononuclear phagocyte activity in a study by researchers from the Montana State University (Schepetkin *et al.* 2005).

Some of the terpenoids in juniper displayed anti-malarial effects (Okasaka *et al.* 2006).

Juniper proved to be toxic to cells infected with HIV-1 and HIV-3 at 50% concentration (Salido *et al.* 2002).

Juniper also showed antimicrobial activity against *Fusobacterium necrophorum, Clostridium perfringens, Actinomyces bovis* and *Candida albicans* in research performed at Oregon State University (Johnston *et al.* 2001).

Juniper's diterpenes and sesquiterpene showed activity against *Mycobacterium tuberculosis* (Topcu *et al.* 1999).

In an *in vivo* study, juniper oil resulted in higher levels of TNF (stimulated immune system) and lower levels of PGE2 and cytokines IL-6 and IL-10 (reduced inflammation) compared to controls (Chavali *et al.* 1998).

In another study, juniper oil reduced liver damage and increased liver microcirculation and bile flow, illustrating that juniper was liver-protective (Jones *et al.* 1998).

Cinnamon

This is *Cinnamomum cassia*, also referred to as *Ramulus cinnamomi cassiae* in traditional Chinese medicine. It is commonly called cinnamon—a delicious culinary spice present in most kitchens.

Cinnamon is used in just about every traditional medicine. The bark is often used, although the twigs are also utilized. Its constituents include limonene, camphor, cineole, cinnamic aldehyde, gums, mannitol, safrole, tannins and oils.

According to Western herbalism, Ayurvedic medicine and traditional Chinese medicine, it is useful for colds, sinusitis, bronchitis, dyspepsia, asthma, muscle tension, toothaches, the heart, the kidneys, and digestion. It is also thought to strengthen circulation in general. Its properties are described as expectorant, diuretic, stimulating, analgesic and alterative. In other words, it is an immune-system modulator. It is also thought to dilate the blood vessels and warm the body according to these traditional disciplines.

Astragalus

Astragalus (*Astragalus mongholicus* or *Astragalus membranaceus*) root is a well-known immune system adaptogen. In other words, it strengthens the immune system, allowing it to become more tolerant. Astragalus has also been proven to be calming, anti-inflammatory and anti-microbial.

In Chinese medicine, Astragalus is known to treat *qi* deficiency. Remember, *qi* (or *chi*) is the vigor of the body, expressed in circulation, heat, detoxification and immunity. Thus, Astragalus invigorates the body. Astragalus is often used to treat exhaustion, adrenal deficiency, spleen deficiency and circulation issues. Laboratory and *in vivo* research has shown it can reduce blood pressure and increase circulatory health.

Astragalus contains a number of constituents, such as astragalosides, isoastragalosides, astramembrannin, afrormosin, catycosin, daucosterol, formononetin, ononin, pinitol, sitosterol, and various flavonoids, including methoxyisoflavone. It also contains two polysaccharide glucans, heteroglycans, and calycosin.

Researchers from China's Sichuan University (Wang *et al.* 2010) found that Astragalus reduced IL-4 cytokines and modulated the Th1/Th2 ratio, reducing pro-inflammatory processes—evidenced by changes in genetic signalling.

Researchers from Shanghai's Huashan Hospital of Fudan University (Xie *et al.* 2006) found that Astragalus reduced the production of TNF-alpha and inhibited NF-kappa B activity. This illustrated its adaptogenic properties and ability to inhibit inflammation.

Rose Hips

Scientific research has determined that rose hips can help a number of conditions. But now we find that rose hips can significantly reduce our chances of catching the common cold.

These mature rose buds can also help reduce the severity of colds and increase general well-being according to a study from the cold north.

In a 2018 study led by Dr. Kaj Winther, a professor at the University of Copenhagen, 120 people were tested over a period of six months during the wintertime.

The people were randomly split into two groups. One group was given two grams of liquid rose hips. The other group was given a placebo. The study was double-blinded, so no one knew who was given what.

During the six winter months in Denmark, the volunteers reported their incidences of colds. They also reported duration and symptoms when they did have a cold.

The researchers found of the 107 volunteers who completed the study, 31 of the 58 people in the placebo group reported having a cold. That is over 53 percent of the group.

During the same period, only 24 out of 54 people in the rose hips group got a cold. That is 43.6 percent compared to 53.4 percent in the placebo group.

But when symptoms were compared, the rose hips group had significantly more mild symptoms compared to the placebo group.

Only 15 of the rose hips group had headaches when they caught a cold, compared to 26 in the placebo group.

Only 15 people had muscle stiffness when they had a cold in the rose hips group, compared to 27 in the placebo group.

Only 20 people had fatigue when they had a cold in the rose hips group, compared to 29 in the placebo group.

The researchers also found that the rose hips liquid boosted general well-being during the test period. The well-being scale for the rose hips group was 0.21. This compared to 0.12 – nearly half – for the placebo group.

The rose hips also boosted muscle flexibility and reduced general stiffness among the rose hips group. The stiffness scale fell from 2.40 to 2.02 in the rose hips group. Muscle stiffness in the placebo group jumped from 2.37 to 2.93 during the same period.

Wintertime does tend to increase muscle stiffness. This relates not only to catching colds, but being cold in general. It also likely relates to decreases in vitamin D from the sun, which tends to increase flexibility.

Jujube

The *Ziziphus ziziphus* plant produces a delicious sweet date that tastes very much like a sweet apple. The fruit has many different properties in traditional medicine. It has been used to stimulate the immune system. It has been used to reduce stress, reduce inflammation, sooth indigestion, and repeal GERD.

Jujube contains a variety of constituents, including mucilage, ceanothic acid, alphitolic acid, zizyberanal acid, zizyberanalic acid, zizyberanone, epiceanothic acid, ceanothenic acid, betulinic acid, oleanolic acid, ursolic acid, zizyberenalic acid, maslinic acid, tetracosanoic acid, kaempferol, rutin, quercetin and others.

Panex Ginseng

Panex ginseng is an immune stimulant with thousands of years of use. Panax ginseng will come in white forms and red forms. The color depends upon the aging or drying technique used.

When Ginseng is cultivated and steamed, it is called 'red root' or Hong Shen. Ginseng root will turn red when it is oxidized or processed with steaming. Some feel that red root is better than white, but this really depends upon its intended use, the age of the root, and how it was processed. Soaking Ginseng in rock candy produces a white Ginseng that is called Bai shen. This soaking seems odd, but this has been known to increase some of its constituent levels such as superoxide and nitric oxide. When the root is simply dried, it is called 'dry root' or Sheng shaii shen. Korean Red Ginseng is soaked in a special herbal broth and then dried.

There are a number of species within the *Panax* genus, most of which also contain most of the same adaptogens, referred to as gensenosides. Most notable in the *Panex* genus is American Ginseng, *Panax quinquefolius.*

Ginseng contains camphor, mucilage, panaxosides, resins, saponins, gensenosides, arabinose and polysaccharides, among others.

Eleutherococcus senticosus, often called Siberian Ginseng, is actually not Ginseng. While it also contains adaptogens (eleutherosides), these are not the gensenoside adaptogens within Ginseng that have been observed for their ability to relieve hypersensitivity.

Researchers from Italy's Ambientale Medical Institute (Caruso *et al.* 2008) tested an herbal extract formula consisting of *Capparis spinosa, Olea europaea, Panax ginseng* and *Ribes nigrum* (Pantescal) on allergic patients. They found that allergic biomarkers, including basophil degranulation CD63 and sulphidoleukotriene (SLT) levels were significantly lower after 10 days. They theorized that these biomarkers explain the herbal formulation's *"protective effects."*

Researchers from Japan's Ehime University Graduate School of Medicine (Sumiyoshi *et al.* 2010) tested *Panax ginseng* on mice sensitized to hen's eggs. After the oral feedings, they found that the Ginseng significantly reduced allergen-specific IgG Th2 levels. It also increased IL-12 production, and increased the ratio of Th1 to Th2 among spleen cells. In addition, it enhanced intestinal CD8, IFN-gamma, and IgA-positive counts. The researchers concluded that, *"Red Ginseng roots may be a natural preventative of food allergies."*

Ginseng has been found to stimulate circulation and improve cognition. It is also known to reduce fatigue, and stress. Herbalists also use it to improve appetite, and as a mild stimulant and potent antioxidant.

Black Plum

Prunus mume (Seib et Zucc) is also referred to as *Fructus pruni mume* in Chinese medicine. It is also called *Omae* in Korea, *Ume* or *Umeboshi plum* in Japan, which translates, quite simply, to 'Dark plum' or 'Black plum.' It is also referred to as Mume. It is, quite simply, the fruit of a special variety of plums.

This plum is treasured for its immune-stimulating properties. The Chinese *Materia Medica* describes it as able to alleviate coughing and lung deficiencies. It has a strongly astringent property, and thus helps to cleanse the digestive tract and halt diarrhea. Research documented in the *Medica* has indicated that it stimulates bile production, is anti-microbial, and has been able to relieve fever, nausea, abdominal pain and vomiting.

Gingko

The extracts or powders from the leaves of the *Gingko biloba* plant are now popular all over the world. Ginkgo's standardized extracts are part of many formulas, from brain tonics to blood purification formulations. It also has a long history of use in Chinese medicine for expanding the airways.

Gingko contains numerous flavonoids and terpenoids, including ginkgolide, amentoflavone, biolobetin, bilobalide, ginkgetin, glycosides, ginkgolic acids, quercetin, isorhamnetins, kaempferol and others. Ginkgolide, for example has been shown to inhibit platelet aggregating factor (PAF). This means it helps prevent clotting events within the arteries.

A study from researchers at Germany's Hannover School of Pharmacy and Medicine (Wilkens *et al.* 1990) found that gingko resulted in an almost immediate reduction in platelet factor 4 (PF4) and beta-thromboglobulin (beta-TBG).

Boswellia (Frankincense)

The medicinal Boswellia species include *Boswellia serratta, Boswellia thurifera,* and *Boswellia spp.* (other species). Boswellia contains a variety of active constituents, including a number of boswellic acids, diterpenes, ocimene, caryophyllene, incensole acetate, limonene and lupeolic acids.

The genus of *Boswellia* includes a group of trees known for their fragrant sap resin that grow in Africa and Asia. Frankincense was extensively used in ancient Egypt, India, Arabia and Mesopotamia thousands of years ago, as an elixir that relaxed and healed the body's aches and pains. The gum from the resin was applied as an ointment for rheumatic ailments, urinary tract disorders, and on the chest for bronchitis and general breathing problems. It is classified in Ayurveda as bitter and pungent.

Over the centuries, boswellia has been used as an internal treatment for a wide variety of inflammatory ailments and a variety of infections. Its properties are described as stimulant, diaphoretic, anti-rheumatic, tonic, analgesic, antiseptic, diuretic, demulcent, astringent, expectorant, and antispasmodic.

In two studies, boswellic acids extracted from Boswellia were found to have significant anti-inflammatory action. The trials revealed that Boswellia inhibited the inflammation-stimulating LOX enzyme (5-lipoxygenase) and thus significantly reduced the production of inflammatory leukotrienes (Singh *et al.* 2008; Ammon 2006).

Another study (Takada *et al.* 2006) showed that boswellic acids inhibited cytokines and suppressed cell invasion using NF-kappaB inhibition.

In *in vivo* studies by researchers from the University of Maryland's School of Medicine (Fan *et al.* 2005), Boswellia extract exhibited significant anti-inflammatory effects. The report also concluded that, *"these effects may be mediated via the suppression of pro-inflammatory cytokines."*

In an *in vitro* study also from the University of Maryland's School of Medicine (Chevrier *et al.* 2005), boswellia extract proved to modulate the balance between Th1 and Th2 cytokines. This illustrated Boswellia's ability to strengthen the immune system and increase tolerance.

A similar-acting anti-inflammatory Ayurvedic herb is **Guggul**. Guggul is another gum derived from the resin of a tree—*Commiphora mukul.*

Black Pepper

In Ayurveda, *Piper nigrum* is considered medicinal. Yet it is probably one of the most common spices used in Western foods. In fact, the world probably owes its use of Black pepper in foods to Ayurveda.

Black pepper is used in a variety of Ayurvedic formulations because of its anti-inflammatory action. Ayurvedic doctors describe Black pepper as a stimulant, expectorant, carminative (expulsing gas), anti-inflammatory and analgesic. It has been used traditionally for rheumatism, arthritis, bronchitis, coughs, asthma, sinusitis, gastritis and other histamine-related conditions. It is also thought to stimulate a healthy mucosal membrane among the stomach and intestines.

Black pepper used as a spice to increase taste is certainly not unhealthy, but it takes a significantly greater and consistent dose to produce its anti-inflammatory effects.

A traditional Ayurvedic prescription for gastroesophageal reflux or GERD, for example, is to take Black pepper in a warm glass of water on an empty stomach first thing in the morning over a period of time. This dose of Black pepper, according to Ayurveda, stimulates mucosal secretion, and purifies the mucosal membranes of the stomach and intestines.

Researchers from South Korea's Wonkwang University (Bae *et al.* 2010) found that the *Piper nigrum* extract piperine significantly inhibited inflammatory responses, including leukocytes and TNF-alpha.

Long Pepper

The related Ayurvedic herb, *Piper longum,* has similar properties and constituents as Black pepper. It is often used in Indian recipes. It is used to inhibit the inflammation and histamine activity that results in lung and sinus congestion. Like Black pepper, Long pepper is also known to strengthen digestion by stimulating the secretion of the mucosal membranes within the stomach and intestines. It is also said to stimulate enzyme activity and bile production. One study by researchers from India's Markandeshwar University (Kumar *et al.* 2009) found that the oil of Long pepper fruit significantly reduced inflammation.

Triphala

Triphala means *"three fruits."* Triphala is a combination of three botanicals: *Terminalia chebula, Terminalia bellirica* and *Emblica officinalis.* They are also termed Haritaki, Bihitaki and Amalaki, respectively. This combination has been utilized for thousands of years to rejuvenate the intestines, regulate digestion and create efficiency within the digestive tract.

The 'three fruits' also are said to produce a balance among the three doshas of *vata, pitta* and *kapha.* Each herb, in fact, relates to a particular *dosha:* Haritaki relates to *vata,* Amalaki relates to *pitta* and Bibhitaki relates to *kapha.* The three taken together comprise the most-prescribed herbal formulation given by Ayurvedic doctors for digestive issues.

This use has been justified by preliminary research. For example, in a study by pharmacology researchers from India's Gujarat University (Nariya *et al.* 2003), triphala was found to significantly reverse intestinal damage and intestinal permeability *in vivo.*

The traditional texts and the clinical use of triphala today in Ayurveda have confirmed these types of intestinal effects in humans.

We might want to elaborate a little further on Haritaki in particular. *Terminalia chebula* has been used by Ayurvedic practitioners specifically for conditions related to inflammation, abdominal issues, skin eruptions, itchiness, and epithelial issues. It is also called He-Zi in traditional Chinese medicine.

Research has found that Haritaki contains a large number of polyphenols, including ellagic acids, which have significant antioxidant and anti-inflammatory properties (Pfundstein *et al.* 2010).

Turmeric

Curcuma longa has been extensively used as a medicinal herb for many centuries, and this predicated its use as a curry food spice—as Ayurveda has long incorporated healing herbs with meals. The roots or rhizomes of Turmeric are used. It is a relative of Ginger in the *Zingiberaceae* family.

Just as we might expect from a medicinal botanical, Turmeric has a large number of active constituents. The most well known of those are the curcuminoids, which include curcumin (diferuloylmethane, demethoxycurcumin, and bisdemethoxycurcumin). Others include volatile oils such as tumerone, atlantone, and zingiberene; as well as polysaccharides and a number of resins.

As stated in a recent review of research from the Cytokine Research Laboratory at the University of Texas (Anand 2008), multiple studies have linked Turmeric with *"suppression of inflammation; angiogenesis; tumor genesis; diabetes; diseases of the cardiovascular, pulmonary, and neurological systems, of skin, and of liver; loss of bone and muscle; depression; chronic fatigue; and neuropathic pain."*

Indeed, Turmeric has been used for centuries for arthritis, asthma, inflammation, gallbladder problems, diabetes, wound-healing, liver issues, hepatitis, respiratory disease, menstrual pain, anemia, and gout. It is described as alterative, antibacterial, carminative and stimulating. It is also known for its wound-healing, blood-purifying and circulatory powers. Studies have illustrated that curcumin has about 50% of the effectiveness of cortisone, without its damaging side effects (Jurenka 2009).

A number of studies have proved over the past decade that Turmeric and/or its key constituents such as curcumin halt or inhibit both inflammatory COX and LOX enzymes. Curcumin has specifically been shown to inhibit IgE signaling processes, and slow mast cell activation (Aggarwal and Sung 2009; Thampithak *et al.* 2009; Sompamit *et al.* 2009; Kulka 2009).

Parsley/Coriander/Cilantro/Italian Parsley

Coriandrum sativum has documented throughout traditional medicines as an anti-allergy and antioxidant herb. The seeds are called Coriander, and the leaves are called Cilantro. Cilantro has been popularly used throughout Central America, Italy, and also Asia—where it is sometimes called Chinese parsley. Cilantro is the backbone ingredient—together with tomatoes and garlic—of salsa. It is related to Italian parsley, with many of the same constituents. Coriander is taken as fresh or juiced fresh, and it has been used by Ayurvedic practitioners primarily for allergic skin rashes and hay fever.

Fresh Italian parsley can readily be found in supermarkets and farmers' markets. While often used as a garnish (for looks and/or to clean the breath), a therapeutic quantity of parsley is about a *bunch*. A bunch of parsley is about two ounces or about ten stalks together with their branches and leaves. A *bunch* can be added to a salad or put into a soup. Parsley can be delicious with tomatoes, vinegar and olive oil. And of course, it can also freshen the breath.

Research proves that parsley boosts the immune system, reduces inflammation and fights off cancer.

Parsley is also rich in numerous antioxidant nutrients, including vitamin A, vitamin C, vitamin E, beta carotene, lutein, cryptoxanthin, zeaxanthin, folate and is one of the greatest sources of vitamin K, with 1640 micrograms per gram – over 12 times the U.S. DRI (dietary reference intake) of 90-120 micrograms per day. One hundred grams of Parsley also contains more than double the RDA for vitamin C and almost triple the RDA of vitamin A.

Other bioactive constituents in Parsley include eugenol, crisoeriol, luteolin and apiin. Eugenol has been used by traditional doctors as an antiseptic and pain-reliever in cases of gingivitis and periodontal disease, and has been shown to reduce blood sugar levels in diabetics.

Cumarins are natural blood thinning agents, as they provide anti-coagulating properties. This can aid circulation, especially in cases of edema (swelling). However, the cumarin content in Parsley is minor, and balanced by its many other nutrients. So it does not come with the side effects known for wayfarin and other isolated anti-coagulants.

Multiple studies show that Parsley (Petroselinum crispum) contains significant anti-inflammatory properties, boosts liver health, is antioxidant and even anti-carcinogenic. It also supplies numerous nutrients and relaxes smooth muscles.

Research from Germany's University of Rostock (Schröder *et al.* 2017) studied parsley root extract. They tested the extract against malignant and benign breast cancer cells.

The researchers found the parsley extract killed the breast cancer cell lines at a rates ranging from 70 percent to 80 percent.

This and other research has connected parsley's apigenin to cancer inhibition. Apigenin is a flavone. A study from Texas A&M University (Lim *et al.* 2016) found that apigenin from parsley inhibited the growth of uterine cancer cells.

Research from China's Jiangsu Polytechnic College of Agriculture and Forestry (Liu *et al.* 2011) found that apigenin also blocked the action of MEK kinase 1, which in turn prevented bladder cancer cells from migrating and thus inhibited tumor growth.

Hungarian researchers (Pápay *et al.* 2012) confirmed that parsley boosted the body's ability to fight inflammation.

The research found that parsley contained numerous nutrients and bioactive constituents, including several flavonoids and cumarins. They found that in addition to its anti-cancer properties, Parsley slows inflammation and neutralizes oxidative radicals (free radicals).

Parsley's ability to encourage healing has also been shown in other studies. For example, a study from Turkey's Hacettepe University Faculty of Medicine (Tavil *et al.* 2012) found that increased parsley consumption was associated with fewer complications after hematopoietic (bone marrow) stem cell transplantation in children.

In this study, the diets of 41 children who underwent the stem cell transplantation were analyzed. Improved outcomes were seen among those eating more Parsley, as well as those children who ate onions, bulgur, yogurt and bazlama (a Turkish yeast bread).

Furthermore, Denmark's Institute of Food Safety and Toxicology (Nielsen *et al.* 1999) conducted a study on 14 people using parsley. In two study periods, the subjects included about four milligrams of parsley every day for one of two weeks.

The researchers found that taking Parsley boosted levels of erythrocyte glutathione reductase and superoxide dismutase in the subjects. These two enzymes increase detoxification efforts of the body, as they help remove oxidization agents that can harm tissues and blood vessels.

The antioxidant nutrients in parsley have been shown in other research to reduce the oxidation of lipids, relating directly to vision disorders, heart disease, dementia and other inflammation-related conditions.

Cumin Seed

Cuminum cyminum has a long history of use among European and Asian herbalists. It is described as antispasmodic and carminative, so it tends to soothe inflammatory responses. Like Fennel, Cumin has been used traditionally to ease abdominal cramping and gas.

Cumin seed contains mucilage, gums and resins. Traditional herbalists consider these constituents primarily responsible for Cumin's ability to help strengthen the mucosal membranes. This makes Cumin part of a strategy to rebuild the mucosal membranes of the airways.

Dandelion

Dandelion species include *Taraxum officinale, Taraxum mongolicum,* and *Taraxum spp.* Dandelion's role is not directly pulmonary, but rather, a strong supporting herb to purify the blood, restore the liver and reduce inflammation and hypersensitivity.

Dandelion contains hundreds of active constituents, which include beta-carboline alkaloids, beta-sitosterol, boron, caffeic acid, calcium, coumaric acid, coumarin, four steroids, furulic acid, gallic acid, hesperetin, hesperidin, indole alkaloids, inulin, iron, lupenol, lutein, luteolin, magnesium, mannans, monoterpenoids, myristic acid, palmitic acid, potassium, quercetins, rufescidride, sesquiterpenes, silicon, steroid complexes, stigmasterol, syringic acid, syringin, tannins, taraxacin, taraxacoside, taraxafolide, taraxafolin-B, taraxasterol, taraxasteryl acetate, taraxerol, taraxinic acid beta-glucopyranosyl, benzenoids, triterpenoids, violaxanthin, vitamin A, Bs, C, D, K and zinc among others (Hu and Kitts 2003; Hu and Kitts 2004; Seo *et al.* 2005; Trojanová *et al.* 2004; Leu *et al.* 2005; Kisiel and Michalska 2005; Leu *et al.* 2003; Michalska and Kisiel 2003; Kisiel and Barszcz 2000).

Taraxum is derived from the Greek words *taraxos* meaning 'disorder' and *akos* meaning 'remedy.' Dandelion is a common weed with a characteristic beautiful yellow flower that assumes a globe of seeds to spread its humble yet incredible medicinal virtues. Its hollow stem is full of milky juice, with a long, hardy root; and leaves that taste good in a spring salad. Dandelion is one of the most well known traditional herbs for all sorts of ailments that involve toxicity within the blood, liver, kidneys, lymphatic system and urinary tract. Dandelion has been listed in a variety of herbal formularies around the world for many centuries.

Dandelion's use was expounded by many cultures from the Greeks to the Northern American Indians—who used it for stomach ailments and infections. It is also used for the treatment of viral and bacterial infections as well as cancer.

The latex or milky sap that comes from the stem has a mixture of polysaccharides, proteins, lipids, rubber, and metabolites such as polyphenoloxidase. The latex has been used to heal skin wounds and protect those wounds from infection—also the sap's function when the plant is injured. For this reason, Dandelion can significantly increase mucosal membrane health.

Dandelion is known to stimulate the elimination of toxins and clear obstructions from the blood and liver. This is thought to be why Dandelion helps clear stones and scarring from kidneys, gallbladder and bladder. It has also been used to treat stomach problems, and has been used to reduce blood pressure.

In ancient Chinese medicine, it has been recommended for issues related to the imbalance between liver enzymes and pancreatic enzymes. It has been used in traditional treatments for hypoglycemia, hypertension, urinary tract infection, skin eruptions, breast cancer, appetite loss, flatulence, dyspepsia, constipation, gallstones, circulation problems, skin issues, spleen and liver complaints, hepatitis and anorexia.

Probably the best indication of Dandelion's purifying benefits is its ability to reduce leukotrienes—the inflammatory mediators that indicate a situation of toxicity. Laboratory testing has showed that leukotriene production is significantly decreased with an extract of Dandelion (Kashiwada *et al.* 2001).

Dandelion also inhibits other inflammatory mediators. A study by researchers at Canada's University of British Columbia (Hu and Kitts 2004) found that Dandelion extract suppressed the inflammatory mediator prostaglandin E2 (PGE2) without causing cell death. Further tests indicated that COX-2 was inhibited by the luteolin and luteolin-glucosides in Dandelion.

In another study by Hu and Kitts (2005), inflammatory nitric oxide levels were inhibited. Reactive oxygen species—free radicals—were also significantly reduced by Dandelion—attributed to the plant's phenolic acid content. This in turn prevented lipid peroxidation—a mechanism in heightened LDL (bad cholesterol) levels and artery inflammation.

In a 2007 study from researchers at the College of Pharmacy at the Sookmyung Women's University in Korea (Jeon *et al.* 2008), Dandelion was found to reduce inflammation, leukocytes, vascular permeability, abdominal cramping, pain and COX levels among exudates.

Dandelion also supports probiotic survival. Dandelion was found to stimulate fourteen different strains of bifidobacteria—important components of the intestinal immune system (Trojanová *et al.* 2004).

Another study found that Dandelion extract significantly prevented cell death in Hep G2 (liver) cells, while stimulating TNF and IL-1 levels—illustrating its ability to boost immunity and liver health (Koo *et al.* 2004).

This was also illustrated in research showing that Dandelion increases the liver's production of superoxide dismutase and catalase, increasing the liver's ability to purify the blood of toxins and allergens (Cho *et al.* 2001).

Other studies have illustrated that Dandelion inhibits both interleukin IL-6 and TNF-alpha—both inflammatory cytokines (Seo *et al.* 2005).

Dandelion has also illustrated the ability to inhibit inflammatory IL-1 cytokines (Kim *et al.* 2000; Takasaki *et al.* 1999), and the ability to stimulate the liver's production of glutathione (GST)—an important antioxidant needed to clear the system of mucous and toxins (Petlevski *et al.* 2003).

Evening Primrose

Another herb known by traditional herbalists to be beneficial for allergic skin responses is Evening primrose, or *Oenothera spp*. The seeds are rich in gamma-linolenic acid (GLA)—a fatty acid known to slow inflammatory responses of prostaglandins, especially those relating to skin hypersensitivity. The oil from Evening primrose can be applied directly onto the skin and/or taken internally. Evening primrose oil has thus been used successfully in cases of allergic eczema, for example.

Fennel

Foeniculum vulgare contains anetholes, caffeoyl quinic acids, carotenoids, vitamin C, iron, B vitamins, and rutins. Ayurvedic and traditional herbalists from many cultures have used Fennel to relieve digestive discomfort, gas, abdominal cramping, bloating and irritable bowels; and to treat inflammation. Fennel stimulates bile production. Bile digests fats and other nutrients, increasing their bioavailability.

One of Fennel's constituents, called anethole, is known to suppress pro-inflammatory tumor necrosis factor alpha (TNF-a). This inhibition slows excessive immune response. The combination of anethole and antioxidant nutrients such as rutin and carotenoids in Fennel also strengthen immune response while increasing tolerance.

Fennel is not appropriate for pregnant moms, because it has been known to promote uterine contractions. As with any herbal supplement, Fennel should be used under the supervision of a health professional. Those with birch allergies should also be aware that they may also be sensitive to Fennel. (The same goes for Cumin, Caraway, Carrot seed and a few others).

Mallow

Malva silvestris is a close relative of the *Malva verticillata* herb used in the Chinese Ravas Napas remedy mentioned earlier.

Mallow grows throughout Europe and has had an extensive and popular reputation among Western and Middle Eastern traditional medicines as a demulcent herb: It soothes irritated tissues. Mallow contains polysaccharides, asparagine and mucilage—which stimulates a balance among the body's mucosal membranes. The leaves are typically used.

The mucilage is primarily composed by polysaccharides. These include beta-D-galactosyl, beta-D-glucose, and beta-D-galactoses.

Mallow has been used for sore throats, heartburn, dry sinuses, and irritable bowels.

This herb has also been used in decoctions by European herbalists for allergic skin responses and eczema. For this reason, Swiss doctors during the World Wars would apply mallow compresses onto skin rashes with good success.

Mallow's leaves, flowers and roots are all used. It is an emollient and demulcent, rendering the ability to soften and coat, while stimulating healthy mucous membranes around the body.

Marsh Mallow

Althaea officinalis, has similar properties and constituents as the *Malva verticillata* L (Mallow). It belongs in the same family, Malvaceaea, and has similar constituents.

Marsh mallow has also enjoyed an extensive and popular reputation among traditional medicines around the world. This is because it contains mucilage, which supports and stimulates a healthy mucosal membrane.

For this reason, Marsh mallow is considered a demulcent: it's leaves soothe irritated sore throats, heartburn, dry sinuses, and irritable bowels.

The leaves, flowers and roots are all used in healing. Marsh mallow is known to be emollient, which gives it properties that soften and coat practically any membrane within the body, including the sinuses, throat, stomach, intestines, urinary tract and of course, the airways.

The root of the Marsh mallow will contain up to 35% mucilage. It also contains a variety of long-chain polysaccharides. Extracts use cold water, so they dissolve the mucilage without the starches. For this reason, tea infusions for drinking and gargling using Marsh mallow often use cold water overnight, although it can also be steeped for 15-20 minutes using hot water.

Mullein

The leaves, flowers and herbs of *Verbascum theapsiforme* and *V. philomoides olanum* have been part of the traditional herbalist repertory for thousands of years. It is classified as a demulcent and expectorant, because it is known to soothe irritated airways and help clear thickened mucous.

Mullein's soothing and demulcent properties are due primarily to its mucilage content, which can be as high as 3%. Other constituents include saponins, which are believed to produce the expectorant properties of this herb.

Mullein has thus been used for centuries for inflammation including respiratory conditions, skin irritations and ear infections. In all these cases, its effects have been considered soothing to epithelial cells.

Pine Bark Extract

Traditional herbalists have used pine bark extracts for respiratory conditions for centuries. The process of extraction is complex, however. Pine bark contains numerous constituents that yield health benefits, but also contains a high-density tannin complex requiring careful purification.

Today's standard for pine bark extracts is an extract of French Maritime Pine (*Pinus pinaster*) called Pycnogenol®. This extract is produced using a process patented by the Swiss company Horphag Research, Ltd. The process renders a number of bioavailable procyanidolic oligomers (PCOs), including catechin and taxifolin, as well as several phenolic acids.

Pycnogenol® has undergone extensive clinical study and laboratory research. Today, Pycnogenol® has been the subject of nearly 100 human clinical studies, testing over 7,000 patients with a variety of conditions. This extract's unique layered proanthocyanidin content has been shown, among other things, to significantly reduce systemic inflammation.

For example, in a German study (Belcaro *et al.* 2008), Pycnogenol® lowered C-reactive protein levels—known to increase during systemic inflammation and allergies—after 156 patients were given 100 milligrams of Pycnogenol® or placebo for three months. The average CRP decrease went from 3.9 to 1.1 following the treatment period. This is a 354% reduction in this important systemic inflammation marker after only three months of use.

In a study from the National Research Institute for Food and Nutrition in Rome, Italy (Canali *et al.* 2009), 150 milligrams of Pycnogenol® were given to six healthy adults for five days. After the five days, blood tests showed that Pycnogenol® interrupted the genetic expression of 5-lipoxygenase (5-LOX) and cyclooxygenase-2 (COX-2). It also inhibited phospholipase A2 (PLA2) activity. The Pycnogenol® supplementation program also reduced leukotriene production and altered prostaglandin levels. As discussed earlier, COX-2 and 5-LOX production is tied to inflammation processes.

Pycnogenol® also reduces histamine, another critical systemic inflammatory mediator as we've discussed. Researchers from Ireland's Trinity College (Sharma *et al.* 2003) found that Pycnogenol® inhibited the release of histamine from mast cells. The researchers commented that this effect appeared to be the result of the significant bioflavonoid content of Pycnogenol®.

Pycnogenol® has also been shown to reduce and inhibit NF-kB by an average of 15%. NF-kB is involved in the expression of inflammatory leukotrienes, as well as adhesion molecules. The matrix metalloproteinase 9 (MMP-9) enzymes known as conducive to inflammatory responses, is also reduced by Pycnogenol® (Grimm *et al.* 2006).

The bottom line is that Pycnogenol®, an extract bark of the French maritime pine tree, has been shown not only to reduce systemic inflammation in general through the radical scavenging abilities of procyanidolic oligomers.

Red Algae

Red algae—from the *Rhodophyta* family—have been used for thousands of years for inflammation-oriented conditions.

Researchers from the National Taiwan Ocean University (Kazłowska *et al.* 2010) studied the ability of the red seaweed *Porphyra dentata*, to halt allergic responses. The researchers found that a *Porphyra dentata* phenolic extract suppressed nitric oxide production among macrophages using a NF-kappa-Beta gene transcription process. This modulated the hypersensitivity immune response on a systemic level. The phenolic compounds within the Red algae have been identified as catechol, rutin and hesperidin.

We discuss red algae at length in the *Herbs for Pandemic Viruses* section of this book.

Mucilage Seeds

A number of seeds are helpful for calming inflammation and increasing the body's gentle purification systems. These include Flax, Safflower, Rapeseed, Caraway, Anise, Fennel, Licorice seed, Black seed and others. Seeds contain basic compounds that offer mucilage, saponins and other polysaccharides that contribute to the health of the mucous membranes.

Not surprisingly, combinations or single versions of these seeds have been used in traditional medicine for centuries.

Herbal Ointments and Inhalants

Certain herbal oils of these compounds can clear congestion and increase respiratory purification when rubbed on the chest and neck. Herb-derived ointments that are applied to the skin of the neck and chest have been traditional treatments for chest congestion due to colds and bronchitis for thousands of years among traditional medicine cultures.

In the nineteenth and early twentieth centuries, these traditions were developed into commercial products, primarily as ointments containing menthol and camphor. They were eventually applied to vaporizers, chest rubs and in inhalants.

Camphor

Camphor oil is derived from the camphor tree, which is native to Asia and Japan. The tree will grow from 50 to 100 feet tall, and will live for many decades. The oil has been used for thousands of years throughout Asia and the Middle East for anointing, healing and embalming.

Camphor oil is steam-extracted from the tree's wood and roots. Its central constituents include camphene, eugenol, cineole, pinene, phellandrene, limonene, terpinene, cymene, terpinolene, sabinene, furfural, safrole, linalool, terpinen, caryophyllene, borneol, piperitone, geraniol and cinnamaldehyde, among others.

This extensive list of components illustrates the complexity of camphor. It thus has many properties. It is considered anti-inflammatory, antiseptic, analgesic, carminative, diuretic, rubefacient and stimulating.

Camphor has been used traditionally for coughs, bronchial infections, colds, muscle pain and arthritis. It is either rubbed onto the skin, put into a compress or vaporized with steam. It is not consumed internally. Some consumed herbal formulations have utilized camphor oil, but these have only very tiny portions of camphor. Care must be taken by breastfeeding mothers applying camphor on the chest not to allow the baby to consume any.

Camphor research has typically concentrated on ointments formulated with camphor and menthol.

Eucalyptus

Eucalyptus is a large fragrant genus of trees that have primarily come from Australia, although they have been migrating to different regions over the past few hundred years. Today, California and many Pacific Rim countries are now home to eucalyptus species, as is the Mediterranean, Africa and many parts of Asia. The tree's bark and leaves are a source of a medicinal sap known for its decongestant and anti-inflammatory properties.

Eucalyptus oil is derived from this sap, and it is the 1.8-cineol called eucalyptol—a monoterpene—that is the key constituent of eucalyptus oil. Eucalyptol has been shown to suppress arachidonic acid metabolism as well as inhibit cytokine release from monocytes.

Research scientists from the University of Cincinnati College of Medicine (Yadav *et al.* 2017) studied the ability of eucalyptus oil to prevent the spread of the mycobacteria that causes tuberculosis.

The researchers tested the oil and its primary compound, eucalyptol (1,8-cineole). They tested these against a similar bacteria called Mycobacterium smegmatis. This mimics the spread of the TB mycobacterium. The researchers utilized lung cells in the laboratory to duplicate lung infections.

The researchers found that the eucalyptus oil helped the cells counteract becoming infected by the mycobacterium.

Research from the University of Illinois' College of Pharmacy (Ramos *et al.* 2014) also found that eucalyptus essential oil can be used to stop the spread of tuberculosis from those who are contagious.

The researchers tested essential oil from the Eucalyptus citriodora – also called Corymbia citriodora – with airborne tuberculosis. The researchers found that the essential oil significantly inhibited the spread of airborne tuberculosis using eucalyptus essential oil with inhalation therapy.

The researchers then quantified 32 different anti-tuberculosis constituents – medicinal compounds that included eucalyptol, spathulenol, linalool, citronellol, isopulegol, terpineol, eudesmol, cadinol and others.

This is not that surprising a result because eucalyptus essential oil has been found to be significantly antibacterial. A study from Germany's Heidelberg University (Mulyaningsih *et al.* 2011) found that Eucalyptus essential oil from the Eucalyptus globules fruit was found to be significantly antibiotic against methicillin-resistant Staphylococcus aureus.

One of the main compounds found in this oil included aromadendrene at 31 percent. The scientists found the eucalyptus leaf oil was not as antibiotic as the fruit essential oil.

In a study from Italy's SOC Microbiology and Virology Clinic (Camporese *et al.* 2013), researchers found the Eucalyptus smithii was strongly antibiotic against biofilms of Staphylococcus aureus and Pseudomonas aeruginosa.

Having some eucalyptus essential oil with us when we are traveling is a good idea that may help us prevent an infection. We can apply some to a tissue and lay the tissue in our close presence. We can also apply some to our skin, but applying eucalyptus essential oil onto our skin should be done with caution, and preceded by first applying a small test drop.

Mints and Menthol

The plants of the mint family include Peppermint (*Mentha piperita*), Watermint (*Mentha aquatica*), Spearmint (*Mentha spicata*), Pennyroyal (*Mentha pulegium*) and several others. They have a variety of common constituents, of which menthol is the most applicable to respiratory issues. Other active constituents of many mints will include menthylacetate, menthone, mentofuran, limonene, cineole, isomenthol, neomenthol, azulenes and rosmarinic acid.

Mint is well-known for its ability to settle digestion and ease flatulence. These effects are due to azulene's ability to relax the smooth muscles around the intestines. Azulene also relaxes the smooth muscles around the airways as well. Note that Chamomile also contains azulene.

Menthol is most known for its ability to clear congestion and expand the airways. It is the expectorant property of menthol that produces this effect. Menthol reduced coughing in a study from Britain's Leicester University Hospitals (Kenia *et al.* 2008) of 42 children.

It should be mentioned that all the mints make delicious herbal teas, a great addition to any breakfast or after-dinner beverage.

Anti-inflammatory Herbal Spices

A number of other herbs also contain anti-inflammatory properties. These work in different ways, and while they may or may not specifically modulate food sensitivities, they can help strengthen the immune system and stimulate our purification processes. Here is a quick overview of some of the most well-known (and most available) of these anti-inflammatory herbs:

Basil

Scientists are confirming that Basil and Holy Basil (*Ocimum sanctum*), has numerous health and medicinal benefits, including boosting the immune system.

Research from the All India Institute of Medical Sciences (Mondal *et al.* 2009) tested 24 healthy people. They gave either a placebo or 300 milligrams of Tulsi each day for four weeks. After the treatment period, those who were given the Tulsi leaf extract showed significantly more T-helper cells, more natural killer cells, and increased IL-4 – indicative of a stronger and more vibrant immune system.

A number of studies have investigated Basil's ability to reduce infections due to bacteria. Much of this antibacterial character of Basil is due to eugenol. Eugenol has undergone study in other venues as a proven antimicrobial substance. For example, a study from Brazil's University Federal de Alfenas (de Souza *et al.* 2015) found that eugenol was antimicrobial against Salmonella typhimurium and Micrococcus luteus – both infective bacteria.

A study from India's Calcutta School of Tropical Medicine tested extracts of Holy Basil against antibiotic-resistant strains of Salmonella Typhi and found the Tulsi significantly reduced these strong contagious bacteria. They stated in their conclusion:

"O. sanctum is potential in combating S. typhi drug resistance, as well promising in the development of non-antibiotic drug for S. typhi infection."

This antibacterial quality of Holy Basil supports the clinical experience of Ayurvedic doctors of ancient times that used Tulsi for conditions related to numerous bacteria infections, including intestinal issues, lung conditions, skin infections and eye infections.

Research from India's Annamalai University found that a whole leaf extract of Holy Basil significantly reduced lipid and protein oxidation. The researchers found that Tulsi exhibited superior antioxidant properties but also lowered phase I enzymes that are found in peroxidation metabolism. The extract also increased the phase II enzymes – which tend to balance and moderate oxidative stress.

Another study from India's DVS College of Arts and Science found that two different extracts of Holy Basil was able to significantly reduce lipid peroxidation activity in a dose-dependent manner.

Research from India's Sharma Post Graduate Institute of Medical Sciences fed rabbits 2 grams of Tulsi leaves for 30 days. After the period, the rabbits showed significantly reduced levels of glutathione and superoxide dismutase – indicating they had reduced levels of oxidative stress.

This ability of Tulsi to reduce oxidative stress is often referred to as an adaptogen. This means that it helps the body cope with the stresses that burden our bodies from various fronts – whether it be physical, chemical, emotional or otherwise.

A couple of studies have investigated Tulsi's ability to halt or treat liver damage. Both studies showed Holy Basil had a positive effect on the liver's health. These and other researchers have thus described Holy Basil as "hepatoprotective."

Research from the All India Institute of Medical Sciences tested 24 healthy people. They gave either a placebo or 300 milligrams of Tulsi each day for four weeks. After the treatment period, those who were given the Tulsi leaf extract showed significantly more T-helper cells, more natural killer cells, and increased IL-4 – indicative of a stronger and more vibrant immune system.

Another study showed that Tulsi stimulated the increase in monocytes – THP-1. This is another sign of a stronger immune system.

Basil contains ursolic acid and oleanolic acid, both shown in laboratory studies to inhibit inflammatory COX-2 enzymes.

Garlic

(*Allium sativum*) probably deserves a larger section, but that information could easily encompass a book in itself—as was well documented by Paul Bergner: *The Healing Power of Garlic* (1996). Garlic is an ancient medicinal plant with a wealth of characteristics and constituents that stimulate the immune system, protect the liver, purify the bloodstream, reduce oxidative species, reduce LDL lipid peroxidation, reduce inflammation, and stimulate immunity systems throughout the body. This is supported by a substantial amount of rigorous scientific research.

Garlic is also one of the most powerful antimicrobial plants known. A fresh garlic bulb has at least five different constituents known to inhibit bacteria, fungi and viruses. Much of this antimicrobial capability, however, is destroyed by heat and oxygen. Therefore, eating freshly peeled bulbs are the most assured way to retain these antimicrobial potencies.

Diallyl trisulfide is a key active compound of garlic, and it is commonly extracted from garlic oil. Other research has found both garlic and diallyl trisulfide to have antimicrobial effects against a variety of infective agents, including both bacteria and fungi. Garlic has also been shown to reduce cholesterol and reduce the risk of thrombosis – the major cause of strokes and heart attacks. Garlic has also been shown to inhibit the growth of other types of cancer cells.

Researchers from Australia's University of Western Australia (Lissiman *et al.* 2014) analyzed 146 people given either a garlic supplement – standardized to 180 milligrams of allicin – or a placebo for 12 weeks. The research found that the placebo group in total had 65 common cold occurrences while the garlic group only had 24 occurrences. This is less than half the number of colds.

Furthermore, when those who were taking the garlic supplement did catch a cold, that cold lasted an average of one day shorter than the colds among the placebo group – some 20-25% shorter.

Another study, from the University of Florida (Nantz *et al.* 2012) tested 120 people. They gave half of the group 2.5 grams per day of an aged garlic extract supplement. The rest were given a placebo. Over a six month period, the garlic group had 61 percent fewer number of days of colds, and 58 percent had few incidences of colds, along with 21 percent fewer cold symptoms when they did catch a cold.

In a 2017 study published in the International Journal of Oncology, scientists (Ling *et al.* 2017) tested a garlic extracted constituent against leukemia cells. The study utilized the extracted compound called diallyl trisulfide, and applied it to human U937 leukemia cells within a laboratory tissue system. The researchers found that diallyl trisulfide stopped the growth and expansion of leukemia cells in the laboratory.

The researchers also tested the compound against growing leukemia systems, and against found that it beat down the leukemia cells and prevented the further growth of the cancer.

Cooked or dehydrated garlic powder also has a variety of powerful antioxidants, but fewer antibiotic abilities of raw garlic.

Garlic is also a tremendous sulfur donor as well. The combination of garlic's antibiotic, antioxidant, anti-inflammatory and immune-building characteristics make it a *must* spice-herb-food for any inflammatory condition.

Oregano

Origanum vulgare contains at least thirty-one anti-inflammatory constituents, twenty-eight antioxidants, and four significant COX-2 inhibitors (apigenin, kaempherol, ursolic acid and oleanolic acid).

Rosemary

Rosmarinus officinalis contains ursolic acid, oleanolic acid and apigenin—a few of the many constituents in this important botanical—shown to inhibit inflammatory enzymes in laboratory studies. Research has also shown that rosemary's volatile oils can halt airway constriction by inhibiting mast cell degranulation.

Adding anti-inflammatory spices to meals

It should be noted that there is a great difference between a spice dose and a therapeutic dose. A therapeutic dose of one or more of these spices will typically be larger than a spice dose. The sign of a therapeutic dose of these spices within a dish is when the spice can be readily tasted. That is, the pungent flavor of the spice stands out in the food. If the amount of spice simply flavors the food a little, then it will probably not be enough to stimulate any immune response. If the spice can be specifically tasted (for example, *"that dish tastes garlicy"* or *"tastes peppery"*) then the spice will likely be enough to stimulate a therapeutic response.

That said, if multiple spices are used, the dose of each spice can be smaller. After all, the meal should also taste good. This, however, is why traditional Chinese and Indian food is so spicy. The recipes come from therapeutic traditions.

Another element of the therapeutic dose is consistency. It is not enough to have one or more of these spices once a week with a particular dish. The spice(s) should be added to at least one meal every day.

In addition, care must be taken to protect therapeutic spices from degradation. This can occur when spices are left in the light or sun for an extended period, or when spices are left open to oxygen. Often spices are left in kitchen racks exposed to the lights of the kitchen and window, or left in unsealed containers or shakers. Oxygen and light degrade the biochemical constituents that give these spices their therapeutic properties.

This latter point is likely one of the main reasons our culinary spices cannot be considered therapeutic. Leaving the spice exposed can take place during processing, packaging and shipping; as well as in the kitchen. Therefore, we should consider purchasing our therapeutic spices from a bulk herb store, or from suppliers or brands that respect their therapeutic nature.

By far the best way to consume or add these foods to our diet is in their fresh form. Many of these herbs can be grown in our garden or purchased from a local farmers' market or grocery store as fresh. As discussed earlier, fresh foods maintain more bioactive nutrients. This is because their beneficial constituents are naturally sealed within the food's peel, shell or cell walls.

Note also that these anti-inflammatory herbal spices (and most of the other natural products contained in this chapter) will typically not stimulate a therapeutic response immediately. Depending upon the status of our immune system, it may take weeks or months before the daily dosing of these natural elements is seen in the form of strengthening our immunity and reducing our toxin levels.

Other Anti-Inflammatory Herbs

The list does not end here. Still other herbs have been used among traditional medicines throughout the world to reverse the toxic, inflammatory metabolism. Many of these are not direct pulmonary herbs, but rather, serve to purify the blood, strengthen the liver, strengthen the adrenals, strengthen the immune system and inhibit inflammation.

Comfrey, Aloe and **Slippery elm,** for example, aid the health of the mucosal membrane with their high mucilage and mucopolysaccharide content—while **Cayenne, Nutmeg** and **Goldenseal** stimulate the body's immunity processes to clear catarrh.

In addition to these bronchial herbs, there are herbs that relax the muscles and support the nervous system in general. This is a common formulation strategy used by herbalists. These types of herbs are called nervines, and they include **Chamomile, Tulsi, Hops, Wild lettuce** and **Skullcap.**

Here are more common anti-inflammatory herbs that are readily available in spice form, herbal tea form or in our garden:

> ➤ Aloe (*Aloe vera*)
> ➤ Anise (*Pimpinella anisum*)
> ➤ Cayenne (*Capsicum* spp.)
> ➤ Chamomile (*Matricaria chamomilla*)
> ➤ Comfrey (*Symphytum officinale*)
> ➤ Green Tea (*Camellia sinensis*)
> ➤ Guggul (*Commiphora mukul*)
> ➤ Lemongrass (*Cymbopogon citratus*)
> ➤ Nutmeg (*Myristica fragrans*)
> ➤ Slippery elm (*Ulmus fulva*)
> ➤ Stinging Nettle (*Urtica dioica*)
> ➤ Thyme (*Thymus serphyllum*)
> ➤ Tulsi (*Ocimum gratissimum*)
> ➤ Wild onion (*Hymenocallis tubiflora*)

There are certainly many more gentle herbs we can to this collection. But these are certainly good candidates to consider for one's garden, tea or spice cupboard.

Dosage and Usage Considerations

As mentioned, most of the herbs mentioned here, with the exception of essential oils, are safest when used as *infusions.* An infusion is simply the steeping of the fresh or dried root, bark, leaf, seed, stem or fruit in water. In the case of most herb leaves and stems, the water is brought to a boil, and the herb can be steeped for 5-10 minutes using a strainer or tea-ball. In the case of most roots, seeds and barks, the root can be steeped a little longer, for 10-20 minutes, depending on the herb. In some cases a seed, root or bark is better when it is soaked overnight in room temperature water.

It is suggested that any herb not readily known be taken as a tea or as a spice in a food following some consultation with an herbalist or medical professional. This is especially the case if we are under the care of a doctor for any reason—in such a case, the doctor should be consulted that we are trying some new spices or herbal teas.

Before we leave this topic let's focus on a few conditions that illustrate the success of herbal medicines.

Antiviral Herbs for Colds, Flu and Herpes

The immunostimulatory effects of probiotics have also been observed among some of the most frequent ailments known to humankind, including rhinovirus (colds), influenza virus (flu), rotavirus (intestinal infection) and even herpes infections.

Viral influenza is now an important topic among medical experts, with the advent of the H1N1 swine flu epidemic that is threatening millions of people. While some have quoted statistics that from 25,000 to 35,000 people die each year of influenza, upon closer examination, well over 90% of those actually are elderly persons who die of pneumonia. Whether the flu or pneumonia is the official cause of death, the reason for these deaths is an overburdened and weakened immune system, not necessarily the flu or pneumonia itself.

Furthermore, despite valiant efforts by so many researchers over many decades, the "cure for the common cold" still eludes modern medicine. For most immune systems, this virus is not such a problem, because we typically can get over a cold within a few days. However, for those who are immunosuppressed, a simple cold can easily turn into pneumonia and other respiratory infections. In fact, many elderly people die from infections that began with a simple cold or the flu as mentioned above.

We are now faced with more risk of virulent influenza and other infectious outbreaks due to transcontinental flights and world travelers.

Researchers from South Korea's Konkuk University (Bae *et al.* 2019) tested three herbs that have been used in traditional Asian medicines to counteract the flu. These are:
   – Brassica juncea (also called brown mustard)

– **Forsythia suspensa (also called forsythia or Lian Qiao)**
– **Inula britannica (also called British yellowhead)**

The researchers made extracts from the three herbs and tested these in the laboratory against influenza infections including H1N1 in tissue cultures. The researchers found that B. juncea (the brown mustard) extracts significantly reduced viral infection. The British yellowhead herb also showed antiviral properties in the study.

These confirmed that the traditional use of at least two of these herbs for influenza were substantiated as being truly antiviral.

Another study from China's Northwest A&F University confirmed the antiviral activity of two herbs used traditionally for influenza – one also studied above. In this study, researchers determined that two medicinal herbs known for clinical success in influenza treatment, and at least fifty phytochemicals contained in them, can inhibit the growth of the flu virus.

The researchers tested Forsythia or Lian Qian (Forsythia suspensa) as studied above, as well as Lonicera japonica (also called Suikazura, Jinyinhua and Japanese Honeysuckle).

The researchers exposed these herbs and their constituents to influenza viruses and human cells within a laboratory setting.

The researchers found that these two herbs, and fifty of their constituents – phytochemicals that were isolated from them – significantly inhibited the replication of the viruses. This study follows other research concluding similar findings with other herbs.

The researchers' findings have unveiled a new dimension among the phytochemicals that nature produces within certain medicinal herbs. This has to do with a two-pronged effect:

1) The ability of these herbs and their phytochemicals to stimulate the body's own immunity, allowing the body to be able to more effectively fight off the infection;

2) The ability of the independent constituents within the herbal medicine to shut off a virus' ability to replicate, even in a sterile environment outside the body.

Clinical research (Yoshino et al. 2019) has supported that the Japanese herbal formulation called **Maoto** can significantly reduce the duration and fever of the flu. A review of research from Japan's Keio University School of Medicine found 12 clinical studies that measured the effectiveness of Maoto against the flu.

The researchers concluded that Maoto significantly reduced fevers and flu duration.

In one of these studies, from Japan's Ohmura Hospital in Chiba (Yoshino et al. 2019) 150 patients with influenza A completed a study whereby the Japanese medicinal combination called Maoto was found to significantly reduce symptoms and influenza duration as compared to those taking Oseltamivir or Zanamivir or patients not receiving any treatment.

The research found that those patients given the Maoto had an average duration of 33 hours, versus 70 hours in the patients given no treatment, versus 61 hours among those patients treated only with Oseltamivir. The marginally shortest flu duration was among those patients given both the Maoto and Oseltamivir, at 31 hours.

Researchers from Japan's Fukuoka University (Toriumi *et al.* 2012) also found that Maoto reduces the duration of influenza.

The researchers randomly gave 28 adults with influenza either the Maoto herbal medicine, or one of two neuraminidase inhibitor pharmaceutical drugs found to reduce influenza duration.

The Japanese herbal combination – taken in granule form – reduced the average flu duration from its typical four to five day duration down to an average of 29 hours. Because the subjects had contracted influenza symptoms within 48 hours of the study, the maximum mean duration totaled about three days, with the average at about two days.

The two neuraminidase inhibitor drugs, known also for reducing influenza duration – but can accompany side effects including vomiting and nausea – had average durations of 43 and 27 hours respectively.

The Maoto herbal treatment caused no side effects and was characterized as "well tolerated."

The Japanese Maoto combination is composed of **Ma Huang (Ephedra), Apricot Kernel, Cinnamon Bark and Licorice** – also called Glycyrrhiza Root. Each of these herbs have been clinically utilized in different combinations by Traditional Japanese and Chinese Medical doctors for stimulating immunity and inhibiting viruses. Ayurveda has also utilized these herbs for boosting the immune system.

Another clinical study found similar results with another plant, Napal smartweed (Polygonum nepalense. Smartweed is also known for effectively treating influenza. The researchers found that six polyphenols within the herb that effectively reduced infective inflammation. These include kaempferol, glucopyranoside, quercetin, pyrogallol, gallic acid and epipinoresinol.

We add to this the Native American legend of Lomatium dissectum. According to the legend, Ernst Krebs, M.D. of Carson City observed that the Washoe Indians of Nevada seemed to recover quickly and avoid the 1918 Spanish Flu plague by taking an herbal medicine called "Toh-sa."

Dr. Krebs named it Balsamea, as it smelled like balsa. It was later named Leptotaenia dissecta and then Lomatium dissectum by botanists.

Consistent with this legend, the root of Lomatium dissectum was tested for antiviral activity at Canada's University of British Columbia (McCutcheon *et al.* 1995). The Lomatium was found to inhibit the "cytopathic effects" of rotavirus.

Lomatium is only one herb from one traditional medicine among hundreds of herbs and hundreds of traditional medicines around the world. The effective inhibition of influenza by fifty constituents isolated from the two herbs in the new laboratory study from China illustrate that there are many anti-influenza herbal medicines, even besides the Maoto combination. Many of the fifty anti-influenza constituents found in Fructus forsythiae and Lonicera japonica also occur in other herbal medicines.

A Cochrane Review of Research from the Beijing University of Chinese Medicine (Chen *et al.* 2011) found among 26 studies that several Chinese herbal medicines "demonstrated a positive effect on fever resolution, relief of symptoms, and global effectiveness rate" for influenza. The research concluded, however, that more clinical research was necessary to confirm certainty.

These herbs studied present only the tip of the iceberg among herbs that have been used among various traditional medicines around the world. There are a variety of herbs that are known to stimulate immunity, giving the immune system a stronger ability to fight off various infections.

What about probiotics? Can probiotics help stave off viral infections such as influenza? The answer lies in the ability of probiotics to specifically stimulate the immune system and attack foreigners.

The evidence from these and other scientific studies from Japan and China considerably advance the level of certainty that herbal medicine can be used successfully to fight the flu.

Herbs for Pandemic Viruses

There are a number of viruses that are unique in that they have the potential to become pandemics. The prominent viruses that have this ability include SARS-CoV-2 coronavirus (COVID-19), SARS-CoV (Severe acute respiratory syndrome), MERS (Middle East respiratory syndrome) and Ebola (Ebola haemorrhagic fever). Other potential contagious viruses include the H1N1 virus, HIV/AIDS and others.

There have been several outbreaks of Ebola, primarily in Africa. After two 1996 Ebola outbreaks in Gabon Africa, medical scientists determined that Ebola causes death among about 70 percent of those who contracted the virus. Since then there have been several other outbreaks. The largest broke out in West Africa between 2013 and 2016. This outbreak caused over 28,000 cases and over 11,000 deaths.

The first outbreak led researchers from Gabon's Franceville International Center of Medical Research to investigate. The questions ensued: Why don't the other 30 percent die? How do 30 percent of those infected recover?

Furthermore, medical researchers found many instances where there were close contacts of those who became infected who never were infected at all. Even though they were in contact with the infected patient while the patient was symptomatic.

Note: An infected patient with Ebola must be symptomatic in order to be contagious – with fever and other flu-like symptoms. A person must also have direct contact with body fluids of an infected person in order to become infected with the virus. This means contact with saliva, urine, semen or blood – which can include contact with needles or other contaminated objects.

Thus, when the researchers investigated "close contact" individuals, they focused upon those who had this sort of exposure.

The research found that nearly half of those who were asymptomatic and seemingly immune developed antibodies (IgM and IgG) to the Ebola virus. This means these individuals certainly were intimately exposed to the virus, but simply naturally developed the immunity tools – including those discussed below – that prevented the infection from replicating out of control.

Severe acute respiratory syndrome (SARS) – more specifically SARS-CoV. SARS is an outbreak that began in China in 2002, infecting people through 2004. More than 700 people died worldwide of SARS.

In 2014, the new Middle East respiratory syndrome coronavirus (MERS-CoV) killed 92 people and infected at least 238 people in Middle Eastern countries, Malaysia and the Philippines.

Both of these viruses are Beta-C coronaviruses, and both produce severe acute respiratory syndrome. And like SARS, some reports have suggested that there is a 50% risk of death for someone in an advanced stage of the condition.

COVID-19 is a second generation SARS coronavirus (SARS-CoV-2) originated in China according to most sources. This is truly a pandemic, as it has infected and killed millions of people around the world.

Sequencing of the virus has determined it to be 75 to 80 percent match to SARS-CoV and more than 85 percent similar to multiple coronaviruses found in bats.

Researchers from the Wuhan Institute of Virology published a paper on January 23, 2020. Their paper informs that COVID-19 has a 96 percent genome match with a bat coronavirus.

They also stated that COVID-19 utilizes the same cell entry receptor as the SARS-CoV of 2002-2004. The receptor is ACE2. We'll discuss the importance of this later.

The elderly have been most at risk of the infection. Fatalities among healthy people and younger people have been lower. This is similar to SARS, though it appears COVID-19 is less lethal than SARS and MERS. About 15 to 20 percent of cases can become severe. The rest are mild and recovery takes between a few days to two weeks.

The COVID-19 virus, just as was SARS and MERS, is an enveloped virus. This means the virus is protected by a glycoprotein shell, with spikes. This is why these viruses are so difficult to treat.

Red algae

An anti-viral extract has been found from the New Zealand red alga species, Griffithsia sp. This protein is called Griffithsin, abbreviated with GRFT.

Griffithsin has proven to fight SARS and MERS infections. Red algae Griffithsin has also proven to be antiviral against HIV-1 (human immunodeficiency virus), HSV-2 (Herpes simplex virus), HCV (Hepatitis C) and the Ebola virus.

What do these viruses have in common? Along with COVID-19, they all have glycoprotein shells around them. According to doctors at the University of California at Davis:

"Griffithsin is a marine algal lectin that exhibits broad-spectrum antiviral activity by binding oligomannose glycans on viral envelope glycoproteins."

The researchers are discussing what is also called a mannose-binding lectin. Mannose-binding lectins have been shown to penetrate and break down the shells that surround this class of viruses – which includes COVID-19 virus.

The red algae extract above was found in the Griffithsia species of red algae. This is not the only species of red algae that contains mannose-binding lectins.

Another mannose-binding lectin found to be antiviral against these viruses is the Scytonema varium red algae, also called Scytovirin. Another one was found in the Nostoc ellipsosporum algae species – called Cyanovirin-N.

A study from France's Institute of Research and Development (Barre *et al.* 2019) tested a number of other species, and found the Ulva pertusa algae species contained lectins that fight these viruses. They also found the Oscillatoria agardhii blue-green algae halt the replication of these viruses.

A study from the University of Louisville School of Medicine (Barton *et al.* 2016) also studied Griffithsin and found it also inhibited SARS-CoV as well as HIV and similar viruses. The researchers wrote:

"These findings support further evaluation of GRFT [Griffithsin] for pre-exposure prophylaxis against emerging epidemics for which specific therapeutics are not available, including systemic and enteric infections caused by susceptible enveloped viruses."

Studies have found that these mannose-binding lectins break down the glycoprotein shells of the viruses mentioned above, including Ebola and SARS. A number of animal tests and human cell laboratory tests have shown that these mannose-binding lectins are successful in halting replication of the virus.

Harvard researchers (Michelow *et al.* 2011) tested a recombinant version of Griffithsin – called rhMBL – against Ebola. Once again, they found the mannose-binding lectins were able to not only breakdown the viral shells of the Ebola, but when given to mice infected with Ebola, the mice became immune to the virus.

In a study on mice with Ebola, researchers found that Griffithsin halted not only replication, but made mice immune to the virus. Similar results were found with SARS and MERS infections.

A study from New York's Center for Biomedical Research (Alam *et al.* 2018) tested the effectiveness of Griffithsin against enveloped viruses. The researchers found that Griffithsin extracts from red algae inhibited HIV infections, HPV (human papillomavirus) and herpes simplex-2 viruses. The researchers also found that Griffithsin protected monkeys from HIV and mice from being infected with HSV-2.

Multiple studies illustrated these effects. Research from the Center for Cancer Research in Frederick, Maryland found that Griffithsin not only stopped HIV-1 virus replication, but stopped cellular intrusion of the virus.

This means that Griffithsin – from red algae – could make an effective vaccine of sorts.

Griffithsin extract is currently being pursued by commercial interests looking for a long term patent with a pharmaceutical model. Thus, this product is not available commercially at this time.

Red algae is a supplement that can be purchased in health food stores and online. Most of the commercial supplements labeled red algae utilize the Gigartina species of red algae (such as Gigartina skottsbergii). This species has been tested against HSV and HIV in laboratory testing, but not on CoVs to date.

These studies indicate that the ability to break down the glycoprotein shell of these enveloped viruses is also a feature of the Gigartina red algae.

Licorice root

Licorice root (Glycyrrhiza spp.) has been used for thousands of years for lung infections with similar symptoms as viral infections.

This is now being confirmed in the research. For example, scientists from Sun Yat-sen University in China studied the antiviral potential of licorice and its triterpenoids. They found that several triterpenoids in licorice can provide "broad-spectrum antiviral medicine."

Their research found glycyrrhizic acid, glycyrrhizin, glycyrrhetinic acid and their derivatives to inhibit viruses that include SARS coronavirus, herpes, HIV, hepatitis, influenza.

We have also published evidence that licorice root (Glycyrrhiza glabra) can fight SARS and MERS CoV infections. Studies have found that licorice root extracts were able to reduce SARS and MERS-CoV replication.

A study from the UK's Luton & Dunstable Hospital NHS Foundation Trust tested licorice root extracts against a number of viruses, including HIV and SARS. They found that the extract broke down the viral envelope and also boosted immune activity.

The researchers stated the research:

"revealed antiviral activity against HIV-1, SARS related coronavirus, respiratory syncytial virus, arboviruses, vaccinia virus and vesicular stomatitis virus."

For the mechanisms, the researchers stated,

"Mechanisms for antiviral activity of Glycyrrhiza spp. include reduced transport to the membrane and sialylation of hepatitis B virus surface antigen, reduction of membrane fluidity leading to inhibition of fusion of the viral membrane of HIV-1 with the cell, induction of interferon gamma in T-cells, inhibition of phosphorylating enzymes in vesicular stomatitis virus infection and reduction of viral latency."

Confirming their findings, researchers from Italy's University of Padua (Fiore *et al.* 2008) studied the mechanisms of licorice for viral respiratory tract infections. They found that licorice showed antiviral action against SARS related coronavirus, respiratory syncytial virus by increasing cell membrane protection against the virus, increasing T-cell activity to fight the virus and helping to prevent a latency – or the ability of the virus to hide from the immune system and resume its attack later.

In 2003 – when the SARS virus was in full infection swing around the world – scientists from Frankfurt University Medical School (Cinatl *et al.*) tested licorice's central antiviral constituent, glycyrrhizin in a study that was published in the British Medical Journal Lancet.

The researchers tested glycyrrhizin along with three conventional antiviral medications on infected cells from two SARS-infected individuals who were admitted into the Frankfurt University clinic. In fact they tested two different infective types of SARS coronavirus: FFM-1 and FFM-2.

Along with glycyrrhizin the researchers tested ribavirin, 6-azauridine, pyrazofurin and mycophenolic acid. Remember, ribavirin was recently tested against MERS in monkeys.

The researchers found that the glycyrrhizin provided the strongest effects against the virus compared to the other medicines. More importantly, they found that glycyrrhizin prevented replication of the SARS-CoV.

Often deglycyrrhizinated licorice (DGL) is recommended for ulcers and other digestive conditions. But in the case of licorice's antiviral properties, deglycyrrhizinated licorice will likely not confer these antiviral abilities. This is clarified by the evidence linking glycyrrhizin to licorice's antiviral properties.

Antiviral plant lectins

In the *Immunity Diet* section of this book we discuss *Lectin Foods*. These are foods that contain mannose-binding lectins. As we discuss in that section, a number of studies have shown that plants that contain mannose-binding lectins can significantly stimulate the immune system and help prevent a number of viral infections.

Another promising form of mannose-binding lectins is a component of the Scytonema varium red algae called Scytovirin. The protein extract was isolated by researchers from the National Cancer Institute at Frederick, Maryland (Bokesch *et al.* 2003). The protein contains 95 amino acids, and was found to bind to HIV-1 viral shells.

A similar antiviral protein was found in Nostoc ellipsosporum – called Cyanovirin-N. Both of these antiviral proteins did similar things – they broke down the glycoprotein shells of HIV and HCV.

Immune Stimulating Mushrooms

Edible and medicinal mushrooms offer a significant tool to boost our immunity. We can include delicious mushrooms like Shiitake, Buttons or Chanterelles into our dishes, and we can also take mushroom supplements with Reishi (*Ganderma lucidum*), Hoelen (*Wolfiporia extensas*), Maitake (*Grifola frondosa*), Shiitake (*Lentinula elodes*), Turkey Tails (*Coriolus versicolor or Trametes versicolor*), Agaricus (*Agaricus blazei*), Cordyceps (*Cordyceps sinensis*) and Lion's Mane (*Hericium erinaceus*). All of these significantly stimulate the immune system, and their constituents bind to toxins within our bodies.

The Agaricus species is the most popular eating mushroom, and this species contains the button mushroom. But there are many, many others. Scientists have cataloged some 50,000 mushrooms, and identified less than 20,000 different mushroom species. Some estimate there may be over 150,000 mushroom species within the Fungi kingdom, which likely encompasses more than 1.5 million total species. Biologists have described less than 5% of Fungi species.

Over 600 mushroom species have been documented to stimulate the immune system. However, the ones mentioned above have received the most attention. Research on these mushrooms have revealed their effects as being antimicrobial, cholesterol-lowering, anti-inflammatory, anti-oxidant, anti-mutagenic, anti-tumor, adaptogenic and immunostimulating.

Cancer has been a significant area of research. A number of these mushrooms have been shown to inhibit cancer cell line growth, for example. American researchers were awakened by Dr. Tetsuro Ikekawa's groundbreaking epidemiological study showing significantly lower cancer rates among Japanese mushroom growers between 1972 and 1986. The research since then has shown significant anticarcinogenic properties among most of the mushrooms mentioned above. While most clinical research to date has been adjunctive to conventional therapies for ethical reasons, human studies have consistently confirmed animal and laboratory models. By August of 2008, there were 4,087 mushroom studies and scientific papers filed with the U.S. National Library of Medicine.

These mushrooms are incredible radical scavengers. For example, lion's mane mushroom has been shown to reduce the risk of Alzheimer's and senility. The mushroom appears to stimulate nerve growth factor, a substance that has can reduce dementia and benefit Alzheimer's patients.

A immune-boosting compound called AHCC—Active Hexose Correlated Compound—has been is derived from shiitake mushroom and their sub-species. This has been shown to stimulate the activity of white blood cells. Further research showed they stimulated interferon (IFN-y) and tumor necrosis factor (TNF-a) as well.

Much of the dramatic immunity effects of mushrooms are due to their polysaccharides and polysaccharide-protein complexes. Laboratory research has isolated multiple polysaccharide types within each species. Twenty-nine unique polysaccharides have been isolated in Maitake, for example.

Mushroom polysaccharides are primarily glucans with different glycosidic linkages, including 1->3 and 1->6 beta glucans, and 1->3 alpha glucans. The complex branching and even helical nature of mushroom glucans appears to be significant. Schizophyllan polysaccharides with (1,3)-b-glucans with 1,3-b-d-linked glucose with 1,6-b-d-glucosyl side groups have been described as "stiff triple-stranded" helices in laboratory research, for example. Schizophyllan (SPG) is an active macrophage stimulator, increasing T cell and NK cell activity and inhibiting various infective agents.

Various immunostimulatory effects have been also attributed to polysaccharide-protein complexes such as PSK (krestin), PSP, lentinan and others. While many varieties contain different levels of the various beta glucans, many researchers believe it is their unique protein sequencing that differentiates effects among species.

Medicinal mushrooms also contain a variety of nutrients. Many mushrooms contain significant amounts of protein. Shiitake can be as much as 17% protein while oyster mushrooms can be 30% protein by weight. Several also contain vitamin B complexes. Most edible mushrooms also contain a variety of macro-minerals and trace elements. Shiitake also can contain as much as 126 mg of calcium, and 247 mg of magnesium per serving, for example. Reishi also contains magnesium, calcium, zinc, iron, copper and trace minerals. Many are good sources of selenium.

Maitake and a number of other mushrooms also contain ergosterols (provitamin D2), along with phosphatidylcholine and phosphatidylserine. Shiitake, Reishi and Maitake have been known to increase from less than 500 IU of D2 in indoor growing conditions to 46,000 IU, 2760 IU, and 31,900 IU respectively, following six to eight hours of sunlight exposure (Stamets 2005).

Various anti-oxidants have been isolated among popular mushroom varieties. Constituents such as ganoderic acid (*G. lucidum*), cordycepic acid (*C. sinensis*), linzhi (*G. frondosa*), agaric acid (several), sizofilan and sizofiran (*S. commune*), galactomannan (*C. sinesis*), and various triterpenoids (several) can actively reduce oxidative radicals and stimulate the immune system.

The density of these in mushrooms is quite incredible. Reishi has over 100 ethanol-soluble triterpenoids. Most of these are antioxidant, and many are anti-inflammatory agents.

Some of the mechanisms of mushrooms to safely stimulate the immune system and produce long-term cleansing benefits are quite complicated. For example, differently branched beta glucans have been observed stimulating immune cells in different ways. For example, certain beta glucans from Maitake will stimulate T-cell production, while differently bonded-chain beta glucans from *Agaricus blazei* stimulate natural killer (NK) cells. Others stimulate B-cells, T-helper cells, lymphokine activated killer cells [LAK], macrophages; and the cytokines interferon gamma, interleukin-2, -12 and tumor necrosis factor [TNF].

Mushrooms significantly detoxify heavy metals inside our bodies, and in their natural environments. Their proteins will bind to certain heavy metals within the soil. These same metabolites become active within the body when eaten, and thus help chelate minerals in our bodies.

For this reason, Cordyceps, reishi, *Agaricus blazei* and maitake have been used in China to treat heavy metal and radiation poisoning.

Mushrooms that aid the liver

When the liver is damaged by toxins such as alcohol, pharmaceuticals, preservatives, pesticides and other toxins, liver cells begin to produce enzymes such as aspartate aminotransferase (AST) and alanine aminotransferase (ALT) in an attempt to heal and remove the toxins. As liver cells become more damaged, fibrosis can occur, which can progress to a complete shutting down of the liver.

A number of studies have shown that extracts from a number of medicinal and edible mushrooms reduce the levels of these enzymes in liver damage situations, and help bring about a healthier liver. Let's look at a few of these.

A study from the Fujian Academy of Agricultural Sciences (Chen *et al.* 2018) studied the ability of **Reishi (Ganoderma lucidum)** to help protect the liver. The researchers found that a number of polysaccharides from Reishi protected against oxidative damage to the liver. Reishi reduced liver enzymes. Reishi also boosted the liver's antioxidant status and provided protection against the liver.

A study from India's National Institute of Technology at Manipur (Wangkheirakpam *et al.* 2018) found that the Auricularia delicata mushroom significantly protected against liver damage from acetaminophen.

In a study from Turkey's Osmangazi University (Soares *et al.* 2013) researchers tested **Agaricus brasiliensis and Phellinus linteus** on alcoholic liver damage. The Agaricus brasiliensis mushroom decreased ALT liver enzyme levels.

Panus giganteus – also called Pteropus giganteus with a common English name of Indian Flying Fox, part of many Malaysian, Chinese, and Indian recipes – was found to reduce AST and ALT levels at similar rates as a standardized extract of Silymarin (Milk Thistle's active liver constituent). In this study, the mushroom was tested against liver injury caused by the drug thioacetamide (Wong *et al.* 2012).

In another study– this from Japan's Osaka University – found that two different fractions of **Shiitake** (hot-water extraction and ethanol extraction) not only decreased AST and ALT levels, but also inhibited the formation of collagen fibrils – which produce liver fibrosis (Akamatsu *et al.* 2004).

According to these studies and others some of the more productive medicinal mushrooms in terms of reducing liver damage include:

- **Lentinula edodes (also known as Shiitake)**

- Cordyceps
- Agaricus blazei
- Ganoderma lucidum (also known as Reishi)
- Ganoderma tsugae (Tsugae Reishi)
- Pleurotus cornucopiae (Oysters)
- Panus giganteus
- Agaricus brasiliensis
- Auricularia delicata

Mushrooms and Influenza

A steady stream of research has confirmed that medicinal mushrooms have antiviral properties. A number of these studies have shown that many medicinal mushrooms can indeed inhibit the influenza virus. In other words, many mushrooms fight the flu.

Agaricus brasiliensis

Researchers from Japan's Azabu University (Eguchi *et al.* 2017) tested the Agaricus brasiliensis against the PB8 strain of influenza A. This is an H1N1 virus. The researchers found that an extract of this mushroom significantly inhibited the influenza strain in a dose-dependent manner.

Dose-dependency means there is a direct association between the mushroom and the inhibition of the flu. The researchers also found the mushroom extract somehow blocked the virus after it invaded cells.

The researchers concluded: "These results demonstrated that it is expected that AE can effectively prevent the spread of the influenza virus."

Confirming this, a 2016 review of research from Russia's State Research Center of Virology and Biotechnology Vector studied the antiviral activity of Agaricomycetes mushrooms, which includes Agaricus brasiliensis. The researchers did confirm the ability of wild mushrooms of this family of mushrooms to inhibit the influenza virus.

Oyster mushroom mycelia

Researchers from Japan's Shinshu University (Kojima *et al.* 2015) found that oyster mushroom mycelia accumulate a substance called shikimic acid. Shikimic acid is a material used to produce the anti-flu drug Tamiflu (oseltamivir). (Mycelia are the underground rooting system of mushrooms.) The researchers concluded that this natural substance gives oyster mushrooms the ability to fight the influenza virus.

Aureobasidium mushroom

Research from Japan's Aureo Science (Muramatsu *et al.* 2012) established that an extract from the mushroom fungus Aureobasidium pullulans significantly inhibits influenza.

The researchers found that the active constituents were the beta-D-glucans and the beta-glycosides of the extract. These have been determined in other research to significantly stimulate the immune system, also giving many mushrooms the reputation of being able to help fight cancer.

In this study, the researchers tested the mushroom extract against the highly contagious and virulent H1N1 influenza strain A (Puerto Rico/8/34). The researchers found that the extract significantly inhibited influenza.

Seven other mushrooms inhibit influenza

A study from Russia's State Research Center of Virology and Biotechnology Vector (Teplyakova *et al.* 2012) tested 11 mushroom species that grow in the Altai Mountains of Russia against two different strains of type A influenza: The H5N1 virus type A (chicken/Kurgan/05/2005) and the H3N2 type A human virus (Aichi/2/68).

The research found that seven of the eleven species of mushrooms provided antiviral activity against these influenza strains.

The researchers found that the antiviral mushrooms were:

- **Trametes versicolor (also called Turkey Tail)**
- **Daedaleopsis confragosa (also called Blushing Bracket and Rauhe Tramete)**
- **Datronia mollis (also called Mazegill)**
- **Ischnoderma benzoinum (also called Benzoin Bracket)**
- **Trametes gibbosa (also called the Lumpy Bracket)**
- **Laricifomes officinalis (also called the Agarikon)**
- **Lenzites betulina (also called the Birch Mazegill)**

Influenza mushroom vaccine

Scientists from Japan's National Institute of Infectious Diseases (Ichinohe *et al.* 2010) found that mycelial extracts from medicinal mushrooms worked so well against influenza that they developed an influenza vaccine adjuvant using the mushroom extracts.

In laboratory studies, they found that a mycelial mushroom extract from the Phellinus linteus mushroom (also called Meshimakobu in Japan and Sang Huang in China) significantly stimulated the body's HA-specific

IgA and IgG antibody responses, and boosted cytokines specific to fighting influenza.

The researchers concluded:

"The use of extracts of mycelia derived from edible mushrooms is proposed as a new safe and effective mucosal adjuvant for use for nasal vaccination against influenza virus infection."

Other flu-fighting mushrooms

Researchers from China's Shandong University of Traditional Chinese Medicine (Wang *et al.* 2011) found that extracts of **Ganoderma lucidum (also called Reishi), Cordyceps militaris, Kuehneromyces mutabilis (also called Woodtuft), Inonotus hispidus (also called Hairy Bracket) and Rhodocollybia maculata (also called Spotted Toughshank)** inhibited influenza in mice studies. The researchers commented that the mushrooms "may provide prophylactic protection against influenza infection via stimulation of host innate immune response."

Researchers from Japan's Sugitani Department of Oriental Medicine (Obi *et al.* 2008) studied an extract from the Grifola frondosa (Maitake) mushroom on the Influenza A virus on canine kidney cells.

The researchers found that the Maitake extract significantly inhibited the virus from replicating, and stimulated the production of antiviral cytokines such as TNF-alpha.

Mushrooms and Cancer

Over three decades of laboratory and clinical research have established that a number of medicinal mushrooms work in a myriad of ways to help our bodies naturally fight cancer.

The science shows that medicinal mushrooms are not all alike. They each work a little differently. Nonetheless, the research does find that most of these medicinal mushrooms help boost the body's own immunity, along with working to kill or weaken cancer cells.

We should note that due to their care for patients, medical researchers are reluctant to test cancer patients by only treating them with mushroom extracts. Most of the research has therefore treated patients with mushroom therapy alongside conventional chemotherapy and/or radiotherapy (radiation).

This is logical, since chemotherapy and radiotherapy have received intensive research focus and have been dramatically improved over the past two decades. Survival rates have therefore increased for these therapies.

At the same time, these therapies are also still wrought with side effects. They also tend to severely depress the immune system. Both of these provide a segue for the use of mushroom therapy in cancer treatment alongside conventional therapy.

At the same time, we should appreciate that mushroom therapy has come a long way over the past three decades. Not so long ago, treating cancer patients with mushroom extracts was unheard of by Western researchers. That left all the research on mushrooms mostly in the territory of laboratory research on human cancer cells or animals.

This preliminary research has yielded significant success. But as some of the research has moved to humans, it has been found that there is a definite place for mushroom therapy in cancer treatment.

But this is only the beginning of this human research. So much more is necessary. It behooves us to encourage medical researchers to put more focus on medicinal mushrooms and their extracts. Yes, it is difficult to patent a natural compound. But we're talking about helping people here, right? Isn't that the goal of medical science? Or at least, shouldn't it be?

For this reason, what you'll find in the research below is a mix of adjunctive clinical research and a summary of some of the laboratory research. Note that in most cases, this follows tens of previous laboratory studies on any of these mushrooms and their extracts.

My focus is to present you the current progress of the science of anticancer mushroom therapy research.

Please note that I will be adding additional species of mushrooms to this article in the weeks ahead. Therefore you might consider returning to this post to read about more anticancer mushrooms.

Here is a summary of the latest medical research on medicinal mushrooms.

Split-gill Mushroom (Schizophyllum commune)

The Split-gill mushroom has been tested clinically and in the laboratory for decades. One of its main anti-cancer compounds is Hydrophobin SC3. In 2013, researchers from The Netherlands injected this compound into growing tumors in the laboratory. The researchers found that after 12 days of daily injections, the compound suppressed the growth of the tumors. This was facilitated by the boosting of natural interleukin-10 and TNF-alpha levels, which naturally fight tumor growth.

Another anti-cancer compound from Split-gill is Schizophyllan. In a 2015 study, researchers from the Chinese Academy of Agricultural Sciences tested Schizophyllan against human breast cancer cells. They found the compound fights tumor growth for breast cancer.

Split-gill mushrooms have also been tested clinically. In a 1991 study, Tokyo's Cancer Institute Hospital tested 40 patients, with 15 cervical cancer patients with benign tumors. Prior to surgery, they administered 20 milligrams of sizofiran, also called SPG – a schizophyllum glucan. After 8 days of injections, the researchers found the patients who received the injections had boosted immune markers such as helper-T cells and IL-2.

In a 1995 study from Japan's Kumamoto University School of Medicine, 312 patients with cervical cancer were tested. In 90 patients given the SPG compound along with radiotherapy, their 5-year survival rates were significantly longer than those of a group of 82 patients treated with radiotherapy alone.

Furthermore, another 60 cervical cancer patients given the sizofiran along with chemotherapy had significantly better 5-year survival rates than those who had chemotherapy alone. And 244 cancer patients who were given the sizofiran compound showed boosted natural anticancer immunity such as CD8+ and CD4+ T-cells.

Huaier (Trametes robiniophila)

The Huaier mushroom has been used in Chinese Medicine for almost two thousand years. The mushroom has been found to help treat liver cancer, breast cancer, stomach cancer, ovarian cancer and others in laboratory research. Studies have shown it helps kill cancer cells, helps prevent tumors, helps inhibit tumor growth, reduces chemo side effects, and activates the immune system.

In a 2018 study, researchers found that a water extract of Huaier inhibited human prostate cancer cell growth. In a 2017 study, researchers found Huaier significantly inhibited cancer growth on human stomach cancer cells. The researchers found it reduced MMP expression while boosting immune markers.

In a 2016 study, researchers tested Huaier against human liver cancer cells. They found the extract inhibited tumor growth potential in this laboratory study.

Similarly, a 2016 study on human breast cancer cells found Huaier extract inhibited tumor growth.

Yunzhi (Coriolus versicolor)

C. versicolor has been tested for more than three decades. Lab and clinical testing finds it boosts the body's natural immunity (including cytokines IL-1, IL-2, IL-6, IL-8, TNF-α, and TNF). The results indicate that the mushroom improves cancer survival.

In a 2017 study from the National Cancer Center in Sinapore, researchers tested 15 acute liver cancer patients who were unable to receive other treatment. Those given the C. versicolor extract did not appear to reduce the disease progression of the patients. But it did significantly increase the quality of live for those patients. Those given the mushroom extract had reduced pain and less appetite loss as a result of the mushrooms.

Other clinical studies have shown even better results. A 2003 study tested 34 patients with non-small cell lung cancer. Part of the group took a PSP extract from Coriolus versicolor for 28 days. The researchers found the extract improved symptoms and improved immune cell counts, along with boosted IgG and IgM. The mushroom extract patients also showed reduced symptoms of disease progression.

A 2005 clinical study tested C. versicolor with 82 breast cancer patients for six months, following their conventional cancer treatment. The researchers found the PSP extract boosted anticancer immunity markers (such as CD4+, CD8_ and B-lymphocytes. They also decreased pro-cancer markers.

A 2013 clinical study on breast cancer patients found that the PSP extract significantly boosted anticancer immune cells. It also downgraded tumor-boosting mechanisms among the cancer patients.

A 1997 study from Japan's Kyushu University tested 224 patients with stomach cancer after they received surgery to remove the cancer. The patients were split into two groups and one group received the PSP extract for a year.

The research found the PSP group had longer survival rates and decreased recurrence rates. They also had lower recurrence rates compared to those who didn't receive the PSP extract.

Maitake (Grifola frondosa)

This ancient medicinal mushroom has been used for thousands of years and has undergone a tremendous amount of cancer research. It has been shown to stimulate anticancer macrophages, and boost the body's immunity against cancer. These include boosting leukocytes, IL-1, IL-6, and IL-8.

In a 2015 clinical study from New York's Memorial Sloan Kettering Cancer Center, researchers tested 21 patients with MDS (Myelodysplastic syndromes). MDS are a group of bone marrow-related cancers.

The researchers found that the Maitake extract boosted basal neutrophils and improved monocyte function. The researchers found the treatment to be beneficial in this relatively short study.

In a 2010 study, researchers tested 72 patients with polycystic ovary syndrome (PCOS). They gave the patients either a Maitake extract called MSX with or without chemo or the chemo therapy alone. The researchers found the mushroom extract boosted ovulation in a majority of the patients (77 percent and 93 percent), while the chemotherapy rates were much lower.

A 2008 study from the Memorial Sloan Kettering Cancer Center tested 34 breast cancer patients in a safety and tolerance study. They were given Maitake liquid extract for three weeks. The researchers found the mushroom extract boosted immune function among the patients. Increasing doses increased some function while depressing other immune function. The researchers noted further testing was required to better understand the extract's effects.

A 1999 clinical study tested 313 patients after being treated with bladder cancer. They were given either mitomycin treatment, Maitake extract, thiotepa chemo or served as controls. The patients were followed for up to 15 years. The researchers found that the control group had a 65 percent recurrence of the bladder cancer. This was compared to only 34.9 percent in the Maitake group. Those in the mitomycin group had a slightly higher recurrence rate, while the thiotepa chemo group had a 42 percent recurrence rate. The Maitake recurrence rate was the lowest, and nearly half of the control group.

A similar study from 1994 tested 146 bladder cancer patients, and found that tumor recurrence rates were 33.3 percent in the Maitake group, 34.3 percent in the conventional group and 65 percent in the control group.

Lentinula edodes AHCC

A series of studies led by Dr. Judith Smith from the University of Texas Medical School and the UT Health Science Center investigated a medicinal mushroom extract called AHCC. Dr. Smith heads up the Women's Health Integrative Medicine Research Program at the University of Texas. The program focuses on investigating the use of natural therapies for women.

AHCC stands for active hexose correlated compound. It is an extract from the mycelia of Shiitake mushroom (Lentinula edodes) along with other medicinal mushrooms. The mycelia is the root-like fingers that weave within the growing medium – whether soil or in the case of AHCC cultivation, within rice bran. Mycelia are like roots of mushrooms. In the wild, the tiny tenticles can spread for miles.

Dr. Smith and her associates conducted studies HPV in the laboratory, then on mice infected with HPV, and then a human study on women with HPV. The results of this study were presented at the 11th International Conference of the Society for Integrative Oncology in Houston.

In the human study, ten women who tested positive for HPV were treated with the mushroom mycelia extract called AHCC. The patients were given three grams (3,000 mg) of the AHCC once a day for at least six months. During that period, eight of the patients tested negative for HPV, including three that were confirmed eradicated after stopping the AHCC treatment.

Reishi (Ganoderma lucidum)

A study from Mexico's National Institute of Public Health and the National Autonomous University of Mexico (Hernández-Márquez *et al.* 2014) tested human cervical cells infected with human papillomavirus together with cervical cancer cells. The cells were tested variously with difference concentrations of Reishi (Ganoderma lucidum) mushroom extract (water extract) for 24 hours each. Different sources of Reishi mushrooms were also tested. One source was China, with two sources from Mexico.

After tested with nuclear DNA fragmentation, the researchers found that all three Reishi mushroom extracts inhibited the growth of the cancer cells and the HPV infection among the cells.

In a 2016 study from China's Xinjiang University, scientists tested an extract from the Ferulae mushroom (Pleurotus ferulae) on HPV cervical cancer. The researchers found the mushroom extract boosted the immune response to the HPV cancer cells and inhibited the cancer cells from growing.

Research from France's Medicine Information Formation conducted a study of 472 gingivitis patients who were swabbed and screened for Human Papillomavirus. They found that 61 of the patients were positive for either HPV16 or HPV18.

The HPV-positive patients were randomized and for two months 20 of these patients were treated with the medicinal mushroom species Laetiporus sulphureus. The other 41 patients were treated with a combination of Trametes versicolor and Reishi (Ganoderma lucidum).

After the two months, the researchers found that 88% of the 41 patients treated with Trametes versicolor and Reishi tested negative for HPV. In the other group, 5% tested negative for HPV.

Mushrooms can be eaten fresh, frozen, drank as teas, cooked with sauces or eaten as supplements. Parts used include the fruiting body (cap and stem) and the mycelia (colonizing rooting network).

While each form will stimulate our immune system, fresh or freeze-dried are preferable. Some supplements are hot-water extracted, and some are alcohol extracted. Hot water extracts likely retain more constituents, although alcohol can extract specific medicinal constituents as well.

Chapter Six

The Immunity Diet

Let's now consider how we can eat our way towards boosting our immune system. The foods that we will discuss in this section may also be taken as supplements in various forms, as well as foods. But we will categorize them as foods here to show how we can add these to our diet with little effort.

Probiotic Foods

We've discussed at length the benefits of consuming foods that naturally contain probiotics that augment our immune system. Here are a few probiotic foods (among many others) to consider adding to our diets:

Traditional Yogurt

Because yogurt is usually produced using *L. bulgaricus, S. thermophilus* and sometimes *L. acidophilus,* it is certainly a good source of probiotics. However, we should clarify again that pasteurization kills many probiotics. This means that commercial yogurts that pasteurize the yogurt after it has been cultured will have killed most or all of those colonies used to convert the milk to yogurt. Some producers pasteurize the milk first and then make the yogurt.

The best yogurt is made using raw milk. It is quite simple to make yogurt: After heating a pot of milk to 180 degrees F (82 C) momentarily, we can add a half-cup of starter (active yogurt from a previous batch or an active commercial yogurt) into the milk after it cools to about 105 degrees F (40 C). After stirring thoroughly, we can put the container in a warm, clean, dry place, with a clean towel or loose seal over the container. The mixture will sour and gel in about six to ten hours depending upon temperature. Then we can jar and refrigerate.

The ideal blend of probiotic species for a yogurt starter—one that was developed over the centuries by the Bulgarians—is a ratio of seven parts *S. thermophilus* to one part *L. bulgaricus.* This ratio produces the ideal sourness that is tasty yet tart. It also prevents the *L. bulgaricus* from outgrowing and overwhelming the *S. thermophilus.*

This later point is one of the reasons why yogurt starters that include *L. acidophilus* often fail to supply any *L. acidophilus* in the end product. *L. bulgaricus* is a hardy organism that will easily overtake *L. acidophilus* in a culture. The use of *L. acidophilus* in yogurt is not only wasteful, but possibly can result in an overly acidic flavor, as *L. bulgaricus* colonies swell with the lactic acid produced initially by *L. acidophilus*. In addition, it appears that *L. bulgaricus* produce small amounts of hydrogen peroxide—which knocks out the *L. acidophilus* colonies.

The moral of this also is not to expect much in the way of *L. acidophilus* in a commercial yogurt that blends *L. acidophilus* with *L. bulgaricus*.

Yogurt and other fermented dairy foods have little or no lactose. This is because the probiotics convert the lactose to lactic acid. The lactic acid is healthy for the intestinal tract, because it renders a medium that helps promote our own probiotic colonies. Lactic acid also offers a pleasing tart flavor to yogurt and other fermented dairy.

Traditional Kefir

Kefir is a traditional drink originally developed in the Caucasus region of what is now considered southern Russia, Georgia, Armenia and Azerbaijan. Here Moslem tribe leaders vigorously protected their kefir recipe, as it was considered an esteemed and regal food with healing properties. The secret recipe was eventually ransomed by a young beautiful female Russian emissary who was kidnapped by a local prince. She wrestled a few kefir grains from the secrecy of the prince's family as a settlement for her abduction. She brought kefir into the Moscow market shortly thereafter and it spread as a highly prized healing food all over Russia and Europe. Kefir also became a focus of Soviet research, discovering some of the surprising benefits of probiotics we have outlined in this book.

Kefir uses fermented milk mixed with kefir grains that resemble little chunks of cauliflower. One tablespoon of kefir grains can be mixed with whole milk and sealed in a jar at room temperature. The milk is fermented overnight in a warm location with the starter grains. Depending upon the temperature, milk and kefir grains, it will take 1-3 days to completely ferment. The jar should be opened and swirled one to two times a day. The grains are screened or filtered out and utilized for the next batch. Cow's milk is most used, but sheep's milk, goat's milk or deer milk can also be used.

Buttermilk

Buttermilk is a soured beverage that was originally curdled from cream. Traditional buttermilk utilized the acids that probiotic bacteria produce for curdling. Today, forced curdling is done using commercially available acidic products. Cream of tartar, lemon juice or vinegar is added to heated and stirred whole milk at a rate of one tablespoon per cup of milk, until the curdling starts. After standing for 15 minutes and stirring another 15, it is refrigerated. See the butter section for the traditional method.

Cultured Butter

Today commercial butter contains no probiotics. Traditionally, butter was made with the cow's natural probiotics. The raw milk sits for a half-day or day depending upon temperature, until the cream rises to the top. The cream is taken from the milk to be churned and aged; letting the probiotics convert lactose to lactic acid. This creates a mix of buttermilk and butter. The buttermilk is strained off, leaving the butter. The butter can be further dried of moisture and mixed with salt for taste. Again, the probiotics from the raw milk will have matured the butter and buttermilk naturally.

Cultured Cottage Cheese

Commercial cottage cheese is now made without probiotics. It was a probiotic process before dairy processors began to pasteurize the product and force the curdling with lactic acids. Again, probiotics also produce the lactic acids that were used to curdle the product in traditional cottage cheese making. Skim milk with cream and buttermilk is probably the easiest way to make cottage cheese at home today, using the curds off the cream separation. The probiotics arising from the buttermilk help curdle the thickened milk and cream before separating the curds. Salt is one of the secrets to making a tasty cottage cheese.

Korean Kimchi

Kimchi is a fermented cabbage with a wonderful history from Korea. Kimchi was considered a ceremonial food served to emperors and ambassadors. It also was highly regarded as a healing and tonic food. There are a variety of different recipes of kimchi, depending upon the region and occasion.

Kimchi can be made by slicing and mixing cabbage with warm water, salt, ginger, garlic, red pepper, green onions, oil and a crushed apple. It is then put into a sealed jar(s) at room temperature for 24 hours, before putting into the refrigerator to continue the fermenting process (*Lactobacillus kimchii* is a typical colonizer). After several weeks of continued fermentation in the fridge, it is ready for eating.

Japanese Miso

Miso is an ancient food from Japan. A well-made miso will contain over 160 strains of aerobic probiotic bacteria. This is because the ingredients are perfect prebiotics for these probiotics.

Miso is produced by fermenting beans and grains. Soybeans are often used, but other types of beans are also used. Equal parts soaked and cooked soybeans and rice are mixed. A fungi spore (koji, or *Aspergillus oryzae*) and salt is added to the rice prior to mixing. The mixture is put into a covered container in a dark, dry, room-temperature location and stirred occasionally. It can take up to a year of aging like this for the fermentation to result in a tasty miso.

When other beans other than soy are used, they will produce different varieties of miso. Shiromiso is white miso, kuromiso is black miso, and akamiso is red miso. They are each made with different beans. There are also various other miso recipes, many of which are highly guarded by their makers.

Japanese Shoyu

Shoyu is a traditional form of soy sauce made by blending a mixture of cooked soybeans and wheat, again with koji, or *Aspergillus oryzae*. The combination is fermented for an extended time. The aging process for shoyu is dependent upon the storage temperature and cooking methods used, and is also guarded.

Traditional Tempeh

Tempeh is an aged and fermented soybean food. It is extremely healthy and contains a combination of probiotics and naturally metabolized soy. Tempeh is made by first soaking dehulled soybeans for 10-12 hours. The beans are then cooked for 20 minutes and strained. The dry, cooked beans are then mixed with a tempeh starter containing *Rhyzopus oryzae, Rhizopus oligosporus* or both. The mixture is shaped and flattened (about a half-inch high) and put into a warm (room temperature) incubation container for a day or two. The cake will be full with white mycelium (fungal roots) when it is ready. It can then be eaten raw, baked, or toasted.

Other beans other than soy are also sometimes used to make tempeh. The trick is in getting good starter colonies.

Indian Lassi

Lassi is a traditional and popular beverage from India—once enjoyed by kings and governors in ancient India. It is quite simple to make, as it is made with yogurt, fruit and spices. Quite simply, it is a blend of diluted yogurt with fruit pulp—often mango is used in the traditional lassi. A little salt, turmeric and sweetener give it a sweet-n-salty taste. Other spices are also sometimes used. Sugar is often added in today's versions, but honey and/or fruit are preferable.

German Sauerkraut

Sauerkraut is a traditional German fermented food. It is made quite simply, by blending shredded cabbage and pickling salt (12:1, or 3 tablespoons of salt per five pounds of cabbage). The mixture is covered with water and put into a covered bowl or container. It is then stored in the dark in this semi-airtight cover for a month to two months at room temperature. Then it should be stored in the refrigerator in an enclosed container for a month or two to complete the fermentation of the cabbage. Probiotic bacteria such as *Lactobacillus plantarum* and *L. brevis* will typically overtake the early-growth bacteria during fermentation. This is a testament to the power of probiotics.

There are a number of other wonderful fermented foods that can be included into a probiotic-rich diet. This sampling illustrates the general techniques of fermentation. As we can see here, bacteria and fungi in our foods are not necessarily bad. To the contrary, if cultured correctly, they can be healthy for us, and may even help prevent infection from their more lethal cousins.

Most of these foods are traditional and even ancient foods that have been passed down through generations over thousands of years. This does not mean that we cannot be creative, however.

For example, there is a lot that can be done with yogurt. We've all heard of frozen yogurt, and certainly that is one. But yogurt in some cultures, such as among Indians, is eaten with every meal. It is eaten with and in salads, and rice dishes. Yogurt is creamy and delicious, and can make for an excellent salad dressing with a little oil and vinegar and dill. It can also be added to nearly every sauce to make the sauce creamy and delicious.

Kefir and lassi cultures can be added to nearly every combination of beverage, including smoothies and shakes.

Just about every vegetable can be pickled. Pickles using brine with probiotics is delicious and healthy. We can pickle peppers, olives and so many other foods.

Fermented beverages are now the rage among healthy foods. There are now many fermented beverages, including kombucha and others.

Raw vs. Pasteurized Milk

This naturally brings us to the topic of milk, since there are many reports that indicate that dairy may not be so healthy—and not conducive to detoxification processes.

To the contrary, numerous experiments have shown that raw milk, and dairy containing probiotics such as yogurt is not only healthy, but stimulates the immune system and fights off disease.

First let's consider a study by researchers at Switzerland's University of Basel (Waser *et al.* 2007). The researchers studied 14,893 children between the ages of five and 13 from five different European countries, including 2,823 children from farms, and 4,606 children attending a Steiner School (known for its farm-based living and instruction). The researchers found that drinking farm milk was associated with decreased incidence of allergies and asthma. Why?

Raw milk from the cow can contain a host of bacteria, including *Lactobacillus acidophilus, L. casei, L. bulgaricus* and many other healthy probiotics. Cows that feed from primarily grasses will have increased levels of these healthy probiotics. This is because a grass diet provides prebiotics that promote the cow's own probiotic colonies. Should the cow be fed primarily dried grass and dried grains, probiotic counts will be reduced, replaced by more pathogenic bacteria. As a result, most non-grass fed herds must be given lots of antibiotics to help keep their bacteria counts low. Probiotics, on the other hand, naturally keep bacteria counts down.

As a result, the non-grass fed cow's milk will have higher pathogenic bacteria counts than grass-fed cows. This means that the milk itself will also have high counts. When the non-grass-fed cow's milk is pasteurized, the heat kills most of these bacteria. The result is a milk containing dead pathogenic bacteria parts. These are primarily proteins and peptides, which get mixed with the milk and are eventually consumed with the milk.

In other words, pasteurization may kill the living pathogenic bacteria, but it does not get rid of the bacteria proteins. This might be compared to cooking an insect: If an insect landed in our soup, we could surely cook it until it died. But the soup would still contain the insect parts—and proteins.

Now the immune system of most people, and especially infants with their hypersensitive immune system, is trained to attack and discard pathogenic bacteria. And how does the body identify pathogenic bacteria? From their proteins.

In the case of pasteurized commercial milk, our immune systems will readily identify heat-killed microorganism cell parts and proteins and launch an immune response against these proteins as if it were being attacked by the microorganisms directly. This was shown in research from the University of Minnesota two decades ago (Takahashi *et al.* 1992).

It is thus not surprising that weak immune systems readily reject pasteurized cow's milk. In comparison, healthy cow raw milk has fewer pathogenic microorganisms and more probiotic organisms. This has been confirmed by tests done by a California organic milk farm, which compared test results of their raw organic milk against standardized state test results from conventional milk farms.

In addition, pasteurization breaks apart or denatures many of the proteins and sugar molecules. This was illustrated by researchers from Japan's Nagasaki International University (Nodake *et al.* 2010), who found that when beta-lactoglobulin is naturally conjugated with dextran-glycylglycine, its allergenicity is decreased. A dextran is a very long chain of glucose molecules—a polysaccharide. The dextran polysaccharide is naturally joined with the amino acid glycine in raw state. When pasteurized, beta-lactoglobulin is separated.

This is not surprising. Natural whole cow's milk also contains special polysaccharides called oligosaccharides. They are largely indigestible polysaccharides that feed our intestinal bacteria. Because of this trait, these indigestible sugars are called prebiotics.

Whole milk contains a number of these oligosaccharides, including oligogalactose, oligolactose, galactooligosaccharides (GOS) and transgalactooligosaccharides (TOS). Galactooligosaccharides are produced by conversion from enzymes in healthy cows and healthy mothers.

These polysaccharides provide a number of benefits. Not only are they some of the more preferred foods for probiotics: Research has also shown that they reduce the ability of pathogenic bacteria like *E. coli* to adhere to our intestinal cells.

These oligosaccharides also provide environments that reduce the availability of separated beta-lactoglobulin. This is accomplished through a combination of probiotic colonization and the availability of the long-chain polysaccharides that keep these complexes stabilized.

This reduced availability of beta-lactoglobulin has been directly observed in humans and animals following consistent supplementation with probiotics (Taylor *et al.* 2006; Adel-Patient *et al.* 2005; Prioult *et al.* 2003).

It is not surprising, given this information, that people with many conditions have benefited from withdrawing from pasteurized milk and cheese. Raw milk, yogurt, kefir, goat's milk and cheese, along with soy and almond milk, are great alternatives.

What About Casein and Beta-lactoglobulin?

In a number of studies, the milk protein casein has been shown to be implicated in a number of conditions, including cancer (Campbell and Campbell 2006).

In addition, beta-lactoglobulin has been implicated in allergies.

For example, Japanese researchers (Nakano *et al.* 2010) found that casein and beta-lactoglobulin were the main allergens in cow's milk—as confirmed by other research. They also found that 97% of 115 milk allergy children had casein-specific IgE antibodies, while 47% had IgE antibodies against beta-lactoglobulin (beta-LG).

However, fermented dairy and probiotic-rich raw dairy presents an altogether different casein and beta-lactoglobulin molecular structure than does pasteurized milk.

When milk is heated to extremely high degrees, the surfaces of casein micelles—minute fat globules about 100 nanometers in diameter—become harder, and more stable. They move within the fluid but remain in a highly rigid state. Other molecules within the milk do not affect these casein micelles. Thus, the consumption of these rigid casein micelles results in a macromolecule—large protein the body does not easily break down.

However, when dairy is fermented, these casein molecules become destabilized by the probiotics. Once a particular acidity is reached in the milk culture, the casein molecules will become sticky, and they will become congealed—observed as "curdling."

As this curdling takes place—driven by the conversion of lactose to lactic acid by probiotic bacteria—an interesting combination occurs. The destabilized casein micelles react with the beta-lactoglobulin whey protein, which produces a *beta-lactoglobulin-kappa-casein complex*. This neutralizes both the effects of separated beta-lactoglobulin molecules and the casein micelles within the body. In other words, both of these proteins—which spawn radicals in the body—become neutralized through the enzymatic processes driven by probiotic bacteria.

As this occurs, another whey protein, called lactoferrin, also undergoes degradation. This process liberates an immune-stimulating derivative called lactoferricin. This lactoferricin released during the degradation of lactoferrins is also produced by probiotic bacteria, most notably *Streptococcus thermophilus* and *Lactobacillus delbrueckii* ssp. *bulgaricus* (Paul and Somkuti 2010).

Thus we find that these whey-casein components and their derivatives create an altogether different combination of elements than pasteurized milk. They also maintain known antimicrobial components such as lactoferricin and other bacteriocins.

Prebiotic Foods

One of the most important factors in establishing a healthy environment for our probiotic colonies is making sure they have the right mix of nutrients available. The nutrients our probiotic families favor are called prebiotics. In other words, some foods are particularly beneficial for *bifidobacteria, lactobacilli* and other probiotic populations. These are the oligosaccharides, fructooligosaccharides, galactooligosaccharides, and transgalactooligosaccharides—also referred to as inulin, FOS, GOS and TOS. Even two or three grams of one of these prebiotics will dramatically increase probiotic populations assuming healthy colonies. Inulin, FOS, GOS and TOS are also antagonistic to toxic microorganism genera such as *Salmonella, Listeria, Campylobacter, Shigella* and *Vibrio*. These and other pathogenic bacteria tend to thrive from refined sugars as opposed to the complex saccharides of inulin, FOS, GOS and TOS.

Oligosaccharides are short stacks of simple yet mostly indigestible sugars (from the Greek *oligos*, meaning "few"). If the sugar molecule is fructose, the stacked molecule is called a fructooligosaccharide. If the sugar molecule is galactose, the stacked molecule is called a galactooligosaccharide. These molecules are very useful for human cells and probiotics because they can be processed directly for energy as well as be combined with fatty acids to create cell wall structures and cellular communication molecules. These nutrients also provide energy and nourishment to our probiotic colonies.

The oligosaccharides inulin and oligofructose are probably the most recognized prebiotics. Inulin is a naturally occurring carbohydrate used by plants for storage. It has been estimated that more than 36,000 plant species contain inulin in varying degrees (Carpita *et al.* 1989). The roots often contain the greatest amounts of inulin.

Commercial sources of inulin include Jerusalem artichoke, agave cactus and chicory. Chicory, the root of the Belgian endive, is known to contain some of the highest levels of both inulin at 15-20%, and oligofructose at 5-10%. Inulin from agave has been described as highly branched. This gives it a higher solubility and digestibility than inulin derived from Jerusalem artichoke or chicory.

Notable prebiotic FOS-containing foods include beets, leeks, bananas, tree fruits, soybeans, burdock root, asparagus, maple sugar, whole rye and whole wheat among many others. Bananas contain one of the highest levels of FOS. Bananas are thus a favorite food for both humans and probiotics.

GOS and TOS are natural byproducts of milk. They are produced as lactose is enzymatically converted or hydrolyzed within the digestive tract. This process can also be done commercially. Before much of the recent research on prebiotics was performed, nutritionists simply thought of GOS and TOS as indigestible byproducts of milk.

Another element in plant foods providing prebiotic nutrition for probiotics is the polyphenol group. Polyphenols are groups of biochemicals produced in plants such as lignans, tannins, reservatrol, and flavonoids. There is some uncertainty as to which of these are most helpful to probiotic populations.

Some prebiotics have interesting side effects. For example, there seems to be a relationship between oligofructose inulin and calcium absorption. Inulin has been shown to improve calcium absorption by 20%, and yogurt supplemented with TOS has increased calcium absorption by 16% (van den Heuvel *et al.* 2000)

Galactooligosaccharides have another side effect that is important to note. Dr. Kari Shoaf and fellow researchers at the University of Nebraska

(Shoaf *et al.* 2006) found in laboratory tests that galactooligosaccharides reduce the ability of *E. coli* to attach to human cells within tissue cultures. This effect was isolated from GOS' ability to nourish probiotics. This means that GOS provides more than nutrition to our probiotic colonies. This once considered useless indigestible nutrient also helps keep *E. coli* and other pathogenic bacteria from attaching to our cells. A nice package deal indeed.

FOS and GOS have been known to cause digestive disturbance in rare cases. Such a digestive disturbance is likely caused by dysbiosis, however.

Conclusively, a preponderance of scientific literature indicates that probiotics thrive from a diet of plant-based natural foods with plenty of phytonutrients, while overly processed, sugary and meat diets tend to promote pathogenic bacteria and their disease-causing endotoxins.

Edible Yeasts

Baking yeast and brewer's yeast are common yeasts that are primarily derived from an organism called *Saccharomyces cerevisiae*. In most applications, the yeast is not eaten alive, however. It is *heat-killed* prior to eating. This simply means that it is cooked to a temperature that kills off the viable organisms. This doesn't mean that living *S. cerevisiae* organisms are toxic or anything. In reasonable colony sizes, they are perfectly docile, and even healthy to our bodies because they produce nutrients that our bodies use.

For baking, brewing and supplementation, the heat-killed version of this organism can be very healthy, because when it is alive, it produces a variety of nutrients and immune factors that are left behind in whatever food it was used to ferment.

Just before these yeasts die during heating or baking, they will release intense immune factors in an attempt to protect themselves. These immune factors also help protect our bodies, by stimulating our body's detoxification processes and boosting our immune system. In addition, some of their nutrients, such as B-vitamins produced by yeasts, will donate methyl groups to our liver's glutathione radical-neutralizing processes.

Furthermore, because the biofactors that yeasts produce tend to be acidic, they will lend a tart flavor to the food. This of course lends the flavoring that we relish among our traditional probiotic foods such as cottage cheese, pickles, and so many other foods as we discussed above.

This is the case for **sourdough bread**, for example. Sourdough bread is not only delicious. It is healthy, even if it is made with white flour (for best results, try whole wheat sourdough bread).

Originally, all the fermented brews such as *ginger ale* and *root beer*, were all made using probiotic fermentation.

Yeast Supplements

Baking yeast and Brewer's yeast, Nutritional Yeast and EpiCor®, are all derived from an organism called *Saccharomyces cerevisiae*. This organism is used in brewing and baking. It is thus considered a healthy organism, and acts in a territorial manner to repel organisms and toxins that are seen as foreign to their territories.

For this reason, EpiCor®, Brewer's Yeast or Nutritional Yeast come in dehydrated forms. In other words, the yeast colonies are killed by heat. This heat-killing preserves their nutrients, yet prevents their overgrowth in the body. (However, a person who has mold allergies might still have a reaction to heat-killed yeast because those proteins are still present.)

So what is the difference between EpiCor®, Brewer's Yeast and Nutritional Yeast? The answer lies in their unique processes of fermentation.

Brewer's Yeast is a byproduct of the brewing industry, thus it typically does not have the higher levels of nutrients that the other two have. Brewer's yeast still has a variety of nutrients, including many trace elements (such as chromium and selenium), B vitamins (but typically not B12 as many assume), many antioxidants and proteins.

Nutritional Yeast will typically produce more of these same nutrients, because it has been prepared in such a way that both stresses the yeasts more, and preserves more of their nutrients. Nutritional yeast will contain chromium and selenium, as well as thiamin, riboflavin, niacin, vitamin B6, folate, vitamin B12, pantothenic acid, magnesium, zinc, and a number of amino acids. It is a great protein source, with 50% protein by weight.

EpiCor® is another yeast derivative that is produced using a proprietary method. EpiCor®, however, may have even more enhanced levels of certain nutrients, which include those mentioned above, along with nucleotides and possibly additional antioxidants and immune factors. The reason that EpiCor® may have additional immune factors is because during fermentation, the yeast is *stressed*. Like any organism, when it is stressed, it produces immune factors to protect itself.

After EpiCor® has been stressed, it is then heat-killed, dehydrated and powdered, rendering those immune factors and nutrients.

EpiCor® has been the subject of focused research, which has found that it significantly lowers systemic inflammation.

In one study (Robinson *et al.* 2009), 500 milligrams of EpiCor® or a placebo was given to 80 healthy volunteers with seasonal grass allergies during pollen season. After six and twelve weeks, the EpiCor® group experienced a significant reduction of allergy symptoms compared to the placebo group.

Other EpiCor® studies have shown that it increases salivary IgA (mucosal immunity), and reduces serum IgE (pro-allergy sensitivity).

Red Yeast Rice: The yeast *Monascus purpureus,* when fermented with rice, becomes what is known as red yeast rice. Red yeast rice has been shown in research to lower LDL cholesterol (Liu *et al.* 2006). The mechanism renders red yeast the ability to help prevent lipid peroxidation in the body. Red yeast rice has been used in China for over a thousand years. However, red yeast rice use as a supplement has been questioned by the FDA and pharmaceutical industry. This might have something to do with the fact that correctly fermented red yeast rice can be a significant source of the constituent monacolin K, the primary active ingredient of the statin drug lovastatin.

While there are others, these yeast products have been shown to maximize the body's antioxidant capacities, increase tolerance, and stimulate detoxification processes. They also have considerable research backing up these claims.

Vinegars

Vinegars are excellent living foods that stimulate the body's living purification systems. Vinegar made from apples, grapes or other fruits also contain a variety of antioxidants, as well as acetic acid, which helps stimulate a good environment for our body's own probiotics, and one that repels pathogenic microorganisms.

Researchers from the School of Food and Biological Engineering at Jiangsu University, Zhenjiang China (Ali *et al.* 2019) tested 76 people who had moderately high levels of cholesterol and inflammation.

The researchers had each test subject consume either 30 milliliters of date vinegar per day or a placebo. They tested their cholesterol levels and their inflammatory markers from their blood.

After only four weeks, the researchers tested the subjects' inflammatory biomarkers. Those who had consumed the date vinegar saw their inflammation markers go down. Average levels of C-reactive protein went from 7.05 to 4.12 mg/L. Nitric oxide went from 31.05 to 27.01 umol/L. And fibrinogen levels went from 272 to 238 mg/dL.

Indeed, the immune systems of the subjects who consumed the date vinegar were strengthened. Their tumor necrosis factor-alpha (TNFa) levels went from 17.2 to 13.5 pg/mL.

As this shows, there are a variety of different types of vinegars, depending upon the raw material used. In all cases, the raw material of a healthy vinegar will be a plant source, fermented by a healthy yeast culture. The yeast culture will convert the sugars of the plant source (and added sugars if used) to alcohol. As the alcohol is fermented further, it is oxidized by the zymase enzymes in the yeast, which convert to alcohol to carboxylic acetic acids. These acetic acids are the main constituent of vinegar, and what gives vinegar its tartness.

To speed up the process, alcohols are often used commercially to make vinegars. These include cheaper or turned wines, distilled alcohol (from wood or grain) and other spirits. The conversion of alcohol to vinegar is much quicker because the first step (sugar to alcohol) has already been made.

Fresh vinegar is typically made by crushing whole apples, grapes, potatoes, barley or other fruits or grains - even pears, bananas and others - into a mash. Sugar can be added to speed up the process, typically at a ratio of one-to-four of mash.

Brewer's yeast (*Saccharomyces cerevisiae*) can then be added for fermentation. One-quarter of a yeast cake will typically inoculate a liter of the mash. Alternatively, a "mother" of fresh vinegar that has been retained from a previous vinegar can be used. Such a "mother" will likely contain more yeast species than just the *S. cerevisiae* yeast, and possibly even some probiotic bacteria. The amount needed depends upon the strength of the "mother," but one cup of the mother (from the top center of the previous batch) per liter should probably do it.

The mix is then put aside in a warm place, with the jar covered by a cloth to let in oxygen. The period of fermentation depends upon the sugar content and the temperature stored. The vinegar may be strained or unstrained. Unstrained retains more living yeasts.

Balsamic vinegars will ferment for years in oak barrels, for example. An apple vinegar might take 60 days to nine months. Care should be taken that the alcohol levels are reduced down to well below .5% (legal alcohol limit). Higher acetic acid levels will mean lower alcohol levels. Testing with a round piece of fine marble (5/6 of marble weight reduction equates to acetic acid levels). Look for 30-32 grams reduction per marble piece, after vinegar loses sour taste for a 5% acetic acid vinegar.

Vinegar can be used in salads, for pickling vegetables and other creative recipes. It can also simply be taken by the teaspoon. A traditional raw cider is the Bragg's brand of apple cider vinegars (no financial affiliation).

Alcohol Warning

A key point to remember regarding fermented beverages is that unless the alcohol level is fermented down to a level below .5%, it will be considered an alcoholic beverage. Alcohol is unhealthy for body. Alcohol is ethanol, which is highly toxic to the liver. Alcohol damages the liver. This means that the liver will produce less enzymes and filter the blood poorly. This leaves the body in a state of increased toxicity. Over time this can produce severe liver disease, which can result in death.

Often people consider that because wines and other spirits are made from natural ingredients, they must be healthy. For example, resveratrol from wine is touted as being healthy. Resveratrol, however, comes from the grapes themselves. While red wine certainly will also contain resveratrol, the alcohol content of the wine can do more damage than the resveratrol can help.

As for those reputed to have been drinking a glass or two of wine every day and remain seemingly healthy, yes, the liver can certainly manage a minimal amount of alcohol every day. This doesn't mean that the alcohol is healthy for the liver. There have been a few studies that have indicated the possibility that a drink or two of wine every day may increase longevity. This type of epidemiological research, however, is highly questionable, notably because those who have a glass or two of wine everyday may also well be doing something else—such as socializing while drinking or reducing stress levels—that might also account for their longevity. Other studies have shown that socializing and reducing stress levels also extend life.

The bottom line is that the research showing that the liver is damaged by alcohol consumption is irrefutable. For example, Canadian scientists (Rehm *et al.* 2010) reviewed seventeen studies that analyzed the relationship between alcohol and cirrhosis of the liver. They found that all of them linked alcohol consumption with liver disease and death from liver disease. They also found that the same amount of alcohol consumption produces a higher incidence of liver disease among women.

Alcohol also damages our probiotic colonies.

Antioxidant Foods

When we harvest a fresh plant-based food and eat it with minimal storage, processing and cooking, we are deriving significant benefits from the living organism that produced the food. Because living organisms defend themselves against toxins throughout their lives, by eating fresh whole foods or whole foods minimally cooked, our bodies can utilize the same elements the plant utilized to protect itself against toxins.

This in turn stimulates our immune systems, and also provides direct free radical protection. This is because antioxidants are designed to neutralize toxins.

As we've discussed, a plethora of research has confirmed that damage from free radicals is implicated in many health conditions. Free radicals from toxins damage cells, cell membranes, organs, blood vessel walls and airways—producing systemic inflammation—as the immune system responds to an overload of tissue damage.

Free radicals are produced by synthetic chemicals, pathogens, trans fats, fried foods, red meats, radiation, pollution and various intruders that destabilize within the body. Free radicals are molecules or ions that require stabilization. They reach stabilization by 'stealing' atoms from the cells or tissues of our body. This in turn destabilizes those cells and tissues—producing damage.

Antioxidants serve to stabilize free radicals before our cells and tissues are robbed—by donating their own atoms. A diet with plenty of fruits and vegetables supplies numerous antioxidants. Although antioxidants cannot be considered treatments for any disease, many studies have proved that increased antioxidant intake supports immune function and detoxification. These effects allow the immune system to respond with greater tolerance.

Antioxidant constituents in plant-based foods are known to significantly repeal free radicals, strengthen the immune system and help detoxify the system. These include *lecithin* and *octacosanol* from whole grains; *polyphenols* and *sterols* from vegetables; *lycopene* from tomatoes and watermelons; *quercetin* and *sulfur/allicin* from garlic, onions and peppers; *pectin* and *rutin* from apples and other fruits; *phytocyanidin flavonoids* such as *apigenin* and *luteolin* from various greenfoods; and *anthocyanins* from various fruits and oats.

Some sea-based botanicals like kelp also contain antioxidants as well. Consider a special polysaccharide compound from kelp called *fucoidan*. Fucoidan has been shown in animal studies to significantly reduce inflammation (Cardoso *et al.* 2009; Kuznetsova *et al.* 2004).

Procyanidins are found in apples, currants, cinnamon, bilberry and many other foods. The extract of *Vitis vinifera* seed (grapeseed) is one of the highest sources of bound antioxidant *proanthocyanidins* and *leucocyanidines* called *procyanidolic oligomers* or PCOs. Pycnogenol® also contains significant levels of these PCOs. Blueberries, parsley, green tea, black currant, some legumes and onions also contain PCOs and similar proanthocyanidins.

Research has demonstrated that PCOs have protective and strengthening effects on tissues by increasing enzyme conjugation (Seo *et al.* 2001). PCOs have also been shown to increase vascular wall strength (Robert *et al.* 2000).

Oxygenated carotenoids such as *lutein* and *astaxanthin* also have been shown to exhibit strong antioxidant activity. Astaxanthin is derived from the microalga *Haematococcus pluvialis,* and lutein is available from a number of foods, including spirulina.

Most of these phytonutrients specifically modulate the immune system. For example, the flavonoids *kaempferol* and *flavone* have been shown to block mast cell proliferation by over 80% (Alexandrakis *et al.* 2003). Sources of kaempferol include Brussels sprouts, broccoli, grapefruit and apples.

Furthermore, *resveratrol* from grapes and berries modulate nuclear factor-kappaB and transcription/Janus kinase pathways—which strengthens immunity. Good sources of resveratrol include peanuts, red grapes, cranberries and cocoa (wine is not advisable for cleansing as we'll discuss later).

Nearly every plant-food has some measure of phytonutrients discussed above and more. These phytonutrients alkalize the blood and increase the detoxification capabilities of the liver. They help clear the blood of toxins.

Foods that are particularly detoxifying and immunity-building include fresh pineapples, beets, cucumbers, apricots, apples, almonds, zucchini, artichokes, avocados, bananas, beans, collard greens, berries, casaba, celery, coconuts, cranberries, watercress, dandelion greens, grapes, raw honey, corn, kale, citrus fruits, watermelon, lettuce, mangoes, mushrooms, oats, broccoli, okra, onions, papayas, parsley, peas, whole grains, radishes, raisins, spinach, tomatoes, walnuts, and many others.

These plant-based foods are also our primary source of soluble and insoluble fiber. Diets with significant fiber help clear the blood and tissues of toxins, and lipid peroxidation-friendly LDL cholesterol. Fiber is also critical to a healthy digestive tract and intestinal barrier. Fiber in the diet should range from about 35 to 45 grams per day according to the recommendations of many diet experts. Six to ten servings of raw fruits and vegetables per day should accomplish this—which is even part of the USDA's recommendations. This means raw, fibrous foods should be present at every meal.

Good fibrous plant sources also contain healthy *lignans* and *phytoestrogens* that help balance hormone levels, and help the body make its own natural corticoids. Foods that contain these include peas, garbanzo beans, soybeans, kidney beans and lentils.

A study from several universities and Spain's Centro de Investigación Biomédica en Red Fisiopatología de la Obesidad y la Nutrición (CIBEROBN) (Papandreou *et al.* 2018) followed 7,216 people for an average of six years. The researchers analyzed their diets, and in particular, their consumption of legumes – including dry beans, chickpeas, lentils and fresh peas.

The researchers found that those who ate more legumes had a half the number of cancer deaths compared to those who ate fewer legumes. Yes, they found a 49 percent lower incidence of death from cancer by eating more legumes.

Plant-based foods provide these immune-stimulating factors because these vary same factors make up the plants' own immune systems. For example, the red, blue and green flavonoid pigments in plants and fruits help protect the plant from oxidative damage from radiation. The proanthocyanidins in grains like oats, for example, help protect the oat plant from crown rust caused by the *Puccinia coronata* fungus. So the same biochemicals that stimulate immunity in humans are part of plants' immune systems.

These same whole food phytonutrients also neutralize oxidative radicals in our bodies—the reason they are called antioxidants. How do we know this? Scientists can measure the ability of a particular food to neutralize free radicals with specific laboratory testing. One such test is called the *Oxygen Radical Absorbance Capacity Test* (ORAC). This technical laboratory study is performed by a number of scientific organizations that include the USDA, as well as specialized labs such as Brunswick Laboratories in Massachusetts.

Research from the USDA's Jean Mayer Human Nutrition Research Center on Aging at Tufts University has suggested that a diet high in ORAC value may protect blood vessels and tissues from free radical damage that can result in inflammation (Sofic *et al.* 2001; Cao *et al.* 1998). These tissues, of course, include the airways. Research has confirmed that consuming 3,000 to 5,000 ORAC units per day can have protective benefits.

ORAC Values (100 grams) of Selected (raw) Fruits (USDA, 2007-2008)

Cranberry	9,382		Pomegranate	2,860
Plum	7,581		Orange	1,819
Blueberry	6,552		Tangerine	1,620
Blackberry	5,347		Grape (red)	1,260
Raspberry	4,882		Mango	1,002
Apple (Granny)	3,898		Kiwi	882
Strawberry	3,577		Banana	879
Cherry (sweet)	3,365		Tomato (plum)	389
Gooseberry	3,277		Pineapple	385
Pear	2,941		Watermelon	142

There is tremendous attention these days on two unique fruits from the Amazon rain forest and China called *açaí* and *goji berry* (or wolfberry) respectively. A recent ORAC test documented by Schauss *et al.* (2006)

gives açaí a score of 102,700 and tests documented by Dr. Paul Gross gives goji berries a total ORAC of 30,300. However, subsequent tests done by Brunswick Laboratories, Inc. gave these two berries 53,600 (açaí) and 22,000 (goji) total-ORAC values.

In addition, we must remember that these are the dried berries being tested in the latter case, and a concentrate of açaí being tested in the former case. The numbers in the chart above are for fresh fruits. Dried fruits will naturally have higher ORAC values, because the water is evaporated—giving more density and more antioxidants per 100 grams.

For example, in the USDA database, dried apples have a 6,681 total-ORAC value, while fresh apples range from 2,210 to 3,898 in total-ORAC value. This equates to a two-to-three times increase from fresh to dried. In another example, fresh red grapes have a 1,260 total-ORAC value, while raisins have a 3,037 total-ORAC value. This comes close to an increase of three times the ORAC value following dehydration.

Part of the equation, naturally, is cost. Dried fruit and concentrates are often more expensive than fresh fruit. High-ORAC dried fruits or concentrates from açaí or goji will also be substantially more expensive than most fruits grown domestically (especially for Americans and Europeans). Our conclusion is that local or in-country grown fresh fruits with high total-ORAC values produce the best value. Local fresh fruit offers great free radical scavenging ability, support for local farmers, and pollen proteins we are most likely more tolerant to.

By comparison, spinach—an incredibly wholesome vegetable with a tremendous amount of nutrition—has a fraction of the ORAC content of some of these fruits, at 1,515 total ORAC. Spinach, of course, contains many other nutrients, including proteins lacking in many high-ORAC fruits.

Dehydrated spices can have incredibly high ORAC values. For example, USDA's database lists ground Turmeric's total ORAC value at 159,277 and oregano's at 200,129. However, while we might only consume a few hundred milligrams of a spice per day, we can eat many grams—if not pounds—of sweet colorful fruit every day.

Quercetin Foods

A number of foods and herbs that reduce inflammation and toxicity contain quercetin. This is no coincidence. Multiple studies have shown that quercetin inhibits the release inflammatory mediators histamine and leukotrienes. Foods rich in quercetin include onions, garlic, apples, capers, grapes, leafy greens, tomatoes and broccoli. In addition, many of the herbs listed earlier contain quercetin as an active constituent. Many of the herbs listed in the herbal section also contain quercetin. Onions, garlic and apples contain some of the highest levels.

Quercetin stimulates and balances the immune system. In an *in vivo* study, four weeks of quercetin reduced histamine levels and allergen-specific IgE levels. More importantly, quercetin inhibited anaphylaxis responses (Shishehbor *et al.* 2010).

Cairo researchers (Haggag *et al.* 2003) found that among mast cells exposed to allergens and chemicals in the laboratory, quercetin inhibited histamine release by 95% and 97%.

Over the past few years, an increasing amount of evidence is pointing to the conclusion that foods with quercetin slow inflammatory response and autoimmune derangement. Researchers from Italy's Catholic University (Crescente *et al.* 2009) found that quercetin inhibited arachidonic acid-induced platelet aggregation. Arachidonic acid-induced platelet aggregation is seen in allergic inflammatory mechanisms.

Researchers from the University of Crete (Alexandrakis *et al.* 2003) found that quercetin can inhibit mast cell proliferation by up to 80%. Onions have also been shown *in vivo* tests to reduce bronchoconstriction.

Organic foods contain higher levels of quercetin. A study from the University of California-Davis' Department of Food Science and Technology (Mitchell *et al.* 2007) tested flavonoid levels between organic and conventional tomatoes over a ten-year period. Their research concluded that quercetin levels were 79% higher for tomatoes grown organically under the same conditions as conventionally-grown tomatoes.

Leafy greens

Leafy greens like lettuce, spinach and cabbage boost the immune system in multiple ways. For example, green leafy vegetables stimulate the immune system within the intestines by donating a gene that regulates the gut's defense mechanisms.

Research from the University of Melbourne (Rankin *et al.* 2013) studied the ingestion of leafy and cruciferous vegetables along with other foods. They measured and analyzed intestinal levels of interleukin 22 – a critical element that regulates intestinal immunity through an immune cell called NKp46+. This is also called an innate lymphoid cell – or ILC.

IL-22 and the innate lymphoid cells play a critical part of the intestine's control of inflammatory conditions and food allergies. Low levels have been seen amongst various inflammatory diseases.

Sprouts

Sprouts and their powders are nutritional powerhouses. They have exponential nutritional value, well above the nutrient content of their seeds or the fully-grown plants. This was confirmed in 1970s experiments by former Hippocrates Health Institute Director of Research, Viktoras Kulvinskas, M.S. Kulvinskas, who found that ascorbic acid levels in soybean sprouts increased from zero to 103 milligrams per 100 grams by day six—about the ascorbic acid content found in lime juice. These levels fall off significantly within days.

Each plant has a different nutrient peak. Ascorbic acid content in broad bean sprouts—used to cure scurvy during World War I—peaks in three days, after which the levels fall off.

Many believe that sprouts produce this greater antioxidant content to defend themselves against threats from the soil.

Great nutritional sprouts include wheat grass sprouts, barley, oats, beans, broccoli and cabbage. The latter two provide a class of nutrients called glucosinolates. These glucosinolates yield sulfur compounds and indole-3 carbinols. Both have shown to have significant anticarcinogenic and anti-inflammatory effects in the body.

Seed selection is critical. A good quality seed will germinate at least 50%. Heirloom seeds often germinate at much higher rates.

Root Foods

It is no coincidence that many antioxidants are roots, such as ginger, turmeric, onions garlic, beets, carrots, turnips, parsnips and others. These root foods are known for their ability to alkalize the bloodstream and stimulate detoxification. They are also known to help rejuvenate the liver and adrenal glands.

Beets, for example, contain, among other nutrients, betaine, betalains, betacyanin and betanin. They also contain generous portions of folate, iron and fiber. One of the primary fibers in beets is pectin, which is also found in apples. Pectin has a unique soluble and insoluble fiber content that maximizes the attachment of radical-producing LDL cholesterol in the intestines. Pectin also attaches to many other toxins, drawing them out of the body as well.

Meanwhile, betaine is known as stimulating liver health. Betaine has been shown to reduce liver injury (Okada *et al.* 2011). Betaine is also considered healthy for the bile ducts, because it helps draw out toxins. Beets are delicious foods that can be grated into salads, juiced, steamed, baked and simply eaten raw. Red beets are typically considered the healthiest, but pink and white beets also contain betaine.

We should note that while beets contain significant amounts of betaine, other betaine-rich foods include broccoli, spinach and some whole grains.

Each of the root foods listed above contain unique constituents that support liver health and detoxification.

Cultured Soy Foods

We discussed a few of these, including tempeh, shoyu and miso. Other cultured soy foods such as tofu have been shown in numerous studies to reduce breast cancer risk, reduce cholesterol, reduce the risk of heart disease, increase artery health, reduce allergies and reduce the risk of bone fractures (Messina 2010).

In addition, several large epidemiological studies done in the 1990s found that those populations that ate higher levels of tofu in their diets had lower levels of heart disease and many cancers.

Washington state researchers (Lerman *et al.* 2010) found that people with higher LDL cholesterol levels and cardiovascular disease experienced a reduction of LDL cholesterol and smaller particle size, greater HDL cholesterol, lower apolipoprotein levels and lower homocysteine levels. Remember that LDL cholesterol is related to lipoperoxidation, which is what causes artery disease leading to heart attacks and strokes. And lower apolipoprotein levels and lower homocysteine levels mean lower levels of systemic inflammation.

These benefits come from one of soy's isoflavones, genistein. Researchers from Northwestern University's Feinberg School of Medicine, in association with the American Lung Association Asthma Clinical Research Centers (Smith *et al.* 2004) studied asthma severity in 1,033 adolescents and adults. They found that 250 micrograms per 1,000 Kcal per day of the soy isoflavone genistein significantly increased forced expiratory volumes and peak expiratory volumes.

Because some soy nutrients (such as raffinose) can be difficult for some to digest, soy's best antioxidant benefits come when soy is cultured or fermented. Cultured soy foods such as tofu and tempeh thus provide easily assimilable sources of soy.

Traditional Antioxidant Food Recipes

This brings us to some traditional food recipes that provide superior antioxidant power. The science on quercetin, enzymes and antioxidants now gives some of these cleansing remedies significant credibility:

> ➤ *Lemon and honey:* This remedy is often blended with an herbal tea such as peppermint or chamomile. The combination of lemon juice and honey provide an alkalizing and cleansing effect.

> ➤ *Super salsa:* This Mexican dish provides cilantro, garlic, cayenne peppers and tomatoes to stimulate blood purification and

> ➤ *Honion syrup:* Equal parts chopped onions and raw honey provides constituents to stimulate the immune system.

> *Horseradish syrup:* Equal parts grated horseradish and honey will clear the sinuses and open the airways, while providing an alkalizing effect.

> *Garlic syrup:* Garlic and raw honey combine two antimicrobials and immune-system boosters.

> *Super pickles:* Jerusalem Artichokes, celery and carrot, pickled in apple cider vinegar provide a great alkalizer and blood purifier.

> *Raw vegetable juices:* Juiced endive, celery and carrots. These feed us with immediate nutrients that stimulate our immune system and alkalize our blood.

> *Super soup:* Barley, celery, carrots, beets and ginger. These also provide significant blood alkalizing effects, liver cleansing and stimulate the immune system.

> *Super fruits:* Raw apricots, blueberries, blackberries, strawberries. These provide significant levels of antioxidants.

> *Miso soup:* Miso provides a fermented form of soybeans that stimulates immunity. This remedy has been a long-time favorite among Asian countries.

> *Turmeric curry dishes:* Ayurvedic cooking provides many traditional dishes steeped in spices that stimulate the immune system and provide antioxidants. Turmeric is a favorite that has shown to reduce cancer risk. This is only one type of spiced dish that Ayurvedic cooking provides. An Ayurvedic cookbook is suggested.

The Importance of Raw, Fresh Foods

Most nutrients are heat-sensitive. Vitamin C, fat-soluble vitamins A, E and B vitamins are reduced during pasteurization. Many fatty acids are transformed by high heat to unhealthy fats. Important plant nutrients, such as anthocyanins and polyphenols, are also reduced during pasteurization, along with various enzymes. Proteins are denatured or broken down when heated for long. While this can aid in amino acid absorption, it can also form unrecognized peptide combinations. In milk, for example, some of the nutritious whey protein, or lactabumin, will denature into a number of peptide combinations that are not readily absorbed.

A 2008 study on strawberry puree from the University of Applied Sciences in Switzerland showed a 37% reduction in vitamin C and a significant loss in antioxidant potency after pasteurization. A 1998 study from Brazil's Universidade Estadual de Maringa determined that Barbados cherries lost about 14% of their vitamin C content after pasteurization. During heat treatment, vitamin C will also convert to dehydroascorbic acid together with a loss of bioflavonoids.

A 2008 study at Spain's Cardenal Herrera University determined that glutathione peroxidase—an important antioxidant contained in milk—was significantly reduced by pasteurization. In 2006, the University also released a study showing that lysine content was significantly decreased by milk pasteurization. A 2005 study at the Universidade Federal do Rio Grande determined that pasteurizing milk reduced vitamin A (retinol) content from an average of 55 micrograms to an average of 37 micrograms. A study at North Carolina State University in 2003 determined that HTST pasteurization significantly reduced conjugated linoleic acid (CLA) content—an important fatty acid in milk shown to reduce cancer and encourage good fat metabolism.

A 2006 study on bayberries at the Southern Yangtze University determined that plant antioxidants such as anthocyanins and polyphenolics were reduced from 12-32% following UHT pasteurization. Polyphenols, remember, are the primary nutrients in fruits and vegetables that render anti-carcinogenic and antioxidant effects.

One of the most important losses from pasteurization is its enzyme content. Diary and plant foods contain a variety of enzymes that aid in the assimilation or catalyzing of nutrients and antioxidants. These include xanthenes, lysozymes, lipases, oxidases, amylases, lactoferrins and many others contained in raw foods. The body uses food enzymes in various ways. Some enzymes, such as papain from papaya and bromelain from pineapples, dissolve artery plaque and reduce inflammation. While the body makes many of its own enzymes, it also absorbs many food enzymes or uses their components to make new ones.

Pasteurization also typically leaves the food or beverage with a residual caramelized flavor due to the conversation of the enzymes, flavonoids and sugars to other compounds. In milk, for example, there is a substantial conversion from lactose to lactulose (and caramelization) after UHT pasteurization. Lactulose can cause intestinal cramping, nausea and vomiting.

In the case of pasteurized juices, pasteurization can leave the beverage in a highly acidic state, which can irritate our mucous membranes and intestines.

As for irradiation, there is little research on the resulting nutrient content outside of a few microwave studies (which showed decreased nutrient content and the formation of undesirable metabolites). There is good reason to believe that irradiation may thus denature some nutrients.

Whole foods in nature's packages are significantly different from pasteurized processed foods. Fresh whole foods produced by plants contain various antioxidants and enzymes that reduce the ability of microorganisms to grow. The Creator also provided whole foods with peels and shells that protect nutrients and keep most microorganisms out. Microorganisms may invade the outer shell or peel somewhat, but the peel's pH, dryness and density—together with the pH of the inner fruit—provide extremely effective barriers to microorganisms and oxidation.

For this reason, most fruits and nuts can be easily stored for days and even weeks without having significant nutrient reduction. Once the peel or shell is removed, the inner fruit, juice or nut must be consumed to prevent oxidation and contamination—depending upon its pH and sugar content.

Peels are also very healthy. An example of this is the research done on citrus pectin from citrus peels.

Research led by anti-aging expert, Dr. Isaac Eliaz (M.D., L.Ac) has found that modified citrus pectin, derived from the peels of citrus fruits, boosts immunity by blocking the destructive Galectin-3.

Dr. Eliaz presented to the 19th Annual World Congress on Anti-Aging Medicine and Regenerative Biomedical Technologies new findings that show citrus pectin blocks the biomarker Galectin-3 – found to increase life-threatening disease incidence and early death.

"MCP offers unprecedented health benefits by binding and blocking excess Galectin-3 molecules throughout the body. With the latest research linking Galectin-3 to the progression of numerous diseases, this presentation felt like a breakthrough moment where a new tool in medicine is being introduced to a whole medical community for the first time," said Dr. Eliaz.

Dr. Eliaz' research data revealed that the modified citrus pectin, derived from the pith of citrus fruit peels, blocked unhealthy levels of Galectin-3 molecules circulating within the body. Elevated levels of Galectin-3 has been shown to be associated with heart disease, tissue fibrosis, cancer, and diseases of other organs. So far, MCP has been found to be the only natural Galectin-3 blocker available today. MCP binds to excess Galectin-3 molecules, preventing them from damaging tissues.

Dr. Eliaz' research has also shown that modified citrus pectin enhances immunity. One of his studies showed that MCP activated B-cells and activated T-cells and natural killer cells. The NK-cells' stimulated activity was found to kill leukemia cancer cells, as published in the journal *BMC Complementary and Alternative Medicine.*

MCP has also been shown to stimulate detoxification. Dr. Eliaz found that MCP reduces heavy metal levels within the body.

"When the toxic burden is high, I recommend a gentle yet highly effective heavy metal detoxification program using Modified Citrus Pectin. MCP is clinically proven to

significantly reduce dangerous heavy metals, including lead, mercury, arsenic, and cadmium, without lowering levels of essential minerals," added Dr. Eliaz.

Other research (Fang *et al.* 2018) has confirmed that MCP significantly inhibited the growth and survival of bladder cancer cells.

Another compound from citrus is nobiletin. Research has found that nobiletin helps the heart and the liver, and fights cancer. Citrus peels also fight bacteria according to other research.

Whole natural foods also contain polysaccharides and oligosaccharides that combine nutrients and sugar within complex fibers. These combinations also help prevent oxidation and pathogenic bacteria colonization. With heat processing, however, the sugars are broken down into more simplified, refined form, which allows microbial growth and oxidation. Why? Because simple sugars provide convenient energy sources for aggressive bacteria and fungi colonies. By contrast, our probiotics are used to eating the complexed oligosaccharides in fibrous foods. In other words, heat-processing produces the perfect foods for pathogenic microorganism colonization.

As we discussed in the last chapter, pathogenic microorganisms provide the fuel for systemic inflammation. They can infect the body's (and airways') tissues directly, and/or their endotoxins—waste products—stream into our bloodstream to max out our immune system and detoxification processes. This causes systemic inflammation, and toxicity.

Healthy Cooking

While raw whole foods are often more wholesome to the body, some foods must be cooked to make them more digestible. These include most grains, beans, and some vegetables. Our section on Chinese medicine earlier illustrated that some herbs also require cooking to eliminate certain toxins.

The question is: how much cooking and processing do we need to do to our foods? How much cooking is necessary? Yes, cooking some foods often increases their digestibility. This is particularly important with grain-based foods and beans. Cooking these foods will help break down their fibers and complex carbohydrates into more digestible forms.

Also, many vegetables are more assimilable when they are cooked—or even better, steamed. Steaming vegetables in a pot with a covered lid will preserve most nutrients, while softening some of fibers that hold the nutrients. Foods such as beets, asparagus, broccoli, rhubarb, squash and many others are delicious and nutritious after being steamed or lightly boiled in clean water.

Other plant foods are best eaten raw. These include lettuce, cucumbers, avocado, onions and many others. Because the nutrients in these foods are not so tightly bound within the cell walls of the plants, they can be destroyed by the heat and/or easily separated during cooking.

While the cell walls of plants do contain nutrients, they must be broken down during mastication and digestion. Some cell walls are tougher than others are, and require cooking or processing to break their cell walls. Chlorella—a blue-green algae—is a good example. Many nutrients in chlorella are bound within tightly-packed cell walls, so chlorella is more nutritious when the cell walls have been broken prior to ingestion.

A healthy diet strikes a balance between raw and cooked foods. A perfect way to accomplish this is a dinner that includes a salad topped with seeds, yogurt, olive oil and apple cider vinegar; and an entrée of cooked grains and/or beans with a nice sauce spiced with antioxidant herbs. Breakfast and lunch can include fresh fruit, nuts, raw cheese and fermented dairy; with lightly cooked grains such as oats and barley. Snacks can go raw with apples, nuts, raisins and seeds for sustained, slow-digesting energy and essential fats.

A plant-based food diet can be extremely creative and varied. It can also be extremely colorful and exotic. This is because there are so many different foods and spices to choose from. A flip through a Mediterranean diet cookbook will confirm this immediately.

Lectin Foods

You've probably been hearing about yet another diet fad – the lectin-free diet. Does this newest fad trailing a host of previous fads have any validity? Will it help you lose weight and reduce inflammation? Are lectins really toxins?

Like the gluten-free fad that preceded it, and the litany of so many other fad diets, the lectin-free diet is a misrepresentation of selective research studies that paint lectins as poisons or toxins.

Promoters of the lectin-free diet have accused foods that are supposedly high in lectins as causing leaky gut syndrome and increased inflammation.

Their claim is that by reducing intake of certain foods, primarily beans, grains, tomatoes, potatoes and "nightshade" vegetables, we can decrease inflammation and lose weight.

Certainly, as the gluten-free diet proved, if we stop eating a good portion of the foods humans have been eating for thousands of years, we might lose some weight. But is the weight loss merely a result of an onerously selective diet, resulting in a reduction of calories?

To answer the questions above about the lectin-free diet, let's look objectively at the facts.

What is a lectin?

Lectins are proteins that exist throughout nature. They are present in practically every animal, practically every unicellular creature, and in most, if not practically all plants. Lectins are parts of plant roots, plant leaves, stems and flowers.

Lectins are complicated, and they are difficult to isolate. Over the past two decades, dozens of lectins have been isolated using complex purifying techniques. But most researchers agree that there are likely thousands of different types of lectins throughout nature.

A general definition of lectins relates to their ability to help bind compounds. These include proteins, carbohydrates, fats and other molecules in the body. Lectins are multifaceted and there are many types of lectins.

Lectins also exist in all animals. In animals – including humans – lectins have many metabolic functions. Lectins help the body's cells in their DNA production and replication. They assist the immune system by fighting inflammation, infections by viruses and bacteria, and protecting organs from outside invaders and toxins.

We have discussed other research showing that lower levels of lectins in humans and animals leads to greater risk of infections.

Lectins are responsible for making sure our blood coagulates so we won't bleed to death. Lectins are responsible for killing cancer cells, which the body produces on a regular basis. Lectins help maintain our blood vessel health and help them expand and contract.

Lectins help the liver function properly in the face of various toxins. Lectins help us process carbohydrates to convert them into energy. Lectins help our immune systems recognize invading viruses, bacteria and other entities that are not healthy.

The list goes on and on. Lectins are critical to the health of our body. Without lectins, our body is not protected.

These include binding proteins to proteins, fats and proteins, carbohydrate processing, DNA activity, and so much more carbohydrates and proteins, structures other than carbohydrates via protein-protein, protein-lipid or protein-nucleic acid interactions.

While animal lectins undoubtedly fulfill a variety of functions, many could be considered in general terms to be recognition molecules within the immune system. More specifically, lectins have been implicated in direct first-line defense against pathogens, cell trafficking, immune regulation and prevention of autoimmunity.

And some lectins are known to bind to bacteria and viruses and other foreign elements – helping to protect cells from their intrusion. We have discussed research showing that lectins fight viruses.

In fact, this is one of the central benefits for these important proteins in plants. They help protect the plants that produce them from being harmed by bacteria and viruses. They do this through molecular affinity, and the binding-reception process that takes place on the surface of most cells.

In plants, lectins also have a variety of other purposes. These including binding to carbohydrates and assisting the plant's immune system deter infections. Lectins in plants help the plant grow strong and stay protected against the elements.

These abilities of immunity-related plant lectins actually make them healthy for humans. Lectins or lectin-produced compounds in plants have proven over and over to aid human health.

Lectins and lectin-produced compounds in plants form most of the protective elements in plants. These relate directly to fibers, antioxidants and so many other health-giving compounds.

In other words, lectins are found everywhere, throughout nature. They conduct so many processes that it is unreasonable to define them as toxins in general, because most are required for survival. Lectins are contained in just about every plant food, including bananas, coconuts, potatoes, beans, nuts, seeds, vegetables and so many other health-promoting foods. To define them as anything but health-promoting is to look at health through a very narrow bandwidth indeed.

Lectins bind with innumerable molecules involved in millions of life-sustaining biological processes. Some of them are particularly healthy. For example, lectins from Wisteria japonica bind with cancer cells but not normal cells, just as lectins from wheat germ do.

This is not to say that all lectins are healthy. Ricin, for example, is a lectin. It is a lectin found within castor beans of the castor plant (Ricinus communis). But then castor beans haven't been part of the human diet either.

Wheat germ, for example, has been shown in several human clinical studies to reduce intestinal inflammation, boost liver health, stimulate immunity and help normalize cholesterol levels. In a study from France's INSERM (National Institute of Health and Medical Research) (Cara et al. 1992) researchers found that lectin-containing wheat germ reduced triglycerides, improving cardiovascular health.

Proteins called lectins can also form a clumping – in this case often to polysaccharides or carbohydrates.

And as far as the agglutinin in wheat germ – yes, a particular type of lectin protein called wheat germ agglutinin (WGA) will bind to a glucose derivative called N-Acetylglucosamine. And note that wheat germ agglutinin – or WGA – is unrelated to gliadin and glutenin proteins termed 'gluten.'

The investigation into WGA's effect upon the intestines has provided some grist for gluten-free advocates. But what must be examined with the science is the context and rationale for studying WGA lectins.

Many food plants produce lectins as a natural part of their immunity, so it is important for food scientists to understand the effects of these lectins from an isolated viewpoint – out of the context of normal dietary use of the foods they are contained within.

Can lectins cause leaky gut syndrome?

This is perhaps the central argument of the lectin-free diet proponents. They claim the research overwhelmingly shows lectins produce leaky gut. Well, certainly not all lectins do this. And under normal conditions, the one lectin shown to bother the gut wall is neutralized by a healthy gut before it even reaches the intestinal walls.

A 2009 laboratory study from Italy's University of Verona is quoted by many lectin-free diet proponents. The study abstract states that wheat germ agglutinin (WGA) "is a toxic compound and an anti-nutritional factor." In the same sentence they add, "but recent works have shown that it may have potential as an anti-tumor drug…"

Besides the question of why WGA lectin is toxic yet it kills cancer, the primary question relates to the setting of the study. The tests that rendered this conclusion was a laboratory that utilized cultured gastrointestinal cells called Caco-2 cells.

Yes, the study found that WGA, at certain doses, can provoke an inflammatory response, specifically by intestinal Caco2 cells. However, in this study, the cells also produced an immune response that balance these effects with cytokines.

The most disturbing thing is that the researchers were not duplicating the gastrointestinal system. They were culturing some intestinal cells in Petri dishes. What about all the other stuff in the human gastrointestinal tract, such as enzymes, probiotics, immunity cells (such as IgA), proteases which break apart proteins such as WGA, and so many other aspects of the human digestive tract?

Cultured intestinal cells within Petri dishes in a laboratory environment is not our gut. It does not duplicate all of the elements involved in human digestion – including the probiotic-rich mucin layer that in a healthy intestinal tract protects the intestinal cells from such exposures.

Rather, the researchers simply exposed isolated intestinal cells to purified WGA and watched the immune response within the laboratory. Such a response, in fact, would occur with many raw food compounds in such isolated conditions.

At the same time, however, other research has illustrated that a vast range of WGA doses are safe and non-inflammatory in a healthy intestinal tract. But when doses are given that dramatically exceed a normal human diet – the equivalent to over 600 grams for an adult male (over a pound of not just wheat germ but a pound of purified WGA lectin in one sitting) – intestinal inflammation can occur if WGA is not broken down before exposure to intestinal cells.

Not only was the quantity far greater than any realm of realism in the lab study above, but the WGA was not within the natural matrix of plant nutrients.

Our bodies produce particular proteases which break apart proteins such as WGA. We also host probiotics that break them down, and have protective layers that help shield the intestinal cells against exposure to undigested proteins.

Cooking inactivates WGA lectins

Furthermore, research has indicated that much of wheat germ agglutinin is neutralized by cooking. A study by researchers from Italy's University of Verona (Matucci *et al.* 2004) determined that WGA lectin is largely deactivated at cooking temperatures of 65 degrees Celsius (about 149 degrees Fahrenheit).

The researchers found WGA in raw flour but found that resulting breads had significantly reduced WGA lectin levels.

This means that baking and fermenting (with yeast) with whole wheat flour will largely inactivate wheat germ agglutinin.

This also goes for many other lectin-containing foods. Especially those such as beans and nightshade foods. Who eats beans raw? No one. Cooking beans will break down most of their lectin content – even if we consider them so bad.

As for other supposedly higher lectin foods such as coconuts, whole grains, tomatoes and nightshades: These foods have been tested in large-scale human diet studies and shown to be seriously healthy. Diets that include these foods have been shown to be extremely heart-healthy and cancer-preventative.

Isolated lectins are not normal foods

But should a lab isolate and purify a huge dose of practically any protein – especially a protein that is a known lectin: There certainly will be intestinal consequences. These would relate to the fact that the protein was not properly broken down, as happens in our intestinal tracts.

Isolated and purified lectins – as found in the above studies – are not normal foods. It is like isolating and purifying sugar from beets. Beets are healthy foods that provide significant nourishment. But when refined sugar is isolated and purified from beets (and cane) – as has been done over the past century: That sugar becomes a cause of diabetes, metabolic disease, heart disease and other conditions.

Should we stop eating whole beets because sugar gets extracted from them?

Even with doses considered healthy, WGA has been shown to be selectively cytotoxic to human colon cancer cells (Pusztai *et al.* 1993 and others). The WGA was able to select, bind to and destroy colon cancer cells while leaving the healthy intestinal cells alone.

So WGA is actually – as many lectins are – pretty smart. And beneficial to humans.

This simply means that within a healthy diet and healthy intestinal tract, food lectins such as WGA are not only safe for human consumption, but help protect against colon cancer.

Wheat germ, for example, has been shown in several human clinical studies to reduce intestinal inflammation, boost liver health, stimulate immunity and help normalize cholesterol levels. In a study from France's INSERM (National Institute of Health and Medical Research) (Cara *et al.* 1992) researchers found that WGA-containing wheat germ reduced triglycerides, improving cardiovascular health.

The Mayo Clinic had this to say about wheat germ in a slideshow of "10 great health foods:"

"Wheat germ is the part of the grain that's responsible for the development and growth of the new plant sprout. Although only a small part, the germ contains many nutrients. It's an excellent source of thiamin and a good source of folate, magnesium, phosphorus and zinc. The germ also contains protein, fiber and some fat. Try sprinkling some on your hot or cold cereal."

Probiotics break down lectins in the gut

Some plant lectins are extremely beneficial for our health. They boost our immunity and offer untold metabolic benefits. Other plant lectins need to be broken down in the gut, and as they are, they are neutralized.

In a study from Argentina's National University of Tucumán (Babot *et al.* 2017) researchers tested WGA lectin consumption in poultry together with probiotic testing. The research found that certain strains of probiotics successfully break down WGA within the gut. The researchers utilized poultry being fed with a mono-diet (wheat).

The researchers tested 14 intestinal probiotics against the lectin. They found that 9 of the Lactobacillus strains and one Enterococcus strain played a role in the breakdown of this lectin.

Furthermore, they found that cultured probiotics significantly broke down the lectin when they were exposed to the probiotics prior to contact with the intestinal cells.

As expected, the study found that some strains were more effective than others. Species such as L. salivarius and L. reuteri were most effective and more efficient at protecting the intestinal walls from exposure to undigested WGA lectins.

Note that poultry farmers often feed their birds with significant antibiotics, which deter the growth of good probiotic populations. This produces a lack of the very probiotics the birds need to digest their wheat feed.

Humans face a similar problem, because so many antibiotics are being prescribed without warrant. These have the effect of killing off the very probiotics we need to break down lectins before our intestinal walls are exposed to them.

Lectins and cancer

Researchers from the University of Tokyo (Soga *et al.* 2013) discovered that a lectin naturally contained in Wisteria japonica seeds selectively binds to several types of cancer. And other plant lectins have been found to have this capability.

The researchers conducted laboratory tests using seeds from three different plants – Wisteria floribunda (Japanese wisteria), Wisteria brachybotrys, and Wisteria japonica (Japonica). The researchers extracted agglutinizing lectins from each of the seeds of these three plants.

What are agglutinizing lectins?

Agglutinizing lectins often play a protective role in nature, where they protect their host from the intrusion of certain molecules or even bacteria or viruses. For this reason practically every plant will contain some lectins.

Agglutinizing lectins appear throughout nature within many different species. The word agglutinin comes from agglutinare, which means "to glue."

Agglutinizing lectins will thus bind with and sometimes "clump" different types of elements. They may bind to bacteria, or they might bind to red blood cells. Or they may simply bind to sugars, or even antibodies.

In the case of the lectins within the Japonica tree, and compared to the other three species of Wisteria, the researchers extracted and purified lectins that were found to bind to N-acetylgalactosamine. This is a galactose sugar combined with an amino acid—a component of living cells involved in intercellular communication and thus a part of most of most living cells.

But in this case, the researchers found these lectins were smart – and one was smarter than the other two. The researchers tested all three against a host of different cells, including human cancer cells that had been collected from cancer patients.

These included human squamous cell carcinoma, cancer cells from the kidney, liver cancer cells and lung cancer cells among others. The researchers also tested the Wisteria lectins against normal (healthy) cells.

The two Wisteria plants were found to bind with all of the cancer cells. But the lectin from the Wisteria japonica was found to bind only with the skin cancer cells, the kidney cells and the lung cancer cells.

The researchers indicated this meant the Wisteria japonica lectin could be used as a diagnostic tool – and possibly even a treatment tool – against these forms of cancer.

The fact that lectins will selectively bind to cancerous cells have been seen among other types of plant lectins, including wheat germ agglutinin (WGA) and others. In a university study from Argentina (Barbeito *et al.* 2013) WGA was found to selectively bind to polycystic ovary cells. Other studies have shown WGA will not only bind but inhibit growth of colon cancer cells in the gut.

In these studies, the WGA and other lectins would selectively differentiate between the cancer cells and the healthy cells around them—leaving the healthy cells intact.

The general take-away relates to utilizing those elements in nature that can help protect us. Lectins within plants help protect the plant from foreign forces that endanger the plant's survival. Now we are finding that these same elements can help us protect our own bodies.

Lectins fight viruses

Scientific research finds that lectins from plants can treat lethal viruses such as Ebola. SARS (severe acute respiratory syndrome) coronavirus and the feline infectious peritonitis virus (FIPV). And low lectin levels have been linked to a number of dangerous diseases.

Other research has found that Ebola virus requires more than contact with a symptomatic patient: It also requires an immune system unable to defend itself against the virus.

This lack of defense can come in the form of immunosuppression, but it can also come from a deficient production of mannose-binding lectins, which may well be the result of a poor diet or other stress factors that erodes the immune system.

As investigators have found over the past decade of research on not just viruses, but many other infectious diseases, part of immunosuppression comes in the form of a lack of production of mannose-binding lectins.

These natural biochemicals are produced by a healthy immune system and they have the distinction of being able to break apart glycoproteins that cover many viruses, as well as certain bacteria and yeasts.

Some of these dangerous microbes use these glycoprotein envelopes to protect themselves from the immune system, and to help them penetrate cell membranes – which also have glycoproteins in their membranes.

As such a glycoprotein enveloped virus or microorganism penetrates the cell membrane, it can wreck its havoc upon the cell.

Viruses do this by inserting genetic information that hijacks the DNA and RNA of the cell – making the cell a clone for the virus to replicate.

The mechanisms mentioned above with regard to mannose-binding lectins are not anecdotal. They come from a flurry of research.

To be precise, researchers have found in numerous studies that deficiencies in mannose-binding lectins in the bloodstream have are associated with the following diseases:

Research from the Graduate School of Dalian Medical University (Gao *et al.* 2014) found that sepsis patients had significantly lower mannose-binding lectin levels in their blood compared to healthy control patients.

University of Ottawa researchers (Chen *et al.* 2014) found that patients with tuberculosis had significantly lower blood levels of mannose-binding lectins.

Research from Copenhagen University Hospital (Hornum *et al.* 2014) found in a study of 98 kidney disease patients that those with higher mannose-binding lectin levels had better cardiovascular health, as measured by pulse wave velocity. Lower pulse wave velocity levels were associated with higher mannose-binding lectin levels. Higher pulse wave velocity levels are associated with less artery elasticity.

Research from Argentina's CONICET and the Laboratorio de Biología Molecular in Buenos Aires (Gravina *et al.* 2014) found that insufficiencies in mannose-binding lectin levels lead to greater risk of severe infantile cystic fibrosis. Even among those with CFTR mutations, higher mannose-binding lectin levels had better outcomes.

University of Liverpool researchers (Swale *et al.* 2014) found that lower mannose-binding lectin levels were associated with a higher risk of recurrent Clostridium difficile infections. MBL did not appear to reduce the risk of initial infection, however.

An Italian review (Nedovic *et al.* 2014) of five studies found that mutations of the MBL2 gene – which can predispose a person to reduced MBL levels – was associated with a greater risk of vulvovaginal candidiasis – Candida infections of the vagina.

Researchers from Italy's Bambino Gesù Children's Hospital (Auriti *et al.* 2014) found that infants with MBL2 gene mutations (resulting in lower levels of mannose-binding lectins) had a greater risk of neurological conditions.

Research from China's General Hospital of Southern Medical University (Luo *et al.* 2014) found that newborns with lower mannose-binding lectin levels had significantly greater risk of contracting neonatal sepsis.

Research from Spain's Hospital University of Bellvitge (Ibernon *et al.* 2014) found that low levels of mannose-binding lectins in the blood are associated with greater inflammation levels in kidney patients.

Researchers from the Duke University School of Medicine (Justice *et al.* 2014) found that low levels of MBL were significantly associated with recurring sinusitis. They found infections of Staphylococcus aureus and Pseudomonas aeruginosa were more evident among low MBL patients.

Research from the Korea University College of Medicine (Song *et al.* 2014) found after reviewing 12 studies that included over 3,500 people with rheumatoid arthritis and primary Sjögren's syndrome that lower MBL levels were associated with higher levels of RA and Sjögren's syndrome – as determined by genotype.

Research from Poland's Institute of Medical Biology (Swierzko *et al.* 2014) found that ovarian cancer was associated with MBL deficiency, as determined by genotype. They concluded that ovarian cancer was associated with alterations in MBL genes.

Research from China's TianJin People's Hospital (Liu *et al.* 2014) found that low levels of mannose-binding lectins were associated with a greater risk of death from pneumonia.

Spanish researchers (Herrera-Ramos *et al.* 2014) found that lower mannose-binding lectin levels were associated with severe respiratory insufficiency in influenza A virus infections.

Research from Australia's Royal Adelaide Hospital (Tran *et al.* 2014) found that lower mannose-binding lectin levels resulted in greater COPD severity.

Research from Brazil and New York's Weill Cornell Medical College (Orsatti *et al.* 2014) found that postmenopausal women with lower MBL levels – found from MBL genotypes (codon 54 polymorphism) – had greater risk of hypertension and insulin resistance.

University of Chieti researchers (Longhi *et al.* 2014) found that higher mannose-binding lectin levels were associated with greater repair following traumatic brain injuries.

Mannose-binding Lectins from Plants

An important study from The Netherlands' University of Gent (Keyaerts *et al.* 2007) studied plant-derived mannose-binding lectins on SARS (severe acute respiratory syndrome) coronavirus and the feline infectious peritonitis virus (FIPV).

The researchers studied known plant lectins from 33 different plants. The researchers utilized Vero E6 cells to determine the ability of these lectins to inhibit the replication of the two viruses.

The cells were infected with SARS and the FIPV viruses with three and four day incubation period to allow for significant replication of the viruses. Then each of the mannose-binding lectins from each plant species – specifically agglutinins that have been shown to be active in humans – were tested against the two viruses.

Of the 33 plant lectins tested, 15 were significantly antiviral against both the SARS and the FIPV coronaviruses. In addition, five lectins were antiviral against only the SARS and two were antiviral against only the FIPV, and only eight of the lectins were not antiviral against any of the viruses.

Those antiviral lectins were successful in inhibiting the replication of the viruses.

Here is the list of the mannose-binding plant lectins that were antiviral against both the SARS and FIPV viruses from the research:

- **Amaryllis (Hippeastrum hybrid)**
- **Snowdrop (Galanthus nivalis)**
- **Daffodil (Narcissus pseudonarcissus)**
- **Red spider lily (Lycoris radiate)**
- **Leek (Allium porrum)**
- **Ramsons (Allium ursinum)**
- **Taro (Colocasia esculenta)**
- **Cymbidium orchid (Cymbidium hybrid)**
- **Twayblade (Listera ovata)**
- **Broad-leaved helleborine (Epipactis helleborine)**
- **Tulip (Tulipa hybrid)**
- **Black mulberry tree (Morus Nigra)**
- **The other plant lectins that were antiviral against both included:**
- **Tabacco plant (Nicotiana tabacum)**

- **Stinging nettle (Urtica dioica)**

Here are the plants whose lectins that were antiviral but not against both viruses:

- **Solomon's Seal (Polygonatum multiflorum)**
- **Mistletoe (Viscum album)**
- **Iris (Iris hybrid)**
- **Yellow wood (Cladastris lutea)**

Note that both of these coronaviruses, SARS and FIPV and extremely virulent because of their envelopment with glycoproteins that protect the virus against many agents as well as provide a means into the cell.

Protecting our body's Mannose-binding Lectin capacity

Research has found that between 7% and 30% of the population among Western countries is deficient in mannose-binding lectins. Interestingly, U.S. research has indicated between 7-10%, while research in the UK has indicated between 10% and 30%.

Does this mean we are born with a MBL deficiency from mutations among the MBL2 gene?

While this is an emerging topic and there is more research to be done, there is clear evidence that our lifestyles have a lot to do with our body's innate ability to produce mannose-binding lectins.

Researchers from the University of Ottawa and China's Central South University tested 205 tuberculosis patients along with 216 control subjects, and found that mannose-binding lectin levels can be reduced by the following:

- Smoking or secondhand smoke exposure
- Exposure to solid cooking fuel exhaust

These relationships are revealed by the study from Australia's Royal Adelaide Hospital that showed high levels of oxidative stress reduced levels of mannose-binding lectins via oxidation – whereby the lectins were oxidized (oxMBL).

The researchers also found the oxidation of MBL created dysfunctional macrophage activity – which decreased the ability of the patients to fight their lung infections.

When we put the pieces together – of MBL being oxidized together with the effects of smoking and carbon monoxide exposure (the result of solid fuel cooking) – which other research has found causes higher levels of oxidative stress – we find a clear relationship between healthy lifestyles and higher MBL levels.

If we then combine in the research laid out above related to the relationships between mannose-binding lectin deficiencies and a number of disease scenarios, we can correlate that diet also has a lot to do with our MBL levels.

The reality is that our diets can be either alkaline or acidic. Alkaline diets are known for their ability to reduce oxidation within the body because they contain more antioxidants.

On the other hand, diets that are more acidic – meaning they have fewer antioxidants and produce more free radicals – would by default also reduce the body's mannose-binding lectin levels.

Sun and vitamin D levels may also predispose higher MBL levels. University of Copenhagen research found in a study of nearly 1,000 children that mannose-binding lectin levels were lower in the wintertime and higher in the summertime.

Greenfoods

A greenfood is a category of foods that are considered nutritionally superior than the typical fruits and vegetables. Greenfoods include the wheat grasses, sprouts, algaes, and sea vegetables.

Greenfoods provide practically every nutrient imaginable, including enzymes, minerals, trace elements, essential and non-essential amino acids, vitamins, antioxidants and various phytonutrients. Many will provide over 1,000 nutrients.

A big benefit of greenfoods is their alkalinity. This gives them the ability to neutralize radicals and lipid peroxides.

Much of this alkalinity comes from greenfoods' bioavailable mineral content. Many of these minerals are also are colloidal. They tend to be hydrophobic, and maintain a positive electrical charge—rendering them alkaline.

Cereal Grasses

Wheat grass is the young grass of the wheat species, *Triticum aestivum*. In addition to a plethora of vitamins, minerals, amino acids, phytonutrients, metabolic enzymes—including superoxide dismutase and cytochrome oxidase—wheat grass maintains up to 70% chlorophyll.

Early research by Dr. Charles Schnabel, Dr. George Kohler and Dr. A.I. Virtanen in the 1925-1950 era found that cereal grasses like wheatgrass achieved their highest nutrient content at around 18 days— right before the first jointing.

Wheat grass can increase blood hemoglobin levels. Wheat grass tablets decreased blood transfusion needs by 25% among 20 children requiring frequent blood transfusions in a recent study.

Barley grass maintains similar properties. Research has found that barley grass is a potent free radical scavenger; significantly reduces total cholesterol and LDL-cholesterol; and inhibits LDL oxidation. Barley grass juice powder can have 14 vitamins, 18 amino acids, 15 enzymes, 10 antioxidants, 18 minerals and 75 trace elements.

Another cereal grass is Kamut grass. The khorasan wheat has higher protein levels than most wheat varieties, and contains higher zinc, selenium and magnesium content. Selenium is known for stimulating glutathione activity as we've discussed.

Sea Grasses

Kelps might be called seaweeds, but these phytonutrient powerhouses are anything but weeds. About 1,500 species of sea kelps flourish, many in the North Pacific and North Atlantic oceans.

Most kelps are stationary, and sustainably harvested in the wild. This means they must be allowed to regrow to guarantee future harvests. *Ascophyllum nodosum* kelp contains an impressive array of vitamins—more than many vegetables. They include over 60 essential minerals, amino acids and vitamins. They also contain growth promoters, according to kelp researchers.

Most kelps also contain fucoidan, a sulfated polysaccharide. Laboratory studies have indicated fucoidan has anti-tumor, anticoagulant and anti-angiogenic effects. It down-regulates Th2 (inhibiting allergic response), inhibits beta-amyloid formation (implicated in Alzheimer's), inhibits proteinuria in Heymann nephritis and decreases artery platelet deposits.

Other kelps include dulse, sargassi seaweed, *Undaria pinnatifida,* sea palm and others.

Spirulina

Spirulina use dates back to the Aztecs. A good source of carotenoids, vitamins (including vegan B12 according to independent laboratory tests) and minerals, spirulina contains all essential and most non-essential amino acids, with up to 65% protein by weight. It also contains antioxidant phytonutrients such as zeaxanthin, myxoxanthophyll and lutein. It also will contain antioxidant carotenoids, vitamins and minerals.

Spirulina also contains phycobiliprotein, a unique blue pigment anti-inflammatory and antioxidant. Research has showed that phycobiliproteins can protect the liver and kidney from toxins. They are also anti-viral, and stimulate the immune system.

Multiple studies were documented in the HIV/AIDS section earlier in this book. These illustrated that spirulina has been proven effective in helping HIV patients. Other research has shown spirulina boosts immunity in other respects.

In a study from the University of California-Davis (Selma *et al.* 2011), 12 weeks of 3,000 milligrams of Hawaiian spirulina per day significantly increased hemoglobin concentration and mean corpuscular hemoglobin among 30 adults over the age of 50. IDO (indoleamine 2,3-dioxygenase) enzyme activity—a sign of increased immune function—was also higher among the subjects.

In a clinical study (Shariata *et al.* 2019), researchers tested 56 obese people. They were between 20 and 50 years old. The subjects were divided into two groups. One group received 1 gram (1,000 milligrams) of Spirulina platensis supplementation daily and the other group received a placebo.

The research determined that the spirulina group had significantly reduced MIC-1 concentrations. They also had significant improvements in their superoxide dismutase levels, and reductions in other oxidative stress markers.

In a study from Poland's Pomeranian Medical University (Juszkiewicz *et al.* 2018), researchers studied 19 members of the Polish Rowing Team. The researchers gave 10 of the rowers 1,500 milligrams of spirulina extract for six weeks. The other 9 rowers were given a placebo.

The researchers tested all the rowers for their a variety of immunity markers. These included:

- T regulatory lymphocytes (Tregs – CD4, CD25, CD127)
- Cytotoxic lymphocytes (CTLs – CD8, CRαβ)
- Natural killer (NK) cells (CD3, D16, CD56)
- TCRδγ-positive cells (Tδγ)

The researchers found that after only six weeks of supplementation with such a small amount (1.5 grams) of spirulina per day, that the spirulina significantly boosted the rowers' immune systems. The placebo group had increased Treg counts and decreased Tδγ counts after their workouts, as is typically.

Researchers from Poland's University of Medical Sciences (Zeinalian, *et al.* 2017) studied 50 obese patients with insulin resistance and poor cholesterol levels in a 2017 study. The patients also experienced higher inflammation levels.

The researchers gave half the patients 2 grams (2,000 milligrams) of spirulina daily. The other half were given a placebo. After three months of supplementation, the researchers retested the patients – for their insulin sensitivity levels, their LDL-cholesterol levels and their interleukin-6 levels to test their inflammation levels.

The researchers found that the spirulina significantly reduced their LDL cholesterol levels, boosted their insulin sensitivity levels, and decreased their inflammation levels. The research also found that spirulina reduced oxidative stress biomarkers.

This means that spiritulina directly boosted their immunity.

Chlorella

More than 800 published studies have verified the safety and efficacy of *Chlorella pyrenoidosa.* Chlorella's reputation of drawing out heavy metals and other toxins make it a favorite among health practitioners.

Chlorella maintains considerable vitamins minerals, and phytonutrients—including chlorella growth factor (CGF), known to stimulate cell growth. It is also a complete protein, with about 60% protein by weight and every essential and non-essential amino acid. Clinical studies have shown that chlorella stimulates T-cell and B-cell activity and contributes to the improvement of fibromyalgia, ulcerative colitis and hypertension. Another study showed that chlorella increases IgA levels and lowers dioxin levels in breast milk.

Chlorella's tough cell wall must be broken down mechanically to allow these nutrients' bioavailability. Our digestive enzymes cannot digest these outer cell walls. For this reason, quality chlorella growers will pulverize this tough outer cell wall.

Haematococcus and Astaxanthin

Another greenfood algae is *Haematococcus pluvialis,* known for its high astaxanthin content. Astaxanthin is a strong carotenoid similar to beta-carotene. For this reason, astaxanthin is one of the most powerful natural antioxidants known. It also has anti-inflammatory effects, and has been used for eye health, joint healthy, muscle soreness, cardiovascular health, and skin health. It can also protect against damage from UV radiation.

Blue-Green Algae from Klamath Lake

Aphanizomenon flos-aquae or AFA, grows on the pristine waters of Klamath Lake in Oregon. Commercial AFA harvesting began in the early 1980s. This rich volcanic Klamath Lake gives AFA a good source of protein and all the essential and non-essential amino acids. It also has many vitamins, minerals and phytonutrients. AFA contains about 60% protein by weight, and at least 58 minerals at ppm levels, along with significant chlorophyll content.

One of the more exciting phytonutrient compounds discovered in AFA is phenylethylamine (PEA). PEA has been called the 'love molecule,' as it serves to increase positive moods. PEA is also found in chocolate. AFA has significantly more PEA, however.

Aloe Vera

While aloe has long been known for its skin irritation and wound healing abilities, science on its internal use is still emerging.

Aloe is now used for gastrointestinal health, immune support and cardiovascular health, as well as the health of the skin and mucosal membranes.

Aloe may also help prevent kidney stones. A study published in the *Journal of the Thailand Medical Association* found that 200 grams of fresh aloe gel a day significantly decreased urinary oxalate excretion.

In addition, a study from London's Queen Mary School of Medicine on 44 active ulcerated colitis patients found that internal aloe use resulted in clinical improvement. And double-blind, randomized research using Aloecorp's Qmatrix processed aloe has shown that it reduces oxidative stress markers and stimulates the immune system.

Aloe can be taken as a juice or a gel.

Immunity Fats

The types of fats we eat relate directly to our immunity because some fats result in more radicals and other fats result in fewer radicals. As a result, some fats are pro-inflammatory while others are anti-inflammatory.

Anti-inflammatory fats come from low-processed plant-sources that maintain high levels of what the plant utilized for its own development and procreation (as most healthy plant fats come from the seeds of plants). A few of the healthy fats come from algae sources, as we'll discuss.

The fat balance of our diet is critical to cleansing because our cell membranes are made of different lipids and lipid-derivatives like phospholipids and glycolipids. An imbalanced fat diet therefore can lead to weak cell membranes, which leads to cells that have restricted or inconsistent pores. The cell membrane pores allow nutrients in to the cells and waste out of the cells. Unhealthy fats also lead to weaker cell membranes that are more prone to damage by oxidative radicals—producing more cell damage and more toxicity in the body.

An example of this is the International Study of Asthma and Allergies in Childhood (ISAAC) conducted among eight Pacific countries, which included Samoa, Fiji, Tokelau, French Polynesia and New Caledonia. The research found that margarine consumption was one of the leading predicating factors in current asthma and wheezing among children.

Furthermore, they found that the risk factors for increased rhinoconjunctivitis included the regular consumption of meat products, butter and margarine among others. Allergic eczema was also associated with regular meat consumption and butter consumption among others.

Here is a quick review of the major fatty acids and the foods they come from:

Major Omega-3 Fatty Acids (EFAs)

Acronym	Fatty Acid Name	Major Dietary Sources

ALA	Alpha-linolenic acid	Walnuts, soybeans, flax, canola, pumpkin seeds, chia seeds
SDA	Stearidonic acid	hemp, spirulina, blackcurrant
DHA	Docosahexaenoic acid	Body converts from ALA; also obtained from certain algae, krill and fish oils
EPA	Eicosapentaenoic acid	Converts in the body from DHA

Major Omega-6/7 Fatty Acids (EFAs)

Acronym	Fatty Acid Name	Major Dietary Sources
LA	Linoleic acid	Many plants, safflower, sunflower, sesame, soy, almond especially
ARA	Arachidonic acid	Meats, salmon
PA	Palmitoleic acid (7)	Macadamia, palm kernel, coconut
GLA	Gamma-linolenic acid	Borage, primrose oil, spirulina

Major Omega-9 Fatty Acids

Acronym	Fatty Acid Name	Major Dietary Sources
EA	Eucic acid	Canola, mustard seed, wallflower
OA	Oleic acid	Sunflower, olive, safflower

Major Saturated Fatty Acids

Acronym	Fatty Acid Name	Major Dietary Sources
Lauric	Lauric acid	Coconut, dairy, nuts
Myristic	Myristic acid	Coconut, butter
Palmitic	Palmitic acid	Macadamia, palm kernel, coconut, butter, beef, eggs
Stearic	Stearic acid	Macadamia, palm kernel, coconut, eggs

Essential fatty acids (EFAs) are fats the body does not form. Eaten in the right proportion, they can also lower inflammation and speed healing. EFAs include the long-chain polyunsaturated fatty acids—and the shorter chain linolenic, linoleic and oleic polyunsaturates. EFAs include omega-3s and omega-6s. The omega-3s include alpha linolenic acid (ALA), docosahexaenoic acid (DHA) and eicosapentaenoic acid (EPA). EPA and DHA are found in algae, mackerel, salmon, herring, sardines, sablefish (black cod). The omega-6s include linoleic acid, (LA), palmitoleic acid (PA), gamma-linoleic acid (GLA) and arachidonic acid (ARA). The term *essential* was originally given with the assumption that these types of fats could not be assembled or produced by the body—they must be taken directly from our food supply.

This assumption, however, is not fully correct. While it is true that we need *some* of these from our diet, our bodies can readily convert LA to ARA, and ALA to DHA and EPA as needed. Therefore, these fats can be considered essential in the sense that they are not generated by the body, but we do not necessarily have to consume each one of them.

Monounsaturated fats are high in omega-9 fatty acids like oleic acid. A monounsaturated fatty acid has one double carbon-hydrogen bonding chain. Oils from seeds, nuts and other plant-based sources have the largest quantities of monounsaturates. Oils that have large proportions of monounsaturates such as olive oil are known to lower inflammation when replacing high saturated fat in diets. Monounsaturates also aid in skin cell health and reduce atopic skin responses.

Monounsaturated fatty acids like oleic acid have been shown in studies to lower heart attack risk, aid blood vessel health, and offer anti-carcinogenic potential. They are typical among Mediterranean diets, which have been shown to reduce heart disease risk and cancer risk—related to their lower levels of lipid peroxidative radicals. The best sources of omega-9s are olives, sesame seeds, avocados, almonds, peanuts, pecans, pistachio nuts, cashews, hazelnuts, macadamia nuts, several other nuts and their respective oils.

Research has found that olives contain good amounts of the monounsaturated fat called oleic acid. In a 2020 review of research (Tutunchi *et al.* 2020), 28 clinical trials were analyzed. The research found that diets rich in oleic acids (rich in olives and olive oil) reduced body weight, body mass and abdominal fat.

Other studies have found that oleic acids change levels of insulin resistance. For example a study from Spain's University of Valladolid (de Luis *et al.* 2017) studied 361 obese adults. They split the group into two diets. They found the monounsaturated fat diet triggered weight loss and lower LDL-cholesterol among the group. It also significantly reduced insulin levels and insulin resistance.

Still other research has shown that olive oil has other benefits, including lowering blood pressure, reducing inflammation, helping prevent stokes and helping to prevent cancer. As researchers from Spain's Epidemiology Research Programme (Buckland and Gonzalez 2015) put it:

"These health benefits are supported by strong mechanistic evidence from experimental studies, demonstrating that specific components of olive oil have antihypertensive, antithrombotic, antioxidant, antiinflammatory and anticarcinogenic action."

Polyunsaturated fats have at least two double carbon-hydrogen bonds. They come from a variety of plant and marine sources. Omega-3s ALA, DHA and EPA simply have longer chains with more double carbon-hydrogen bonds. ALA, DHA and EPA are known to lower inflammation and increase artery-wall health. These *long-chain* omega-3 polyunsaturates are also considered critical for intestinal health.

The omega-6 fatty acids are the most available form of fat in the plant kingdom. Linoleic acid is the primary omega-6 fatty acid and it is found in most grains and seeds.

Saturated fats have multiple fatty acids without double bonds (the hydrogens "saturate" the carbons). They are found among animal fats, and tropical oils such as coconut and palm. Milk products such as butter and whole milk contain saturated fats, along with a special type of healthy linoleic fatty acid called CLA or *conjugated linoleic acid.*

The saturated fats from coconuts and palm differ from animal saturates in that they have shorter chains. This actually gives them—unlike animal saturates—an antimicrobial quality.

Medium chain fatty acids like coconut and palm oils have been shown in human studies to lower lipoprotein-A concentrations in the blood while having fibrinolytic (plaque and clot reduction) effects (Muller *et al.* 2003).

Trans fats are oils that either have been overheated or have undergone hydrogenation. Hydrogenation is produced by heating while bubbling hydrogen ions through the oil. This adds hydrogen and repositions some of the bonds. The "trans" refers to the positioning of part of the molecule in reverse—as opposed to "cis" positioning. The cis positioning is the bonding orientation the body's cell membranes work best with. Trans fats have been known to be a cause for increased radical species in the system; damaging artery walls; contributing to inflammation, heart disease, high LDL levels, liver damage, diabetes, and other metabolic dysfunction (Mozaffarian *et al.* 2009). Trans fat overconsumption slows the conversion of LA to GLA.

Conjugated linolenic acid (CLA) is a healthy fat that comes from primarily from dairy products. CLA is also a trans fat, but this is a trans fat the body works well with—it is considered a healthy trans fat.

Researchers from St Paul's Hospital and the University of British Columbia (MacRedmond *et al.* 2010) gave 28 overweight adults 4.5 g/day of CLA or a placebo for 12 weeks in addition to their medications. After the twelve weeks, those in the CLA group experienced significantly better lung function compared to the placebo group. The CLA group also experienced a significant reduction of weight and BMI compared with the control group. The CLA group also had lower leptin/adiponectin ratios—associated with balanced metabolism.

Other research has also found that CLA can to reduce lipid peroxidation and provide better balance among lipids (Noone *et al.* 2002).

Arachidonic acid (ARA): ARA is considered an essential fatty acid, and research has shown that it is vital for infants while they are building their intestinal barriers. However, ARA is pro-inflammatory and stimulates pro-inflammatory mediators like leukotrienes. Too much of it as we age thus burdens our immune systems, pushing our bodies towards systemic inflammation and slower detoxification.

Red meats provide the highest levels of arachidonic acid. Because arachidonic acid stimulates the production of pro-inflammatory prostaglandins and leucotrienes in an enzyme conversion process, too much ARA leads to a greater level of toxicity, producing more inflammation.

Interestingly, carnivorous animals cannot or do not readily convert linoleic acid (found in many common plants) to arachidonic acid, but herbivore animals do convert linoleic acid to arachidonic acid, as do humans. This conversion—on top of a red meat-heavy diet—produces high arachidonic acid levels. In contrast, a diet that is balanced between plant-based monounsaturates, polyunsaturates and some saturates (such as the Mediterranean diet) will balance arachidonic acids with the other fatty acids.

Gamma linoleic acid (GLA): A wealth of studies have confirmed that GLA reduces or inhibits the inflammatory response. Leukotrienes produced by arachidonic acid stimulate inflammation, while leukotrienes produced by GLA block the conversion of polyunsaturated fatty acids to arachidonic acid. This means that GLA lowers inflammation, and promotes a healthy immune system.

A healthy body will convert linoleic acid into GLA readily, utilizing the same delta-6 desaturase enzyme used for ALA to DHA conversion. From GLA, the body produces *dihomo-gamma linoleic acid,* which cycles through the body as an eicosinoid. This aids in skin health, healthy mucosal membranes, and down-regulates inflammatory hypersensitivity.

In addition to conversion from LA, GLA can also be obtained from the oils of borage seeds, evening primrose seed, hemp seed, and from spirulina. Excellent food sources of LA include chia seeds, seed, hempseed, grapeseed, pumpkin seeds, sunflower seeds, safflower seeds, soybeans, olives, pine nuts, pistachio nuts, peanuts, almonds, cashews, chestnuts, and their respective oils.

The conversion of LA to GLA (and ALA to DHA) is reduced by trans fat consumption, smoking, pollution, stress, infections, and various chemicals that affect the liver.

Docosahexaenoic acid (DHA) obtained from algae, fish and krill, has significant therapeutic and anti-inflammatory effects according to the research. DHA is also associated with stronger cell membranes, and lower levels of lipid peroxidation.

It appears that the anti-inflammatory effects of DHA in particular relate to a modulation of a gene factor called NF-kappaB. The NF-kappaB is involved in signaling among cytokine receptors. With more DHA consumption, the transcription of the NF-kappaB gene sequence is reduced. This appears to reduce inflammatory signaling (Singer *et al.* 2008).

DHA readily converts to EPA by the body. EPA degrades quickly if unused in the body. It is easily converted from DHA as needed. Our bodies store DHA and not EPA.

Because much of the early research on the link between fatty acids and inflammatory disease was performed using fish oil, it was assumed that both EPA and DHA fatty acids reduced inflammation. Recent research from the University of Texas' Department of Medicine/Division of Clinical Immunology and Rheumatology (Rahman *et al.* 2008) has clarified that DHA is primarily implicated in reducing inflammation. DHA was shown to inhibit RANKL-induced pro-inflammatory cytokines, and a number of inflammation steps, while EPA did not.

The process of converting ALA to DHA and other omega-3s requires an enzyme produced in the liver called delta-6 desaturase. Some people— especially those who have a poor diet, are immune-suppressed, or burdened with toxicity such as cigarette smoke—may not produce this enzyme very well. As a result, they may not convert as much ALA to DHA and EPA.

For those with low levels of DHA—or for those with problems converting ALA and DHA—low-environmental impact and low toxin content DHA from microalgae can be supplemented. Certain algae produce significant amounts of DHA. They are the foundation for the DHA molecule all the way up the food chain, including fish. This is how fish get their DHA, in other words. Three algae species—*Cryptheodinium cohnii, Nitzschia laevis* and *Schizochytrium spp.*—are in commercial production and available in oil and capsule form.

Microalgae-derived DHA is preferable to fish or fish oils because fish oils typically contain saturated fats and may also—depending upon their origin—contain toxins such as mercury and PCBs (though to their credit, many producers also carefully distill their fish oil). However, we should note that salmon contain a considerable amount of arachidonic acid as well (Chilton 2006).

Thus, the DHA derived from fish sources, because it requires increased levels of filtering and processing to remove PCBs and mercury, would not be considered a living source of DHA, as it is too far removed from the living source. Algae-derived DHA is a wholesome source, as it is derived directly from living algae. Algae-derived DHA also does not strain sensitive fishery populations.

Algal-DHA also decreases pro-inflammatory arachidonic acid levels. One study (Arterburn *et al.* 2007) measured pro-inflammatory arachidonic acid levels within the body before and after supplementation with algal

DHA. It was found that arachidonic acid levels decreased by 20% following just one dose of 100 milligrams of algal DHA.

For those who consider fish the superior source of DHA: In a study by researchers from The Netherlands' Wageningen University Toxicology Research Center (van Beelen *et al.* 2007), all three species of commercially produced algal oil showed equivalency with fish oil in their inhibition of cancer cell growth. Another study (Lloyd-Still *et al.* 2007) of twenty cystic fibrosis patients concluded that 50 milligrams of algal DHA was readily absorbed, maintained DHA bioavailability immediately, and increased circulating DHA levels by four to five times.

In terms of DHA availability, algal-DHA is just as good as fish. In a randomized open-label study (Arterburn *et al.* 2008), researchers gave 32 healthy men and women either algal DHA oil or cooked salmon for two weeks. After the two weeks, plasma levels of circulating DHA were bioequivalent.

Alpha-linolenic acid (ALA) is the primary omega-3 fatty acid the body can most easily assimilate. Once assimilated, the healthy body will convert ALA to omega-3s, primarily DHA, at a range of about 7-40%, depending upon the health of the liver. One study of six women performed at England's University of Southampton (Burdge *et al.* 2002) showed a conversion rate of 36% from ALA to DHA and other omega-3s. A follow-up study of men showed ALA conversion to the omega-3s occurred at an average of 16%.

We should include that ALA, which comes from plants, has been shown to halt or slow inflammation processes, similar to DHA. In studies at Wake Forest University (Chilton *et al.* 2008), for example, flaxseed oil produced anti-inflammatory effects, along with borage oil and echium oil (the latter two also containing GLA).

Furthermore, flaxseed has been recommended specifically for toxicity and inflammation for centuries. This is not only because of its omega-3 levels: it is also because flaxseed contains mucilage, which helps strengthen our mucosal membranes.

The healthy fat balance: In a meta-study by researchers from the University of Crete's School of Medicine (Margioris 2009), numerous studies showed that long-chain polyunsaturated omega-3s tend to be anti-inflammatory while omega-6 oils tend to be pro-inflammatory.

This, however, simplifies the equation too much. Most of the research on fats has also shown that most omega-6s are healthy oils. Balance is the key.

Research has illustrated that reducing animal-derived saturated fats reduces inflammation, cardiovascular disease, high cholesterol and diabetes (Ros and Mataix 2008). All of these relate to toxicity, because as we've discussed, lipid peroxidation lies at the root of these conditions.

The relationships became clearer from a study performed at Sydney's Heart Research Institute (Nicholls *et al.* 2008). Here fourteen adults consumed meals either rich in saturated fats or omega-6 polyunsaturated fats. They were tested following each meal for various inflammation and cholesterol markers. The results showed that the high saturated fat meals increased inflammatory activities and decreased the liver's production of HDL cholesterol; whereas (good) HDL levels and the liver's anti-inflammatory capacity were increased after the omega-6 meals.

What this tells us is that the omega-3/omega-6 story is complicated by the saturated fat content of the diet and subsequent liver function. High saturated fat diets increase (bad) LDL (lipid peroxidation) content and reduce the anti-inflammatory and antioxidant capacities of the liver. Diets lower in saturated fat and higher in omega-6 and omega-3 fats encourage antioxidant and anti-inflammatory activity.

We also know that diets high in monounsaturated fats—such as the Mediterranean diet—are also associated with significant anti-inflammatory effects. Mediterranean diets contain higher levels of monounsaturated fats like oleic acids (omega-9) from foods like olives and avocados (and their oils); as well as higher proportions of fruits and vegetables, and lower proportions of saturated fats.

High saturated fat diets are also associated with increased obesity, and a number of studies have shown that obesity is directly related to inflammatory diseases—including allergies as we've discussed. High saturated fat diets and diets high in trans fatty acids have also been clearly shown to accompany higher levels of inflammation—illustrated by increases in inflammatory factors such as IL-6 and CRP (Basu *et al.* 2006).

To maximize anti-inflammatory factors, the ideal proportion of omega-6s to omega-3s is recommended at about two to one (2:1). The western diet has been estimated by researchers to up to thirty to one (30:1) of omega-6s to omega-3s. This large imbalance (of too much omega-6s and too little omega-3s) has also been associated with inflammatory diseases, including asthma, arthritis, heart disease, ulcerative colitis, Crohn's disease, and others. When fat consumption is out of balance, the body's metabolism will trend towards inflammation. This is because in the absence of omega-3s and GLA, omega-6 oils convert more easily to arachidonic acid. And remember, ARA is pro-inflammatory (Simopoulos 1999).

Noting the research showing the relationships between the different fatty acids and inflammation, and the condition of the liver (which can be burdened by too much saturated fat), scientists have logically arrived at a model for dietary fat consumption for a person who is either dealing with or wants to prevent inflammation-oriented conditions and toxicity:

Omega-3	20%-25% of dietary fats
Omega-6+Omega-9	40%-50% of dietary fats
Saturated	5%-10% of dietary fats
GLA	10%-20% of dietary fats
Trans fats	0% of dietary fats

Nuts, seeds, grains, beans, olives and avocados can provide the bulk of these healthy fats in balanced combinations. Walnuts, pumpkin seeds, flax, chia, soy, canola and algal-DHA can fill in the omega 3s. Healthy saturated fats can be found in coconuts, palm and dairy products. These foods are typical of the Mediterranean diet.

Immunity Enhancing Supplements

As we've discussed, antioxidant nutrition can significantly lighten our body's inflammatory load, and stimulate our detoxification processes. For example, researchers from the Human Nutrition Research Center on Aging at Tufts University (Tucker *et al.* 2004) studied the relationships between homocysteine and B vitamins. They studied 189 healthy volunteers between 50 and 85 years old. They gave the subjects either one cup daily of fortified cereal (with 440 micrograms of folic acid, 1.8 milligrams of vitamin B-6, and 4.8 micrograms of vitamin B-12) or an unfortified cereal (placebo). After twelve weeks, the fortified cereal eaters had significantly less homocysteine levels than did the placebo cereal.

A diet with a variety of plant-based fresh foods of sufficient quantity requires minimum supplementation, assuming organically-grown foods and/or foods grown in healthy soils. This said, there is a great likelihood that our diets are lacking in some nutrients, especially if we suffer from systemic inflammation.

In such a condition, we are likely eating a narrow range of foods and/or exposed to a significant amount of toxins or infections. In other words, because toxins and infections 'burn up' nutrients—as the body requires these to neutralize radicals and produce enzymes—a person with systemic inflammation living in a toxic environment will likely require more nutrients than a healthy person living in a natural environment.

There are a number of isolated nutrients that have been shown to help reduce toxins. A few, like antioxidant vitamins C, A, D, and E and others have been shown to reduce inflammation by modulating inflammatory mediators and balancing Th1 and Th2 (Mainardi *et al.* 2009). Others, such as selenium, directly relate to the liver's glutathione processes for reducing toxins and radicals.

When a person's diet is lacking in an important nutrient, the body sometimes responds with critical weaknesses in immunity and inflammation. This can produce a greater tendency for toxin accumulation, simply because the body's supply of radical-neutralizing nutrients is decreased.

Many people are deficient in some or many nutrients, depending upon their diet. Even people who regularly take multi-vitamins become deficient in some nutrients. Why is this? This is an extremely complicated subject—one that could take an entire book to fully explore. To summarize, there are a number of reasons why people don't get the nutrients their body needs. These range from the more obvious—of poor diet choices—to the less obvious—of not being able to absorb certain nutrients due to enzyme issues, probiotic deficiencies and/or intestinal defects.

As has been shown in a number of studies, especially regarding B vitamins, a person may take a good multivitamin yet still be deficient because they lack the intrinsic factors that help assimilate those nutrients. In other cases, there is a chelation problem, where the nutrient is not absorbed because it doesn't have the right intestinal biofactors available within either the diet or the intestines. In still other cases, a nutrient may not be in a form that the body recognizes. This is often the case with synthetic multivitamins. In some cases, the body might treat the particular nutrient as a foreign molecule, and decide to break it down and expel it!

For those who are deficient in one or more nutrients, a good food-source supplement or change in the diet can immediately help their inflammatory hypersensitivity. Yet for another person, who may not be deficient in that nutrient, the nutrient supplement may not offer a significant change in toxicity and/or inflammation.

If a person is not deficient in the nutrient, taking more of the nutrient may not help them at all. Furthermore, overloading on isolated nutrients that have been shown to help those who are deficient can lead to a worsening of inflammation. This is due to the fact that synthesized, isolated nutrients can overload the liver and detoxification systems, as they have to be broken down. Some vitamins, such as vitamin A, can be toxic if over-supplemented. The bottom line is that for the most part, more is not necessarily better when it comes to nutrients.

So it is essential that we engage in a supplement strategy very logically. First, we need to have a healthy amount of plant-based foods in our diet, with raw, fresh foods with plenty of fiber and phytonutrients. This will create a solid foundation.

Secondly, we can add a food-based multivitamin as a sort of insurance policy to make sure we get enough of the most important nutrients. A food-based multivitamin is one where the nutrients are sourced directly from foods, or grown on food substrates such as spirulina. These sorts of multivitamins are more recognized by the body.

Thirdly, we can pay closer attention to certain nutrients that have been shown in some research to decrease inflammation. For these nutrients, we may decide to take a focused combination or isolated nutrient. But here we need to understand that many isolated nutrients can imbalance our body and create other deficiencies. Therefore, we need to approach isolated nutrient supplementation with caution. Best to err on the side of nature's balance of whole food sources, in other words.

For example, if we are taking more vitamin C, we can use a food-based or mineral ascorbate vitamin C supplement that offers chelated versions, and bioflavonoids that help the body assimilate and utilize the vitamin C.

If we are taking a mineral supplement like magnesium, we can take one that offers a chelated version together with calcium and trace minerals—offered by coral or mined sources, for example. The point here is that taking excess magnesium without the supporting and balancing minerals can exhaust the body of calcium, zinc and other essential, supporting elements.

We can also consult with a nutritionally-oriented health professional who can test our body's nutrient levels. Tests range from urine tests to blood tests and hair analyses—the latter of which may be appropriate to establish cellular mineral levels (Wilson 1998). This can be very helpful when trying to determine if we have a particular nutrient deficiency.

What is a Food-Source Supplement?

A food-source supplement is one where the nutrients have been produced by a living organism. The three key sources of natural nutrients are those produced by plants, those produced by probiotics, those produced by yeasts or those produced by the earth. These are nature's nutrients. Living organisms produce nutrients to protect themselves from the environment or other species. Thus, the nutrients they produce stimulate our immune system.

Our immune system also readily recognizes the nutrients, and our body and liver can readily metabolize these nutrients. They can be easily broken down and utilized, in other words.

Nutrients that are produced in a lab or manufacturing facility using synthesized substrates and catalysts can be recognized as a nutrient by the body, but many may not, especially if the immune system is already subject to inflammation. Such an immune system may not tolerate many synthetic nutrients.

As a result, the best nutrients on the market are:

> ➢ Nutrients that have been grown by yeasts or probiotics
> ➢ Nutrients that have utilized natural substrates (many use spirulina)
> ➢ Nutrients that have been derived directly from plant sources (vitamin C from acerola, for example)
> ➢ Nutrients that have been gathered from mines or dead coral (magnesium and calcium carbonate, for example)

Because these types of nutrients are produced by living organisms, they are well-recognized by the body, and well-utilized by the body.

A Few Cleansing Nutrients

With that said, we should know that nearly every nutrient has a role in the body's immune system and/or the liver's detoxification process. Thus we can really list practically every nutrient here. Instead, we'll just list a few "heavy-hitters" that are known to significantly stimulate cleansing. Remember, however, that the body needs a balance of nutrients. Therefore, it is advisable to not focus on isolated nutrients, but rather on living nutrients combined (chelated) within natural supplement substrates.

Quercetin: We also discussed quercetin foods previously. Quercetin supplements may be appropriate if the diet is lacking in plant-based foods. As mentioned earlier, this flavonoid inhibits histamine and leukotrienes—inflammatory mediators—in the body.

Vitamin C is considered by researchers as one of the "first line of defense" antioxidants, because it is readily available to neutralize free radicals at mucosal membranes and tissue fluids. A number of studies have shown that vitamin C can reduce inflammation.

Vitamin C supplement doses aimed at reducing inflammation typically range from one to three grams per day. As mentioned, chelated versions and versions with bioflavonoids help the potency of vitamin C.

A Cochrane review (Hemilä *et al.* 2013) of 29 clinical trials that including 9,676 cold episodes found a "consistent" benefit of 8 percent reduction of cold duration among adults and 14 percent reduction of cold duration among children. The large metadata calculation utilized vitamin C doses over 200 milligrams per day.

With regard to higher doses, better results were found. Children given between 1,000 and 2,000 milligrams of vitamin C a day had an average of 18 percent shorter colds.

This review also found that regular vitamin C supplementation reduced the severity of colds.

Some health researchers have also noted that vitamin C and quercetin tend to work well together. This is why apples and onions are so healthy. While fruits and many vegetables offer readily-assimilable doses of vitamin C with bioflavonoids, vitamin C drink powders with chelated ascorbates also provide a good way to supplement extra vitamin C.

Lycopene: This phytonutrient, usually isolated from tomatoes, has been shown in some research to reduce inflammation. Best approach here is to consume tomatoes, which have been found to contain about 10,000 different nutrients.

Beta-carotene and other Carotenoids: These vitamin A precursors are essential antioxidants often lacking in many diets. Some research has shown that carotenoids can reduce radical damage to the eyes and other organs.

Vitamin E: Vitamin E supplementation has been shown to provide significant antioxidant benefits. As a result, studies have shown that vitamin E can help prevent cardiovascular disease, respiratory diseases and cognitive impairment.

A few recent studies on vitamin E have shown inconclusive findings, however. What is going on here?

Most people consider vitamin E a single nutrient. But there are actually at least eight forms of vitamin E. Four of them are tocopherols, which include alpha-tocopherol, beta-tocopherol, gamma-tocopherol, and delta-tocopherol. There are also four tocotrienol forms of vitamin E. This includes alpha-tocotrienol, beta-tocotrienol, gamma-tocotrienol, and delta-tocotrienol. The primary vitamin E form in most supplements is alpha-tocopherol.

Most of the research on vitamin E has utilized only alpha-tocopherols. Ongoing research has established that alpha-tocopherols do provide some benefits, but a mix of tocotrienols provide more benefit—especially with regard to cardiovascular health.

Diets can vary in terms of their vitamin E forms. Western diets are typically restricted to alpha-tocopherols and gamma-tocopherols. However, a mixed plant-based diet that includes coconut and palm foods, whole grain rice and other whole grains will render more of the tocotrienol forms.

The bottom line is that the E vitamins are essential antioxidants that help prevent lipid peroxidation—as discussed earlier.

Vitamin Bs: All the vitamin Bs are important to the body's detoxification systems. They are most known for donating methyl groups, used by the liver and glutathione to scavenge free radicals. We should also note that toxins and pharmaceuticals will reduce our stores of Bs. Also, many people lack the intrinsic factor that allows for B vitamin—especially B12—assimilation. For these people, many doctors have advised B12 shots.

Research has recently illustrated, however, that sublingual (under the tongue) B12 is absorbed just as readily into the blood as a B12 shot. There are several sublingual B vitamin supplements on the market today.

Magnesium, Sulfur, Zinc and Other Minerals

Minerals are critical to our detoxification and cleansing processes because they donate ions that neutralize radicals, and are part of key enzymes. Without enough of these important minerals, the body's metabolic systems slow down, due to the lack of enzymes.

Magnesium deficiency has been found to be at the root of a number of conditions, especially those related to anxiety, spasms and muscle cramping. Not surprisingly, inflammation can be significantly reduced with magnesium supplementation.

Magnesium, along with calcium, is critical for smooth muscle tone and nerve conduction. Magnesium is part of the calcium ion channel system. Magnesium regulates calcium infusion into the nerves, which helps keep them stabilized and balanced. This is why magnesium deficiencies within the calcium ion channel system causes overstrain among muscles. This translates to spasms, cramping and muscle fatigue.

If magnesium levels are low, the ion channels will be unstable, stimulating nerve hyperactivity. This nerve hyperactivity can cause changes in the flow of nutrients into cells and toxins out of cells. In other words, magnesium deficiency can result in toxemia.

Magnesium is also a critical element used by the immune system. A body deficient in magnesium will likely be immunosuppressed. Animal studies have illustrated that magnesium deficiency leads to increased IgE counts, and increased levels of inflammation-specific cytokines. Magnesium deficiency is also associated with increased degranulation among mast/basophil/neutrophil cells, which stimulates the allergic response.

Dr. Jabar from the State University of New York Hospital and Medical Center, notes the blood magnesium levels can help determine if magnesium supplements can help. Magnesium levels among red blood cells indicate whether magnesium will likely have any effects.

It is no surprise that magnesium has also been shown to benefit anxiety, as it helps balance nerve firing. Magnesium has also been shown to have anti-inflammatory effects when combined with dosing with larger (one gram or more) doses of vitamin C.

Foods high in magnesium include soybeans, kidney beans, lima beans, bananas, broccoli, Brussels sprouts, carrots, cauliflower, celery, cherries, corn, dates, bran, blackberries, green beans, pumpkin seeds, spinach, chard, tofu, sunflower seeds, sesame seeds, black beans and navy beans, mineral water and beets.

Calcium is also critical for the functioning of nerves and muscles. Every cell utilizes calcium, evidenced by calcium ion channels present in every cell membrane. Therefore, calcium is necessary for healthy lungs and airways. Thus, calcium deficiency results in more than bone problems. Muscle cramping and airway constriction are also side effects of calcium deficiency. Low calcium levels also result in deranged nerve firing, which can produce anxiety and depression. Supplementing calcium should also be accompanied by magnesium supplementing. For example, a supplement with 1,000 mg of calcium can be balanced by 600 mg of magnesium along with trace minerals.

Good calcium foods include dairy, bok choy, collards, okra, soy, beans, broccoli, kale, mustard greens and others.

Zinc is another important mineral for immunity.

A study from Germany's Aachen University (Rosenkranz *et al.* 2016) found that zinc supplementation increased autoimmune tolerance. In particular, Th17 cells significantly decreased, and autoimmunity symptoms were reduced in laboratory research.

Another study from Aachen University (Maywald *et al.* 2016) found that zinc supplementation reduced T cell expansion and stabilized cytokines typically involved in autoimmune responses.

A study from Germany's Otto-von-Guericke-University (Stoye *et al.* 2012) found that zinc aspartate supplementation reduced T cell proliferation and reduced autoimmune reactions in laboratory research. The scientists duplicated autoimmunity and found that 1.5 milligrams per kilo of body weight (about 2.2 lbs) was able to significantly alter T cell proliferation.

Researchers from Italy's INRAN National Research Institute on Food and Nutrition (Devirgiliis *et al.* 2007) have investigated the relationship between zinc and chronic diseases. Their research determined that an "imbalance in zinc homeostasis" can impair protein synthesis, cell membrane transport and gene expression. These factors, they explained, stimulate imbalances among hormones and tissue systems, producing inappropriate inflammation.

As zinc ions pass through the cell membrane, they assist the cell in the uptake of nutrients. Zinc transporters interact with genes to regulate the transmission of nutrients within the cell, and the pathways in and out of the cell. Zinc concentration within the cell is balanced by proteins called metallothioneins. These proteins require copper and selenium in addition to zinc. Metallothioneins are critical to the cell's ability to scavenge various radicals and heavy metals that can damage the cells. Deficiencies in metallothioneins have been seen among chronic inflammatory conditions, and even fatal diseases such as cancer.

A Cochrane database review (Singh *et al.* 2013) analyzed 16 therapeutic studies that included 1,387 people, plus two prevention trials. The research found that zinc taken within 24 hours of the appearance of cold symptoms significantly reduced the duration of a cold.

There was a 55 percent reduction in the number of people symptomatic of a cold after seven days compared to those not taking zinc. And the incidence of colds among those taking zinc regularly was 36 percent less than those who were not.

The researchers also noted that significant cold duration occurred when doses were 75 milligrams per day or greater.

Not surprisingly, research has also shown that zinc modulates T-cell activities (Hönscheid *et al.* 2009).

Good zinc foods include cowpeas, beans, lima beans, milk, brown rice, yogurt, oats, cottage cheese, bran, lentils, wheat and others.

Selenium: Research has shown that greater levels of lipid peroxidation (due to greater consumption of poor fats and fatty foods) decrease our body's levels of selenium. This is because selenium is a critical component of , glutathione peroxidase—which reduces lipid peroxidation. Those with higher levels of lipid peroxidation tend to require more selenium because they exhaust this nutrient more readily, as we discussed earlier. While selenium supplements might offer generous amounts of selenium, one brazil nut will supply about 120 micrograms of selenium. This is 170% of the recommended daily value.

Sulfur: Research has also confirmed that dietary sulfur can significantly relieve inflammation and hypersensitivity. In a multi-center open label study by researchers from Washington state (Barrager *et al.* 2002), 55 patients with allergic rhinitis were given 2,600 mg of methylsulfonylmethane (MSM)—a significant source of sulfur derived from plants—for 30 days. Weekly reviews of the patients reported significant improvements in allergic respiratory symptoms, along with increased energy. Other research has suggested that sulfur blocks the binding of histamine among receptors.

Another study (Kim *et al.* 2006) of 50 patients with knee osteoarthritis given either 6 grams per day of MSM) or a placebo for 12 weeks found that after 12 weeks, the MSM group had significantly less pain and significantly more mobility than the placebo group.

Supplemental MSM is typically derived from plant sources. Good food sources of sulfur include avocado, asparagus, barley, beans, broccoli, cabbage, carob, carrots, Brussels sprouts, chives, coconuts, corn, garlic, leafy green vegetables, leeks, lentils, onions, parsley, peas, radishes, red peppers, soybeans, shallots, Swiss chard and watercress.

Potassium is lowered by many pharmaceutical medications, toxins and sweating. Low potassium levels will contribute to imbalances in blood pressure and the kidneys. These issues reduce our ability to cleanse toxins.

Good potassium foods include bananas, spinach, sunflower seeds, tomatoes, pomegranates, turnips, lima beans, navy beans, squash, broccoli and others.

Trace minerals: These should not be ignored in this discussion. Trace elements are important to nearly every enzymatic reaction in the body.

While minerals have been shown to provide therapeutic results, we must be careful about mineral supplements, especially those that provide single or a few minerals. Minerals co-exist in the body, and a dramatic increase in one can exhaust others as the body depletes the oversupply. Thus, an isolated macro-mineral supplement can easily produce a mineral imbalance in the body, which can produce a variety of hypersensitivity issues.

Better to utilize natural sources of minerals. These include, first and foremost, mineral-intensive vegetables. Nearly all vegetables contain generous mineral content in the combinations designed by nature. Best to eat a mixed combination of vegetables to achieve a healthy array of trace minerals.

Whole food mineral sources also contain many trace minerals in their more-digestible *chelated* forms. Chelation is when a mineral ion bonds with another nutrient, providing a ready ion as the body needs it.

Most organically-grown plant-based foods provide a rich supply of trace minerals, assuming we are eating enough of them. Other good sources of full spectrum trace minerals include natural mineral water, whole (unprocessed) rock salt, coral calcium, spirulina, AFA, kelp and chlorella. These sources will typically have from 60 to 80 trace elements, all of which are necessary for the body's various enzymatic functions. See the author's book, *Pure Water.*

We should also note that research by David Brownstein, M.D. (2006) has illustrated that whole unprocessed salt does not affect the body—high blood pressure, cardiovascular disease, diabetes and so on—as do refined salts (often called sodium).

These naturally-chelated mineral sources also prevent the side effects known for mineral supplements. For example, magnesium can easily produce diarrhea in the 2,000-5,000 milligram level. While this might be considered a minor side effect, diarrhea can also produce dehydration.

Numerous holistic doctors now prescribe full-spectrum mineral combinations for inflammatory conditions. Many have attested to their clinical successes in recommending minerals to balance the inflammatory response and stimulate healthy mucosal membranes. Full range supplements that have RDA levels of the macrominerals combined with trace levels of the other minerals can provide a good foundation. Eating more than 5-6 servings a day of fruits and vegetables can provide the rest.

Micronutrients: These trace minerals, along with some low-dose vitamins, are called micronutrients. This is because they are not needed in the body in large amounts.

Research carried out by the Department of Nutrition of Beijing's PLA General Hospital (Liu *et al.* 2011) studied 196 type 2 diabetic outpatients. They were randomly divided into two groups of 97 and 99 persons. One group was given micronutrient supplements in tablets for six months, while the other group was given a placebo.

Before the study began, the researchers recorded blood and other health measurements, as well as infection incidence among the patients. They documented their diet, exercise and incidence of infections – including respiratory, skin, urinary and genital infections along with others – for a month before the study began, and throughout the study.

In every type of infection area, the micronutrient group had fewer infections; and when there was infection, the duration of fevers were significantly lower in the micronutrient group than among the placebo group.

Superfood Supplements

Isolated nutrients in large doses can also throw off the body's balance of other nutrients, as we've discussed. Many nutrients are called cofactors because their effectiveness requires the presence of other nutrients. This sort of cooperative character of nutrients is simply because the body's processes are heavily related to each other. As opposed to a lot of research, very little occurs in the body within a vacuum.

Superfood supplements are quite simply, extremely nutritious foods. Many—such as wheatgrass, spirulina, chlorella, barley grass and others—also typically contain generous levels of chlorophyll—which alkalizes the blood, stimulates more red blood cells, and helps neutralize radicals.

Many of these are available as supplements, as they may be dehydrated and encapsulated or pressed into tablets—or simply taken as a powder. Many superfood supplements—primarily nutritious fruits and vegetables such as noni, mangosteen and wheat grass—may also be eaten raw as we've discussed.

We've covered a number of these earlier, but we'll summarize some of them again to underscore their importance to stimulating our immune system and reducing inflammation. We'll also cover introduce some new superfoods as well:

Chlorella: A virtually complete food. This microalgae is cultivated in pools or tanks under controlled conditions. Chlorella contains numerous antioxidant nutrients, B vitamins, lots of chlorophyll, beta-carotene, trace minerals, and is an excellent source of protein. It also contains Chlorella Growth Factor, (CGF) which helps stimulate growth and immunity.

Spirulina: This is a microalgae, grown in hot climates; also in pools or tanks. It contains most of the antioxidant vitamins, prebiotics, beta-carotene, every essential amino acid, GLA, phycocyanin, B12 and many other nutrients.

Wheatgrass: This is the young plant of the wheat, picked when it is several inches high. Wheatgrass is a concentrated source of greenfood nutrients, and contains many of the phytonutrients and trace minerals found in vegetables. Wheatgrass is also known to help detoxify the blood and liver due to its high levels of chlorophyll and alkalizing mineral content.

Sprouts: Sprouts from beans and wheats contain numerous enzymes, along with high levels of phytonutrients. Sprouts can be homegrown easily, but can now also be found in powder form.

Aloe: *Aloe vera* has been used traditionally for inflammation, constipation, wound healing, skin issues, ulcers and intestinal issues for at least five thousand years. Aloe's constituents include anthraquinones and mucopolysaccharides, which help replenish the mucosal membranes.

Mushrooms: We discussed most of the major mushrooms earlier. Some of the better superfood mushrooms are Reishi and Hoelen mushroom (*Wolfiporia extensas*), Maitake (*Grifola frondosa*), Shiitake (*Lentinula elodes*), Turkey Tails (*Coriolus versicolor or Trametes versicolor*), Agaricus (*Agaricus blazei*), Cordyceps (*Cordyceps sinensis*) and Lion's Mane (*Hericium erinaceus*). These have the distinction of stimulating the immune system and increasing tolerance. Blends of mushrooms are readily available in encapsulated supplement form.

Lecithin: This is derived primarily from brewer's yeast and soy, and is known to contain choline and inositol—two nutrients beneficial for cell membranes and nerve cells. Lecithin has been shown to relax nerves and help smooth muscle function.

Kelp is a macroalgae that contains a host of nutrients and phytonutrients, including fucoidan—shown to be a significant antioxidant. Kelp is also a good source of iodine—a critical trace element for thyroid health. Kelp powder is salty, and can replace refined salt as a condiment.

Green Papaya: This superfood has been used to help rebuild weakened mucosal membranes. It contains a special enzyme called papain, as well as vitamins A, C, E and Bs. In fact, it contains more vitamin A than carrots and more vitamin C than oranges on a per-content basis.

Fermented papaya: A study from Japan's Kyushu University (Fujita *et al.* 2017) studied elderly patients who were on tube feeding in the hospital. They separated the patients into three groups. They gave one group fermented papaya (Carica papaya Linn.) at different doses to each group. Before and after the trial, they tested the patients' blood levels for immunity markers.

After 30 days, the patients had increased levels of immunity. This was detected with lower levels of peripheral blood mononuclear cell (PBMC) dieoffs. Those patients given the greater levels of fermented papaya also had greater levels of immunity.

Italian researchers (Marotta *et al.* 2012) also found eating fermented papaya significantly increases immune function. Six weeks of fermented papaya, they also found, stimulates the body's ability to detoxify. This occurs through detoxification enzymes such as superoxide dismutase.

The researchers, from Italy's ReGenera Research Group for Aging Intervention Group in Milan, studied 90 healthy but sedentary human subjects. They divided the subjects into three groups by age (20-40 years old, 41-65 years old and over 65). They tested the subjects' blood and saliva together with questionnaires prior to and after the papaya protocol.

The researchers then gave half of each of the subjects from each group either a placebo or nine grams per day of fermented papaya.

After the six weeks, the subjects were again tested and given a month break (washout period). Then the the placebo group was given the fermented papaya while the previous papaya group was given the placebo. This research method is called a crossover.

Before and after each testing period the researchers performed blood analysis on the patients, checked for white blood cells count, checked saliva flow rates and secretary IgA activity. They also checked lysozymes and redox gene expression for Phase II enzymes and superoxide dismutase secretion from upper airway cells.

Immunoglobulin-A is an antibody produced by the body to help identify invaders and guard the body from infections.

The researchers found that those taking the fermented papaya had significantly greater IgA (immunoglobulin-A) levels than the placebo groups.

Bee Pollen has been recommended by traditional practitioners for inflammatory conditions because it contains a variety of antioxidant nutrients, enzymes, and proteins—many of which are derived from pollen. Clinicians have documented observing that bee pollen can increase tolerance and immunity in many of their patients. Bee pollen is best used from hives and honeybees harvesting pollens from the local plants if possible.

Royal Jelly: This superfood, made by the Queen, supplies similar nutrients as bee pollen, along with others. Royal jelly supplies vitamins A, C, D, E, Bs, enzymes, steroid hormones, trace minerals and all the essential amino acids. Royal jelly is also a rare source for natural acetylcholine. Royal jelly has been recommended for inflammatory conditions for many centuries. It is also reputed to stimulate the adrenal and thyroid glands.

Manuka Honey: Raw honey in general has been shown to be anti-microbial and soothing to the mucosal membranes. Thus, it is often used in cough syrups and sore throat remedies as we've described. Manuka honey is a special honey that comes from honeybees that harvest from the flowers of the Manuka bush (*Leptospermum scoparium*). This particular honey is thought to exert stronger health properties than normal raw honey. It is also reputed to be a remedy for ulcers, sinus infections and irritable bowels. Most of the world's supply comes from New Zealand, where the Manuka tree flourishes. This honey is also typically treated very gently to preserve its antioxidant and antimicrobial properties.

Dehydrated Vegetables: Extraordinary vegetables include parsley, broccoli, spinach, kale and cabbage. Cabbage is also excellent for rebuilding mucosal membranes, supplying what is now termed vitamin U. See the discussion on mucosal membrane strategies for more information on vitamin U.

Super Brans, Fibers and Seeds: These include psyllium seed, oat bran, rice bran, fennel seed, flax seed, sesame seed, sunflower seeds and others. These supply mucilage, lignans and important plant fibers that stimulate mucosal membrane health and decrease levels of lipid peroxidation-sensitive LDL cholesterol.

Plant Gums: These include guar gum and glucomannan. Most gums derived from plants provide mucilage and glucuronolactone, and other special polysaccharides. These constituents help maintain the health of our mucosal membranes. They also bind to toxins. Glucuronolactone is also a key component in many of the body's flexible connective tissues, which include the lungs.

Juicing for Immunity

Many of the above-mentioned nutrients and superfoods can be added to our diet by making smoothis, or simply by juicing raw veggies and fruits. Juicing has been advocated for many years by a number of health experts and nutritionists. Many have promoted juicing for detoxification and cleansing. This is not the case here.

However, juicing is a suboptimal way to glean the benefits of fruits and vegetables. This is because it is the combination of the antioxidant nutrients and the soluble and insoluble fibers in fruits and vegetables that give them their true cleansing benefits.

The moral here is that natural fiber with antioxidants renders more cleansing benefits than do antioxidants alone. While antioxidants do attach and bind to toxins and neutralize radicals such as lipid peroxides, fiber attaches to LDL cholesterol in the intestines, which prevents them from becoming lipid peroxides in the first place. Fibers also attach to numerous other radicals and toxins within the intestines, flushing them out through the colon. *This prevents their entry into the bloodstream.*

While juicing is somewhat practical for hard fiber vegetables like carrots, the best strategy for most other fruits and vegetables is to make smoothies. This is basically putting the whole fruit or vegetable into a blender (after peeling in the case of oranges and the like, although orange peels are also a great cleansing nutrient), mixing with some water, a greenfood powder, and perhaps some kefir or yogurt, and then blending them up into a fruit/vegetable smoothie. For thinner consistency, simply add more water, and for thicker consistency, less water.

While juice can also be added to our smoothies, juice made from concentrates can be problematic for boosting immunity. This is because concentrated juices are often separated from their fibers, and this makes the juice less wholesome, imparting large doses of sugar into our system. Furthermore, many commercial juices are pasteurized, rendering many of the enzymes and antioxidants useless, and often denatured. Furthermore, the sugars in concentrated and pasteurized juices can turn to more simplified versions, producing spikes in our blood sugar levels. This can produce increased amounts of radicals within the body, and increased acidity.

This denaturing can easily be observed. Simply pour some pasteurized filtered orange juice into a glass. Now peel an orange and put into the blender. Pour that into a glass next to the juice glass. Now take a gulp of the juice, and then take a gulp of the orange smoothie. You will taste the difference. As you let the juice slide past your throat, take an extra swallow and see if you do not sense the acidification of the juice on the epithelia of the throat/esophagus. Now do the same with the smoothie. The smoothie will go down, uh, okay, *smooth.*

Problems with Processed Foods

Food processing consists of one or a combination of the following actions on food:

> ➢ chopping or pulverizing

> ➢ heating to high temperatures
> ➢ distilling or extracting its constituents
> ➢ otherwise isolating some parts by straining off or filtering
> ➢ clarifying or otherwise refining

Most consider food processing a good thing, because we humans like to focus on one or two characteristics or nutrients within a food. The idea is that we want the essence of the food, and don't want to fool around with the rest. In most cases—in terms of commercial food—it is a value proposition, because all the energy and work required to produce the final food product must equal or be greater than the increase in the processed food's financial value. Therefore, the more concentrated or isolated the attractive portion is, the more financial value is added.

Typically, this increase in financial value is due to the food being sweeter, smoother or simply easier to eat or mix with other foods. In the case of oils or flours, the food extract is used for baking purposes, for example. In the case of sugar—which is extracted and isolated from cane and beets—it is added to nearly every processed food recipe.

Ironically, what is left behind in this extraction is the food's real value. The healthy fiber and nutrients are stripped away in most cases. Plant fiber is a necessary element of our diet, because it renders sterols that aid digestion and reduce LDL cholesterol. Many nutrients are also attached to and protected by the plant's fibers. Once the fiber is stripped away, the remaining nutrients are damaged by sunlight, air, and the heat of processing.

What is being missed in the value proposition of food processing is that nature's whole foods have their greatest value—nutritionally—prior to processing. When a food is broken down, the molecular bonds that attach nutrients to the food's fibers and complex polysaccharides are lost. As these bonds are lost, the remaining components can become unstable in the body. When these components—such as refined sugar and simple polysaccharides (starches)—become unstable, they can form free radicals in the body. They thus add to our body's toxic burden because they can damage our cells.

In other words, whole foods provide the nutrients our bodies need in the combinations our bodies recognize. Nutrients are bonded within a matrix of structure and fiber, rendering their benefits as our bodies require them.

In some cases, we might need to physically peel a food to get to the edible part. In other cases, such as in the case of beans and grains, we may need to heat or cook them to soften the fibers to enable chewing and digestion. In the case of wheats, we can mill the whole grain (including the bran) to deliver the spectrum of fibrous nutrients. In other words, the closer we match the way our ancestors ate foods, the more our bodies will recognize them, and the better our bodies will utilize them.

Because many of our processed foods have been in our diet for many decades, it is difficult to prove that our modern diet of overly-processed foods produces greater levels of systemic inflammation. This doesn't mean that it is impossible, however.

To test this hypothesis, French researchers (Fremont *et al.* 2010) studied the effects of processed flax. Foods containing processed flax are a new addition to our diet—although our ancestors certainly ate raw or cooked whole flax. So they studied the introduction of modern processed flax into the French diet. In a study of 1,317 patients with allergies, they found that those who were allergic to flax could be identified by their sensitivity to extruded, heated flax, rather than raw flax seed. This of course indicates that the increase in flax allergies among the French is due to the increase in *processed flax* rather than the increased availability of flax. Certainly, over time, as flax allergies proceed, there will be more crossover allergies to raw flax. But now, while flax exposure is fairly recent, allergies to processed flax but not raw flax indicate that it is the extrusion processing that causes the identification of flax protein as an allergen.

What does processing do to create more inflammatory sensitivity? Our digestive enzymes and probiotics have evolved to break down (or not) certain types of molecules. Imbalanced or denatured molecules can be considered foreign.

We can also see how processing increases diseases when we compare the disease statistics of developing countries with those of developed countries.

For example, like many developing countries, India has more heart disease in recent decades because of increased consumption of processed and fried foods. In the same way, the Chinese thrived for thousands of years on a rice-based diet. But when modern processing machines introduced white dehulled rice, malnutrition diseases began to occur. This is because the dehulling process results in the loss of important lignans, B vitamins E vitamins and others.

Processed and refined foods damage intestinal health and promote free radicals. They are nutrient-poor. They burden and starve our probiotics. Frying foods also produces a carcinogen called acrylamide (Ehling *et al.* 2005).

Refined Salt

Salt is included in this section because not only is it refined: Processed salt is stripped of important mineral nutrients. And processed foods typically contain incredible amounts of refined salt.

Salt is sometimes also referred to as sodium. However, it is not technically sodium. It is actually sodium chloride. Sodium is an essential trace element that helps balance blood pressure and the kidneys. Guidelines for maximum salt levels range from 2,200 milligrams a day to 2,300 milligrams. Adults who eat processed foods at every meal can consume from 3,000 milligrams to 5,000 mg per day.

An overload of processed salt has been implicated in high blood pressure, cardiovascular disease, kidney disorders and lung disorders.

Researchers from Indiana University (Mickleborough *et al.* 2005) found that dietary salt among 24 patients caused higher levels of pro-inflammatory neutrophils, eosinophils, eosinophil cationic protein (ECP), leukotrienes, prostaglandins, and inflammatory cytokines interleukin (IL)-1beta and IL-8 among the high-salt diet group, compared with the lower-salt diet group.

As we discussed earlier, the earth provides natural living salts in the form of rock salts and unprocessed sea salts. These provide a matrix of up to 80 different trace elements in addition to sodium. This broad spectrum of trace elements, according to some clinical findings as discussed earlier, lower the imbalances created by processed sodium chloride salts.

Glycation

The rates of peanut allergies nearly doubled during the 1990s (Sicherer *et al.* 2003), and have continued to slowly rise among industrialized nations. As discussed earlier, peanut allergies are associated with inflammation, and cause one of the deadliest forms of inflammation—anaphylaxis.

So what changed during the 1990s? Did industrialized counties eat more peanuts during the 1990s? There is no evidence of that.

What changed during this period was the way peanuts are produced and packaged. Dry-roasted and sugar-coated ("honey roasted") peanuts became more popular among consumers in Western industrialized countries due to the fact that manufacturers developed new technologies for dry-roasting processing.

While trying to understand the associations, researchers from the Mount Sinai School of Medicine (Beyer *et al.* 2001) determined that even though the Chinese also eat a significant amount of peanuts, there are significantly fewer peanut allergies in China. Since the Chinese primarily eat boiled or minimally fried peanuts—while Western countries are now eating mostly dry-roasted peanuts—the researchers decided to compare the allergenicity of dry-roasted peanuts with boiled and fried versions.

First they found that the *Ara h1* protein content in peanuts—a primary allergen—was significantly reduced when peanuts are fried or boiled, as compared with the dry-roasted. Secondly, they found that the

IgE binding ability of the *Ara h2* and *Ara h3* proteins was reduced when peanuts were boiled or fried—again compared with dry-roasting. This protein-IgE binding affinity is directly associated with the allergenicity of a food, as we discussed earlier.

A couple of years later, researchers from the USDA's Agricultural Research Service (Chung *et al.* 2003) confirmed these findings when their tests revealed that mature dry-roasted peanuts produced an increase in IgE binding—along with glycation end products.

This research was also duplicated later by other USDA researchers (Schmitt *et al.* 2004). However, in this study, the researchers also established that all three methods—frying, boiling and dry-roasting—increase the allergenicity of peanuts when compared to raw peanuts.

One of the leading researchers in the 2001 Mount Sinai study was Dr. Hugh Sampson. Dr. Sampson has since commented:

> *"The Chinese eat the same amount of peanut per capita as we do, they introduce it early in a sort of a boiled/mushed type form, as they do in many African countries, and they have very low rates of peanut allergies. All the countries that have westernized their diet are now seeing the same problem with food allergy as we see. Countries that have introduced peanut butter are now starting to see a rise in the prevalence of peanut allergies akin to the high rates already found in the UK, Australia, Canada and some European countries."*

We would add to his point regarding peanut butter that many peanut butter producers use dry-roasted peanuts. Additionally, there are generally two ways to manufacture peanut butter. Many commercial peanut butters are produced through a complex heating and blending process that includes blending the peanut butter with sugar and hydrogenated oils.

Alternatively, peanut butter can simply be made using a natural grinding process where the whole peanuts are ground and packed into jars without heating or blending. This process typically produces a separation of the oil on top, which is why so many manufacturers over-process and blend their peanut butters. However, the oil stirs back in quite easily.

Researchers from France's University of Burgundy (Rapin and Wiernsperger 2010) have confirmed that protein or lipid glycation produced by modern food manufacturers is linked to allergies.

In general, food manufacturing glycation is produced when sugars and protein-rich foods are combined and heated to extremely high temperatures. This is a typical process used for the manufacture of many commercial packaged foods on the grocery shelves today. During the process, sugars bind to protein molecules. This produces a glycated protein-sugar complex and glycation end products, both of which have been implicated in cardiovascular disease, diabetes, some cancers, peripheral neuropathy and Alzheimer's disease (Miranda and Outeiro 2010).

With regard to Alzheimer's disease, one of the end products of the glycation reaction is amyloid protein. Amyloid proteins have been found among the brain tissues and cerebrospinal fluids of Alzheimer's disease patients. Glycation is implicated in the amyloid plaque buildup found in Alzheimer's.

Glycation also takes place within the body. This occurs especially with diets with greater consumption of refined sugars and cooked or caramelized high-protein foods.

Too Much Protein

The western diet contains extraordinary levels of processed protein compared to traditional diets. Americans eat far beyond the amount of protein required for health. Studies indicate that Americans eat an average of 80-150 grams of protein a day. This is significantly higher than the 25-50 grams of protein recommended by nutritionists and health experts (Campbell 2006; McDougall 1983).

This amount of protein in the American diet is also significantly higher than even U.S. RDA levels. The U.S. recommended daily allowance for protein is 0.8 grams per 2.2 lbs of body weight. This converts to 54 grams for a person weighing 150 pounds. Americans eat on average nearly double that amount.

Too much protein produces a state of proteinuria. This produces excess uric acid in the tissues and joints, leading to a state of acidosis toxemia. Remember that amino acids are acids, and too many of them can overload the body. Conditions that have been linked with proteinuria include gout, bile stones, kidney stones and others.

Too Much Refined Sugar

The western diet is also laden with refined sugars. Today, nearly every pre-cooked recipe found in mass market grocery stores contains refined sugar. Many brands now try to white-wash the massive sugar content of their products by calling their sugar content "all natural." This is a deception, because nature in the form of fiber has been unnaturally stripped away from their refined sugars. This is hardly a "natural" proposition.

Research has linked refined sugars to diabetes, obesity, kidney diseases, Candida and many other conditions. This is hardly news to those who have investigated natural health literature.

Nature attaches sugars to complex fibers, polysaccharides and nutrients in such a way that prevents them from easily attaching to proteins. Sugars that are cooked and stripped of these complexes are assimilated too quickly, and drive the pancreas to produce and even overproduce insulin. This has the effect of stressing the pancreas. Refined sugars also stress the liver that feeds the pancreas, and stresses the detoxification processes that must metabolize the insulin, glucose and glycogen byproducts. All of this slows down the body's immunity and detoxification processes.

Refined sugars also feed pathogenic microorganisms. While our probiotics feed on oligosaccharides such as FOS, GOS and others, pathogenic microorganisms tend to feed on refined sugars. This is the case for *Candida albicans,* a virtual sugar fiend.

Refined sugars also become immediate unnatural glycation candidates within the body.

As our digestive system combines refined sugars with proteins, many of the glycated proteins are identified as foreign by IgA or IgE antibodies in immune-burdened physiologies. Why are they considered foreign? Because glycated proteins and their AGE end products damage blood vessels, tissues and brain cells. In this case, the immune system is launching an inflammatory attack in an effort to protect us from our own diet!

There is no surprise that glycation among foods and in the body is connected with systemic inflammation. It is also no accident that the increased consumption of overly-processed foods and manufacturing processes that pulverize and strip foods of their fiber; and blend denatured proteins and sugars using high-heat processes has increased as our rates of inflammatory diseases have increased over the past century.

In fact, this connection between inflammatory diseases and processed foods has been observed clinically by natural physicians over the years. They may not have understood the precise mechanics, however. Many of these reputable health experts have categorized the effect of processed foods as one of acidifying the bloodstream. The concept was that denatured and over-processed foods produced more acids in the body.

This thesis did not go over too well among scientific circles, because the acidification mechanism was not scientifically confirmed, and there was no concrete mechanism.

Well this can now change, as we are providing the science showing both the mechanism and the evidence that glycation end products do produce acidification in terms of peroxidation radicals that damage cells and tissues.

We should note that a healthy form of natural glycation also takes place in the body to produce certain nutrient combinations. Unlike the radical-forming glycation formed by food manufacturing and refined sugar intake, this type of glycation is driven by the body's natural enzyme processes, resulting in molecules and end products the body uses and recognizes. When glycation is driven by the body's own enzyme processes, it is termed *glycosylation,* however.

Hydrolyzed Proteins

Proteins are composed of very long chains of amino acids. Sometimes hundreds and even thousands of amino acids can make up a protein. The body typically breaks apart these chains through an enzyme reaction called *proteolysis.*

Proteolysis breaks down proteins into amino acids and small groups of aminos called polypeptides. This is also called *cleaving.* As enzymes break off these polypeptides or individual amino acids from proteins, they replace the protein chain linkages with water molecules to stabilize the peptide or amino acid. This process is called *enzymatic hydrolysis.* Breaking away the peptides or amino acids allows the body to utilize the amino acid or polypeptide to make new proteins within the body.

The body then assembles its own proteins from these amino acids and small polypeptide combinations. The body's protein assembly is programmed by DNA and RNA. For this reason, the body must recognize the aminos and polypeptide combinations. The body produces a variety of enzymes to naturally break apart multiple proteins and polypeptides. Protein-cleaving enzymes are called *proteases.*

For this reason, strange or large polypeptide combinations can burden the body, especially if the body does not have the right enzymes to break those peptide chains apart.

Food manufacturers can synthetically break down proteins by extrusion, heating and blending with processing aids—including commercially produced enzymes. These enzymes force the break down of the proteins in the food. As water is integrated into the process, synthetic hydrolysis occurs. This produces foods that contain hydrolyzed proteins. These synthetically hydrolyzed protein foods may not be recognized by the body's immune system, and may stimulate an inflammatory response.

Illustrating this, French laboratory researchers (Bouchez-Mahiout *et al.* 2010) found by using immunoblot testing that hydrolyzed wheat proteins from skin conditioners produced hypersensitivity, which eventually crossed over to wheat protein food allergies. In other words, hydrolyzed wheat proteins in skin treatments are not necessarily recognized by the immune system. Once the body becomes sensitized to these hydrolyzed wheat proteins from skin absorption, this sensitivity can cross over to sensitivity to similar wheat proteins in foods.

Researchers from France's Center for Research in Grignon (Laurière *et al.* 2006) tested nine women who had skin contact sensitivity to cosmetics containing hydrolyzed wheat proteins (HWP). Six were found to react with either skin hives or anaphylaxis to different products (including foods) containing HWP. The whole group also had IgE sensitivity to wheat flour or gluten-type proteins. The tests showed that they had become sensitive to HWP, and then later to unmodified grain proteins. As they tested further, they found that reactions often occurred among larger wheat protein peptide aggregates. The researchers concluded that the use of HWP in skin products can produce hypersensitivity to HWP, followed by a crossover to inflammatory responses to the wheat proteins in foods.

Spanish researchers (Cabanillas *et al.* 2010) found that enzymatic hydrolysis of lentils and chickpeas produced allergens for four out of five allergic patients in their research.

The commercial enzymes used by many food manufacturers can also stimulate allergic responses. Danish researchers (Bindslev-Jensen *et al.* 2006) tested 19 commercially available enzymes typically used in the food industry on 400 adults with allergies. It was found that many of the enzymes produced histamine responses among the patients.

Hydrolyzing proteins through manufacturing processes can create epitopes that the immune system does not recognize. Once the immune system launches an immune response to the epitope, it will remember those as foreigners, and possibly allergens, even if they are part of foods once accepted by the body.

The Ultimate Immunity Diet

We know that humans certainly did eat living foods for much of our existence. For well over a million years, humanoids ate nuts, berries, fruits, roots and leaves directly off the trees. They also harvested some of these and stored and cooked or dried them later.

Humans also ate raw milks from goats, cows, donkeys and other animals. These raw milks contained many probiotic bacteria—as does all raw milk, including human breast milk. Our ancestors also made various cultured foods from these raw milks, and the passed on 'mother' cultures to make kefirs, yogurts and other ancient foods. We'll discuss all these momentarily.

There are a number of debates ongoing with respect to whether humans were meant to eat meat and whether meat is healthy. There has been a growing population of medical experts and consumers who have problems with eating meat, and the research overwhelmingly supports this. After reviewing a multitude of studies, the American Dietetic Association and the Dietitians of Canada published an extensive report in 2003 regarding vegetarian diets.

The report found that vegetarians have lower body mass indices, lower levels of prostate and colorectal cancer, healthier cholesterol levels, lower blood pressure, lower levels of type 2 diabetes, and lower death rates from heart disease. Other studies have revealed that people on vegetarian diets experience lower cancer levels, lower osteoporosis, lower rates of urinary diseases, less dementia, lower rates of diverticulosis, fewer gallstones, and lower rates of rheumatoid arthritis (Leitzmann 2005). In a twelve year mortality study of 6115 vegetarians and 5015 meat-eaters, vegetarians had a 40% less mortality rate for cancer, and 20% less likely to die before the age of 65 than meat-eaters. (Thorogood *et al.* 1994; West 1994).

According to the World Cancer Research Fund and the American Institute for Cancer Research, in a report *Food, Nutrition and the Prevention of Cancer: A Global Perspective* (1997), 25-50% of all cases of cancer can be prevented by a vegetarian diet.

Medical researchers from Britain's University of Nottingham (McKeever *et al.* 2010) researched the relationship between diet and respiratory symptoms, including forced expiratory volumes. Their data was derived from 12,648 adults from the Monitoring Project on Risk Factors and Chronic Diseases in The Netherlands. They also included dietary patterns and lung function decline over a five-year basis.

They found that diets with higher intakes of meat and potatoes, and lower levels of soy and cereals, was linked to reduced lung function and lower expiratory levels (FEV1) levels. They also found that the heavy meat-and-potatoes diet produced higher levels of chronic obstructive pulmonary disease. They also found that a "cosmopolitan diet" with heavier intakes of fish and chicken (both of which are commonly fried) produced higher levels of wheeze and asthma.

In three studies of approximately 11,000 subjects each done at the University of Oxford, death rates among vegetarians were significantly lower than the general population (Key *et al.* 2003). Research has also confirmed that vegetarians have higher levels of circulating antioxidants such as lutein, xanthins, carotenoids, and corresponding higher levels of glutathione and superoxide dismutase (Rauma 2003).

In a study of 460 children and their mothers on Menorca—a Mediterranean island—medical researchers from Greece's Department of Social Medicine and the University of Crete (Chatzi *et al.* 2008) found that children of mothers eating primarily a Mediterranean diet (a predominantly plant-based diet) produced significantly lower rates of asthma among the children.

They found that mothers with a high Mediterranean Diet Score during pregnancy reduced the incidence of persistent wheeze among their children by 78%. Their children also had 70% lower incidence of allergic wheezing; and a 45% reduction in allergies among their children at age six (after removing other possible variables).

The list goes on. Study after study confirms that those who eat vegetarian diets are healthier, have better cholesterol levels, have lower body mass indices, have less disease, live longer and get more nutrients in their diet. The choice between vegetarianism and meat-eating is clear based on these facts alone. However, there are many more reasons.

Nutritionally there are several problems with meat. In order to eat meat, we must substantially overcook it. Should we not cook meat enough, we risk the ingestion of so many different bacteria and parasites, which quickly accumulate in dead animal flesh. This is a natural occurrence, as formerly living tissue undergoes biological decomposition. This is very difficult to curtail, even with refrigeration. After the long haul between the slaughterhouse and the market, the process will surely begin. Dead flesh is, well, dead flesh. It rots. It attracts various scavenger insects and pathogenic bacteria that want to eat it.

As a result, meat typically has to be cooked intensely for quite some time. This process destroys many of the heat-sensitive nutrients available in meat. For many meat-eaters, cooking means charbroiling or frying, both of which create various trans-fats, altered saturated fats, nitrites and various other toxic byproducts such as the deadly heterocyclic amines (or HCA). In a number of studies, HCA was notable in its connection with higher cancer risk. HCA works as a mutagen—altering the DNA of cells. This type of DNA alteration is connected with cancer.

The connection between cancer and red meats have also been made among recent European research studying the Mediterranean diet. The Med diet is known for its reduced intake of red meats, and increased intakes of fruits, vegetables, monounsaturated fats and low levels of saturated fats.

For example, a study by researchers from Spain's Programme of Epidemilogical Cancer Research in Barcelona (Gonzalez and Riboli 2010) conducted an analysis of 519,978 human participants from 23 centers among 10 European countries in Denmark, France, Germany, Greece, Italy, the Netherlands, Norway, Spain, Sweden and the United Kingdom. They found that gastric cancer was associated with higher consumption of red and processed meats, and lower risk was evident among those with higher phytonutrient (plant nutrients) plasma levels.

They also found that lung cancer was lower among those who ate more fruits and vegetables, even among smokers. And they found that higher breast cancer incidence was related to higher saturated fat consumption.

Researchers from the International Agency for Research on Cancer in Lyon, France found that the Mediterranean diet reduced overall cancer risk. The researchers studied 142,605 men and 335,873 women. They graded adherence to the Med diet with a 0-9 score. Among the whole population, 9,669 men contracted cancer and 21,062 women contracted cancer. They found that a two point better Med diet score resulted in a 4% reduction in cancer. The results cancelled out cancers relating to smoking.

The nutrient level of meat is dubious at best. Studies have shown that vegetarians, especially lacto-vegetarians, have higher circulating levels of many important vitamins and minerals, and red meat eaters have fewer of these nutrients. While meat typically has higher levels of protein, animal proteins are typically complex, with amino acids bound tightly into complex and lengthy molecules.

The bonds of these molecules are quite difficult for our peptidase enzymes to break down into the more digestible amino acids. As a result, the digestive system must work extra hard to break down those complex proteins. This significantly slows down the digestive process. As a result, a meat meal takes about twice the amount of time to digest than a vegetarian meal.

Yes—at least twice as long. This means a meat diet will result in a greater tendency of constipation, diverticulosis, colorectal cancer and irritable bowel syndrome. In a study published in the *Journal of the American Medical Association,* those who ate more red meat had twice the risk of colon cancer and 40% chance of rectal cancer (Chao 2005). While a typical vegetarian meal takes 24-36 hours to turn around food from meal to stool, a meat meal may take from 48-72+ hours to complete the cycle.

What happens to food matter sitting for this long in the intestines or colons? It putrefies. It stagnates. It rots. We might compare the process of decomposition through a 2-3 day cycle to a compost heap. During the composting process, various species of pathogenic bacteria accumulate. As the composting time increases, pathogenic bacteria accumulate in larger numbers, causing dysbiosis. As a result, not only do meat-eaters have more colon cancers, but they burden their immune systems and are thus more susceptible to infections.

When we compare animal proteins to vegetable proteins, we find a vast difference in terms of digestive affinity. The amino acid composition in plants is far easier to assimilate. The peptidase enzymes easily break down the various peptides available from plants. Because the body builds its own protein complexes from amino acids and simple peptides, plant protein is easier to utilize for the body. A healthy vegetarian diet will easily supply every essential and non-essential amino acid. Contrary to

320

information presented several decades ago, the body does not require every amino acid is present in each meal to form the appropriate proteins. The body does store and utilize various amino acids and peptides, and as long as all are available in the diet the body will make the appropriate protein molecules just fine.

Ironically, while Americans have been fixated on getting enough protein in the diet, research has been revealing that typical meat-eating diets contain too much protein. The overloading of amino acids into the bloodstream creates an acidic environment. To counter this situation, the body releases calcium from bones and tissues to neutralize this overly acidic situation. The loss of calcium contributes to osteoporosis, weakened bones, joints, and muscles. This precious body calcium is excreted out through the kidneys.

Unusable protein is broken down in the liver and converted to urea. Urea stimulates urination, which works the kidneys harder and stimulates the excessive loss of water. This can cause sub-clinical dehydration and kidney disorders. The combination of excess calcium and urea can also create painful and even lethal kidney stones.

Animal foods also contain high levels of purines. Purines are part of RNA and DNA. Purines are converted to uric acid by the body. Circulating uric acid can cause a common problem among heavy meat-eaters: Gout. Circulating uric acid will find its way into the joints, where it can cause extreme pain and stiffness.

Nutritional experts like James McDougall, M.D. state that healthy protein consumption should range from 30 to 60 grams per day. The average American consumes more than 100 grams a day. Populations who eat greater quantities of meat (Eskimos and Americans, for example) have shown higher levels of many of the illnesses discussed above (McDougall and McDougall 1983) than lower-protein consuming regions such as Africa and Asia.

Indeed, the complications provided by a number of other constituents in meat such as saturated fats, the animal's own hormones, and the accumulation of environmental toxins, antibiotics and hormones fed to the animal add to the complications and risks of meat in the diet.

Dr. Walter Willett, a professor at the Harvard School of Public Health puts it clearly: *"At most, it [meat] should be eaten only occasionally. And it may be maximally effective not to eat red meat at all."*

The slow movement of meat through the digestive tract is compounded by the fact that meats contain higher levels of various infectious agents before then land on our kitchen counters. Dangerous bacteria such as *E. coli* and *L. monocytogenes* (listeria) are common and prevalent in most red meats. Salmonella and campylobacter are also quite common infectious agents found in meat. *Consumer Reports* found 50-75% contamination levels among meat and chicken and 25% of meat had listeria between two studies done in 1997 and 2003 in 60 U.S. cities. To make matters worse, one study showed that 42% of meat-eaters did not cook their meat enough to remove these sorts of pathogens.

Processed meats also contain sodium nitrite, now a known precursor for *nitrosamine*. Nitrosamine has been identified as a carcinogen. One recent study of 200,000 people showed that consumers of the most processed meats had a 67% increased risk for pancreatic cancer. Nitrosamines are also mutagenic, especially in cells around the colon. Some say this effect is related to the high levels of nitrites and iron found in many meats.

The levels of iron found in meat can be dangerous for other reasons. The body does not need the quantity of iron present in many meats. About 3 or 4 grams is probably the max that a healthy adult body should retain. Meanwhile the body probably loses about 1 gram a day in sweat or through the kidneys. Healthy systems should absorb just enough to replace that amount. Any more has the possibility of accumulating in the tissues. Should we have an iron-absorption disorder such as *hemochromatosis,* we may find our iron overloading synovial membranes, organs and other tissues of the body.

Most meats have about 50% of their calories as fat—much of it saturated. A number of studies have confirmed meat-eaters suffer more heart disease. One study showed that meat-eating four or more times a week had twice the risk of congestive heart disease. This reduces the heart's ability to circulate blood throughout the body, causing various functional organ and tissue problems stemming from a build-up of blood and a lack of circulation and nutrition. Today close to 5 million people live with this condition, with over a half million new cases developing each year.

Various pro-meat advocates have proclaimed the benefits of meat-eating, saying that the human body has a genetic disposition for meat. They also claim vegetarians are missing necessary nutrients and propose that the human body evolved from cavemen, who supposedly ate lots of meat.

This later point runs contrary to historical evidence. Evidence from the 'Old World,' dating back to 10,000 years ago, indicates the population was primarily agricultural. Most evidence confirms that meat was rarely eaten more than once per week, and even then during celebrations or festivals (Flandrin 1999). Even as larger domesticated livestock farming enterprises took hold in the late Middle Ages, meat consumption in Northern Europe provided less than fifteen percent of protein consumption among the pre-industrial humans. For those households with domesticated animals and even for households without animal husbandry; milk, butter and cheese were regarded as staples.

Among the more populated regions of the Middle East, Asian Minor and Africa, meat eating took even less of a position. In these regions, meat eating was frowned upon as a diet for lower-class citizens, and was considered as unclean. Meat eating was either forbidden or highly regulated by religious culture. Regulations regarding meat eating included restrictions on animal species, draining the blood, and special offering sequences. Frankly, the unrestricted killing and eating of animals was discouraged by most religions. These cultures were for the most part crop and dairy farmers, and gatherers. Grains, tubers, berries, nuts, dairy, and fruit have formed the majority of historical humanity's diet.

It is presumptuous to find a few bones at campsites and a few cave drawings and conclude that early humans predominantly ate meat. While primitive drawings in colder climates may illustrate men who hunted on occasion, key evidence points to a large part of the diet being gathered or harvested. Research has pointed to the fact that early hominids were foragers and scavengers much like the primates (Whiten and Widdowson 1991). While some primates like chimpanzees are omnivores, the majority of primates have primarily fruit and plant-based diets.

Indeed, it is difficult to ascertain the difference between a spear used in self-defense from a hunting spear. It is likely spears were weapons of self-defense. In fact, highly intellectual writings from ancient times from Mesopotania and the Hundus valleys—where much of early man lived—illustrated a well-thought out and organized diet of milk, grains, fruits and vegetables. An everyday diet of meat for much of ancient man outside of the northernmost and colder regions appears highly debatable.

The proposal that the human body has a genetic disposition towards meat eating is drastically short sighted. Quite simply, if the human body was genetically disposed for hunting and eating meat, our bodies would have claws for ripping and tearing rather than fingers and nails able to accurately and precisely unpeel fruits, crack nuts and open plant fibers. Operations human hands and feet are most equipped for include gathering and preparing roots; picking and prying open vegetables; cracking apart nutshells and pulling out nut meats; and climbing up trees to harvest seeds or honey. Certainly if we were meat eaters, we would have legs that could run at faster speeds. Our legs cannot even keep up with a rabbit or squirrel let alone catch an antelope or other larger "game." As opposed to carnivores, our mouths would be full of incisors instead of mostly bicuspids and molars. Our teeth are primarily designed for grinding. Our two incisors are perfectly positioned to tear apart fleshy fruits and vegetables. To propose these two dull incisors positioned in the middle of grinding teeth make a case for humans being carnivores is quite a reach. Meanwhile tigers, sharks, wolves and other hunters have a mouth full of razor-sharp ripping teeth and incredibly strong jaws. Seriously, can we really expect to rip apart and fully chop up an animal's flesh and organs into small enough pieces to eat with our two rounded incisors and our weak jaws?

Furthermore, if we were carnivores, our feet would have claws for tearing apart our victims instead of soft toes to run and balance on while we reach or climb into the trees for our fruits and berries. Our eyes would be equipped with night-vision, allowing us to track the majority of animals that roam the earth after sunset. Rather, we have day-only vision with retinal cells equipped to distinguish bright colors of ripening fruits and vegetables. This vision allows us not only to find those fruits and vegetables ready to eat, but to distinguish between poisonous ones. We have ears that pick up the medium spectrum of sounds, focused on our own voices and the sounds of more dangerous animals like wolves and tigers. Our ears are not equipped to listen to the very high- and very-low pitched rhythms of the animals we are able to catch and beat up with our blunt fingers and toes, such as squirrels, mice, moles, deer and rabbits. Because of our narrow auditory skills, we have great difficulty tracking these animals.

As hunters, humans are poorly equipped all over. Humans have longer and slower muscles. Our leg muscles make us one of the slowest specimens on the planet. What kind of creature could we catch? Almost every creature can outrun us, from squirrels to birds to fish to wolves, tigers, horses, etc. On foot, it would be difficult for us to even catch one of the largest vegetarians, the elephant.

If we consider the physical characteristics of species that hunt, we can easily see other drastic differences. Hunters can travel at tremendous speeds. They either are equipped to fly and swoop; jump and leap; run and snatch; or sneak up and pounce on their prey. They usually have sharp ripping claws, night vision, very quick coordination, and response, allowing them to out-maneuver or surprise other creatures during the hunt. The human body is slow; dull; soft; gangly; rounded; obvious; and stupid when it comes to the element of surprise. Our muscles are inflexible in comparison. We have little ability to quickly leap or jump. In comparing the length and width of our appendages, we are quite weak and slow. About the only thing we have going for us besides our problem-solving nature is a misplaced sense of pride, thinking we are so smart that we can control nature and do whatever we want without restriction.

When it comes to digestion, we can hardly eat meat without cooking it. Even if when we cook it we can hardly digest it. If we examine and compare the intestinal tract of hunters, tigers or other meat-eating animals, we find they have short, fat colons to move the unfibrous meat through faster. Most herbivores have long digestive tracts, ranging from ten to twelve times our body length. Meat eating animals typically have shorter tracts, averaging only about three times their body length. We also find meat eating animals secrete incredibly strong hydrochloric acid to enable the break down of the more complex proteins and peptides of meat. Humans and other herbivores have hydrochloric acid strengths about twenty times weaker than meat eaters have. Humans, like most herbivores, have developed salivary glands that produce amylase, which facilitates the digestion of plant starches. Meat eating animals do not have salivary glands.

The human body was equipped with the perfect tools for harvesting fruits, vegetables, roots and nuts. We can eat them raw or they can easily be dried in the sun without difficulty. We have the fingers and thumb to pull the husks or peels off, or crack the hulls. Then we can just pop them into our mouths and move on. We do not have to cook vegetables, fruits and nuts. We have the digestive tools to handle these foods without any complications. Can you imagine a tiger trying to peel an orange? Certainly not. The tiger's body is not equipped for eating fruits. Its claws would shred the fruit into a mangled juicy lump.

In order to logically assess our genetic eating traits, the focus should be on our physical traits. There are obvious foods the body can handle without advanced or complex preparation. These are the foods we were genetically designed to eat. Meat would naturally fall off of this list, because raw meat will make most human bodies ill. Our teeth are not sharp enough to tear raw meat (reason why we need steak knives). Our digestive tracts are too long for meat. Our digestive enzymes are too weak and not designed for meat. Our nails are too soft to kill an animal with. Our legs are too weak to catch most animals. Our vision is too daylight oriented to see most animals.

The famous physician and botanist Dr. Carl Linnaeus (1707-1778), considered the "father of taxonomy," once stated that *"Man's structure, external and internal, compared with that of the other animals, shows that fruit and succulent vegetables constitute his natural food."*

We might note that the human hands and fingers are perfectly equipped to milk a cow or a goat. Most healthy individuals also produce a prolific amount of enzyme lactase, an enzyme specifically designed to digest lactose—the sugar of cow's milk. Those rare humans who do not produce enough lactase can easily eat naturally cultured milk like cheese and yogurt, because bacteria in these cultured foods produce enough lactase to allow assimilation. These cultured foods also secret *bacteriocins*, which exhibit otherwise antimicrobial activity. We should also be aware that lactobacilli—the most prevalent probiotics of our intestinal tract—produce lactase as well. As we age, our probiotic colonies should be blossoming with lactase. The antibiotic use of modern society is largely responsible for our lack of healthy probiotics, and the subsequent lack of lactase available. We should note that some cultures, like Africans, have less experience with cow milk and thus produce less lactase.

Bovine milk supplies a number of oligosaccharides and glycoconjugates, which promote the growth of probiotics in the intestinal tract. These are referred to as probiotics because they encourage the growth of probiotics, which assist our bodies digest food and fight infection.

Cows and goats produce prolific quantities of these wonderfully healthy foods. Naturally, these animals produce more than their large families supply. The key to obtaining good nutrition from the milk of animals like cows and goats is to treat them with care. Should we torture these poor animals by trapping them into cages while punching them with injections of antibiotics and growth hormones, we will certainly experience the backlash of those acts when we consume the milk.

So while we are not arguing that hungry humans in desolate places have not eaten meat, we know from the research that red meats are more toxic to our bodies than plant-based and cultured foods. This fact is not in dispute when the research involving cancer, intestinal diseases and others are examined carefully. Let's look at a few reasons why this is the case:

> *Fatty acid imbalances:* Animal foods provide increased levels of saturated fats, which lead to greater levels of LDL cholesterol. LDL, remember, is more susceptible to lipid peroxidation.

> *Arachidonic acid overload:* Red meats and oily fish provide higher levels of arachidonic acid. Increased arachidonic acid levels in the body push the immune system towards inflammation.

> *Nitrites:* Red meats have greater levels of nitrites. This is especially true for processed and fried meats. As nitrites enter the body, they produce reactive nitrogen species. These damage cells and cell membranes, producing inflammatory peroxidation.

> *Dysbiosis:* Animal foods facilitate the growth of colonies of pathogenic microorganisms in the intestines. These produce

endotoxins that damage cell membranes and tissues, stimulating inflammation, again through peroxidation.

> *Beta-glucuronidase:* Omnivore diets result in higher levels of beta-glucuronidase and other mutagenic enzymes. These enzymes directly damage cells and increase systemic inflammation.

> *Toxemia:* Animal foods typically contain a greater number of toxins compared to plant foods. This is because animals are *bioaccumulators:* They accumulate toxins. Many toxic chemicals are fat-soluble: The toxins thus accumulate among fat cells. Animals also produce and circulate various waste products, and their waste production increases during slaughter. Plant-based foods, by contrast, provide various antioxidants.

> *Protein metabolic stress:* Animal proteins require significant effort by the body to break them down into useable amino acid and smaller peptide form. The body utilizes single amino acids and small amino acid chains (peptides). Animal proteins contain hundreds, even thousands of amino acids in a single molecule. This requires significantly more energy and enzyme production to break down and process these complex proteins.

> *Acidic plasma:* The excess proteins in animal foods produce greater levels of acids in the bloodstream and tissues, which can lead to toxemia. Remember, amino acids are acidic.

Let's review some of the science supporting these points:

Nitrites

Researchers from the Harvard School of Public Health (Varraso *et al.* 2007) studied the effects of nitrites in the diet and lung health. They analyzed 111 diagnosed cases of COPD between 1986 and 1998 among 42,915 men who participated in the Health Professionals Follow-up Study. The average consumption of high-nitrite meats (processed meats, bacon, hot dogs) was calculated from surveys conducted in 1986, 1990, and 1994. They found that consuming these meats at least once a day increased the incidence of COPD by more than 2-½ times over those who rarely ate high-nitrite meats.

These same Harvard researchers used a similar analysis of 42,917 men, but with more dietary parameters. This research found that the *"western diet"* consisting of refined grains, sugary foods, cured and red meats, and fried foods, increased COPD incidence by more than four

327

times. Meanwhile, a *"prudent"* diet, rich in fruits, vegetables and fish, halved COPD incidence.

The same researchers from the Harvard School of Public Health studied lung function, COPD and diet among 72,043 women between 1984 and 2000 in the Nurses' Health Study. Diets that had more fruit, vegetables, fish and whole-grain products reduced the incidence of COPD by 25%. Meanwhile, a diet heavy in refined grains, cured and red meats, desserts and French fries increased the incidence of COPD by 31%.

Pathogenic Enzymes

In the early 1980s, Dr. Barry Goldin, a professor at the Tufts University School of Medicine, led a series of studies that found that certain diets promoted a group of cancer-causing enzymes. These included beta-glucuronidase, nitroreductase, azoreductase, and steroid 7-alpha-dehydroxylase. The enzymes were linked with cancer in previous studies. (Cancer is caused by the same types of cell damage that also stimulates systemic inflammation.)

A number of studies on vegetarians found lower levels of these mutagenic enzymes, while those eating animal-based diets had greater levels. Apparently, these cancer-related enzymes originate from a group of pathogenic bacteria that tend to occupy the intestines of those with diets rich in animal-based foods. It was discovered that the cancer-producing enzymes are actually the endotoxins (waste products) of these pathogenic bacteria.

Dr. Goldin and his research teams studied the difference between these enzyme levels in omnivores and vegetarians. In one study, the researchers removed meat from the diets of a group of omnivores for 30 days. An immediate reduction of steroid 7-alpha-dehydroxylase was found. When the probiotic *L. acidophilus* was supplemented to their diets, this group also showed a significant reduction in beta-glucuronidase and nitroreductase.

In other words, two dietary connections were found regarding these disease-causing enzymes: animal-based diets and a lack of intestinal probiotics. The two are actually related, because probiotics thrive in prebiotic-rich plant-based diets and suffer in animal-rich diets.

Two years later, Dr. Goldin and associates (Goldin *et al.* 1982) studied 10 vegetarian and 10 omnivore women. He found that the vegetarian women maintained significantly lower levels of beta-glucuronidase than did the omnivorous women.

The association between colon cancer and diets heavy in red meat has been shown conclusively in a multiple studies over the years. For example, an American Cancer Society cohort study (Chao *et al.* 2005) examined 148,610 adults between the ages of 50 and 74 living in 21 states of the

U.S. They found that higher intakes of red and processed meats were associated with higher levels of rectal and colon cancer after other cancer variables were eliminated.

Other studies have confirmed that vegetarian diets result in a reduction of these carcinogenic enzymes produced by pathogenic bacteria. Researchers from Finland's University of Kuopio (Ling and Hanninen 1992) tested 18 volunteers who were randomly divided into either a conventional omnivore diet or a vegan diet for one month.

The vegan group followed the month with a return to their original omnivore diet. After only one week on the vegan diet, the researchers found that fecal urease levels decreased by 66%, cholylglycine hydrolase levels decreased by 55%, beta-glucuronidase levels decreased by 33% and beta-glucosidase levels decreased by 40% in the vegan group. These reduced levels continued through the month of consuming the vegan diet. Serum levels of phenol and p-cresol—also inflammation-producing endotoxins of pathogenic bacteria—also significantly decreased in the vegan group.

Within two weeks of returning to the omnivore diet, the formerly-vegan group's pathogenic enzyme levels returned to the higher levels they had before converting to the vegan diet. After one month of returning to the omnivore diet, serum levels of toxins phenol and p-cresol returned to their previously higher levels prior to the vegan diet. Meanwhile, the higher levels of inflammation-producing enzymes remained among the conventional omnivore diet (control) group.

A study published two years earlier by Huddinge University researchers (Johansson et al. 1992) confirmed the same results. In this study, the conversion of an omnivore diet to a lacto-vegetarian diet significantly reduced levels of beta-glucuronidase, beta-glucosidase, and sulphatase (more tumor-implicated, inflammation-producing enzymes) from fecal samples.

Another study illustrating this link between vegetarianism, pathogenic bacterial enzymes and cancer was conducted at Sweden's Huddinge University and the University Hospital (Johansson et al. 1998) almost a decade later. Dr. Johansson and associates measured the effect of switching from an omnivore diet to a lacto-vegetarian diet and back to an omnivore diet with respect to mutagenicity—by testing the body's fluid biochemistry to determine the tendency for tumor formation.

In this extensive study, 20 non-smoking and normal weight volunteers switched to a lacto-vegetarian diet for one year. Urine and feces were examined for mutagenicity (cancer-causing bacteria and their endotoxins) at the start of the study, at three months, at six months and at twelve months after beginning the vegetarian diet. Following the switch to the lacto-vegetarian diet, all mutagenic parameters significantly decreased among the urine and feces of the subjects. The subjects were then followed-up and tested three years after converting back to an omnivore diet (four years after the study began). Their higher mutagenic biochemistry levels had returned.

In another of Dr. Johansson's studies (Johansson and Ravald 1995)—this from Sweden's Karolinska Institute—29 vegetarians and 28 omnivores were tested. The tests revealed that the vegetarians secreted more salivary juices than did the omnivores. Salivation is critical to the health of the mucosal membranes among the oral cavity and airways.

Arachidonic Acid

To add to these issues is the problem of consuming too much arachidonic acid in the diet. Arachidonic acid is an essential fatty acid naturally converted from other fatty acids by the body. However, diets rich in red meats can directly overload the body with arachidonic acid, producing a pro-inflammatory condition.

This subject has been studied extensively by researchers from Wake Forest University School of Medicine, led by Professor Floyd Chilton, Ph.D. Dr. Chilton has published a wealth of research data that have uncovered that foods high in arachidonic acid can produce a pro-inflammatory metabolism, especially among adults. Dr. Chilton's research also confirmed that a pro-inflammatory metabolism is trigger-happy and hypersensitive: creating the systemic inflammatory conditions prevalent in many degenerative diseases.

In research headed up by Dr. Darshan Kelley from the Western Human Research Center in California, diets high in arachidonic acid stimulated four times more inflammatory cells than diets low in arachidonic acid content. And this problem increases with age. In other words, the same amount of arachidonic acid-forming foods will cause higher levels of arachidonic acid as we get older (Chilton 2006).

According to the USDA's Standard 13 and 16 databases, red meats and fish produce the highest levels of arachidonic acid in the body. Diary, fruits and vegetables produce little or no arachidonic acid. Grains, beans and nuts produce none or very small amounts. Processed bakery goods produce a moderate amount of arachidonic acid.

Phytanic Acid

Another association we can make between inflammation and diets rich in animal-based foods relates to phytanic acid. Phytanic acid (tetramethylhexadecanoic acid) is a byproduct of plant food digestion inside the intestinal tracts of ruminating animals such as cows, goats, sheet and so on. While phytanic acid can be derived from plant-based foods, greater concentrations of nonesterified phytanic acid are formed in animals when chlorophyll is degraded within the stomachs of ruminants, along with mammalian peroxisomes. This is the result of these animals' unique multiple-stomach digestion process of grasses and other plant material. Humans, of course, do not digest food in the same manner, so we do not produce these concentrated levels of nonesterified phytanic acid from plant-based diets.

Otto-von-Guericke University (Germany) professor Dr. Peter Schönfeld has showed that the nonesterified phytanic acids from ruminants directly damage the membranes of our cell's mitochondria. The end result, his research found, is a corruption of the mitochondrial ATP energy production process (Schönfeld 2004).

This corruption in turn damages cell function, stimulating inflammation.

Obesity and Toxicity

Obesity is also associated with a disorder now called *metabolic syndrome.* According to the American Heart Association, metabolic syndrome is related to the following conditions:

> ➤ Blood sugar issues (diabetes, insulin resistance, hypoglycemia)
> ➤ Obesity (most specifically abdominal obesity)
> ➤ Cholesterol issues (high LDL, low HDL, high triglycerides)
> ➤ High blood pressure
> ➤ Chronic inflammation markers (including C-reactive protein, high white blood cell count, high eosinophils)
> ➤ Atherosclerosis (damage and hardening to the arteries—indicated by fibrinogen, circulation problems and so on.)

Metabolic syndrome is characterized by cholesterol problems, high blood pressure, diabetes or hypoglycemia, chronic inflammation, cardiovascular disease, high CRP levels, and heart disease. All of these issues add up to the same issue: systemic inflammation. Furthermore, each of these conditions have the same underlying issues: Poor dietary choices, high levels of reactive oxygen species, increased infections, an overburdened immune system, lack of exercise and other poor lifestyle choices.

Currently about 72 million Americans—nearly one-third of the population—are obese according to the 2005-2006 National Health and Nutrition Examination.

Research from the National Center for Chronic Disease and Prevention discussed in the first chapter (Cory *et al.* 2010) determined that Americans among communities across the country were 52% to 74% were obese or overweight in 2006, with a nationwide average of 62%. In 2007—just one year later—estimated rates of being overweight or obese ranged up to 77%, with an average of 63%—nearly 1% greater than a just a year earlier.

And what is the prevailing diet of Americans—who make up the most obese country in the world? The western diet, composed primarily of red meats, fried poultry and seafood, processed starchy foods, and sugary foods. Could this possibly be a coincidence that these foods produce more obesity? Nada. Numerous Universities and Governmental agencies have been studying the relationship between obesity and diet for many years, and have concluded that the western diet is by far the most fattening diet.

Most of us realize that diet and obesity are related. But do we know that toxicity and obesity are related? As we discussed earlier, many toxins—especially many dangerous ones—are fat soluble. This means that they will build up among our fat cells. This also means that the more and larger fat cells we have, the more build up of toxicity we can have.

It is thus not an accident that the relative intake of our fats is specific to our levels of toxicity. This has been studied by a number of researchers, who have concluded that obesity and inflammation are irreparably tied.

It is a well-known fact that obese people have higher rates of cardiovascular disease, diabetes, kidney disorders, liver diseases, arthritis, asthma, hay fever, dementia, intestinal disorders and many, many other conditions. Just about every medical condition is worsened by obesity, and we need no scientific reference for this fact, simply because the research is so widely known.

In a recent study from Boston University's School of Medicine, led by cardiologist and medical professor Noyan Gokce, MD, fat tissues from 109 obese and lean people provided clear evidence. Tissue from none of the lean patients illustrated any signs of inflammation. In comparison, fat tissues from the obese patients showed "significant" signs of inflammation.

In addition, the lean patients showed "no sign" of poor vascular function while the obese patients showed significantly poor vascular function. This of course relates to inflammation, as we've discussed. When the blood vessel walls become damaged by free radicals and lipid peroxides, they are damaged. This damage results in scarring and artery deposit build-up, which inhibits healthy circulation and releases clots that block other arteries.

The research also illustrated that the obese persons exhibited varying degrees of inflammation, indicating that a toxic environment and intake of toxins is also associated with the extent of inflammation. Obesity simply allows for a better 'net' to capture more filters within the fat cells.

The Practical Approach

This text does not assume that every reader is prepared to completely give up eating red meat. We are simply laying out the facts showing the connection between the western diet and greater levels of inflammation and toxicity, together with the evidence that a diet with more plant-based foods will present less toxicity and systemic inflammation. A diet with more plant-based foods and less red meat will enable a stronger immune system and faster detoxification. We can each make our own decisions with regard to how to incorporate this information with our diet. For some, it will simply mean eating less red meat, which will have the effect of reducing our toxin levels. For others, it might mean adopting the Mediterranean diet.

Alkaline Nutrition

This discussion of nutrients should also include the reflective effects of a healthy diet: The proper acid-alkaline balance among the blood, urine and intercellular tissue regions. The reference to acidic or alkaline body fluids and tissues has been made by numerous natural health experts over the years. Is there any scientific validity to this?

Many nutritionists condemn an acidic metabolism and loosely call appropriate metabolism as a *state of alkalinity*. Strictly speaking, however, an alkaline environment is not healthy. The blood, interstitial fluids, lymph and urine should be *slightly acidic* to maintain the appropriate mineral ion balance. Let's dig into the science.

Acidity or alkalinity is measured using a logarithmic scale called pH. The term pH is derived from the French word *pouvoir hydrogene,* which means 'hydrogen power' or 'hydrogen potential.' pH is quantified by an inverse log base-10 scale. It measures the proton-donor level of a solution by comparing it to a theoretical quantity of hydrogen ions (H+) or H_3O+.

The scale is pH 1 to pH 14, which converts to a range of 10^{-1} (1) to 10^{-14} (.00000000000001) moles of hydrogen ions. This means that a pH of 14 maintains fewer hydrogen ions. It is thus *less acidic* and *more alkaline* (or basic).

The pH scale has been set up around the fact that water's pH is log-7 or simply pH 7—due to water's natural mineral content. Because pure water forms the basis for so many of life's activities, and because water neutralizes and dilutes so many reactions, water was established as the standard reference point or neutral point between what is considered an acid or a base solution. In other words, a substance having greater hydrogen ion potential (but lower pH) than water will be considered acidic, while a substance with less H+ potential (higher pH) than water is considered a base (alkaline).

Now the solution with a certain pH may not specifically maintain that many hydrogen ions. But it has the same *potential* as if it contained those hydrogen ions. That is why pH is hydrogen power or hydrogen potential.

In human blood, a pH level in the range of about 6.4 is considered healthy because this state is slightly more acidic than water, enabling the bodily fluids to maintain and transport minerals. It enables the *potential* for minerals to be carried by the blood, in other words. Minerals are critical to every cell, every organ, every tissue and every enzyme process occurring within the body. Better put, a 6.4 pH offers the appropriate *currency* of the body's fluids: This discourages acidosis and toxemia, maintaining a slight mineralized status.

Acidosis is produced with greater levels of carbonic acids, lactic acids, and/or uric acids among the joints and tissues. These acids are readily oxidizing, which produces free radicals. However, an overly alkaline state can precipitate waste products from cells, which also floods the system with radicals. For this reason, *toxemia* results from either an overly acidic blood-tissue content or an overly alkaline blood-tissue content. In other words, pH *balance* is the key.

Ions from minerals like potassium, calcium, magnesium and others are usually positively oriented—with alkaline potential. But to be carried through a solution, the solution must have the pH potential to carry them.

Besides being critical to enzymatic reactions, these minerals bond with lipids and proteins to form the structures of our cells, organs and tissues—including our airways, nerves and mucosal membranes.

Natural health experts over the past century have observed among their patients and in clinical research that an overly acidic environment within the body is created by a diet abundant in refined sugars, processed foods, chemical toxins and amino acid-heavy animal foods. More recently, research has connected this acidic state to toxemia. The toxemia state is a state of free radical proliferation, which damages cells and tissues. It is also a state that produces systemic inflammation, because the immune system is over-worked as it tries to remove the cell and tissue damage.

As mentioned earlier, animals accumulate toxins within their fat tissues. They are bioaccumulators. Thus, animals exposed to the typical environmental toxins of smog and chemical pollutants in their waters and air—along with pesticides and herbicides from their foods—will accumulate those toxins within their fat cells and livers. And those who eat those animals will inherit (and further accumulate) these accumulated toxins. In addition, animals secrete significant waste matter as they are being slaughtered.

Plants are not bioaccumulators. While they can accumulate some pesticides and herbicide chemicals within their leaves and roots, they do not readily absorb or hold these for long periods within their cells. This is because many environmental toxins are, as mentioned, fat soluble. Because plants have little or no fat, they can more easily systemically rid their tissues of many of these toxins over time.

Further, as the research has shown, a diet heavy in complex proteins—which contain far more amino acids than our bodies require—increases the risk and severity of inflammation. Amino acids are the building blocks of protein. A complex protein can have tens of thousands of amino acids. While proteins and aminos are healthy, a diet too rich in them will produce deposits in our joints and tissues, burdening our immune system.

As we discussed in the last chapter, research also reveals that diets rich in red meats discourage the colonization of our probiotics, and encourage the growth of pathogenic microorganisms that release endotoxins that clog our metabolism and overload our immune system. Diets rich in red meats also produce byproducts such as phytanic acid and beta-glucuronidase that can damage our intestinal cells and mucosal membranes within the intestines. Greater levels of cooked saturated fats also raise cholesterol levels, especially lipid peroxidation-prone low-density lipoproteins (LDL).

The complexities of digesting complex proteins produce increased levels of beta-glucuronidase, nitroreductase, azoreductase, steroid 7-alpha-dehydroxylase, ammonia, urease, cholylglycine hydrolase, phytanic acid and others. These toxic enzymes deter our probiotics and produce systemic inflammation. Not surprisingly, they've been linked to colon cancer.

By contrast, plant-based foods contain many antioxidants, anti-carcinogens and other nutrients that strengthen the immune system and balance the body's pH. Plant-based foods also discourage inflammatory responses. Plant-based foods feed our probiotics with complex polysaccharides called prebiotics. They are also a source of fiber (there is little fiber in red meat)—critical for intestinal health.

The Mediterranean diet does not completely eliminate meat, but it is focused on more plant-based foods, healthier oils and less red meat. However we configure our diet, there are choices we can make at every meal. The research shows that the greater our diet trends toward the Mediterranean diet, the lower our toxic load will be and the stronger our immunity will be. This will allow us to better combat and eventually lower systemic inflammation.

This also not a condemnation of dairy. Milk is a great food, assuming it contains what nature intended: probiotics. Real milk is inseparable from probiotics, and when probiotics are killed off by pasteurization, milk becomes a dubious food. We'll talk about this more later.

Chapter Seven

Other Immunity Strategies

In this chapter we'll discuss a variety of other strategies to increase our immunity. These include avoiding toxins, drinking enough water, getting outside and getting enough sunshine, exercising, sweating, skin brushing, sleeping and others.

Hydration

The fact that dehydration (lack of sufficient fluid intake) can contribute to systemic inflammation and toxicity has been confirmed by research.

The mucosal membranes are made primarily of water. In a dehydrated state, our mucosal membranes thin. It is for this reason that other research has found that many ulcerated conditions can be cured simply by drinking adequate water (Batmanghelidj 1997).

Water is directly involved in inflammatory metabolism. Research has revealed that increased levels of inflammatory mediators such as histamine are released during periods of dehydration in order to help balance fluid levels within the bloodstream, tissues, kidneys and other organs.

Inadequate water intake will dehydrate the mucosal membranes. This produces irritation and hypersensitivity. Research by Dr. Batmanghelidj (1987; 1990) led to the realization that the blood becomes more concentrated during dehydration. As this concentrated blood enters the capillaries of the respiratory system, histamine is released in an attempt to balance the blood dilution.

The immune system is also irrevocably aligned with the body's water availability. The immune system utilizes water to produce lymph fluid. Lymph fluid circulates immune cells throughout the body, enabling them to target specific intruders. The lymph is also used to escort toxins out of the body.

Intracellular and intercellular fluids are necessary for the removal of nearly all toxins—and pretty much every metabolic function of every cell, every organ and every tissue system.

Water also increases the availability of oxygen to cells. Water balances the level of free radicals. Water flushes and replenishes the digestive tract. Thus, water is necessary for the proper digestion of food, as well as nutrition utilization. The gastric cells of the stomach and the intestinal wall cells require water for proper digestive function. The health of every cell depends upon water.

There is certainly reason to believe that dehydration is a key factor for toxicity and inflammation.

337

As Dr. Jethro Kloss pointed out decades ago (1939), the average person loses about 550 cubic centimeters of water through the skin, 440 cc through the lungs, 1550 cc through the urine, and another 150 cc through the stool. This adds up to 2650 cc per day, equivalent to a little over 2-½ quarts (about 85 fluid ounces).

Meanwhile many have suggested drinking eight 8-oz glasses per day. This 64 ounces would result in a state of dehydration. In 2004, the National Academy of Sciences released a study indicating that women typically meet their hydration needs with approximately 91 ounces of water per day, while men meet their needs with about 125 ounces per day. This study also indicated that approximately 80% of water intake comes from water/beverages and 20% comes from food. Therefore, we can assume a minimum of 73 ounces of fresh water for the average adult woman and 100 ounces of fresh water for the average adult man should cover our hydration needs. That is significantly more water than the standard eight glasses per day—especially for men.

The data suggests that 50-75% of Americans have chronic dehydration. Fereydoon Batmanghelidj, M.D., probably the world's foremost researcher on water, suggests a ½ ounce of water per pound of body weight. Drinking an additional 16-32 ounces for each 45 minutes to an hour of strenuous activity is also a good idea, with some before and some after exercising. More water should accompany temperature and elevation extremes, and extra sweating or fevers. Note also that alcohol is dehydrating.

A glass of room-temperature water first thing in the morning on an empty stomach can significantly help our mucosal membranes. Then we should be drinking water throughout the day. Our evening should accompany reduced water consumption, so our sleep is not disrupted by urination.

There are easy ways to tell whether we are dehydrated. A sensation of being thirsty indicates that we are already dehydrated. A person with toxicity and/or inflammation should thus be drinking enough water to not ever feel thirsty. Dark yellow urine also indicates dehydration. Our urine color should be either clear, or bright yellow if after taking multivitamins.

Drinking just any water is not advised. Municipal water and even bottled water can contain many contaminants that can burden the immune system, and trigger inflammation. Care must be taken to drink water that has been filtered of most toxins yet is naturally mineralized. Research has confirmed that distilled water and soft water are not advisable. Natural mineral water is best. Please refer to the author's book,

Pure Water for more information on water content, filters and water treatment options.

Hydrotherapy

The ancient physician Hippocrates was a proponent of hydrotherapy for respiratory conditions, and there have been many treatment successes among the many hydrotherapy treatment centers all over Europe, Asia and the U.S. over the centuries. Early nineteenth century physician Vincent Priessnitz from Austria popularized many types of modern water treatments, as did Father Sebastian Kneipp—a 19th century German monk. These included water compresses, cold-water therapy, contrast baths, hot baths, and warm baths.

Dr. Wilhelm Winternitz, an Austrian neurologist, observed one of Priessnitz's treatment centers and became one of the most celebrated proponents of water treatment in modern times. Dr. Winternitz designed a number of different water treatments and influenced American physicians such as Dr. John Harvey Kellogg, Dr. Jethro Kloss and Dr. Simon Baruch. Dr. Kellogg operated the famous Michigan Battle Creek Health Center for many years until it burnt down in 1902. The center utilized hydrotherapy as a key healing agent. Dr. Kloss ran his own clinic and also worked closely with the Battle Creek Center.

Despite its history of success, opposition to hydrotherapy came from pharmaceutical medicine circles in the decades that followed. Water cures became targeted by the new medical establishment, and many hydrotherapy treatment centers were shut down between 1920 and 1950. Hydrotherapy experienced a resurgence in the U.S. following World War II, when physical therapists found success in whirlpool treatment. Today hydrotherapy is widely used in various modalities, treatments, and physical therapy centers. Many hot springs and wellness spas are unmistakably similar to the hydrotherapy centers of years past. Today these centers draw millions of people seeking therapy and relaxation.

Hot and Cold Water Techniques

Hot and warm water therapy increases circulation, relaxation and detoxification efforts. Let's review some of the techniques recommended:

Cold water showers or a quick cold water rinse off after a warm water shower is invigorating and stimulating to the immune system and nervous system. It also helps balance the body's thermoregulation systems, cool the body in hot weather, as well as heat the body (through muscle contraction) in cold weather.

These actions are produced by our blood vessels' response to cold water. Cold water constricts the blood vessels and leads to involuntary muscle contraction. This type of muscle contraction increases the body's immune function by pumping the lymphatic vessels. In other words, lymph flow is circulated by movement and muscle contraction.

The mechanism works like this: As cold water hits the skin, internal muscles autonomically contract. This effectively pumps or squeezes lymphatic vessels. When the lymph vessels are pumped, the lymphatic fluid speed is increased—much like our heart's pumping increases blood circulation.

Lymph circulation distributes macrophages, T-cells, B-cells and other immune factors throughout the body, enabling them to break down invading bacteria, viruses, and chemical toxins. This effectively speeds up our immune response. As our immune system is responding faster, our toxic load is decreased and our infective burden lightens.

Blood vessel constriction from cold water also stimulates the health of our blood vessels. This serves to increase blood vessel wall elasticity, especially when the cold shower follows a warm or hot shower.

German researchers (Goedsche et al. 2007) studied the treatments used of Dr. Kneipp on twenty patients with chronic obstructive pulmonary disease. Cold-water hydrotherapy was tested for immunostimulation, maximal expiratory flow, quality of life, and respiratory function. After ten weeks of three cold effusions and two cold washings on the upper body per day, IFN-gamma lymphocytes increased, quality of life increased, lung function improved and the frequency of respiratory infections decreased.

Many traditional healers have used cold water therapy with great success for many inflammatory conditions. Additional cold water strategies include walking in a few inches to a few feet of cold water by a lake, river or ocean for at least a few minutes, building to up to 30 minutes a day.

Contrast baths reference a therapy of alternating hot water and cold water bathing. This therapy has been used with great success, and can be easily practiced at home by simply following a hot shower with a short cold one before toweling off.

Besides constricting blood vessels and stimulating lymph flow, a cold rinse at the end of a shower causes the skin pores to close. This leaves the body prepared to step out of the shower or bath. A cold rinse also reduces the potential of a basal cell chilling, which can stress the body. In other words, a cold rinse will better prepare the body for the temperature change.

Wet Sock hydrotherapy has been used for respiratory issues for centuries. The feet are soaked in hot water for 10-30 minutes while a pair of thin socks are soaked in cold, icy water. The feet are taken out of the hot water and the cold socks are wrung out and put on, with a pair of thick wool socks over top. This is followed by lying down or sitting with the feet up for an hour or two while relaxing.

Finnish sauna and plunge system: The Fins are famous for their wooden saunas, often built outside near a cold-water plunge. A vigorous sweat in the sauna immediately followed by the cold plunge stimulates the immune system dramatically. This ritual has also been a part of other cultures, including many North American Indian tribes, who used *sweat lodges* with great success. These cultures are known for their long lives and strengthened immunity. Infrared saunas are great modern devices for this purpose. Infrared saunas have the added benefit of quickly and safely dilating blood vessels.

Hot baths also have a great tradition of success among those with respiratory ailments. Hippocrates, known to western medicine as the father of medicine, stated that the hot bath *"...promotes expectoration, improves the respiration, and allays lassitude; for it soothes the joints and the outer skin, and is diuretic, removes heaviness of the heat and moistens the nose."*

Hot water calms the body and slows the heart rate, as the body's blood vessels relax and dilate in response to thermal radiation. A hot bath will open skin pores, allowing a detoxification and exfoliation of skin cells and their contents. For sore or damaged muscle tissues, the dilation of capillaries and micro-capillaries speeds up the process of cleansing the muscle cells of lactic and carbonic acids—the byproducts of inadequate respiration.

Recovery times from strenuous activity are typically reduced by the use of hot water therapy. Hot water is also *hydrostatic*—it gently massages the dermal layers. Hot water also slows internal organ activity, and relaxes the airway smooth muscles. This provides a soothing effect upon the innervations to these areas. The result is reduced stress and widened airways. This effect is increased when hot water is in motion—for example a hot tub.

Hot baths can also be medicated with a variety of anti-inflammatory herbs, as listed earlier. Simply make an infusion tea and pour it into the bath.

It should be noted that too much hot water for too long of a period can lead to cardiovascular stress. Hot water can also lead to heat exhaustion. For best results, hot water applications or saunas should be limited to about 10-15 minutes at the hotter levels.

Also, care should be taken to prevent chlorine and chlorine byproduct overload. The byproducts of chlorine breakdown are trihalomethanes (TTHM) and haloacetic acids (TAA5). Over-exposure to these can increase our toxin burden. Today there are healthier alternatives to chlorine, including bromine and salt water blends.

Hot Mineral Springs: From deep within the earth's surface come special waters of a thermal nature. Geothermal heat from volcanic magma creates a rich environment for charging aquifers with high temperatures and a variety of minerals. Many hot springs have a wholesome mixture of bicarbonates, iron, boron, silica, magnesium, copper, lithium, and many trace elements. Some contain exotic elements such as arsenic—believed to help heal skin issues and digestive issues. In other words, not all hot springs are alike.

Due to the earth's sulfur conveyor system, many of these hot spring waters are rich in sulfur in the form of hydrogen sulfide or sulfate. These can loosen phlegm and relax the airways.

Other mineral ions in hot springs have beneficial effects. Magnesium baths have been shown in studies to relax muscles and ease tension. Magnesium also strengthens arteries and relaxes the airway smooth muscles. Iron in hot springs has been associated with strengthening the immune system. Bicarbonates in hot springs—also called "soda springs"—have been associated with easing tension and aiding digestion.

Epson Salt Bath: For those without a nearby hot springs, a simple bath can be easily turned into therapeutic waters. At home, we can duplicate a magnesium and sulfur mineral springs bath by adding natural mineral salts such as Epson salts to our bath water. Epson salts—originally named after the magnesium-rich waters of Epson, England—are primarily magnesium sulfate, which will ionize in the water into magnesium ions and sulfur ions. As mentioned, ionic magnesium is beneficial to body tissues—relaxing the skin, reducing muscle tension, and lowering stress. Sulfur was also discussed above.

The Epson salt bath can be supplemented with the addition of rock salt. Natural rock salt contains upwards of 80 minerals and trace elements, which can make the bath a nourishing soak for the entire body.

A drop or two of an essential oil such as lavender or rose oil into the bath will further support relaxation. Lavender oil in particular can significantly calm the nerves.

The skin is said to be the largest organ of the body and absorbs water quite readily. The skin is similar to a mucous membrane. Ancient seamen understood this fact well. When out to sea and dehydrated, seamen would soak their garments in seawater for survival.

For this same reason, our bath waters should not contain toxic chemical bubble baths, chemical-laden perfumed soaps, or heavily chlorinated water. The skin will readily absorb these toxins, putting an extra burden upon the liver and immune systems. Best to use clean water and only natural additives.

Steam baths are especially helpful for most inflammatory conditions. The steam bath can be accomplished with a formal steam room, by the use of a humidifier, or simply with a hot bath in an enclosed room. A cool or coldwater rinse after is helpful for immune stimulation and temperature adjustment. Eucalyptus can be added to increase the expectoration effect. With this and all hot baths, water intake should be increased dramatically, depending upon duration.

Steams can also be done with a pan of boiled water steeped with anti-inflammatory herbs, or boiled potatoes. Just put a towel over the head and over the pan to breathe in the steam.

Sweating to Cleanse

The adult body has about 2.6 million sweat glands located throughout the body's skin cells. This makes the skin the body's greatest outlet for the elimination of toxins. As exposure to chemicals has increased, our need for regular sweat is even greater. Our ancestors worked and sweated daily in order to survive. Today, many of us sit in our heat-controlled environments all day without ever breaking a sweat. This trend has suspiciously increased with the prevalence of inflammatory and autoimmune diseases. University of Alberta researchers (2010) concluded in a study published in the *Archives of Environmental Contamination and Toxicology* that, *"induced sweating appears to be a potential method for elimination of many toxic elements from the human body."*

Typical methods of sweating include exercise, saunas and steam rooms. However, most people overlook the fact that outdoor work, walking or manual labor can produce a healthy sweat. Most people crank on the air conditioning at the slightest sign of heat. Sweating to cool off is a better strategy, as this will stimulate the turnover of toxins that burden our immune system.

Sweating outdoors in the summer heat also makes our body more heat tolerant, which allows us to live in warmer conditions in general. This means we can use the air conditioner less, which is better for our lungs and sinuses in the long run.

Strengthening our Mucosal Membranes

As we've illustrated in this text, our ability to cleanse and avoid new toxins is dependent upon the health of our mucosal membranes. Here is why:

> ➤ Toxins and microorganisms come into closer contact with epithelia that have damaged mucosal membrane layers. This

allows those toxins more access to our tissues and bloodstream.

➢ The cilia within the airways do not have the right basement fluid to operate effectively. Either they are overwhelmed by too much mucous or don't have enough basement membrane to effectively 'sweep' out toxins, cell parts and mucous.

➢ Defects in the mucosal membranes stimulate inflammation due to the decreased protection they offer those parts of the body they normally protect.

Foods and Beverages that Deplete Our Mucosal Membranes

The foods and beverages that deplete our mucosal membranes also increase systemic inflammation because they contribute free radicals and other toxins, stimulating systemic inflammation.

These include:

➢ Alcohol

➢ Foods/beverages high in refined sugars

➢ Highly processed foods/beverages

➢ Foods/beverages high in refined salt

➢ Foods high in saturated fats

➢ Fried foods and fast foods

➢ Foods that are burnt or overcooked

➢ Foods containing chemical additives

These foods and beverages serve to irritate the mucous membranes. This is because they either directly contribute free radicals to the body, or the oxidation occurs as they make contact with the mucosal membranes and body cells.

Other Things that Deplete Our Mucosal Membranes

A number of activities also reduce our mucosal health. These include:

➢ Stress

➢ Anxiety

➢ Anger

➢ Pharmaceuticals

➢ Illicit drugs

➢ Tobacco smoke (primary and secondary)

➢ Air pollution

➢ Lack of sunshine

➢ Infections (fungal, bacterial, viral)

➢ Lack of hydration

As for anger and stress, when our body is stressed, our body switches to fight-or-flight metabolic mechanisms that pull energy away from the processes of the sub-mucosal glands and gastric glands—which produce our mucosal membrane fluids. This is why a person who is nervous or anxious will also often have dry mouth and an upset stomach. They are not producing enough mucosal secretions to protect those epithelial cells.

The others on the list are either toxins that directly alter the pH of our mucosal membranes, or simply infect them.

Most pharmaceuticals are toxic to the mucosal membranes. This is why a significant side effect of most medications is dry mouth and an upset stomach. These chemicals can deplete our mucosal membranes and/or block mucosal secretions by virtue of inhibiting the COX-2 process. This also goes for other drugs, chemicals, pollutants, and so on.

Methylmethionine and Cabbage

Nature also provides nutrients from whole foods that can help rebuild our mucosal membranes. One of the more productive whole foods applicable to rebuilding our body's mucosal membranes is cabbage. Cabbage contains a unique constituent, s-methylmethionine, also referred to as vitamin U. Through a pathway utilizing one of the body's natural enzymes, called Bhmt2, s-methylmethionine is converted to methionine and then to glutathione in several steps.

In this form, glutathione has been shown to stimulate the repair of the mucosal membranes within the stomach, intestines and airways. Glutathione has also been shown to increase the health and productivity of the liver.

Raw cabbage or cabbage juice has been used as a healing agent for ulcers and intestinal issues for thousands of years among traditional medicines, including those of Egyptian, Ayurvedic and Greek systems. The Western world became aware of raw cabbage juice in the 1950s, when Garnett Cheney, M.D. conducted several studies showing that methylmethionine-rich cabbage juice concentrate was able to reduce the pain and bleeding associated with ulcers.

In one of Dr. Cheney's studies, 37 ulcer patients were treated with either cabbage juice concentrate or a placebo. Of the 26-patient cabbage juice group, 24 patients were considered "successes"—achieving an astounding 92% success rate.

Medical researchers from Iraq's University Department of Surgery (Salim 1993) conducted a double-blind study of 172 patients who suffered from gastric bleeding caused by nonsteroidal anti-inflammatory drugs (NSAIDs). They gave the patients either cysteine, methylmethionine sulfonium chloride (MMSC) or a placebo. Those receiving either the cysteine or the MMSC stopped bleeding. Their conditions became *"stable"* as compared with many in the control group, who continued to bleed.

Plants use s-methylmethionine to help heal cell membrane damage among their leaves and stems. This is reminiscent of antioxidants: Plants produce antioxidants to help to protect them from damage from the sun, insects and diseases. In other words, the very same biochemicals that protect plants also help heal our bodies.

Note that MMSC or cabbage juice does not inhibit the flow of gastric juices in the stomach to produce these effects as do acid blocking medications. Rather, they stimulate the body's natural production of mucous, which serves to protect the stomach's cells from the effects of acids.

Herbs that Stimulate Mucosal Health

A number of the herbs help revitalize the mucous membranes. Some of these, such as Aloe, Slippery elm, Marsh mallow and Mallow, specifically contribute mucopolysaccharides in the form of mucilage. These constituents supplement the mucosal membranes, providing protection. At the same time, they contain nutrients that stimulate submucosal gland secretions, which include the glycoproteins and mucopolysaccharides that form the foundation for our mucous membranes.

Most will also exert antioxidant effects and, in the case of aloe, will exert an antimicrobial effect upon the mucosal membranes. This of course, helps remove infective microorganisms, which in turn helps lighten the burden on our immune system.

Other gentle herbs that can help stimulate our mucosal membrane health include:

➤ Triphala (*Terminalia chebula, Terminalia bellirica* and *Emblica officinalis*)
➤ Black Pepper (*Piper nigrum*)
➤ Mallow (*Malva sylvestris*)
➤ Marsh Mallow (*Althaea officinalis*)
➤ Cumin Seed (*Cuminum cyminum*)
➤ Aloe (*Aloe vera*)
➤ Comfrey (*Symphytum officinale*)
➤ Chamomile (*Matricaria chamomilla*)
➤ Slippery elm (*Ulmus fulva*)
➤ Flaxseed (*Linum usitatissimum*)

All of these contain constituents that specifically help stimulate mucosal membrane health.

There are several ways to incorporate these herbs into our daily regimen. We can add more freshly ground Black pepper to our foods. We can add a teaspoon of Aloe to a smoothie or juice. We can spice our foods with fresh Cumin seed (also a spice used in many curries). We can make teas (infusions) from one of the Mallows, some Comfrey and Chamomile. Flaxseeds may be steeped into tea, eaten raw, baked into breads, or sprinkled directly on foods.

We can also take a teaspoon of Triphala in a glass of warm water each day or every few days. Reputable Triphala formulations are available at health food stores and online. A teaspoon can be stirred into a glass of water or a healthy fruit smoothie.

Gentle Fasting

Fasting can quickly reduce our toxic burden and systemic inflammation, because it allows the body's liver, kidneys and immune system to clear waste with a lower dietary workload.

However, fasting must be done cautiously. Fasting too aggressively may stimulate too much detoxification too fast, which can overload the bloodstream with toxin byproducts as the tissues clear waste. For this reason, it may be safer to do short, one-day fasts once or twice a week, or fast with soups, juices or fruits.

Fasting with healthy but limited food selections also allows the liver, kidneys and immune system to do a deep cleanse, yet adds some energy nutrients to sustain blood sugar levels.

A systematic approach to fasting is recommended. Here are a few optional approaches to consider:

> ➤ Fast for one afternoon with lemon juice.
> ➤ Water fast from morning until dinner time once or twice a week
> ➤ Fast for one day with only vegetable soups and fresh juices of carrot and celery.

Any of these fasts should be accompanied by the following:

> ➤ Increased water consumption: 3/4-ounce per pound of weight.
> ➤ Increased relaxation and rest (days off work are suggested).
> ➤ Only light exercise, such as walking or swimming.
> ➤ Peaceful environments (no parties or shouting matches).

This formula will guarantee that the fast is productive and thoroughly detoxifying.

Strategies to Reduce Toxin Exposure

By reducing our toxin exposure, we can dramatically lighten the burden on our immune systems, allowing our body's own detoxification systems to work more effectively. While this is not the total solution, reducing toxin exposure should not be overlooked. Below are some strategies to reduce our incoming toxins.

Know Your Toxins

One of the first things we can do is find out precisely what toxins are in our immediate environment. This means inspecting tags, reading labels and in general getting to know that materials that surround us in our home and work environments.

We should understand what is in our local drinking water. If on a municipal water supply, our local water district will likely list the results of their periodic tests. The EPA mandates that municipalities make this information available to the public, so there should be a website for our local water district.

We should also investigate the makeup and levels of our local air pollution levels are important. We might also find out what times of day the smog levels are higher and lower. Coordinating our exercise times and outdoor activities with lower smog periods is not a bad idea. A good place to start for those in the U.S. is the Environmental Protection Agency's local pollutant website:

http://www.epa.gov/epahome/commsearch.htm

By typing in our zip code into this database, we will be able to investigate the following information about our area:

Air pollution contents, levels and comparison to averages.

Locations of toxic spills, hazardous waste sites, or other areas, and any sites that have been categorized as an NPL—on the National Priorities List.

> Notifications of water quality issues.
> Sites of oil, natural gas or other mining operations nearby.
> Any toxic releases in area.
> Any sites subject to Superfund, Brownfields or other cleanup projects.
> Sites that have been subject to environmental enforcement nearby.

Outdoor Air Pollution Strategies

The best recommendation we find in some texts is simply to shut all the windows as much as possible. Is this really a solution? As we mentioned earlier, research has confirmed that indoor pollution is generally worse than outdoor pollution. What are we to do, then?

As we've discussed, ozone, particulate matter (soot) and carbon monoxide can contribute to and worsen toxicity.

Fresh Air

There is little doubt that city living increases toxicity. For example, a study done by the Arizona Health Care Cost Containment System (Smith *et al.* 2010) found that among 3,013 people, urban residents had a 55% greater likelihood of respiratory disorders than did rural residents.

Living around or at least visiting a natural setting such as a forest or beach has many advantages. For example, researchers from Japan's Chiba University (Park *et al.* 2010) conducted 24 field experiments using 280 subjects among 24 forests throughout Japan. In each of the tests, six subjects walked through a forest, while another six walked through a city. The next day the six that walked the city would walk the forest and vice versa. The research concluded that forest environments reduce stress-related cortisol levels, lower heart rate, reduce blood pressure, lower anxiety and increase reaction time. The researchers concluded that: *"These results will contribute to the development of a research field dedicated to forest medicine, which may be used as a strategy for preventive medicine."*

Other studies have confirmed these results. One study found that people living in natural environments had lower levels of stress than those living in urban environments (Ulrich *et al.* 1991). Another, from Emory University, found that natural environments improve health conditions (Frumkin 2001).

City Strategies

As much as we may want to, not everyone can pick up and move away from the city. In this case, focus can turn towards reducing immediate air pollutant exposure. We can make logical choices to reduce our exposure. This doesn't mean staying inside and closing all the windows either. It is important that we get enough sunshine and "fresh" air, and this requires us to go outside. We can simply use some common sense. For example, we can *avoid* the following:

- ➢ Running, walking or biking next to a freeway where soot and carbon monoxide levels are greatest.
- ➢ Hanging out downwind of a smokestack of an industrial plant known to throw toxins into the air.
- ➢ Sitting or standing downwind, or next to, an outdoor fire or gas stove for an extended period.
- ➢ Standing, sitting or walking next to someone spraying pesticides, herbicides or other chemicals.
- ➢ Frequenting tobacco-filled bars or other smoky places.
- ➢ Avoiding dusty areas such as construction sites, runways, racetracks, rodeos and other events that stir up lots of airborne particulates.

In addition, there are a number of proactive things we can do to reduce our airborne toxins. As discussed earlier, breathing in through the nose helps to filter out some particulates and other foreigners. This also warms the air. As we discussed, cold air can dry the mucous membranes, and thinned mucous membranes expose our airways to more airborne toxins.

If we live in an urban area with poor air quality we might consider exercising or getting outside during the morning, when the air quality is typically better. As temperatures rise, immediate ozone levels increase. We might also consider exercising near a lake, river, or ocean. Polluted air around water tends to disperse more quickly in the presence of wind, humidity, pressure gradients, and temperature differences around the water.

Out and out wearing of a facemask is typically not practical—although during an extreme situation, it is not a bad idea. More subtle strategies include wearing a scarf during winter months, and covering our mouth and nose with it when outside. In colder climates, a fleece ski mask could also help filter out some particulates.

These are but a few ways to prevent burdening our immune system with airborne toxins—but again, these cannot be our only strategy. We must also undertake reducing the *other, more controllable* immune system burdens to the greatest degree possible. This may also mean increasing the amount of antioxidants we consume in our diet. And let's not forget that the more antioxidants we eat, the better our ability to remove toxins will be. We can add to this the other strategies discussed—herbs, diet, detoxification and so on.

Home Pollution Strategies

Americans spend over 90% of their lives indoors, and indoor air pollution averages double to five times worse than outdoor pollution levels. In some cases, indoor pollution can be tens, even hundreds of times higher than outdoor pollutant levels.

The issue here is ventilation. While older homes might exchange all the air in the house every couple of hours—even up to twice an hour—modern energy-efficient homes exchange air well over five times slower. The average, in fact, is about .25 times per hour, meaning that it would take four hours to exchange all the air in the home. This problem has been termed the *tight building syndrome.*

Previously, we discussed *sick building syndrome.* Tight building syndrome can result in sick building syndrome, assuming that a tight building is not properly ventilated, or ventilated with a clean ventilation system. Or, quite simply, keeping windows open throughout the house. While this might be frowned upon by city dwellers, most indoor air is still quite worse than even big city air. Plus, as we'll explain further, circulating air removes particulates and other toxins as it moves.

For example, University of Glasgow researchers (Wright *et al.* 2009) found that ventilation increases lung function, but does little to reduce dust mite populations. They tested the homes of 120 asthmatic adults—who were allergic to *Dermatophagoides pteronyssinus* dust mites—using mechanical heat recovery ventilation systems (MHRV). This was in addition to conventional allergen avoidance measures in an attempt to reduce dust mite populations. After one year, the peak expiratory flow among the ventilator group was significantly better than the non-ventilator group. However, the ventilation systems *did not* reduce the mite levels within the houses.

So it is not the number of dust mites: It is the composition of the air itself, determined by circulation. A good ventilation system will circulate air while sending it through a filter. A good filter can remove endotoxins that mites produce, as well as the molds, bacteria, soot and other debris that commonly reside in our indoor air.

As we discussed in depth earlier, indoor air pollution is caused by fungi-laden basements, formaldehydes from furniture, asbestos and other building chemicals, household chemicals, volatile organic compounds, smoking, moldy ventilation systems, moldy dust-mite ridden carpets, and so on.

Air Filtration

These toxins can help overload our immune systems, especially if overloaded by other toxins and/or pathogens. In other words, it would be better to remove as many of these as possible before we breathed them in.

Air purifiers: These can significantly remove toxins from the air, as they draw air through a filter and then push the air out. Studies have shown that air purifiers can significantly increase the quality of life among asthmatics (Brodtkorb *et al.* 2010).

Electric ion generating machines generate negative ions. Ionizers have been reputed to remove dust and bacteria, yet this remains controversial. While dust and soot may be attracted to negative ions, they are likely to remain airborne, or possibly end up on floors or furniture to be picked up again.

The amount of ions generated by these machines may also be of concern. While outdoor air may range from 500 to 5,000 negative ions per cubic centimeter, and indoor air may only have a couple hundred per cubic centimeter, negative ion generators can easily pump out from ten thousand to ten million negative ions per cubic centimeter. At these higher levels—especially over a million—negative ions can become irritating to mucous membranes. They can irritate the throat, the eyes, and the lungs. Quite simply, our bodies were not designed for this level of negative ions.

Furthermore, a Cochrane review (Blackhall *et al.* 2003) of six good quality studies concluded that ionizers exerted no significant effects upon respiratory health.

Ozone generators may be effective at removing bacteria, because bacteria require oxygen to live, and ozone depletes their oxygen levels. For this reason, a good ozone generator will often create a fresher smelling indoor environment. While ozone is not the same as smog, which has carbon or sulphur molecules connected to the molecules, ozone is an atmospheric response to smog, as ozone helps stabilize oxygen levels and clear out other molecules.

At the same time, higher ozone levels may also result in lung irritation and allergic response. As mentioned earlier, the FDA limits ozone generating machines in medical devices (used in hospitals and clinics) to emit no more than 50 parts per billion. The bottom line with both ionizers and ozone generators is that the atmosphere contains a fragile balance of components: It is not a random mixture. The level of ozone present in outdoor pollution reflects the atmosphere's cleansing process. In other words, the decision to use these machines should be made carefully, and the composition of fresh air is likely healthier than any machine-driven composition.

High-Efficiency Particular Arresting (HEPA) filters: It might be noted that neither the ozone nor ion generator systems have been shown to effectively remove dust, dander or allergens (unless the allergens are bacteria, which can be removed with ozone). A HEPA filter is a better strategy for removing dust, dander and other particulates. HEPA filters are designed to pick up over 99.9% of particulate sized .3 micron in size. Putting a HEPA filter on a simple air ducting system with a fan or heater will thus do wonders for removing dust, dander, and allergens.

Electrostatic air filters for forced air systems can be a good choice. These HEPA filters typically filter between ninety and a hundred percent of dander, mold, mites, dust, soot, and bacteria. Many of these filters come with the ability to clean and reuse, allowing us to clean them as often as needed—which should be at least monthly if use is constant.

Environmental filters are good alternatives, especially for cold urban environments. These draw in, filter and heat outdoor air. This maximizes circulation, ventilation and temperature control: The best of all worlds.

Pillowcase filters: This air filtration device is designed to filter the nighttime air through the pillowcase. One study (Stillerman *et al.* 2010) tested this with 35 adults who had allergic rhinoconjunctivitis and sensitivities to either dander or dust mites. The device was found to reduce 99.99% of allergen particulates greater than .3 microns within the patients' breathing zones. The patient group using the filtration device was found to have significantly fewer symptoms and better quality of lie than the placebo group.

Natural Air Sanitation

We can also restrict the level of indoor pollutants by choosing to use household products with natural ingredients free as possible from chemical preservatives. This means using natural flooring and furniture, natural fragrance-free soaps and cosmetics, and cotton clothing. This also means buying fewer plastic household goods and more natural fiber goods. Should we change our purchasing behavior, we may also alter the behavior of those companies manufacturing these items.

When it comes to freshening up stale indoor air, pressurized aerosol air fresheners are not the way to go. They may contain various synthetic fragrances, benzyl ethanols, naphthalene, and formaldehydes among other undesirables. Various micro-particles are also created by these aerosols.

As mentioned in the trigger chapter, many aerosols and pump sprays also contain noxious propellants—many of which are also volatile organic compounds (VOCs). These include butane and propane. Despite their demand in the marketplace, aerosols are not required for survival: Humankind did just fine without them for thousands of years. An effective disbursing method is a simple spray bottle. An active ingredient—say lemon juice—can be diluted with water and lightly sprayed through a room to freshen it up nicely. There are, of course, many other uses for such a common spray bottle—effectively replacing propellant aerosols.

Beware of perfumes and colognes that may reside in the bathroom or on family members. And be careful of fashion magazines and men's magazines that insert fragrances into their pages and advertisements. These perfumes might smell nice, but they can also contain toxins that can burden the immune system.

Candles may smell nice, but they are often made with synthetic fragrances, hydrocarbon-based paraffin waxes, and lead or other heavy metal wicks. The combination often releases unhealthy black soot into our air. Beeswax candles with essential oils can provide good alternatives for the candle-loving household, combined, of course, with fresh air.

Healthy alternatives to toxic household cleaners include lemon, vinegar, borax and/or baking soda. Borax is a great scrubbing detergent for heavy household and yard cleaning jobs. Olive oil, lemon oil or beeswax make for good natural furniture polishes.

Cleaning surfaces with these will also significantly freshen indoor air as well. Rotting food and unclean surfaces create mildew and bacteria quite quickly. Fresh air is quite easy to achieve with clean surfaces. Dusting and wiping down flooring and walls with vinegar can be a good strategy. A small cup of vinegar or a box of baking soda placed in a corner can also absorb odors and airborne toxins. Non-septic friendly chlorine bleach or rubbing alcohol can be used sparingly to remove mold or other microorganisms.

As far as pesticides, there are also natural alternatives. These include clove oil, mints, orange oil, borax and others. Many pest control companies will now apply these alternatives upon request.

House Plants

A house full of indoor plants will do wonders for improving our indoor air quality. Placing between two and five plants in a hundred square foot room—depending upon the outside air—can significantly remove carbon and raise oxygen levels. Research from the *Mississippi Stennis Space Center* concluded that indoor plants absorbed and broke down formaldehydes, trichloroethylenes, benzenes and zylenes.

Better performing plants included the lady palm, the rubber plant, English ivy, and the areca palm plants. Toxin removal rates can range from 1,000 to 1,800 micrograms per hour. One study done in Norway (Fjeld *et al.* 1998) found 23% fewer complaints of fatigue and sinus congestion among workers working around plants.

Studies performed in Texas and at Washington State University found that cognition response and problem-solving were also significantly higher among people working around plants (Wolverton 1997).

It should be noted that potting soils of indoor plants can also harbor some molds, so care can be taken to dry out the soil between waterings, and keep some sunlight on the soil surface.

We can also create forests around our homes. This means planting and maintaining indigenous trees that provide oxygen, shade and soil health: Soils without good plant life and rooting systems become loose and dusty. Nearby outdoor plants can significantly decrease the carbon and toxins in our immediate circulating environment. This also means instead of tearing out trees and paving our courtyards, we can leave the trees or replant them. Living in a space surrounded by trees can also render more privacy, allowing us to keep our windows open more often.

Pros and Cons on Air Conditioning

Air conditioning offers benefits and downsides. On the benefit side, a good one can filter out particulates and some pollutants. This of course depends on the type of filter inside the air conditioner, and how often it is cleaned. And filters not cleaned frequently can build up with fungi and bacteria that can significantly infect our airspace.

Most air conditioners reduce humidity as well. The problem with this massive reduction in humidity is that it can dry out the mucosal membranes in our airways. This, along with the cold air provided by many air conditioners, can lead to or worsen respiratory disorders.

Swamp coolers provide filtering and cooling, but add humidity. This can help keep the airways and skin hydrated. However, swamp coolers can easily get infected with molds and bacteria: So they have to be cleaned periodically, at least seasonally.

Practically every air conditioner creates condensation, which results in small droplets of water dripping around the unit or inside the unit. This can encourage fungi and bacteria growth around the walls and ventilation ducts of the system.

Air conditioning artificially cools down body temperature and airways. While this might be considered a good thing when it is hot outside, artificially cooling the body also stresses the body and the airways. The body must work harder to heat and humidify the air before it hits the lungs. This can stress the turbinates, the airway mucosal membranes, and the immune system. Remember the research we laid out earlier that confirms colder, dryer air can increase airway hypersensitivity.

Also note that car air-conditioning systems typically intake air from around the car—full of traffic exhaust. The air can also contain exhaust from the car itself, or combustion byproducts from the engine. While screened through a filter, this air still contains toxins. We can periodically refresh the car's indoor air by stopping and rolling down the car windows.

Air filters in car air conditions can also become filled with fungi and bacteria, so they can be periodically cleaned. Generally, people do not clean their car air filters. So it is safe to say that any older car has a significant build up of mold and other toxins within its air conditioner system and filters.

Noting these issues, it is probably more sustainable to simply minimize air conditioning and utilize fans when possible. Opening the car windows while driving also provides a fan of sorts. Fanned air on the skin helps cool the skin down without chilling the air. Remember that circulated air is typically cleaner than the same type of air when stagnant.

A fan strategy also allows our bodies to better acclimate to the outdoor temperatures. This is healthier for the body. Our bodies have cooling mechanisms that include sweating and relaxing. Both of these are healthy strategies. Sweating removes waste and toxins from the body, and relaxing takes pressure off the adrenal glands. We can conclude that sweating a little and relaxing a bit can reduce toxicity.

Natural Materials

Using nature's materials for floors, walls and furniture is also a good strategy. This means using stone, ceramic, wood, wool, cotton and so on. Practically every synthetic piece of furniture, wall covering or floor covering contains a host of chemicals, including formaldehyde, VOCs, insecticides, asbestos and fire retardants. While retarding fires is certainly commendable, these can also make us sick in the worst case, and add to our toxin load in the best case. Besides, stone can be a pretty good fire retardant.

Stone, ceramic tile or wooden floors can also be easily cleaned with vinegar and baking soda to safely eliminate dust and allergens. Wood can also be polished and cleaned with olive oil. Nowadays, most walls are sheet rock, which often contains chalks and asbestos that can slowly build up in the airways. Replacing them with wood siding is a possible strategy.

Outgassing

Outgassing (or off-gassing) any new materials we buy is a good idea, regardless. To outgas a material, we can simply set it in the sun for a day before using it. This is a good idea for any new piece of furniture, wall covering, and anything else that may have been coated in VOCs or formaldehydes during manufacturing. Plastics may also be outgassed, but outgassing plastic in direct sunlight can also release additional monomer plasticizers.

Outgassing a new car might also be considered. That "new car smell" is more than just a nice smell. Leave the car in the sun for a few days or weeks with the windows open. For best results, always keep car windows cracked.

Ventilation

Air travels in currents. These currents are electromagnetic. Airflows will thus grab hold of air pollutants and channel them away. Air works much as water does, as it uses electrostatic forces to remove toxins. This means that our freshest air will be the air that flows through our environment. Stagnated air is polluted air. Moving air is typically cleaner and provides the best means to minimize toxicity. Circulating air also has the greatest tendency of maintaining normal atmospheric composition, humidity and pressure values.

Therefore, if possible, we might consider keeping our windows open at all times, even in the wintertime. When it is cold outside, we can crack the window barely—just enough to allow for some airflow. Fans can do the rest.

Work and School Pollution Strategies

Work and school environments are toxin traps. Why? Because they bring people and limited ventilation systems together under the same roof. They also host a number of toxins in building materials, carpets, desks, chairs, production materials, manufacturing exhaust, and whatever anyone brings in to work or school. This of course includes animal dander, dust mites, microorganisms and mold attached to people's clothing, hair and skin as they venture into the building.

This was illustrated in the New Zealand research discussed earlier, where cat allergens were found throughout schools, workplaces, theaters and airplanes.

While there is no way to eliminate these potential toxins, we can certainly take measures to lower our exposure, since as a whole, toxins from the workplace and school do contribute to our overall toxic load and burden upon our immune system. Furthermore, exposure to workplace toxicity in the form of manufacturing wastes, cleaners, gases and other chemical toxins can single-handedly make a person downright sick.

A number of policies and strategies that can reduce our toxin exposure among workplaces and schools:

Hazardous Materials: Workplaces and schools typically utilize various chemicals and cleaning materials. Some workplaces use hazardous materials on a daily basis. These should be handled with care, to make sure that exposures are minimized.

According to United States Occupational Safety Code, *Manufacturer's Safety Data Sheets* (MSDS) are required for every chemical used by consumers, workers or cleaning professionals. These should be carefully read over to make sure that the material is being used in accordance with the MSDS. This means that enough ventilation is supplied. For most hazardous materials, this is the greatest risk: Hazardous materials are frequently used without the proper ventilation. These toxins can also cause illness and death, depending upon the chemical and exposure level.

HVAC: Our school and workplace should have a heating, ventilating and air conditioning system (also called HVAC) that is adequate for the population, space and environmental conditions. The more people, space and toxins present, the better the HVAC system needs to be. In the United States, these are typically determined by local, state or county building codes. When a building is designed, its HVAC must comply with the building code in place.

The standard codes are determined by The *American Society of Heating, Refrigerating and Air Conditions Engineers* (ASHRAE), who have developed the standards that most municipalities abide by. For example, the 1989 standards (6.2-1989) called for 15-20 cubic feet of fresh air to be brought in per minute (CFM) and per person occupying an indoor space. This means, for example, that an office with 10 people must have a system that pumps in 150-200 cubic feet of fresh air per minute.

This same calculation can be done for any school or other space.

In addition, building codes have changed over the years with respect to insulation. This means that if the building has been built in the past few decades, the building codes are tighter, and there will be likely less ventilation in general. This puts an extra strain on the HVAC system.

Windows are certainly a form of ventilation, but they should not be included in this calculation, because during cold or hot weather, the windows are often closed (though they should not be).

Any building needs to be checked with current code to make sure that the HVAC system matches the use and occupancy of the building. The building specifications designed by the architect before the building was built can easily be different from the building's current use. There may be many more workers or children in the building than originally specified for example. Or if the HVAC was designed for office space, but the building is now used as manufacturing space, for example, the HVAC requirements will be different—depending upon what is being produced, and the municipality. So the company owners or school administrators must be reminded to assure their workers or parents that the workplace's/school's HVAC systems are compliant with current codes. This should also be reviewed for any apartment or condominium.

HVAC systems also should also be periodically cleaned. This includes the drip pans and ducting. These can build up with molds and other microorganisms, and infect their occupants. As we discussed earlier, cases have shown that extreme weather changes (from cold to warm or wet) can dramatically affect the HVAC system ducting in terms of mold and microorganisms—significantly infecting the building's occupants.

Flooring: Carpeting in workplaces and schools is particularly problematic. This is because they attract bacteria, molds, dander, allergens and other toxins quickly. Cleaning carpets is typically expensive and difficult. Wood, stone or concrete floors clean easier and can be disinfected more easily, as we've discussed.

Furniture: Chairs and sofas in the work place are susceptible to mold, toxin and allergen build-up as they age, and formaldehydes when newer. Therefore, they need to be periodically cleaned or replaced. Wooden furniture or furniture with cleanable surfaces and moisture barriers are preferred.

Windows: From an individual perspective, sitting or working close to an openable window is suggested in any workplace or school classroom. Any time there is an offensive odor or concern about indoor air quality, the window should be opened and left open until the risk has subsided. Hotel rooms can also be checked for openable windows before they are reserved. A closed-in room with a dirty HVAC system can practically produce illness in itself.

Keeping the house on the dry side. Water feeds molds and fungi. Look for leaks into the windowsills, basements and house corners.

Chemicals: Our houses and work places are best clear of pesticides, fragrances, incense, and other chemicals. If bugs are a problem, try borax or traps.

Household and workplace cleaners should be natural. These include baking soda, vinegar, lemon and borax. These are all, to relative degrees, also antimicrobial.

Tubs and bathrooms should be cleaned of molds and fungi frequently, before mold forms. Mold grows in moist, dark places, so those areas of the bathroom should be cleaned more frequently than areas exposed to sunshine.

Fans: Fans are a valuable and inexpensive addition to any room. These can help blow offensive air out the door or window, for example. Fans, in fact, are better strategies than air conditioning, because they do not artificially cool the body down—as we've discussed. In the opinion of this author, every workplace and school should be equipped with fans.

Carbon monoxide and NO_2 strategies include venting any gas appliance to the outdoors, making sure there are no leaks, using the right fuels for each appliance; using an exhaust fan over a gas appliance; using certified wood stoves; having stoves inspected and cleaned; opening fireplace flues (vents to the outside); and opening the garage door before starting the car.

Air purifiers: Small air purifiers can significant help a person working in a workplace with questionable air. These can be placed right on the desk. These can significantly help remove particulates, mold and allergens from our immediate breathing airspace.

Regular Cleaning: This is a requisite for any workplace, school or apartment building. Common areas should be cleaned at least weekly. Floors and walls should be sanitized. Good natural cleaners include vinegar, lemon, borax and baking soda. Chlorine or rubbing alcohol can be used sparingly to disinfect. Furniture requires regular dusting and sanitization, and HVAC systems and ducts require regular cleaning.

Wearing a mask when we are using any chemical that might contain VOCs or other breathable toxins. Best strategy is to not use these types of chemicals at all, but sometimes we might have to. The mask should have an outside rubber seal. Paper masks do very little to prevent breathing in toxins.

Strengthened Immunity: No matter how clean we get our workplaces and schools, there will always be lots of toxins. While these strategies can help remove toxin exposure, we still need to strengthen our immunity and tolerance. Hygiene, after all, has its place. But it cannot replace a strong immune system. This means following through with other strategies outlined in this text.

Mucosal (Oral) Probiotics

Research documented in the last chapter shows that our probiotics are critical elements in the health of our mucosal membranes. This is because they inhabit and police our mucosal membranes. They are defenders and facilitators for the recycling of mucous, and they help break down toxins and pathogens.

They also secrete very important biochemicals—which contribute to the ionic and nutrient makeup of the mucosal membranes. Without healthy probiotic colonies, our mucosal membranes are subject to pathogen attack and inflammatory alteration.

For the health of our mouth, throat and airway mucosal membranes, we can take oral probiotics. These are particular species of probiotic bacteria, such as *Lactobacillus reuteri* and *L. salivarius,* which (among others) line the mucosal membranes of our mouths, sinuses, pharynx, larynx and bronchial airways. Research has illustrated—as we showed earlier—that oral probiotics help clean, prevent infection and maintain the strength and flexibility of our mucosal passages.

Skin Brushing

Brushing the skin lightly with a natural fiber brush can also stimulate the immune system by stimulating the lymphatic system and opening skin pores. This can also stimulate circulation in general, which increases immunity.

Skin brushing is best accomplished by brushing toward our heart, along the lymphatic vessels and blood vessels. Light but steady pressure is best. It should stimulate circulation and stimulate the skin. This will be readily felt and even seen by more skin color. We likely will not feel an increase in lymph flow, but our immune system will.

Sun Exposure/Vitamin D

Multiple studies have found that inflammatory diseases are significantly greater among regions further from the equator and those with less sunlight exposure. In both Europe and the U.S.—with the exception of urban areas with greater air pollution—those living in Southern regions have shown significantly lower incidence of many degenerative diseases, along with fewer hospital visits.

Vitamin D induces cathelicidin production (Grant 2008). Cathelicidins are proteins found within the lysosomes of macrophages and polymorphonuclear cells (PMNs). These immune cells are intensely antiviral and antibacterial in nature. They are also stimulated and regulated by vitamin D within the body.

Many conditions have been shown to be improved or prevented by therapeutic sunlight and/or vitamin D. These include, lupus vulgaris, small pox, Pick's disease, tuberculosis, asthma, nervous diseases, adrenal insufficiency, hormone imbalances, congestive heart failure, cardiovascular disease, multiple sclerosis, rheumatoid arthritis, Crohn's disease, irritable bowel syndrome, acne, psoriasis, jaundice, depression, eczema, high blood pressure, heart disease, diabetes, hypothyroidism, angina, prostate cancer, lung cancer, colon cancer, ovary cancer, kidney disease, hyperparathyroidism, uterine cancer, stomach cancer, kidney cancer, lymphoma, pancreatic cancer, ovarian cancer, tooth loss, bone loss, obesity, joint inflammation, insomnia, Parkinson's disease, fibromyalgia and a variety of immune- and autoimmune-related diseases.

In all, research over the past ten years has found that sunlight and/or vitamin D deficiency is implicated in over 70 disease conditions.

The sun's ultraviolet-B rays stimulate our bodies to synthesize vitamin D_3. Vitamin D is more of a hormone than a vitamin. It is a critical biochemical for the body. The cholesterol derivative *7-dehydrocholesterol* undergoes a *conrotatory electrocyclic reaction* to produce a pre-vitamin D. The pre-vitamin D molecule undergoes hydroxylation in the liver and kidneys to convert to the final D_3 structure— 1,25 dihydroxyvitamin D (or 25-OHD).

Within a 7-dehydrocholesterol-saturated biomolecular environment of the epidermis, specialized cells called *melanocytes* produce a protective biochemical called *melanin*. Skin melanocytes are primarily located at the lower strata of the epidermis. Other melanocytes located around the body produce specialized forms of melanin. Melanocytes within the uvea, which contains the iris, produce the melanin that gives the color to our irises. Melanocytes around our hair follicles give color to our hair. Melanocytes within the leptomeninges residing within our brain and spinal cord produce a type of melanin thought to support cerebrospinal fluid circulation.

Once produced in skin melanocytes, melanin is transferred to the keratinocytes, which lie on the external skin barrier. Melanin is the biochemical pigment that makes the skin turn brown. Melanin also provides a natural sunscreen for the skin: The greater the melanin level, the fewer ultraviolet-B rays reach the 7-dehydrocholesterol molecules, and the less vitamin D_3 is produced. Vitamin D is used in thousands of metabolic processes around the body. What is not used is stored within fat cells for later use.

Vitamin D is considered a cell membrane antioxidant. It specifically inhibits the lipid peroxidation process. Research has found that vitamin D inhibits lipid peroxidation better than cholesterol—a typical inhibitor. One study found its lipid peroxidation properties have anti-cancer benefits (Wiseman 1993).

Additional effects and mechanisms of sunlight and vitamin D are discussed in the author's book, *Healthy Sun.*

Getting Outdoors

Outdoor therapy – including forest walking, gardening and yoga meditation – not only will increase well-being and quality of life: It will also strengthen the immune system.

Researchers from Japan's Kyoto University (Nakau *et al.* 2013) tested 22 cancer patients for four months. The patients were given weekly sessions of four central protocols: They worked in the garden, planting seeds and caring for plants – termed horticultural therapy. They engaged in walking in the forest. They were engaged in yoga meditation exercises. And they attended weekly support group therapy sessions.

The researchers assessed the patients before and after the therapy using several assessments. Quality of life was assessed using the Short Form-36 Health Survey Questionnaire. Fatigue was assessed using the Cancer Fatigue Scale. Psychological moods and state of mind was assessed using the Profile of Mood States index and State-Trait Anxiety Inventory. Spiritual well-being was assessed using the Functional Assessment of Chronic Illness Therapy-Spiritual. And their immune system was assessed through testing for natural killer cell (NK cells) activity.

The researchers found that the therapy significantly increased quality of life scores. They also found reduced cancer-related fatigue and increased functional well-being scores among the patients. The outdoor therapy also improved moods and emotions among the patients after the twelve week testing period.

The researchers found the outdoor therapy also increased natural killer cell activity among the patients.

Other research has shown the success of some of these measures. Other evidence shows that forest walking has heart benefits and improves quality of life.

Meditation has been found to relieve anxiety, depression and even pain. Researchers from St. Mary's College (Ando *et al.* 2009) found in a study of 28 cancer patients that mindfulness meditation reduced pain scores as well as depression and anxiety after only two weeks of meditation therapy – which included yoga postures, breathing and meditation.

Being outdoors has a number of benefits, ranging from sunshine to increased negative ions to better air quality. Nature's colors also improve moods and wellness.

Sleep Strategies

Sleep is critical to our immune system and our ability to purge toxins. This is especially true when it comes to deep sleep and REM-stage cycles.

When we sleep, our immune system moves into overdrive. Like microscopic elves, our probiotics become more active, taking out pathogenic microorganisms and breaking down toxins. Our T- and B-cells help coordinate the process, and participate in breaking down pathogens and toxins. Our liver will produce more antioxidant enzymes during sleep. The body's purification systems all move into overdrive. When we sleep deeply, we also breathe deeper, which removes more toxins from the lungs and the airway mucosal membranes. Our intestinal probiotics switch into high gear, and our cells dump more toxins into intercellular fluids.

This was illustrated by researchers from Chicago's Rush University Medical Center (Ranjbaran *et al.* 2007), who studied sleep abnormalities and their association with *"chronic inflammatory conditions (CIC)."* They found that changes in the *"sleep-wake cycle"* stimulate an increased systemic inflammation response. Their research also showed that slow wave (deep) sleep can curb inflammation and strengthen immunity.

They also found that sleep disturbances can cause greater levels of inflammatory pain and fatigue, while reducing quality of life. This scenario is often seen amongst those with toxemia. The researchers commented that the underlying mechanism causing a lack of sleep to spurn systemic inflammation relates to the *"dysregulation of the immune system."*

A key strategy for deep sleep is to spend time outside everyday. This helps regulate our light-dark cycles. This means getting outside early in the daytime to stimulate the pineal gland and the SCN cells. Then as the night proceeds towards bedtime, we should turn the lights low and then off. This will regulate the circulation of melatonin and cortisol, allowing us to fall asleep at the right time of the cortisol-melatonin cycle—allowing us to sleep deeper through the night.

If we are consistently tired during the day, we can have someone watch us sleep, looking for irregular breathing, stopping breathing for a short period and/or partial wakening while sleeping. These may be signs of sleep apnea. If someone close says that they see some of these symptoms, we should see a sleep specialist.

Before retiring to bed, we might consider clearing our nose and throat. Going to bed with a stuffy nose and phlegm can inhibit our breathing, and disturb sleep. See the discussion on nasal lavages to clear the sinuses. Deep gargling with slightly salty water can help clear the throat. To gargle deeply, we can try humming while gargling.

We can keep the bedroom clear of dust, mold and other possible allergens. We can consider the bedroom a "safe room" as discussed in the chapter on triggers. Inflammatory symptoms during or following sleeping may indicate toxic exposures from the bedroom or bedroom air.

We can avoid eating late. Food may back up into the esophagus if the sphincter is weak and we are lying down. If the mucous membranes are weak, this may cause acid reflux, which can prevent a good night's sleep. If experiencing some reflux at night, we can raise the head of the bed to help keep stomach contents down, at least while working on mucosal membrane strategies outlined earlier.

For more information on sleep, including many lifestyle, dietary and herbal strategies that promote deep sleep, please refer to the author's book, *Natural Sleep - Insomnia Solutions*.

Exercise Strategies

A plethora of research has shown that sedentary lifestyles dramatically increase the risk of systemic inflammation.

This is based on the fact that exercise increases circulation and detoxification, stimulates the immune system, pumps the lymphatic system and increases lung capacity. Exercise is one of the most assured ways to strengthen the immune system and thus increase tolerance. When we exercise, we contract muscles. Again, muscle contraction is what circulates (or pumps) lymph around the body through the lymph vessels. This is because the lymphatic system does not have a heart like the circulatory system has. The lymphatic system relies on muscle contraction for circulation—as we've discussed.

Lymph circulation is critical for systemic inflammation because immune cells circulating through the blood and lymph break down and carry out of the body those broken-down toxins and cell parts.

And of course, exercise also circulates oxygen and nutrients throughout the body. Exercise also stimulates the thymus gland, and speeds up healing of the intestinal cell walls. In all, exercise is one of the best and cheapest therapies available to boost immunity and tolerance.

All of these effects and more are produced by daily exercise and activity.

Choosing the Routine

Choosing the right type of exercise depends greatly upon the individual and situation. Good forms of exercise include swimming, walking, running, tennis, golf, baseball, basketball, softball, volleyball, surfing, racquetball and squash.

Working out in a warmer, slightly humid environment is probably best for immunity, but exercising in any weather is better than no exercise. If running or working out outside during the winter, we can wear a ski mask or scarf over the nose and mouth to reduce the cold air, for example. Breathing in through the nose will also help warm the air before it hits the lungs. This will allow our lungs to empty more and work more effectively.

The morning also typically contains less air pollutants because the night usually clears out the air a bit. So early morning exercise is worth considering.

Warming up before exercising is also important. A routine of stretching, jumping jacks, push-ups, knee bends and so on will increase circulation and prepare the body for rigorous exercise.

Days with strenuous shorter-burst exercise activity can be alternated with lighter activity. Shorter-burst activity increases lung function and increases tolerance. Long walks are great. But extremely long strenuous exercise like running long distance can sometimes lower current immunity because of a greater load of metabolic waste products being produced.

One of the best forms of exercise utilizing shorter bursts is called HIIT – **high intensity interval training**. This basically consists of sprints with periods of jogging or walking in between. This can be done with swimming, biking and many other forms of exercise. Surfing is a great example of this, because surfing requires bursts of paddling alternating with rest in between waves.

For example, a person might alternate between walking, taking a hike in the woods, or slow swimming on one day, and play some basketball, soccer or do wind sprints the next. This can further be supplemented with abdominal and even weight (or isometric) training—both of which can increase immunity.

The bottom line that the type of exercise depends upon the individual. If a person enjoys a particular sport, they ought to pursue that sport. They will be better for it because they will more likely to continue that sport.

Manual Activity

Manual labor is shunned in modern western society, yet it is one of the best means to stay healthy. Manual labor works many muscle groups and stimulates immunity. For most of us, there is always the choice of doing it ourselves or otherwise. A good example is weeding. While pulling weeds by hand or using the hoe to remove them requires virtually no expense or special skill, most westerners elect to spray the weeds with toxic chemicals. The election to spray not only eliminates the potential for exercise: It also exposes us to chemicals that add to our body's toxin load.

Active choices can also be as easy as taking the stairs instead of the elevator; walking to the next store rather than driving the car to the next parking lot; biking to work instead of driving; raking the leaves instead of using a leaf-blower—and so many other choices.

Breathing and Airway Strategies

Relearning to Breathe

Deep breathing is one of the best ways to purify the blood and strengthen the immune system. It can also increase lung capacity and respiration efficiency. Deep breathing will strengthen and enlarge the diaphragm, strengthen the supporting abdominal muscles, relaxes the smooth muscles of the airways, and helps reduce stress.

We will discuss a number of methods here, but we focus on two established techniques for healthy deep breathing:

Deep core breathing:
> ➢ Slowly push out the abdomen around the belly button. As the lungs fill, push out the upper abdomen. If lying down, a book may be placed on the abdomen to feel and see it rise.
> ➢ Continue pushing out until the lungs are full and the abdomen is fully pushed out.
> ➢ Top it off by expanding the rib cage to completely fill the lungs.
> ➢ Hold in position and relax for 3-7 seconds.
> ➢ Then push the air out by slowly contracting the upper abdominal muscles followed by contracting the lower abdomen as the lungs are completely emptied. This last step is called *flooring*.

Deep diaphragm breathing:
> ➢ Slowly push out at the top of the abdomen, enlarging the diaphragm to its capacity as the lungs fill.
> ➢ Follow by expanding the rib cage to fill out the lungs. Hold for 2-5 seconds.

> Then begin contracting the upper abdominal muscles to contract the diaphragm. This will begin pushing the air out.
> Slowly contract the diaphragm completely to force out as much air as possible.

Diaphragm breathing does not as completely fill or empty the lungs as deep core breathing does, but it is often more practical while sitting, walking or exercising. Core breathing can result in sleepiness, so it is best used at home in bed or on a comfortable sofa. Either method, if practiced daily for at least 15 minutes, can significantly increase our lung cavity capacity. We may begin to breathe deeper without trying. Placing a hand on the abdomen to feel its rise and fall can also help us center ourselves on our breathing.

In both methods, good breathing posture can be maintained. If sitting, the lower back can be arched slightly with the upper spine fairly straight and relaxed, and the back of the head in line with our lower spine. We can sit on the front of our 'sit bones' at the base of the pelvis, rather than the backside of our sit bones where the lower spine tends to curve outward. When we are sitting on the right part of our sit bones, our lower back will naturally arch.

If lying down on our back, a large pillow can be put under the knees, with the spine straight and a comfortable neck pillow that keeps the crown of the head aligned with the lower spine. Most *hatha-yoga* postures are also conducive to deep breathing exercises.

Keeping the Lungs Clear

Remember that the sinus cavity, pharynx, larynx, trachea and bronchi are all lined with epithelial cells covered with a thin fluid of mucous membrane and tiny hairs called cilia. Cilia trap foreign particles in the sticky, immune cell-rich mucous before they can enter the lungs. This should clear out most soot, debris, bacteria and viruses before they proceed further.

When toxic air (air pollution) or bacteria sneak past these defenses, the bronchial tree, alveoli and pleural cavity will swell with inflammation. The pleural cavity will also often leak fluids into the lung. These fluids, together with the swollen airways, effectively decrease lung capacity and air clearance.

For many, swollen and irritated air passages and pleura is constant, due to an overloading of air pollution, airborne chemicals, dust and microorganisms. Strategies to increase lung capacity and maintain healthy mucosal membranes are thus tantamount to reducing the impact of modern toxins.

Keeping the Sinuses Clear

This brings us to the logical conclusion that we need to keep the nasal passages clear. Obviously, keeping the sinuses and nasal passages clear is the key to breathing comfortably if we plan to breathe in through the nose. When the sinuses are clogged, our mucous membranes are not draining properly. Mucous needs to be swept out, and if the mucous is too thick or crustified with waste matter, it will narrow our available airways.

So how do we accomplish keeping the sinuses clear? Well, besides breathing in through the nose and general hygiene to help keep them clean—we might consider periodic nasal irrigation.

Nasal lavage is the first consideration. This can utilize a special Ayurvedic lavage device called the neti pot. Neti has been in practice for thousands of years. The pot is simply filled with warm weakly-salty water, and poured through each nostril. A small teapot can also be used.

The technique is to first mix about a quarter-teaspoon of non-iodized, refined salt to about a cup of lukewarm water. A pinch of baking soda may also be added, especially if the salt is iodized or otherwise burns in any way.

Lean forward, over the sink. With the chin level with the nose, turn the head sideways so the nose on a plane parallel with the ground as much as possible.

The water is lightly poured into one nostril, traveling around the septum and out the other nostril. There is no force or pressure involved. There is no snuffing in or pulling in. The solution is simply poured into one nostril, and out through the other. Just hold the head still while it pours out.

Nasal Irrigation: This can also be accomplished by gently pushing warm saline (water and salt) into each nostril using a soft squeeze bottle. Soft squeeze bottles designed for cleaning the nostrils are often available at most drug stores. After using the saline in the bottle, the bottle can be refilled. Care must be taken not to forcefully squirt the water through, which can get water into the upper sinuses.

Another technique is to sniff the water up the nose and back down through to the pharynx and throat, where it is spit out into the sink. This can provide a more complete cleansing of the pharynx and sinuses, but should not be overdone, and only if the sinuses are at least partially clear.

Nasal irrigation has been proven in research to aid in allergic conditions and sinusitis. For example, researchers from Taiwan's Chung Shan Medical University Hospital (Wang *et al.* 2009) gave nasal irrigation or not to 69 children with acute sinusitis. The saline irrigation group improved significantly better than the other group with regard to symptoms and quality of life.

Nasal irrigation was also effective in reducing sinus congestion, rhinorrhea, sneezing and nasal itching in a study by medical researchers from Italy's University of Milano (Garavello *et al.* 2010). In this study, 23 pregnant women with seasonal allergic rhinitis underwent either nasal irrigation or not for six weeks.

In another study, presented at the 50th Scientific Assembly of the American Academy of Family Physicians, Dr. Richard Ravizza and Dr. John Fornadley of Pennsylvania State University divided 294 students into three groups, one of which did nasal irrigation with salt water and the other two groups either took a placebo pill or did nothing. The nasal irrigation group experienced fewer colds during the treatment period compared to the other two groups.

To be fair, some have questioned whether daily regular nasal irrigation for long periods is necessarily good. In a study presented at a the American College of Allergy, Asthma and Immunology (Nsouli 2009), researchers tested 68 patients with a history of sinusitis, who had been using nasal irrigation daily. Of the total, 44 patients discontinued the irrigation while 24 continued the daily treatment. After a year, those who had discontinued the irrigation had 62% less sinusitis infections than the group who continued to use nasal irrigation daily. Dr. Tamal Nsouli commented that daily irrigation may deplete healthy mucous from the sinuses. As we've discussed, healthy mucous membranes also cover the sinuses, helping protect us from infection. Dr. Nsouli also commented that he is not opposed to irrigation for three or four times a week, but suggested avoiding daily irrigation for long periods.

We should note that the study details and protocol have yet to be published, and was only presented in abstract form at the conference. Diane Heatley, M.D., a Professor at the University of Wisconsin School of Medicine, questioned the report, stating, *"nasal irrigation has previously been proven safe and effective for treatment of sinus symptoms in both adults and children in a number of studies already published in peer-reviewed journals."*

An appropriate conclusion here is that regular nasal irrigation should still include some moderation. Using it during periods of congestion and sensitivity is certainly appropriate. Use after or during environmental conditions where there is an increased level of pollution and/or infectious agents is also appropriate. But we can remember that our mucous membranes also house important immune cells and probiotics, which help protect us. We don't want to flush those away needlessly.

Boosting the Liver

The liver is the primary organ involved in removing toxins that burden the immune system—and contribute to systemic inflammation. In other words, liver health is crucial. The liver produces a number of enzymes that help break down toxins and endotoxins (waste material from microorganisms). The liver also filters blood through its hepatocytes to remove toxins, while breaking apart pathogens using its kuppfer cells.

There are several strategies we can utilize to increase the liver's health. Here are a few:

> ➤ Reducing or eliminating our intake of chemical preservatives, food dyes and synthetic sweeteners. All of these require the liver's resources to break them down.

> ➤ Reducing or eliminating our exposure to formaldehydes, cleaning chemicals, pesticides, herbicides, benzenes, VOCs and other harsh chemicals that the liver must work hard to break down once absorbed into the skin or lungs.

> ➤ Drinking enough water (as outlined earlier). Water nourishes and helps the liver flush and detoxify the blood and lymph.

> ➤ Eliminating unnecessary pharmaceuticals, as pharmaceuticals are typically rough on the liver—as is alcohol. This requires that we work closely with those doctors who have prescribed our pharmaceuticals, while asking the doctor a clear question: *"Do I really need to continue taking this pharmaceutical?"* Most pharmaceuticals are intended and tested for short-term use. Most were never intended for long-term use, and many studies have shown that long-term use of medications can severely damage the liver. Note also that some pharmaceuticals are worse than others. Acetaminophen is particularly harsh on the liver, for example. For a more complete list of pharmaceuticals that aggravate or cause toxemia, see the list in Chapter Two.

> ➤ Correcting the fatty acid balance in our diet to comply more closely to that outlined earlier. The liver must work hard to accommodate our fats. High levels of the wrong fats can put a strain on the liver.

> ➤ Keeping our cholesterol levels in balance through wise dietary choices. Foods that produce high levels of low-density lipoproteins (such as fried foods, saturated fats, grilled meats and so on) will strain the liver as it seeks to balance cholesterol and reduce lipid peroxidation.

> Liver strengthening foods include beets, carrots, turnips, radishes, onions, leafy-green vegetables, spirulina, chlorella, squash, celery and other plant-based foods.
> Liver restoring herbs include Milk Thistle, Turmeric, Garlic, Dandelion, Goldenseal, Ginger, Bupleurum and Guduchi.
> Healthy probiotic colonies are critical for liver health. Consider these studies:

Researchers from Russia's Northern State Medical University (Kirpich *et al.* 2008) studied 66 adult Russian males admitted to a psychiatric hospital with a diagnosis of alcoholic psychosis. They gave the patients standard therapy (abstinence plus vitamins) with *Bifidobacterium bifidum* and *Lactobacillus plantarum* 8PA3 or standard therapy alone without probiotics for five days. Stool cultures and liver enzymes were examined and compared with 24 healthy, matched non-drinker controls. The alcoholic patients had significantly fewer bifidobacteria, lactobacilli, and enterococci than did the healthy non-drinkers. The average starting levels of liver enzymes alanine aminotransferase (ALT), aspartate aminotransferase (AST), and gamma-glutamyl transpeptidase (GGT) were significantly greater in the alcoholic group compared to the healthy non-drinkers.

After 5 days of daily probiotics, alcoholic patients had significantly more bifidobacteria and lactobacilli populations compared to the control group. The probiotic group also had significantly lower AST and ALT levels at the end of treatment than the standard therapy control group. Of the 26 patients with mild alcoholic hepatitis, probiotic therapy significantly reduced liver enzymes ALT, AST, GGT, lactate dehydrogenase and total bilirubin. The researchers concluded that, "Short-term oral supplementation with *B. bifidum* and *L. plantarum* 8PA3 was associated with restoration of the bowel flora and greater improvement in alcohol-induced liver injury than standard therapy alone."

Scientists from Italy's University of Catania (Malaguarnera *et al.* 2007) gave 60 cirrhotic patients *Bifidobacterium longum* plus fructo-oligosaccharides (FOS) or placebo. After 90 days, fasting NH(4) serum levels significantly decreased among the probiotic patients. Other liver tests, including MMSE, Trail Making Test-A and Test-B also significantly improved among the probiotic group as compared with the placebo group.

Researchers from the Liver Failure Group and The Institute of Hepatology at the University College London's Medical School (Stadlbauer *et al.* 2008) studied neutrophil function and cytokine responses in alcoholic cirrhosis patients in an open-label study. Twenty patients with alcoholic cirrhosis were treated with a placebo or *Lactobacillus casei* Shirota for 4 weeks. The data were also compared to 13 healthy control subjects who did not receive probiotics.

The cirrhosis patients' starting neutrophil phagocytic capacity was significantly lower than healthy controls (73% versus 98%) before probiotic treatment. Neutrophil phagocytic capacities after the probiotic treatments were equal among the cirrhosis patients and healthy volunteers at the end of the study—while the placebo group's neutrophil capacity did not change.

In addition, endotoxin-stimulated TNF-receptor-1, TNFR-2 and interleukin IL10 levels were significantly lower among the probiotic group. The researchers concluded that, "Our data provide a proof-of-concept that probiotics restore neutrophil phagocytic capacity in cirrhosis, possibly by changing IL10 secretion and TLR4 expression."

China's Capital University of Medical Sciences and the Beijing Friendship Hospital (Zhao *et al.* 2004) studied fifty patients with liver cirrhosis. They tested and graded the entire group for intestinal probiotic content and severity of liver disease. The researchers found that the cirrhosis was directly associated with intestinal probiotic content.

The more severe the cirrhosis, the more imbalanced the intestinal probiotic content was. The patients were randomized and given *Bifidobacterium, Lactobacillus acidophilus* and *Enterococcus faecium;* or *Bacillus subtilis* and *Enterococcus faecium* for 14 days. Fecal flora, pH and ammonia content, and plasma endotoxin levels were tested before and after. All levels improved after both probiotic treatments. In addition, those given *B. subtilis* and *E. faecium* showed a reduction in endotoxin levels among endotoxemia cirrhosis cases.

Researchers from the Department of Surgery at Japan's Nagoya University Graduate School of Medicine (Kanazawa *et al.* 2005) investigated the effects of *L. casei* with 54 patients following hepatectomy. Infection complications were 19% in the probiotic group and 52% in the placebo group.

Forty cirrhosis patients with hepatic encephalopathy were studied by researchers from the University of Naples (Loguercio, *et al.* 1987). They were given either *Enterococcus* probiotic strain SF68 or lactulose (standard treatment) for 10 days. The probiotics were as effective as lactulose in lowering blood ammonia and improving mental state. The beneficial effects of the probiotics persisted significantly longer after treatment was discontinued

Adrenal Strengthening

The adrenal glands respond to stress by way of biochemical signals from the hypothalamus and pituitary gland. These biochemical signals come in the form of adrenocorticotropic hormone (or ACTH). This master hormone signals nerve centers, and stimulates the adrenal glands to produce cortisol and other glucocorticoids. This is called the *hypothalamic-pituitary-adrenal axis stress response.*

Remember that the adrenals are critical to the production of cortisol, and it is cortisol and other glucocorticoids that control inflammation. Therefore, the adrenals are necessary to balance inflammation and immunity. This is why cortisone is used for inflammation: It blocks and controls the inflammatory response by interrupting the interleukin-1 and IL-2 cytokine communications.

However, cortisone medications over longer periods also depress adrenal function. Because they provide corticoids directly, the adrenal gland begins to switch off its corticoid production. This adrenal switching off has been linked to adrenal insufficiency and systemic inflammation (Polito *et al.* 2007).

For this very reason, withdrawing from or reducing cortisone medications after their long-term use can result in a dramatic rise in uninhibited inflammation throughout the body. This is because inflammatory cytokines such as the interleukins are allowed to act without adequate corticoid control.

This can be compounded by a situation called adrenal exhaustion. Under stressful situations, the healthy adrenal gland is stimulated to produce cortisol. This trigger effect is natural and supports our ability to respond to dire circumstances. However, should we become stressed too often, this automatic adrenal response begins the wear out the adrenals. They become exhausted because they have been over-stimulated.

In other words, healthy adrenals should be balancing inflammatory responses by supplying natural corticoids. In the case of adrenal exhaustion and in the absence of sufficient natural corticoids (and/or inflammatory episodes that have gone way out of control) physicians prescribe synthetic cortisone to achieve what our body's adrenal glands should have: Shutting down inflammation before it got out of control.

Relaxation is critical to the adrenal glands. As the system relaxes more, the adrenal glands are allowed some time to refresh, enabling them to better respond to small inflammatory episodes—before they get out of control.

But what about adrenal glands that are already exhausted? Can we do anything to rebuild and strengthen them? Absolutely.

In fact, many of the strategies we have outlined in this chapter, including many of the herbs, foods and exercises will directly or indirectly strengthen the adrenal glands. This is accomplished because they can:

> ➢ Reduce inflammation—unburdening the adrenal glands.

> ➤ Stimulate relaxation—allowing the adrenals to recuperate.
> ➤ Directly stimulate healthy adrenal activity.
> ➤ Supply adrenals with the raw materials to produce corticoids and androgens.

With regard to the latter point, the adrenal glands do more than simply produce cortisol. They also produce androgens, glucocorticoids and many other hormones that stabilize and balance the body's metabolism. Without a strong and active adrenal complex, the body's hormone and steroid system becomes unbalanced and out of whack. This encourages inflammatory responses to become uncontrolled, producing a number of possible symptoms.

What are some of the more immediate ways to increase adrenal capacity? Here are a few of the many that either unburden or strengthen the adrenals:

> ➤ Decreased toxin consumption, and detoxification efforts.
> ➤ Greenfoods, fruits and vegetables that provide antioxidants.
> ➤ Plenty of water, as defined earlier.
> ➤ Relaxation: Letting things roll off the back, so to speak. Not sweating inconsequential things. This is particularly important for those who drive everyday. Driving is highly stressful. It can help, therefore, to listen to soothing music while driving. Or take public transportation.
> ➤ Deep breathing: This is important for relaxation, as we discussed above. Breathing not only nourishes the adrenals with oxygen and alkalinity: It also stimulates the VNO nerves.
> ➤ Visual imagery: Looking at scenes of nature, or imagining natural settings.
> ➤ Higher sounds: Consider what we hear. Are we hearing a lot of chatter about what other people are stressed about? (This includes television.) Hearing stressful language can stimulate our adrenals. In fact, a dramatic movie or TV program has been shown to stimulate the adrenals and increase cortisol levels. This may be okay periodically, but not constantly. For those with already over-stimulated adrenals, being around uplifting sounds and discussions is a better strategy.
> ➤ Foods particularly good for the adrenals include onions, garlic, peppers, papaya, mango, apricots, squash and broccoli.
> ➤ Herbs that help strengthen and revitalize the adrenals include Shizandra, Tylophora, Astragalus, Dandelion and Licorice.

We might add that the Licorice mentioned here should not be deglycyrrhized licorice, as in the DGL used primarily for stomach ulcers.

This is because glycyrrhizin and its triterpenoid, glycyrrhizinic acid, are considered primary adrenal-restorative constituents.

This said, a 2003 European Commission suggested that a person should not consume more than 100 milligrams of glycyrrhizinic acid per day. Note, however, that even concentrated extracts of licorice herb will contain only 4-25% glycyrrhizinic acid. This means that 400-500 mg a day of *raw, unconcentrated* licorice root will contain far less than the maximum levels documented by the European Commission. Natural licorice root, in fact, has been used safely by Western and Eastern traditional herbalists for many centuries.

Conclusion

Living Immunity

This book has thoroughly investigated what makes up our immune system and how we can stimulate it. Stimulating the immune system means to sharpen it and prepare it for protecting us from the most serious invasions.

Now that we understand what the immune system is, we can go about stimulating and strengthening our immune system. The methods we have discussed utilize improvements in our daily activities, including:

- Avoiding toxins to the extent possible to lighten the burden on our immune system.
- Supplementing our body's probiotic colonies with probiotic foods and supplements.
- Eating prebiotic foods to bolster our probiotic colonies.
- Eating fermented foods that help provide an environment that invites probiotic growth and deters the growth of their competitors.
- Eating a diet rich in antioxidants and nutrients that nourish our blood, liver and immune cells
- Supplementing with immune-boosting herbs, mushrooms and essential oils.
- Consuming antioxidant immune-stimulating greenfoods.
- Exercising regularly.
- Drinking plenty of water.
- Sweating on a regular basis.
- Brushing the skin periodically to stimulate skin health.
- Stimulating our adrenals and liver health.
- Fasting periodically, even if just for a day or part of a day.
- Getting regular sun exposure
- Getting outdoors on a daily basis, even if the weather is bad.
- Doing breathing exercises to breathe deeper and more productive.

Each of these strategies will help stimulate our immune system. For someone who is immunosuppressed, these should be undertaken gradually and carefully, and under the guidance of your health professional.

As we navigate these serious times of pandemic infections and autoimmunity, we come to the conclusion that the natural world has

377

prepared our physical bodies with the tools to help us survive through a variety of bacterial and viral attacks. How does the natural world do this?

Probiotics that naturally inhabit our skin, mouths, sinuses, oral cavity, mucosal membranes and intestinal systems serve to help protect the body from numerous types of invaders.

The various plants and mushrooms that inhabit this world have to protect themselves against these invading forces. So they have developed mechanisms to fight these invasions on the front lines, which we can utilize by consuming them.

Think about how the roots of plants (or the mycelia of mushrooms) lie within the soil, full of so many bacteria and viruses. These roots develop biochemical tools that inhibit those invaders.

The same with the stems and leaves of the plant. They will inhibit airborne viruses and bacteria, again by manufacturing chemicals that inhibit those same viruses and bacteria that can threaten our survival.

Since these plants and mushrooms remain healthy despite these invasions, we know can safely utilize their biochemicals to also help our bodies fight off these same viruses and bacteria.

You see, nature is smart.

Antibiotic Logic

The problems come when we think that we are smarter than nature. This is the case that has been presented with isolated antibiotics developed by good-intentioned scientists and their companies. Yes, antibiotics have been very helpful in preventing many deaths from infections. But the majority of these were already available in nature.

The problem came when we isolated them outside of nature and overused them.

The seemingly unbridled growth in microorganisms and infectious diseases has continued despite the fact that our use of prescriptive and over the counter antibiotics, antifungals, antivirals, antiseptic soaps, and cleaning disinfectants has dramatically increased over the past few decades.

Microbes are considered enemy number one by the Centers for Disease Control and government anti-terrorism officials. This concern for outbreaks and pandemics has put microbial diseases on the front pages of many newspapers and news broadcasts.

At the same time, the use of antibiotics has soared over the past few decades. Today, over 3,000,000 pounds of pure antibiotics are taken by humans annually in the United States. This is complemented by the approximately 25,000,000 pounds of antibiotics given to animals each year.

Meanwhile, many of these antibiotics either are given in vain or are ineffectual. The Centers for Disease Control states that, *"Almost half of patients with upper respiratory tract infections in the U.S. still receive antibiotics from their doctor."* This said, the CDC also warns that *"90% of upper respiratory infections, including children's ear infections, are viral, and antibiotics don't treat viral infection. More than 40% of about 50 million prescriptions for antibiotics each year in physicians' offices were inappropriate."*

Indeed, the growing use of antibiotics has also created a Pandora's box of *superbugs*. As bacteria are repeatedly hit with the same antibiotic, they learn to adapt. Just as any living organism does (yes, bacteria are alive), bacteria learn to counter and resist repeatedly utilized antibiotics. As a result, many bacteria today are resistant to a variety of antibiotics. This is because bacteria tend to adjust to their surroundings. If they are attacked enough times with a certain challenge, they are likely to figure out how to avoid it and thrive despite it.

This has been the case for a number of other new antibiotic-resistant strains of bacteria. They have simply evolved to become stronger and more able to counteract these antibiotic measures.

This phenomenon has created *multi-drug resistant organisms*. Some of the more dangerous MDROs include species of *Enterococcus, Staphylococcus, Salmonella, Campylobacter, Escherichia coli*, and others. Superbugs such as MRSA are only the tip of the bacterial iceberg.

Another growing infectious bacterium is *Clostridium difficile*. This bacterium will infect the intestines of people of any age. Among children, this is one of the world's biggest killers—causing acute, watery diarrhea. It is also a growing infection among adults. Every year *C. difficile* infects tens of thousands of people in the U.S. according to the Mayo Clinic. Worse, *C. difficile* are increasingly becoming resistant to antibiotics and infections from clostridia are growing in incidence each year.

The question is: Are antibiotics helping us or hurting us?

The reason there are so many antibiotics now is the same reason that many pathogens are becoming resistant to many of our antibiotics: They are *static* strategies being used within a *living* system. Living systems are adaptive. They *learn* to work around whatever is thrown at them. Meanwhile, each antibiotic we have developed deters microorganisms with the same strategy every time. Some will interfere with the microorganism's cell wall. Others will interfere with the RNA within the cell—at least until they adapt.

With time, a microorganism can learn to adapt to practically any threat to its survival. In order to protect itself and its colony, a microorganism will gradually learn how to evade the threat. Over many generations, these strategies are passed on and perfected by successive generations.

To illustrate how bacteria become resistant, let's say that that a burglar broke into a house while the family was home. The man of the house grabs a baseball bat and clubs the burglar on the head, and the burglar runs off. A month later, the burglar breaks into the same house again. What do you think the burglar will be wearing this time? A helmet of course!

We should understand that bacteria—even pathogenic bacteria—are living organisms that simply want to survive. Therefore, when they see a mass threat such as an antibiotic, over several generations they will figure out how to work around that antibiotic. They do this through the development of subtle and successive variations to their genes.

We might wonder how bacteria spread their antibiotic resistance. The interesting thing is that bacteria don't only create a genetic variation: They also create a small suitcase-like package of genetic make-over matter called a *plasmid,* with which they can pass on their genetic variation to other bacteria.

The plasmid is often called a *replicon,* because it can be transferred to another bacterium, who will automatically assimilate it into its genetic information. This allows the new bacterium to perfectly replicate the strategies of the source bacterium. Once inside the new bacterium, the plasmid allows the bacterium to perform the workaround to the antibiotic, and be able to pass the plasmid on to yet another bacterium.

Our broad-spectrum antibiotics might be compared to the baseball bat in the analogy above. Once used, bacteria may adapt to that static (antibiotic) tool. Any number of different species can figure out a way around the antibiotic. Once learned, that trick is passed on to other species of bacteria, and soon the antibiotic will be useless against many different species. This ability to learn on an inter-species level provides one of the scariest features about bacteria infections: The ability for different species to grow beyond our ability to control entire legions of many species of cooperative fungi and bacteria.

This also means that antibiotic resistance is not the same in all geographical regions. Plasmid transfer requires direct contact between bacteria. This was illustrated in a 2007 study on antibiotic resistance among several pathogenic bacteria. Gram-positive bacteria isolates were collected from 76 medical centers among nine regions across the U.S. The results indicated that vancomycin resistance in *Enterococcus faecium* ranged from 45.5% in New England to 85.3% in the East South Central U.S. Methicillin-resistant *Staphylococcus aureus* (MRSA) varied from 27.4% in New England to 62.4% in East South Central. Penicillin-resistant

Streptococcus pneumoniae ranged from 23.3% in the Pacific region to 54.5% in the East South Central region (Denys *et al.* 2007).

This also means that as bacteria continue to travel on animals, humans, trains, buses, and airplanes, they will continue to exchange their learned resistance to our antibiotics. This will inevitably lead to most of our antibiotics becoming useless.

Probiotics provide the solution to this conundrum. How so? Probiotics are also smart living organisms. They are also the sworn enemies to these pathogenic species. In fact, the probiotics and the pathogenic bacteria have been battling it out for billions of years, and the probiotics have been winning! This is evidenced, of course, by the fact that the human race is still alive. This means that probiotics have figured out how to identify each new plasmid, and respond by developing their own strategies and plasmids to combat pathogenic bacteria.

In our burglary analogy, when the burglar comes back in his helmet, the man of the house pulls out another weapon to scare off the burglar. If he comes back again prepared for that weapon, the man devises a new one. This is what living organisms do as they protect their territories. As pathogenic and probiotic bacteria battle it out, they are both creating new strategies to resist each other. As one develops a new strategy, the other will develop yet another one. They both throw their naturally developed antibiotics at each other, and they each respond in kind.

Research has confirmed that probiotics have the same sorts of tools at their disposal. Probiotics can also develop antibiotic resistance just as pathogenic bacteria like MRSA can. Researchers from Sweden's University of Agricultural Sciences (Rosander *et al.* 2008) found that not only could the *Lactobacillus reuteri* probiotic strain easily develop antibiotic resistance: *L. reuteri* also developed plasmids. In their study, they observed *L. reuteri* carrying *two* plasmids that created and passed on antibiotic resistance to tetracycline and lincosamide.

The bottom line, and the issue at hand is that a course of antibiotics, while it might provide a life-saving prescription for someone deathly sick, can also seriously damage our colonies of probiotics. Worse, repeated courses of antibiotics, especially among a youngster, can damage their immunity for life. Why? Because their resident colonies are decimated.

After about age five, our resident colonies become established and cannot be replaced. In some cases, probiotic supplements later on can populate to some extent, for the most part, supplemented probiotics are temporary residents. They can help our permanent residents regrow, but they will rarely if ever replace them.

Therefore, it is critical that antibiotics not be used without good reason. Many studies have shown, for example, that children's ear infections heal no faster with antibiotics than without.

There are also a variety of antibiotic botanicals (mentioned in the herb section earlier) that can repel and help eliminate many infections without destroying all of our probiotic populations. Some of these may well interrupt our probiotics (such as fresh garlic) but they are less toxic to our probiotics than many antibiotics.

The Living Defense Model

Conventional medicine has presented us a model of the immune system as a castle with no castle guards. Their castle has elaborate walls and a strong gate with a great big lock. Their castle has a good moat surrounding it. Their model has a big watchtower and a big storehouse full of weapons.

However, this model has no one manning the watchtower to alert others when there is an incoming enemy. There are no guards lining the inside of the walls to shoot arrows and fight off the invaders. There are no warriors inside the gate in case the invading army burns down the gate and swarms the inside of the castle.

In fact, the immune system presented by conventional medicine is like a castle ghost town. There are lots of buildings, structures and weapons, but no one around to use those weapons.

The living immune system provides the realistic picture of the immune system. It also clarifies that our body's immunity is dependent upon the health of those probiotic colonies that line our mouths, ears, sinuses, throats, intestines, vaginas, belly buttons and skin. Without these 'castle guards,' 'warriors' and 'watchtower attendants' we will suffer from an avalanche of invading microorganisms, toxins and the oxidative radicals—free radicals that are ready to burst in where ever we go and what ever we do.

This text does more than teach this new model of the immune system clearly. It also goes a step further and presents those strategies that can increase the strength of the living immune system. We have included dietary strategies, supplementation strategies, exercise, breathing, sun exposure and so much more.

Does this mean we have to apply all of these strategies to boost our immunity? Actually, the research indicates that any of these strategies will serve to boost our immunity in specific ways. But this doesn't mean that we only need to incorporate one of these strategies into our lives. In fact, the more we apply, the stronger our immune system will become. The less burden we will pile onto our immune system, and the more it will be prepared to fight against invaders.

One aspect of immunity should also be added to this list. That the immune system does best when it is naturally stressed. This doesn't mean that we throw all kinds of synthetic toxins at it. Synthetic toxins, in fact, do not build immunity—they only weaken it. Natural toxins, on the other hand, stress our immune system and strengthen it, as long as they don't overload it.

This of course is the concept behind the vaccine. A vaccine is a weakened dose of the precise biological pathogen that could infect us. As the immune system identifies this, it builds the defense strategies to repel it in a bigger way should the pathogen present itself in real life.

Synthetic toxins don't work like vaccines do, however. We cannot give our body a small dose of benzene and expect that it will build the defenses against a huge dose of benzene in the future.

Why? This is because our immune system is biological, and it is set up for biological toxins. Our defense mechanisms have learned over millions of years to adapt to nature's typical invaders—biological toxins. They are not equipped to handle the new toxic invaders presented by modern chemistry.

We might compare this to how the body might adapt. If we go to the gym every day and lift weights, our muscles will adapt by getting stronger. Eventually they will be able to lift some heavy weights, because they have adapted.

But the body would never adapt to getting hit by a truck. If the body got hit by a truck, the body would not adapt. It would become irreparably harmed by the hard steel and weight of the train. The body would never adapt to getting hit by a truck because the body would likely not survive such an accident. And if it did, it would likely heal slowly, with lots of broken bones. After such a healing, the body would be no more prepared to handle getting hit by a truck than it was the first time—and probably less able to handle it because of the broken bones.

What is different about training with weights versus getting hit by a truck? The body was designed to get stronger as it lifted heavier weights, but the body was not designed to be hit by a truck.

Synthetic toxins are the same as the truck because the body was never designed to deal with these types of toxins. It simply is not in our genes. This does not mean that after another century or two of living in a toxic world, we might become more adapted to some of these toxins. That is, if we survive this century. But for now, they are still like the truck: Our bodies aren't prepared to handle them.

One of the main reasons we cannot handle synthetic toxins is because our body's probiotics cannot deal with them. They annihilate our probiotics, in other worlds. And without probiotics, we lose our defenses.

So better to avoid as many synthetic toxins as we can, and bolster our living defenses by naturally stressing our immunity.

And how do we naturally stress our immunity? By making contact with nature's elements. This means more contact with the soil, the sand, the rocks, nature's water sources, the outdoors in general and nature's other living organisms.

Coming into contact with our earth exposes our body to biological organisms that strengthen our probiotics. This is because our probiotics are territorial, and they will increase in numbers and adapt to the challenges of potential invaders when they come into contact with those invaders. So when we get outside, the wind blows nature's microorganisms into our mouths and noses.

When we sink our hands in the soils of our gardens, our probiotics get exposed to the probiotics on our skin surface, as well as our noses and mouths. Here our probiotic corps get a small sampling of the potential invaders, and build the appropriate defense systems (their own antibiotics) to defend themselves from a potential threat.

We also come into contact with natural threats to our probiotics and immune systems in our work environments and our play environments. Assuming our workmates or schoolmates are not coming to work or school at the peak of their infective stages, we will gain contact to a reasonable amount of potential invaders, arming our probiotics with defensive tools. But should our schoolmates or workmates come to work at the peak of their infective stages, this can overload our immunity defenses. This might force an inflammatory immune response: the cold or flu.

The inflammatory immune response is not necessarily bad, however. An occasional cold or flu can help strengthen our immunity significantly. During this inflammatory process, our body will kick out many toxins and invaders, leaving our body's toxin load lightened and our immune system strengthened.

The bottom line is to keep active, avoid toxins, eat a balanced diet rich in antioxidants and nutrients, and utilize nature's healing tools and resources to the greatest extent possible. This will not only boost our immunity. It will also boost our consciousness and gratefulness for what the Creator has provided.

References and Bibliography

Abdureyim S, Amat N, Umar A, Upur H, Berke B, Moore N. Anti-inflammatory, immunomodulatory, and heme oxygenase-1 inhibitory activities of ravan napas, a formulation of uighur traditional medicine, in a rat model of allergic asthma. *Evid Based Complement Alternat Med.* 2011;2011. pii: 725926.

Aberg N, Hesselmar B, Aberg B, Eriksson B. Increase of asthma, allergic rhinitis and eczema in Swedish schoolchildren between 1979 and 1991. *Clin Exp Allergy.* 1995;25:815-819.

Adel-Patient K, Ah-Leung S, Creminon C, Nouaille S, Chatel JM, Langella P, Wal JM. Oral administration of recombinant Lactococcus lactis expressing bovine beta-lactoglobulin partially prevents mice from sensitization. *Clin Exp Allergy.* 2005 Apr;35(4):539-46.

Adoga AS, Otene AA, Yiltok SJ, Adekwu A, Nwaorgu OG. Cervical necrotizing fasciitis: case series and review of literature. *Niger J Med.* 2009 Apr-Jun;18(2):203-7.

Agache I, Ciobanu C. Risk factors and asthma phenotypes in children and adults with seasonal allergic rhinitis. *Phys Sportsmed.* 2010 Dec;38(4):81-6.

Agarwal KN, Bhasin SK, Faridi MM, Mathur M, Gupta S. *Lactobacillus casei* in the control of acute diarrhea—a pilot study. *Indian Pediatr.* 2001 Aug;38(8):905-10.

Agarwal SK, Singh SS, Verma S. Antifungal principle of sesquiterpene lactones from Anamirta cocculus. *Indian Drugs.* 1999;36:754-5.

Agerholm-Larsen L, Raben A, Haulrik N, Hansen AS, Manders M, Astrup A. Effect of 8 week intake of probiotic milk products on risk factors for cardiovascular diseases. *Eur J Clin Nutr.* 2000 Apr;54(4):288-97.

Aggarwal BB, Harikumar KB. Potential therapeutic effects of curcumin, the anti-inflammatory agent, against neurodegenerative, cardiovascular, pulmonary, metabolic, autoimmune and neoplastic diseases. *Int J Biochem Cell Biol.* 2009 Jan;41(1):40-59.

Aggarwal BB, Sung B. Pharmacological basis for the role of curcumin in chronic diseases: an age-old spice with modern targets. *Trends Pharmacol Sci.* 2009 Feb;30(2):85-94.

Agostoni C, Fiocchi A, Riva E, Terracciano L, Sarratud T, Martelli A, Lodi F, D'Auria E, Zuccotti G, Giovannini M. Growth of infants with IgE-mediated cow's milk allergy fed different complementary feeding period. *Pediatr Allergy Immunol.* 2007 Nov;18(7):599-606.

Agustina R, Lukito W, Firmansyah A, Suhardjo HN, Murniati D, Bindels J. The effect of early nutritional supplementation with a mixture of probiotic, prebiotic, fiber and micronutrients in infants with acute diarrhea in Indonesia. *Asia Pac J Clin Nutr.* 2007;16(3):435-42.

Ahmed M, Prasad J, Gill H, Stevenson L, Gopal P. Impact of consumption of different levels of *Bifidobacterium lactis* HN019 on the intestinal microflora of elderly human subjects. *J Nutr Health Aging.* 2007 Jan-Feb;11(1):26-31.

Ahmed, AA, McCarthy RD, Porter GA. Effectof of milk constituents on hepatic cholesterogenesis. *Atherosclerosis.* 1979;32:347-57.

Aho K, Koskenvuo M, Tuominen J, Kaprio J. Occurrence of rheumatoid arthritis in a nationwide series of twins. *J Rheumatol.* 1986 Oct;13(5):899-902.

Ahola AJ, Yli-Knuuttila H, Suomalainen T, Poussa T, Ahlström A, Meurman JH, Korpela R. Short-term consumption of probiotic-containing cheese and its effect on dental caries risk factors. *Arch Oral Biol.* 2002 Nov;47(11):799-804.

Aihara K, Kajimoto O, Hirata H, Takahashi R, Nakamura Y. Effect of powdered fermented milk with *Lactobacillus helveticus* on subjects with high-normal blood pressure or mild hypertension. *J Am Coll Nutr.* 2005 Aug;24(4):257-65.

Akamatsu S, Watanabe A, Tamesada M, Nakamura R, Hayashi S, Kodama D, Kawase M, Yagi K. Hepatoprotective effect of extracts from Lentinus edodes mycelia on dimethylnitrosamine-induced liver injury. Biol Pharm Bull. 2004 Dec;27(12):1957-60.

Akanbi MH, Post E, van Putten SM, de Vries L, Smisterova J, Meter-Arkema AH, Wösten HA, Rink R, Scholtmeijer K. The antitumor activity of hydrophobin SC3, a fungal protein. Appl Microbiol Biotechnol. 2013 May;97(10):4385-92. doi: 10.1007/s00253-012-4311-x.

Akil I, Yilmaz Y, Kurutepe S, Degerli K, Kavukcu S. Influence of oral intake of *Saccharomyces boulardii* on *Escherichia coli* in enteric flora. *Pediatr Nephrol.* 2006 Jun;21(6):807-10.

Akinbami LJ, Moorman JE, Garbe PL, Sondik EJ. Status of childhood asthma in the United States, 1980-2007. *Pediatrics.* 2009;123:S131-45.

Albert RK, Connett J, Curtis JL, Martinez FJ, Han MK, Lazarus SC, Woodruff PG. Mannose-binding lectin deficiency and acute exacerbations of chronic obstructive pulmonary disease. Int J Chron Obstruct Pulmon Dis. 2012;7:767-77. doi: 10.2147/COPD.S33714.

Aldinucci C, Bellussi L, Monciatti G, Passàli GC, Salerni L, Passàli D, Bocci V. Effects of dietary yoghurt on immunological and clinical parameters of rhinopathic patients. *Eur J Clin Nutr.* 2002 Dec;56(12):1155-61.

Alemán A, Sastre J, Quirce S, de las Heras M, Carnés J, Fernández-Caldas E, Pastor C, Blázquez AB, Vivanco F, Cuesta-Herranz J. Allergy to kiwi: a double-blind, placebo-controlled food challenge study in patients from a birch-free area. *J Allergy Clin Immunol.* 2004 Mar;113(3):543-50.

Alexander DD, Cabana MD. Partially hydrolyzed 100% whey protein infant formula and reduced risk of atopic dermatitis: a meta-analysis. *J Pediatr Gastroenterol Nutr.* 2010 Apr;50(4):422-30.

Alexandrakis M, Letourneau R, Kempuraj D, Kandere-Grzybowska K, Huang M, Christodoulou S, Boucher W, Seretakis D, Theoharides TC. Flavones inhibit proliferation and increase mediator content in human leukemic mast cells (HMC-1). *Eur J Haematol.* 2003 Dec;71(6):448-54.

Alfvén T, Braun-Fahrländer C, Brunekreef B, von Mutius E, Riedler J, Scheynius A, van Hage M, Wickman M, Benz MR, Budde J, Michels KB, Schram D, Ublagger E, Waser M, Pershagen G; PARSIFAL study group. Allergic diseases and atopic sensitization in children related to farming and anthroposophic lifestyle—the PARSIFAL study. *Allergy.* 2006 Apr;61(4):414-21. PubMed PMID: 16512802.

Al-Harrasi A, Al-Saidi S. Phytochemical analysis of the essential oil from botanically certified oleogum resin of Boswellia sacra (Omani Luban). *Molecules.* 2008 Sep 16;13(9):2181-9.

Ali Z, Ma H, Wali A, Ayim I, Sharif MN. Daily date vinegar consumption improves hyperlipidemia, β-carotenoid and inflammatory biomarkers in mildly hypercholesterolemic adults. J Herb Med 2019 Sep-Dec; 17-18.

Allen SJ, Okoko B, Martinez E, Gregorio G, Dans LF. Probiotics for treating infectious diarrhea. *The Cochrane Library.* 2004;3. Chichester, UK: John Wiley & Sons, Ltd.

Alleva R, Tomasetti M, Bompadre S, Littarru GP. Oxidation of LDL and their subfractions: kinetic aspects and CoQ10 content. *Mol Aspects Med.* 1997;18 Suppl:S105-12.

Allingstrup M, Afshari A. Selenium supplementation for critically ill adults. Cochrane Database Syst Rev. 2015 Jul 27;(7):CD003703. doi: 10.1002/14651858.CD003703.pub3.

Almqvist C, Garden F, Xuan W, Mihrshahi S, Leeder SR, Oddy W, Webb K, Marks GB; CAPS team. Omega-3 and omega-6 fatty acid exposure from early life does not affect atopy and asthma at age 5 years. *J Allergy Clin Immunol.* 2007 Jun;119(6):1438-44.

Amato R, Pinelli M, Monticelli A, Miele G, Cocozza S. Schizophrenia and Vitamin D Related Genes Could Have Been Subject to Latitude-driven Adaptation. *BMC Evol Biol.* 2010 Nov 11;10(1):351.

Amenta M, Cascio MT, Di Fiore P, Venturini I. Diet and chronic constipation. Benefits of oral supplementation with symbiotic zir fos (*Bifidobacterium longum* W11 + FOS Actilight). *Acta Biomed.* 2006 Dec;77(3):157-62.

American Conference of Governmental Industrial Hygienists. *Threshold limit values for chemical substances and physical agents in the work environment.* Cincinnati, OH: ACGIH, 1986.

American Dietetic Association; Dietitians of Canada. Position of the American Dietetic Association and Dietitians of Canada: vegetarian diets. *Can J Diet Pract Res.* 2003 Summer;64(2):62-81.

Ammon HP. Boswellic acids (components of frankincense) as the active principle in treatment of chronic inflammatory diseases. *Wien Med Wochenschr.* 2002;152(15-16):373-8.

Ammon HP. Boswellic acids in chronic inflammatory diseases. *Planta Med.* 2006 Oct;72(12):1100-16.

Anand P, Thomas SG, Kunnumakkara AB, Sundaram C, Harikumar KB, Sung B, Tharakan ST, Misra K, Priyadarsini IK, Rajasekharan KN, Aggarwal BB. Biological activities of curcumin and its analogues (Congeners) made by man and Mother Nature. *Biochem Pharmacol.* 2008 Dec 1;76(11):1590-611.

Anderson JL, May HT, Horne BD, Bair TL, Hall NL, Carlquist JF, Lappé DL, Muhlestein JB; Intermountain Heart Collaborative (IHC) Study Group. Relation of vitamin D deficiency to cardiovascular risk factors, disease status, and incident events in a general healthcare population. *Am J Cardiol.* 2010 Oct 1;106(7):963-8.

Anderson JW, Gilliland SE. Effect of fermented milk (yogurt) containing *Lactobacillus acidophilus* L1 on serum cholesterol in hypercholesterolemic humans. *J Am Coll Nutr.* 1999 Feb;18(1):43-50.

Anderson M., Grissom C. Increasing the Heavy Atom Effect of Xenon by Adsorption to Zeolites: Photolysis of 2,3-Diazabicyclo[2.2.2]oct-2-ene. *J. Am. Chem. Soc.* 1996;118:9552-9556.

Anderson RC, Anderson JH. Acute respiratory effects of diaper emissions. *Arch Environ Health.* 1999 Sep-Oct;54(5):353-8.

Anderson RC, Anderson JH. Acute toxic effects of fragrance products. *Arch Environ Health.* 1998 Mar-Apr;53(2):138-46.

Anderson RC, Anderson JH. Respiratory toxicity in mice exposed to mattress covers. *Arch Environ Health.* 1999 May-Jun;54(3):202-9.

Anderson RC, Anderson JH. Respiratory toxicity of fabric softener emissions. *J Toxicol Environ Health.* 2000 May;60(2):121-36.

Anderson RC, Anderson JH. Respiratory toxicity of mattress emissions in mice. *Arch Environ Health.* 2000 Jan-Feb;55(1):38-43.

Anderson RC, Anderson JH. Sensory irritation and multiple chemical sensitivity. *Toxicol Ind Health.* 1999 Apr-Jun;15(3-4):339-45.

Anderson RC, Anderson JH. Toxic effects of air freshener emissions. *Arch Environ Health.* 1997 Nov-Dec;52(6):433-41.

Anderson SD, Charlton B, Weiler JM, Nichols S, Spector SL, Pearlman DS; A305 Study Group. Comparison of mannitol and methacholine to predict exercise-induced bronchoconstriction and a clinical diagnosis of asthma. *Respir Res.* 2009 Jan 23;10:4.

Ando M, Morita T, Akechi T, Ito S, Tanaka M, Ifuku Y, Nakayama T. The efficacy of mindfulness-based meditation therapy on anxiety, depression, and spirituality in Japanese patients with cancer. J Palliat Med. 2009 Dec;12(12):1091-4. doi: 10.1089/jpm.2009.0143.

Andoh T, Zhang Q, Yamamoto T, Tayama M, Hattori M, Tanaka K, Kuraishi Y. Inhibitory Effects of the Methanol Extract of Ganoderma lucidum on Mosquito Allergy-Induced Itch-Associated Responses in Mice. *J Pharmacol Sci.* 2010 Oct 8.

André C, André F, Colin L. Effect of allergen ingestion challenge with and without cromoglycate cover on intestinal permeability in atopic dermatitis, urticaria and other symptoms of food allergy. *Allergy.* 1989;44 Suppl 9:47-51.

André C. Food allergy. Objective diagnosis and test of therapeutic efficacy by measuring intestinal permeability. *Presse Med.* 1986 Jan 25;15(3):105-8.

Andre F, Andre C, Feknous M, Colin L, Cavagna S. Digestive permeability to different-sized molecules and to sodium cromoglycate in food allergy. *Allergy Proc.* 1991 Sep-Oct;12(5):293-8.

Anim-Nyame N, Sooranna SR, Johnson MR, Gamble J, Steer PJ. Garlic supplementation increases peripheral blood flow: a role for interleukin-6? *J Nutr Biochem.* 2004 Jan;15(1):30-6.

Annweiler C, Schott AM, Berrut G, Chauviré V, Le Gall D, Inzitari M, Beauchet O. Vitamin D and ageing: neurological issues. *Neuropsychobiology.* 2010 Aug;62(3):139-50.

Antczak A, Nowak D, Shariati B, Król M, Piasecka G, Kurmanowska Z. Increased hydrogen peroxide and thiobarbituric acid-reactive products in expired breath condensate of asthmatic patients. *Eur Respir J.* 1997 Jun;10(6):1235-41.

Anukam K, Osazuwa E, Ahonkhai I, Ngwu M, Osemene G, Bruce AW, Reid G. Augmentation of antimicrobial metronidazole therapy of bacterial vaginosis with oral probiotic *Lactobacillus rhamnosus* GR-1 and *Lactobacillus reuteri* RC-14: randomized, double-blind, placebo controlled trial. *Microbes Infect.* 2006 May;8(6):1450-4.

Anukam KC, Osazuwa E, Osemene GI, Ehigiagbe F, Bruce AW, Reid G. Clinical study comparing probiotic Lactobacillus GR-1 and RC-14 with metronidazole vaginal gel to treat symptomatic bacterial vaginosis. *Microbes Infect.* 2006 Oct;8(12-13):2772-6.

Anukam KC, Osazuwa EO, Osadolor HB, Bruce AW, Reid G. Yogurt containing probiotic *Lactobacillus rhamnosus* GR-1 and *L. reuteri* RC-14 helps resolve moderate diarrhea and increases CD4 count in HIV/AIDS patients. *J Clin Gastroenterol.* 2008 Mar;42(3):239-43.

Aoki T, Usuda Y, Miyakoshi H, Tamura K, Herberman RB. Low natural killer syndrome: clinical and immunologic features. *Nat Immun Cell Growth Regul.* 1987;6(3):116-28.

Apáti P, Houghton PJ, Kite G, Steventon GB, Kéry A. In-vitro effect of flavonoids from Solidago canadensis extract on glutathione S-transferase. *J Pharm Pharmacol.* 2006 Feb;58(2):251-6.

APHA (American Public Health Association). Opposition to the Use of Hormone Growth Promoters in Beef and Dairy Cattle Production. Policy Date: 11/10/2009. Policy Number: 20098. http://www.apha.org/advocacy/policy/id=1379. Accessed Nov. 24, 2010.

Araki K, Shinozaki T, Irie Y, Miyazawa Y. Trial of oral administration of Bifidobacterium breve for the prevention of rotavirus infections. *Kansenshogaku Zasshi.* 1999 Apr;73(4):305-10.

Araujo AC, Aprile LR, Dantas RO, Terra-Filho J, Vianna EO. Bronchial responsiveness during esophageal acid infusion. Lung. 2008 Mar-Apr;186(2):123-8. 2008 Feb 23.

Arbes SJ Jr, Gergen PJ, Vaughn B, Zeldin DC. Asthma cases attributable to atopy: results from the Third National Health and Nutrition Examination Survey. *J Allergy Clin Immunol.* 2007 Nov;120(5):1139-45. 2007 Sep 24.

Argento A, Tiraferri E, Marzaloni M. Oral anticoagulants and medicinal plants. An emerging interaction. *Ann Ital Med Int.* 2000 Apr-Jun;15(2):139-43.

Arif AA, Delclos GL, Colmer-Hamood J. Association between asthma, asthma symptoms and C-reactive protein in US adults: data from the National Health and Nutrition Examination Survey, 1999-2002. *Respirology.* 2007 Sep;12(5):675-82. .

Arif AA, Shah SM. Association between personal exposure to volatile organic compounds and asthma among US adult population. *Int Arch Occup Environ Health.* 2007 Aug;80(8):711-9.

Armstrong BK. Absorption of vitamin B12 from the human colon. *Am J Clin Nutr.* 1968;21:298-9.

Armuzzi A, Cremonini F, Bartolozzi F, Canducci F, Candelli M, Ojetti V, Cammarota G, Anti M, De Lorenzo A, Pola P, Gasbarrini G, Gasbarrini A. The effect of oral administration of Lactobacillus GG on antibiotic-associated gastrointestinal side-effects during Helicobacter pylori eradication therapy. *Aliment Pharmacol Ther.* 2001 Feb;15(2):163-9.

Arrigo G, D'Angelo A. Achromycin and anaphylactic shock. *Riv Patol Clin.* 1959 Oct;14:719-22.

REFERENCES AND BIBLIOGRAPHY

Arshad SH, Bateman B, Sadeghnejad A, Gant C, Matthews SM. Prevention of allergic disease during childhood by allergen avoidance: the Isle of Wight prevention study. *J Allergy Clin Immunol.* 2007 Feb;119(2):307-13.

Arslanoglu S, Moro GE, Schmitt J, Tandoi L, Rizzardi S, Boehm G. Early dietary intervention with a mixture of prebiotic oligosaccharides reduces the incidence of allergic manifestations and infections during the first two years of life. *J Nutr.* 2008 Jun;138(6):1091-5.

Arterburn LM, Oken HA, Bailey Hall E, Hamersley J, Kuratko CN, Hoffman JP. Algal-oil capsules and cooked salmon: nutritionally equivalent sources of docosahexaenoic acid. *J Am Diet Assoc.* 2008 Jul;108(7):1204-9.

Arterburn LM, Oken HA, Hoffman JP, Bailey-Hall E, Chung G, Rom D, Hamersley J, McCarthy D. Bioequivalence of Docosahexaenoic acid from different algal oils in capsules and in a DHA-fortified food. *Lipids.* 2007 Nov;42(11):1011-24.

Arunachalam K, Gill HS, Chandra RK. Enhancement of natural immune function by dietary consumption of *Bifidobacterium lactis* (HN019). *Eur J Clin Nutr.* 2000 Mar;54(3):263-7.

Arvaniti F, Priftis KN, Panagiotakos DB. Dietary habits and asthma: a review. *Allergy Asthma Proc.* 2010 Mar;31(2):e1-10.

Arvola T, Laiho K, Torkkeli S, Mykkänen H, Salminen S, Maunula L, Isolauri E. Prophylactic Lactobacillus GG reduces antibiotic-associated diarrhea in children with respiratory infections: a randomized study. *Pediatrics.* 1999 Nov;104(5):e64.

Asero R, Antonicelli L, Arena A, Bommarito L, Caruso B, Colombo G, Crivellaro M, De Carli M, Della Torre E, Della Torre F, Heffler E, Lodi Rizzini F, Longo R, Manzotti G, Marcotulli M, Melchiorre A, Minale P, Morandi P, Moreni B, Moschella A, Murzilli F, Nebiolo F, Poppa M, Randazzo S, Rossi G, Senna GE. Causes of food-induced anaphylaxis in Italian adults: a multi-centre study. *Int Arch Allergy Immunol.* 2009;150(3):271-7.

Asero R, Mistrello G, Roncarolo D, Amato S, Caldironi G, Barocci F, van Ree R. Immunological cross-reactivity between lipid transfer proteins from botanically unrelated plant-derived foods: a clinical study. *Allergy.* 2002 Oct;57(10):900-6.

Ashrafi K, Chang FY, Watts JL, Fraser AG, Kamath RS, Ahringer J, Ruvkun G. Genome-wide RNAi analysis of Caenorhabditis elegans fat regulatory genes. *Nature.* 2003 Jan 16;421(6920):268-72.

Aso Y, Akaza H, Kotake T, Tsukamoto T, Imai K, Naito S. Preventive effect of a *Lactobacillus casei* preparation on the recurrence of superficial bladder cancer in a double-blind trial. *The BLP Study Group. Eur Urol.* 1995;27(2):104-9.

Aso Y, Akazan H. Prophylactic effect of a *Lactobacillus casei* preparation on the recurrence of superficial bladder cancer. *BLP Study Group. Urol Int.* 1992;49(3):125-9.

Ataie-Jafari A, Larijani B, Alavi Majd H, Tahbaz F. Cholesterol-lowering effect of probiotic yogurt in comparison with ordinary yogurt in mildly to moderately hypercholesterolemic subjects. *Ann Nutr Metab.* 2009;54(1):22-7.

Atkinson W, Harris J, Mills P, Moffat S, White C, Lynch O, Jones M, Cullinan P, Newman Taylor AJ. Domestic aeroallergen exposures among infants in an English town. *Eur Respir J.* 1999 Mar;13(3):583-9.

Atsumi T, Tonosaki K. Smelling lavender and rosemary increases free radical scavenging activity and decreases cortisol level in saliva. *Psychiatry Res.* 2007 Feb 28;150(1):89-96.

Auriti C, Prencipe G, Caravale B, Coletti MF, Ronchetti MP, Piersigilli F, Azzari C, Di Ciommo VM. MBL2 gene polymorphisms increase the risk of adverse neurological outcome in preterm infants: a preliminary prospective study. Pediatr Res. 2014 Aug 13. doi: 10.1038/pr.2014.118.

Azabji-Kenfack M, Dikosso SE, Loni EG, Onana EA, Sobngwi E, Gbaguidi E, Kana AL, Nguefack-Tsague G, Von der Weid D, Njoya O, Ngogang J. Potential of Spirulina Platensis in Malnourished HIV-Infected Adults in Sub-Saharan Africa: A Randomised, Single-Blind Study. Nutr Metab Insights. 2011 May 2;4:29-37. doi: 10.4137/NMI.S5862.

Babot JD, Argañaraz Martínez E, Lorenzo-Pisarello MJ, Apella MC, Perez Chaia A. Lactic acid bacteria isolated from poultry protect the intestinal epithelial cells of chickens from in vitro wheat germ agglutinin-induced cytotoxicity. Br Poult Sci. 2017 Feb;58(1):76-82. doi: 10.1080/00071668.2016.1251574.

Backster C. *Primary Perception: Biocommunication with Plants, Living Foods, and Human Cells.* Anza, CA: White Rose Millennium Press, 2003.

Bacopoulou F, Veltsista A, Vassi I, Gika A, Lekea V, Priftis K, Bakoula C. Can we be optimistic about asthma in childhood? A Greek cohort study. *J Asthma.* 2009 Mar;46(2):171-4.

Badar VA, Thawani VR, Wakode PT, Shrivastava MP, Gharpure KJ, Hingorani LL, Khiyani RM. Efficacy of Tinospora cordifolia in allergic rhinitis. *J Ethnopharmacol.* 2005 Jan 15;96(3):445-9.

Bae GS, Kim MS, Jung WS, Seo SW, Yun SW, Kim SG, Park RK, Kim EC, Song HJ, Park SJ. Inhibition of lipopolysaccharide-induced inflammatory responses by piperine. *Eur J Pharmacol.* 2010 Sep 10;642(1-3):154-62.

Bafadhel M, Singapuri A, Terry S, Hargadon B, Monteiro W, Green RH, Bradding PH, Wardlaw AJ, Pavord ID, Brightling CE. Body mass and fat mass in refractory asthma: an observational 1 year follow-up study. *J Allergy*. 2010;2010:251758. 2010 Dec 1.

Bai AP, Ouyang Q, Xiao XR, Li SF. Probiotics modulate inflammatory cytokine secretion from inflamed mucosa in active ulcerative colitis. *Int J Clin Pract*. 2006 Mar;60(3):284-8.

Baik HW. Nutritional therapy in gastrointestinal disease. *Korean J Gastroenterol*. 2004 Jun;43(6):331-40.

Baize S, Leroy EM, Georges-Courbot MC, Capron M, Lansoud-Soukate J, Debré P, Fisher-Hoch SP, McCormick JB, Georges AJ. Defective humoral responses and extensive intravascular apoptosis are associated with fatal outcome in Ebola virus-infected patients. Nat Med. 1999 Apr;5(4):423-6.

Baker SM. *Detoxification and Healing*. Chicago: Contemporary Books, 2004.

Bakkeheim E, Mowinckel P, Carlsen KH, Håland G, Carlsen KC. Paracetamol in early infancy: the risk of childhood allergy and asthma. Acta Paediatr. 2011 Jan;100(1):90-6.

Balch P, Balch J. *Prescription for Nutritional Healing*. New York: Avery, 2000.

Balimane P, Yong-Haen H, Chong S. Current Industrial Practices of Assessing Permeability and P-Glycoprotein Interaction. *J AAPS* 2006; 8(1).

Ballentine R. *Diet & Nutrition: A holistic approach*. Honesdale, PA: Himalayan Int., 1978.

Ballentine RM. *Radical Healing*. New York: Harmony Books, 1999.

Balli F, Bertolani P, Giberti G, Amarri S. High-dose oral bacteria-therapy for chronic non-specific diarrhea of infancy. *Pediatr Med Chir*. 1992 Jan-Feb;14(1):13-5.

Ballmer-Weber BK, Holzhauser T, Scibilia J, Mittag D, Zisa G, Ortolani C, Oesterballe M, Poulsen LK, Vieths S, Bindslev-Jensen C. Clinical characteristics of soybean allergy in Europe: a double-blind, placebo-controlled food challenge study. *J Allergy Clin Immunol*. 2007 Jun;119(6):1489-96.

Ballmer-Weber BK, Vieths S, Lüttkopf D, Heuschmann P, Wüthrich B. Celery allergy confirmed by double-blind, placebo-controlled food challenge: a clinical study in 32 subjects with a history of adverse reactions to celery root. *J Allergy Clin Immunol*. 2000 Aug;106(2):373-8.

Banno N, Akihisa T, Yasukawa K, Tokuda H, Tabata K, Nakamura Y, Nishimura R, Kimura Y, Suzuki T. Anti-inflammatory activities of the triterpene acids from the resin of Boswellia carteri. *J Ethnopharmacol*. 2006 Sep 19;107(2):249-53.

Bant A, Kruszewski J. Increased sensitization prevalence to common inhalant and food allergens in young adult Polish males. *Ann Agric Environ Med*. 2008 Jun;15(1):21-7.

Barbeito CG, Ortega HH, Matiller V, Gimeno EJ, Salvetti NR. Lectin-binding pattern in ovarian structures of rats with experimental polycystic ovaries. Reprod Domest Anim. 2013 Oct;48(5):850-7. doi: 10.1111/rda.12174.

Barnes M, Cullinan P, Athanasaki P, MacNeill S, Hole AM, Harris J, Kalogeraki S, Chatzinikolaou M, Drakonakis N, Bibaki-Liakou V, Newman Taylor AJ, Bibakis I. Crete: does farming explain urban and rural differences in atopy? *Clin Exp Allergy*. 2001 Dec;31(12):1822-8.

Barnetson RS, Drummond H, Ferguson A. Precipitins to dietary proteins in atopic eczema. *Br J Dermatol*. 1983 Dec;109(6):653-5.

Barnett AG, Williams GM, Schwartz J, Neller AH, Best TL, Petroeschevsky AL, Simpson RW. Air pollution and child respiratory health: a case-crossover study in Australia and New Zealand. *Am J Respir Crit Care Med*. 2005 Jun 1;171(11):1272-8.

Baron M. A patented strain of Bacillus coagulans increased immune response to viral challenge. *Postgrad Med*. 2009 Mar;121(2):114-8.

Barrager E, Veltmann JR Jr, Schauss AG, Schiller RN. A multicentered, open-label trial on the safety and efficacy of methylsulfonylmethane in the treatment of seasonal allergic rhinitis. *J Altern Complement Med*. 2002 Apr;8(2):167-73.

Barros R, Moreira A, Fonseca J, de Oliveira JF, Delgado L, Castel-Branco MG, Haahtela T, Lopes C, Moreira P. Adherence to the Mediterranean diet and fresh fruit intake are associated with improved asthma control. *Allergy*. 2008 Jul;63(7):917-23.

Barton C, Kouokam JC, Lasnik AB, Foreman O, Cambon A, Brock G, Montefiori DC, Vojdani F, McCormick AA, O'Keefe BR, Palmer KE. Activity of and effect of subcutaneous treatment with the broad-spectrum antiviral lectin griffithsin in two laboratory rodent models. Antimicrob Agents Chemother. 2014;58(1):120-7. doi: 10.1128/AAC.01407-13.

Bartram HP, Scheppach W, Gerlach S, Ruckdeschel G, Kelber E, Kasper H. Does yogurt enriched with *Bifidobacterium longum* affect colonic microbiology and fecal metabolites in health subjects? *Am J Clin Nutr*. 1994 Feb;59(2):428-32.

Basu A, Devaraj S, Jialal I. Dietary factors that promote or retard inflammation. *Arterioscler Thromb Vasc Biol*. 2006 May;26(5):995-1001.

Basu S, Chatterjee M, Ganguly S, Chandra PK. Effect of *Lactobacillus rhamnosus* GG in persistent diarrhea in Indian children: a randomized controlled trial. *J Clin Gastroenterol*. 2007 Sep;41(8):756-60.

REFERENCES AND BIBLIOGRAPHY

Basu S, Chatterjee M, Ganguly S, Chandra PK. Efficacy of *Lactobacillus rhamnosus* GG in acute watery diarrhoea of Indian children: a randomised controlled trial. *J Paediatr Child Health*. 2007 Dec;43(12):837-42.

Bateman B, Warner JO, Hutchinson E, Dean T, Rowlandson P, Gant C, Grundy J, Fitzgerald C, Stevenson J. The effects of a double blind, placebo controlled, artificial food colourings and benzoate preservative challenge on hyperactivity in a general population sample of preschool children. *Arch Dis Child*. 2004 Jun;89(6):506-11.

Bates DW, Cullen DJ, Laird N, Petersen LA, Small SD, Servi D, Laffel G, Sweitzer BJ, Shea BF, Hallisey R, *et al*. Incidence of adverse drug events and potential adverse drug events. Implications for prevention. ADE Prevention Study Group. *JAMA*. 1995 Jul 5;274(1):29-34.

Batista R, Martins I, Jeno P, Ricardo CP, Oliveira MM. A proteomic study to identify soya allergens—the human response to transgenic versus non-transgenic soya samples. *Int Arch Allergy Immunol*. 2007;144(1):29-38.

Batmanghelidj F. Neurotransmitter histamine: an alternative view point, *Science in Medicine Simplified*. Falls Church, VA: Foundation for the Simple in Medicine, 1990.

Batmanghelidj F. Pain: a need for paradigm change. *Anticancer Res*. 1987 Sep-Oct;7(5B):971-89.

Batmanghelidj F. *Your Body's Many Cries for Water*. 2nd Ed. Vienna, VA: Global Health, 1997.

Beasley R, Clayton T, Crane J, von Mutius E, Lai CK, Montefort S, Stewart A; ISAAC Phase Three Study Group. Association between paracetamol use in infancy and childhood, and risk of asthma, rhinoconjunctivitis, and eczema in children aged 6-7 years: analysis from Phase Three of the ISAAC programme. *Lancet*. 2008 Sep. 20;372(9643):1039-48.

Beaulieu A, Fessele K. Agent Orange: management of patients exposed in Vietnam. *Clin J Oncol Nurs*. 2003 May-Jun;7(3):320-3.

Beausoleil M, Fortier N, Guénette S, L'ecuyer A, Savoie M, Franco M, Lachaine J, Weiss K. Effect of a fermented milk combining *Lactobacillus acidophilus* Cl1285 and *Lactobacillus casei* in the prevention of antibiotic-associated diarrhea: a randomized, double-blind, placebo-controlled trial. *Can J Gastroenterol*. 2007 Nov;21(11):732-6.

Becker KG, Simon RM, Bailey-Wilson JE, Freidlin B, Biddison WE, McFarland HF, Trent JM. Clustering of non-major histocompatibility complex susceptibility candidate loci in human autoimmune diseases. *Proc Natl Acad Sci U S A*. 1998 Aug 18;95(17):9979-84.

Beddoe AF. *Biologic Ionization as Applied to Human Nutrition*. Warsaw: Wendell Whitman, 2002.

Beecher GR. Phytonutrients' role in metabolism: effects on resistance to degenerative processes. *Nutr Rev*. 1999 Sep;57(9 Pt 2):S3-6.

Belcaro G, Cesarone MR, Errichi S, Zulli C, Errichi BM, Vinciguerra G, Ledda A, Di Renzo A, Stuard S, Dugall M, Pellegrini L, Gizzi G, Ippolito E, Ricci A, Cacchio M, Cipollone G, Ruffini I, Fano F, Hosoi M, Rohdewald P. Variations in C-reactive protein, plasma free radicals and fibrinogen values in patients with osteoarthritis treated with Pycnogenol. *Redox Rep*. 2008;13(6):271-6.

Bell IR, Baldwin CM, Schwartz GE, Illness from low levels of environmental chemicals: relevance to chronic fatigue syndrome and fibromyalgia. *Am J Med*. 1998;105 (suppl 3A).:74-82. S.

Bell SJ, Potter PC. Milk whey-specific immune complexes in allergic and non-allergic subjects. *Allergy*. 1988 Oct;43(7):497-503.

Ben, X.M., Zhou, X.Y., Zhao, W.H., Yu, W.L., Pan, W., Zhang, W.L., Wu, S.M., Van Beusekom, C.M., Schaafsma, A. (2004) Supplementation of milk formula with galactooligosaccharides improves intestinal micro-flora and fermentation in term infants. *Chin Med J*. 117(6):927-931, 2004.

Benard A, Desreumeaux P, Huglo D, Hoorelbeke A, Tonnel AB, Wallaert B. Increased intestinal permeability in bronchial asthma. *J Allergy Clin Immunol*. 1996 Jun;97(6):1173-8.

Bengmark S. Curcumin, an atoxic antioxidant and natural NFkappaB, cyclooxygenase-2, lipooxygenase, and inducible nitric oxide synthase inhibitor: a shield against acute and chronic diseases. *JPEN J Parenter Enteral Nutr*. 2006 Jan-Feb;30(1):45-51.

Bengmark S. Immunonutrition: role of biosurfactants, fiber, and probiotic bacteria. *Nutrition*. 1998 Jul-Aug;14(7-8):585-94.

Benlounes N, Dupont C, Candalh C, Blaton MA, Darmon N, Desjeux JF, Heyman M. The threshold for immune cell reactivity to milk antigens decreases in cow's milk allergy with intestinal symptoms. *J Allergy Clin Immunol*. 1996 Oct;98(4):781-9.

Bennett WD, Zeman KL, Jarabek AM. Nasal contribution to breathing and fine particle deposition in children versus adults. J Toxicol Environ Health A. 2008;71(3):227-37.

Ben-Shoshan M, Harrington DW, Soller L, Fragapane J, Joseph L, St Pierre Y, Godefroy SB, Elliot SJ, Clarke AE. A population-based study on peanut, tree nut, fish, shellfish, and sesame allergy prevalence in Canada. *J Allergy Clin Immunol*. 2010 Jun;125(6):1327-35.

Ben-Shoshan M, Kagan R, Primeau MN, Alizadehfar R, Turnbull E, Harada L, Dufresne C, Allen M, Joseph L, St Pierre Y, Clarke A. Establishing the diagnosis of peanut allergy in children never exposed to peanut or with an uncertain history: a cross-Canada study. *Pediatr Allergy Immunol.* 2010 Sep;21(6):920-6.

Bensky D, Gable A, Kaptchuk T (transl.). *Chinese Herbal Medicine Materia Medica.* Seattle: Eastland Press, 1986.

Bergner P. *The Healing Power of Garlic.* Prima Publishing, Rocklin CA 1996.

Berin MC, Yang PC, Ciok L, Waserman S, Perdue MH. Role for IL-4 in macromolecular transport across human intestinal epithelium. *Am J Physiol.* 1999 May;276(5 Pt 1):C1046-52.

Berkow R., (Ed.) *The Merck Manual of Diagnosis and Therapy.* 16th Edition. Rahway, N.J.: Merck Research Labs, 1992.

Berman TA, Schiller JT. Human papillomavirus in cervical cancer and oropharyngeal cancer: One cause, two diseases. Cancer. 2017 Jun 15;123(12):2219-2229. doi: 10.1002/cncr.30588.

Bernstein DI, Epstein T, Murphy-Berendts K, Liss GM. Surveillance of systemic reactions to subcutaneous immunotherapy injections: year 1 outcomes of the ACAAI and AAAAI collaborative study. *Ann Allergy Asthma Immunol.* 2010 Jun;104(6):530-5. .

Berseth CL, Mitmesser SH, Ziegler EE, Marunycz JD, Vanderhoof J. Tolerance of a standard intact protein formula versus a partially hydrolyzed formula in healthy, term infants. *Nutr J.* 2009 Jun 19;8:27.

Berteau O and Mulloy B. 2003. Sulfated fucans, fresh perspectives: structures, functions, and biological properties of sulfated fucans and an overview of enzymes active toward this class of polysaccharide. *Glycobiology.* Jun;13(6):29R-40R.

Beyer K, Morrow E, Li XM, Bardina L, Bannon GA, Burks AW, Sampson HA. Effects of cooking methods on peanut allergenicity. *J Allergy Clin Immunol.* 2001;107:1077-81.

Bielory BP, Perez VL, Bielory L. Treatment of seasonal allergic conjunctivitis with ophthalmic corticosteroids: in search of the perfect ocular corticosteroids in the treatment of allergic conjunctivitis. *Curr Opin Allergy Clin Immunol.* 2010 Oct;10(5):469-77.

Bielory L, Lupoli K. Herbal interventions in asthma and allergy. *J Asthma.* 1999;36:1-65.

Bielory L, Russin J, Zuckerman GB. Clinical efficacy, mechanisms of action, and adverse effects of complementary and alternative medicine therapies for asthma. *Allergy Asthma Proc.* 2004;25:283-91.

Bielory L. Complementary and alternative interventions in asthma, allergy, and immunology. *Ann Allergy Asthma Immunol.* 2004 Aug;93(2 Suppl 1):S45-54.

Billoo AG, Memon MA, Khaskheli SA, Murtaza G, Iqbal K, Saeed Shekhani M, Siddiqi AQ. Role of a probiotic (*Saccharomyces boulardii*) in management and prevention of diarrhoea. *World J Gastroenterol.* 2006 Jul 28;12(28):4557-60.

Bindslev-Jensen C, Skov PS, Roggen EL, Hvass P, Brinch DS. Investigation on possible allergenicity of 19 different commercial enzymes used in the food industry. *Food Chem Toxicol.* 2006 Nov;44(11):1909-15.

Bin-Nun A, Bromiker R, Wilschanski M, Kaplan M, Rudensky B, Caplan M, Hammerman C. Oral probiotics prevent necrotizing enterocolitis in very low birth weight neonates. *J Pediatr.* 2005 Aug;147(2):192-6.

Birch EE, Khoury JC, Berseth CL, Castañeda YS, Couch JM, Bean J, Tamer R, Harris CL, Mitmesser SH, Scalabrin DM. The impact of early nutrition on incidence of allergic manifestations and common respiratory illnesses in children. *J Pediatr.* 2010 Jun;156(6):902-6, 906.e1. 2010 Mar 15.

Bisgaard H, Loland L, Holst KK, Pipper CB. Prenatal determinants of neonatal lung function in high-risk newborns. *J Allergy Clin Immunol.* 2009 Mar;123(3):651-7, 657.e1-4. 2009 Jan 18.

Bisset N.. *Herbal Drugs and Phytopharmaceuticals.* Stuttgart: CRC, 1994.

Bjarnason I, MacPherson A, Hollander D. Intestinal permeability: an overview. *Gastroenterology.* 1995 May;108(5):1566-81.

Blackhall K, Appleton S, Cates FJ. Ionisers for chronic asthma. *Cochrane Database Syst Rev* 2003;(3):CD002986.

Blackley, CH. *Experimental Researches on the Causes and Nature of Catarrhus Aestivus (Hay Fever or Hay-Asthma).* London, 1873.

Bliakher MS, Fedorova IM, Lopatina TK, Arkhipov SN, Kapustin IV, Ramazanova ZK, Karpova NV, Ivanov VA, Sharapov NV. Acilact and improvement of the health status of sickly children. *Vestn Ross Akad Med Nauk.* 2005;(12):32-5.

Blood AJ, Zatorre RJ, Bermudez P, Evans AC. Emotional responses to pleasant and unpleasant music correlate with activity in paralimbic brain regions. *Nat Neurosci.* 1999;2:382-7.

Blumenthal M (ed.) *The Complete German Commission E Monographs.* Boston: Amer Botan Council, 1998.

Blumenthal M, Brinckmann J, Goldberg A (eds). *Herbal Medicine: Expanded Commission E Monographs.* Newton, MA: Integrative Med., 2000.

Boccafogli A, Vicentini L, Camerani A, Cogliati P, D'Ambrosi A, Scolozzi R. Adverse food reactions in patients with grass pollen allergic respiratory disease. *Ann Allergy.* 1994 Oct;73(4):301-8.

Bode C, Bode JC. Effect of alcohol consumption on the gut. *Best Pract Res Clin Gastroenterol.* 2003 Aug;17(4):575-92.

Bodinier M, Legoux MA, Pineau F, Triballeau S, Segain JP, Brossard C, Denery-Papini S. Intestinal translocation capabilities of wheat allergens using the Caco-2 cell line. *J Agric Food Chem.* 2007 May 30;55(11):4576-83.

Boehm, G., Lidestri, M., Casetta, P., Jelinek, J., Negretti, F., Stahl, B., Martini, A. (2002) Supplementation of a bovine milk formula with an oligosaccharide mixture increases counts of faecal bifidobacteria in preterm infants. *Arch Dis Child Fetal Neonatal Ed.* 86: F178-F181

Boivin DB, Czeisler CA. Resetting of circadian melatonin and cortisol rhythms in humans by ordinary room light. *Neuroreport.* 1998 Mar 30;9(5):779-82.

Boivin DB, Duffy JF, Kronauer RE, Czeisler CA. Dose-response relationships for resetting of human circadian clock by light. *Nature.* 1996 Feb 8;379(6565):540-2.

Bokesch HR, O'Keefe BR, McKee TC, Pannell LK, Patterson GM, Gardella RS, Sowder RC 2nd, Turpin J, Watson K, Buckheit RW Jr, Boyd MR. A potent novel anti-HIV protein from the cultured cyanobacterium Scytonema varium. *Biochemistry.* 2003 Mar 11;42(9):2578-84.

Bolhaar ST, Tiemessen MM, Zuidmeer L, van Leeuwen A, Hoffmann-Sommergruber K, Bruijnzeel-Koomen CA, Taams LS, Knol EF, van Hoffen E, van Ree R, Knulst AC. Efficacy of birch-pollen immunotherapy on cross-reactive food allergy confirmed by skin tests and double-blind food challenges. *Clin Exp Allergy.* 2004 May;34(5):761-9.

Bolleddula J, Goldfarb J, Wang R, Sampson H, Li XM. Synergistic Modulation Of Eotaxin And Il-4 Secretion By Constituents Of An Anti-asthma Herbal Formula (ASHMI) In Vitro. *J Allergy Clin Immunol.* 2007;119:S172.

Bonfils P, Halimi P, Malinvaud D. Adrenal suppression and osteoporosis after treatment of nasal polyposis. *Acta Otolaryngol.* 2006 Dec;126(11):1195-200.

Bongaerts GP, Severijnen RS. Preventive and curative effects of probiotics in atopic patients. *Med Hypotheses.* 2005;64(6):1089-92.

Bongartz D, Hesse A. Selective extraction of quercetrin in vegetable drugs and urine by off-line coupling of boronic acid affinity chromatography and high-performance liquid chromatography. *J Chromatogr B Biomed Appl.* 1995 Nov 17;673(2):223-30.

Bonsignore MR, La Grutta S, Cibella F, Scichilone N, Cuttitta G, Interrante A, Marchese M, Veca M, Virzi' M, Bonanno A, Profita M, Morici G. Effects of exercise training and montelukast in children with mild asthma. *Med Sci Sports Exerc.* 2008 Mar;40(3):405-12.

Borchers AT, Hackman RM, Keen CL, Stern JS, Gershwin ME. Complementary medicine: a review of immunomodulatory effects of Chinese herbal medicines. *Am J Clin Nutr.* 1997 Dec;66(6):1303-12.

Borchert VE, Czyborra P, Fetscher C, Goepel M, Michel MC. Extracts from Rhois aromatica and Solidaginis virgaurea inhibit rat and human bladder contraction. *Naunyn Schmiedebergs Arch Pharmacol.* 2004 Mar;369(3):281-6.

Borresen EC, Brown DG, Harbison G, Taylor L, Fairbanks A, O'Malia J, Bazan M, Rao S, Bailey SM, Wdowik M, Weir TL, Brown RJ, Ryan EP. A Randomized Controlled Trial to Increase Navy Bean or Rice Bran Consumption in Colorectal Cancer Survivors. *Nutr Cancer.* 2016 Nov-Dec;68(8):1269-1280.

Böttcher MF, Abrahamsson TR, Fredriksson M, Jakobsson T, Björkstén B. Low breast milk TGF-beta2 is induced by *Lactobacillus reuteri* supplementation and associates with reduced risk of sensitization during infancy. *Pediatr Allergy Immunol.* 2008 Sep;19(6):497-504.

Böttcher MF, Jenmalm MC, Voor T, Julge K, Holt PG, Björkstén B. Cytokine responses to allergens during the first 2 years of life in Estonian and Swedish children. *Clin Exp Allergy.* 2006 May;36(5):619-28.

Bottema RW, Kerkhof M, Reijmerink NE, Thijs C, Smit HA, van Schayck CP, Brunekreef B, van Oosterhout AJ, Postma DS, Koppelman GH. Gene-gene interaction in regulatory T-cell function in atopy and asthma development in childhood. *J Allergy Clin Immunol.* 2010 Aug;126(2):338-46, 346.e1-10.

Bouchez-Mahiout I, Pecquet C, Kerre S, Snégaroff J, Raison-Peyron N, Laurière M. High molecular weight entities in industrial wheat protein hydrolysates are immunoreactive with IgE from allergic patients. *J Agric Food Chem.* 2010 Apr 14;58(7):4207-15.

Bougault V, Turmel J, Boulet LP. Bronchial challenges and respiratory symptoms in elite swimmers and winter sport athletes: Airway hyperresponsiveness in asthma: its measurement and clinical significance. *Chest.* 2010 Aug;138(2 Suppl):31S-37S. 2010 Apr 2.

Boyce JA, Assa'ad A, Burks AW, Jones SM, Sampson HA, Wood RA, Plaut M, Cooper SF, Fenton MJ, Arshad SH, Bahna SL, Beck LA, Byrd-Bredbenner C, Camargo CA Jr, Eichenfield L, Furuta GT, Hanifin JM, Jones C, Kraft M, Levy BD, Lieberman P, Luccioli S, McCall KM, Schneider LC, Simon RA, Simons FE, Teach SJ, Yawn BP, Schwaninger JM. Guidelines for the diagnosis and management of food allergy in the United States: report of the NIAID-sponsored expert panel. *J Allergy Clin Immunol.* 2010 Dec;126(6 Suppl):S1-58.

Boylan R, Li Y, Simeonova L, Sherwin G, Kreismann J, Craig RG, Ship JA, McCutcheon JA. Reduction in bacterial contamination of toothbrushes using the Violight ultraviolet light activated toothbrush sanitizer. *Am J Dent.* 2008 Oct;21(5):313-7.

Bråbäck L, Breborowicz A, Julge K, Knutsson A, Riikjärv MA, Vasar M, Björkstén B. Risk factors for respiratory symptoms and atopic sensitisation in the Baltic area. *Arch Dis Child.* 1995 Jun;72(6):487-93.

Bråbäck L, Kjellman NI, Sandin A, Björkstén B. Atopy among schoolchildren in northern and southern Sweden in relation to pet ownership and early life events. *Pediatr Allergy Immunol.* 2001 Feb;12(1):4-10.

Bradette-Hébert ME, Legault J, Lavoie S, Pichette A. A new labdane diterpene from the flowers of Solidago canadensis. *Chem Pharm Bull.* 2008 Jan;56(1):82-4.

Brandtzaeg P. The mucosal immune system and its integration with the mammary glands. *J Pediatr.* 2010 Feb;156(2 Suppl):S8-15.

Brasseur JG, Nicosia MA, Pal A, Miller LS. Function of longitudinal vs circular muscle fibers in esophageal peristalsis, deduced with mathematical modeling. *World J Gastroenterol.* 2007 Mar 7;13(9):1335-46.

Braun-Fahrländer C, Gassner M, Grize L, Neu U, Sennhauser FH, Varonier HS, Vuille JC, Wüthrich B. Prevalence of hay fever and allergic sensitization in farmer's children and their peers living in the same rural community. SCARPOL team. Swiss Study on Childhood Allergy and Respiratory Symptoms with Respect to Air Pollution. *Clin Exp Allergy.* 1999 Jan;29(1):28-34.

Brehm JM, Schuemann B, Fuhlbrigge AL, Hollis BW, Strunk RC, Zeiger RS, Weiss ST, Litonjua AA; Childhood Asthma Management Program Research Group. Serum vitamin D levels and severe asthma exacerbations in the Childhood Asthma Management Program study. *J Allergy Clin Immunol.* 2010 Jul;126(1):52-8.e5. 2010 Jun 9.

Brighenti F, Valtueña S, Pellegrini N, Ardigò D, Del Rio D, Salvatore S, Piatti P, Serafini M, Zavaroni I. Total antioxidant capacity of the diet is inversely and independently related to plasma concentration of high-sensitivity C-reactive protein in adult Italian subjects. *Br J Nutr.* 2005 May;93(5):619-25.

Brinkhaus B, Witt CM, Jena S, Liecker B, Wegscheider K, Willich SN. Acupuncture in patients with allergic rhinitis: a pragmatic randomized trial. *Ann Allergy Asthma Immunol.* 2008 Nov;101(5):535-43.

Brisman J, Torén K, Lillienberg L, Karlsson G, Ahlstedt S. Nasal symptoms and indices of nasal inflammation in flour-dust-exposed bakers. *Int Arch Occup Environ Health.* 1998 Nov;71(8):525-32.

Brodtkorb TH, Zetterström O, Tinghög G. Cost-effectiveness of clean air administered to the breathing zone in allergic asthma. *Clin Respir J.* 2010 Apr;4(2):104-10.

Brody J. *Jane Brody's Nutrition Book.* New York: WW Norton, 1981.

Broekhuizen BD, Sachs AP, Hoes AW, Moons KG, van den Berg JW, Dalinghaus WH, Lammers E, Verheij TJ. Undetected chronic obstructive pulmonary disease and asthma in people over 50 years with persistent cough. *Br J Gen Pract.* 2010 Jul;60(576):489-94.

Brostoff J, Gamlin L, Brostoff J. *Food Allergies and Food Intolerance: The Complete Guide to Their Identification and Treatment.* Rochester, VT: Healing Arts, 2000.

Brownstein D. *Salt: Your Way to Health.* West Bloomfield, MI: Medical Alternatives, 2006.

Brown-Whitehorn TF, Spergel JM. The link between allergies and eosinophilic esophagitis: implications for management strategies. *Expert Rev Clin Immunol.* 2010 Jan;6(1):101-9.

Bruce S, Nyberg F, Melén E, James A, Pulkkinen V, Orsmark-Pietras C, Bergström A, Dahlén B, Wickman M, von Mutius E, Doekes G, Lauener R, Riedler J, Eder W, van Hage M, Pershagen G, Scheynius A, Kere J. The protective effect of farm animal exposure on childhood allergy is modified by NPSR1 polymorphisms. *J Med Genet.* 2009 Mar;46(3):159-67. 2008 Feb 19.

Bruneton J. *Pharmacognosy, Phytochemistry, Medicinal Plants.* Paris: Lavoisier, 1995.

Bruton A, Lewith GT. The Buteyko breathing technique for asthma: a review. *Complement Ther Med.* 2005 Mar;13(1):41-6. 2005 Apr 18.

Bruton A, Thomas M. The role of breathing training in asthma management. *Curr Opin Allergy Clin Immunol.* 2011 Feb;11(1):53-7.

Bryborn M, Halldén C, Säll T, Cardell LO. CLC- a novel susceptibility gene for allergic rhinitis? *Allergy.* 2010 Feb;65(2):220-8.

Bu LN, Chang MH, Ni YH, Chen HL, Cheng CC. *Lactobacillus casei* rhamnosus Lcr35 in children with chronic constipation. *Pediatr Int.* 2007 Aug;49(4):485-90.

Bublin M, Pfister M, Radauer C, Oberhuber C, Bulley S, Dewitt AM, Lidholm J, Reese G, Vieths S, Breiteneder H, Hoffmann-Sommergruber K, Ballmer-Weber BK. Component-resolved diagnosis of kiwifruit allergy with purified natural and recombinant kiwifruit allergens. *J Allergy Clin Immunol.* 2010 Mar;125(3):687-94, 694.e1.

Buchanan TW, Lutz K, Mirzazade S, Specht K, Shah NJ, Zilles K, *et al.* Recognition of emotional prosody and verbal components of spoken language: an fMRI study. *Cogn Brain Res.* 2000;9:227-38.

Bucher X, Pichler WJ, Dahinden CA, Helbling A. Effect of tree pollen specific, subcutaneous immunotherapy on the oral allergy syndrome to apple and hazelnut. *Allergy.* 2004 Dec;59(12):1272-6.

Budzianowski J. Coumarins, caffeoyltartaric acids and their artifactual methyl esters from Taraxacum officinale leaves. *Planta Med.* 1997 Jun;63(3):288.

Bueso AK, Berntsen S, Mowinckel P, Andersen LF, Lødrup Carlsen KC, Carlsen KH. Dietary intake in adolescents with asthma - potential for improvement. *Pediatr Allergy Immunol.* 2010 Oct 20. doi: 10.1111/j.1399-3038.2010.01013.x.

REFERENCES AND BIBLIOGRAPHY

Bundy R, Walker AF, Middleton RW, Booth J. Turmeric extract may improve irritable bowel syndrome symptomology in otherwise healthy adults: a pilot study. *J Altern Complement Med.* 2004 Dec;10(6):1015-8.

Burdge GC, Jones AE, Wootton SA. Eicosapentaenoic and docosapentaenoic acids are the principal products of alpha-linolenic acid metabolism in young men. *B J Nutr.* 2002 Oct;88(4):355-63.

Buret AG. How stress induces intestinal hypersensitivity. *Am J Pathol.* 2006 Jan;168(1):3-5.

Burgess CD, Bremner P, Thomson CD, Crane J, Siebers RW, Beasley R. Nebulized beta 2-adrenoceptor agonists do not affect plasma selenium or glutathione peroxidase activity in patients with asthma. *Int J Clin Pharmacol Ther.* 1994 Jun;32(6):290-2.

Burks W, Jones SM, Berseth CL, Harris C, Sampson HA, Scalabrin DM. Hypoallergenicity and effects on growth and tolerance of a new amino acid-based formula with docosahaexaenoic acid and arachidonic acid. *J Pediatr.* 2008 Aug;153(2):266-71.

Burney PG, Luczynska C, Chinn S, Jarvis D. The European Community Respiratory Health Survey. *Eur Respir J.* 1994;7: 954-960.

Burr ML, Butland BK, King S, Vaughan-Williams E. Changes in asthma prevalence: two surveys 15 years apart. *Arch Dis Child.* 1989;64:1452-1456.

Busse PJ, Wen MC, Huang CK, Srivastava K, Zhang TF, Schofield B, Sampson HA, Li XM. Therapeutic effects of the Chinese herbal formula, MSSM-03d, on persistent airway hyperreactivity and airway remodeling. *J Allergy Clin Immunol.* 2004;113:S220.

Byrne AM, Malka-Rais J, Burks AW, Fleischer DM. How do we know when peanut and tree nut allergy have resolved, and how do we keep it resolved? *Clin Exp Allergy.* 2010 Sep;40(9):1303-11.

Cabanillas B, Pedrosa MM, Rodríguez J, González A, Muzquiz M, Cuadrado C, Crespo JF, Burbano C. Effects of enzymatic hydrolysis on lentil allergenicity. *Mol Nutr Food Res.* 2010 Mar 19.

Caglar E, Cildir SK, Ergeneli S, Sandalli N, Twetman S. Salivary mutans streptococci and lactobacilli levels after ingestion of the probiotic bacterium *Lactobacillus reuteri* ATCC 55730 by straws or tablets. *Acta Odontol Scand.* 2006 Oct;64(5):314-8.

Caglar E, Kavaloglu SC, Kuscu OO, Sandalli N, Holgerson PL, Twetman S. Effect of chewing gums containing xylitol or probiotic bacteria on salivary mutans streptococci and lactobacilli. *Clin Oral Investig.* 2007 Dec;11(4):425-9.

Caglar E, Kuscu OO, Cildir SK, Kuvvetli SS, Sandalli N. A probiotic lozenge administered medical device and its effect on salivary mutans streptococci and lactobacilli. *Int J Paediatr Dent.* 2008 Jan;18(1):35-9.

Caglar E, Kuscu OO, Selvi Kuvvetli S, Kavaloglu Cildir S, Sandalli N, Twetman S. Short-term effect of ice-cream containing *Bifidobacterium lactis* Bb-12 on the number of salivary mutans streptococci and lactobacilli. *Acta Odontol Scand.* 2008 Jun;66(3):154-8.

Cahn J, Borzeix MG. Administration of procyanidolic oligomers in rats. Observed effects on changes in the permeability of the blood-brain barrier. *Sem Hop.* 1983 Jul 7;59(27-28):2031-4.

Calder PC. Dietary modification of inflammation with lipids. *Proc Nutr Soc.* 2002 Aug;61(3):345-58.

Camargo CA Jr, Ingham T, Wickens K, Thadhani R, Silvers KM, Epton MJ, Town GI, Pattemore PK, Espinola JA, Crane J; New Zealand Asthma and Allergy Cohort Study Group. Cord-blood 25-hydroxyvitamin D levels and risk of respiratory infection, wheezing, and asthma. *Pediatrics.* 2011 Jan;127(1):e180-7.

Caminiti L, Passalacqua G, Barberi S, Vita D, Barberio G, De Luca R, Pajno GB. A new protocol for specific oral tolerance induction in children with IgE-mediated cow's milk allergy. *Allergy Asthma Proc.* 2009 Jul-Aug;30(4):443-8.

Campbell TC, Campbell TM. *The China Study.* Dallas, TX: Benbella Books, 2006.

Campieri C, Campieri M, Bertuzzi V, Swennen E, Matteuzzi D, Stefoni S, Pirovano F, Centi C, Ulisse S, Famularo G, De Simone C. Reduction of oxaluria after an oral course of lactic acid bacteria at high concentration. *Kidney Int.* 2001 Sep;60(3):1097-105.

Camporese A. In vitro activity of Eucalyptus smithii and Juniperus communis essential oils against bacterial biofilms and efficacy perspectives of complementary inhalation therapy in chronic and recurrent upper respiratory tract infections. *Infez Med.* 2013 Jun;21(2):117-24.

Canakcioglu S, Tahamiler R, Saritzali G, Alimoglu Y, Isildak H, Guvenc MG, Acar GO, Inci E. Evaluation of nasal cytology in subjects with chronic rhinitis: a 7-year study. *Am J Otolaryngol.* 2009 Sep-Oct;30(5):312-7.

Canali R, Comitato R, Schonlau F, Virgili F. The anti-inflammatory pharmacology of Pycnogenol in humans involves COX-2 and 5-LOX mRNA expression in leukocytes. *Int Immunopharmacol.* 2009 Sep;9(10):1145-9.

Canani RB, Cirillo P, Terrin G, Cesarano L, Spagnuolo MI, De Vincenzo A, Albano F, Passariello A, De Marco G, Manguso F, Guarino A. Probiotics for treatment of acute diarrhoea in children: randomised clinical trial of five different preparations. *BMJ.* 2007 Aug 18;335(7615):340.

394

Canducci F, Armuzzi A, Cremonini F, Cammarota G, Bartolozzi F, Pola P, Gasbarrini G, Gasbarrini A. A lyophilized and inactivated culture of *Lactobacillus acidophilus* increases *Helicobacter pylori* eradication rates. *Aliment Pharmacol Ther.* 2000 Dec;14(12):1625-9.

Canducci F, Cremonini F, Armuzzi A, Di Caro S, Gabrielli M, Santarelli L, Nista E, Lupascu A, De Martini D, Gasbarrini A. Probiotics and Helicobacter pylori eradication. *Dig Liver Dis.* 2002 Sep;34 Suppl 2:S81-3.

Canonica GW, Passalacqua G. Noninjection routes for immunotherapy. *J Allergy Clin Immunol.* 2003 Mar;111(3):437-48; quiz 449.

Cantani A, Micera M. Natural history of cow's milk allergy. An eight-year follow-up study in 115 atopic children. *Eur Rev Med Pharmacol Sci.* 2004 Jul-Aug;8(4):153-64.

Cantani A, Micera M. The prick by prick test is safe and reliable in 58 children with atopic dermatitis and food allergy. *Eur Rev Med Pharmacol Sci.* 2006 May-Jun;10(3):115-20.

Cao G, Alessio HM, Cutler RG. Oxygen-radical absorbance capacity assay for antioxidants. *Free Radic Biol Med.* 1993 Mar;14(3):303-11.

Cao G, Shukitt-Hale B, Bickford PC, Joseph JA, McEwen J, Prior RL. Hyperoxia-induced changes in antioxidant capacity and the effect of dietary antioxidants. *J Appl Physiol.* 1999 Jun;86(6):1817-22.

Caramia G. The essential fatty acids omega-6 and omega-3: from their discovery to their use in therapy. *Minerva Pediatr.* 2008 Apr;60(2):219-33.

Carey DG, Aase KA, Pliego GJ. The acute effect of cold air exercise in determination of exercise-induced bronchospasm in apparently healthy athletes. J Strength Cond Res. 2010 Aug;24(8):2172-8.

Carpita N. C., Kanabus J., Housley T. L. Linkage structure of fructans and fructan oligomers from Triticum aestivum and Festuca arundinacea leaves. *J. Plant Physiol.* 1989;134:162-168

Carroccio A, Cavataio F, Montalto G, D'Amico D, Alabrese L, Iacono G. Intolerance to hydrolysed cow's milk proteins in infants: clinical characteristics and dietary treatment. *Clin Exp Allergy.* 2000 Nov;30(11):1597-603.

Carroll D. *The Complete Book of Natural Medicines.* New York: Summit, 1980.

Caruso M, Frasca G, Di Giuseppe PL, Pennisi A, Tringali G, Bonina FP. Effects of a new nutraceutical ingredient on allergen-induced sulphidoleukotrienes production and CD63 expression in allergic subjects. *Int Immunopharmacol.* 2008 Dec 20;8(13-14):1781-6.

Casale TB, Amin BV. Allergic rhinitis/asthma interrelationship. *Clin Rev Allergy Immunol.* 2001;21:27-49.

Cats A, Kuipers EJ, Bosschaert MA, Pot RG, Vandenbroucke-Grauls CM, Kusters JG. Effect of frequent consumption of a *Lactobacillus casei*-containing milk drink in *Helicobacter pylori*-colonized subjects. *Aliment Pharmacol Ther.* 2003 Feb;17(3):429-35.

Caughey AB, Nicholson JM, Cheng YW, Lyell DJ, Washington AE. Induction of labor and Cesarean delivery by gestational age. *Am J Obstet Gynecol.* 2006 Sep;195(3):700-5.

Celakovská J, Vaněčková J, Ettlerová K, Ettler K, Bukac J. The role of atopy patch test in diagnosis of food allergy in atopic eczema/dermatitis syndrom in patients over 14 years of age. *Acta Medica (Hradec Kralove).* 2010;53(2):101-8.

Celikel S, Karakaya G, Yurtsever N, Sorkun K, Kalyoncu AF. Bee and bee products allergy in Turkish beekeepers: determination of risk factors for systemic reactions. *Allergol Immunopathol (Madr).* 2006 Sep-Oct;34(5):180-4.

Centers for Disease Control and Prevention (CDC). Obesity prevalence among low-income, preschool-aged children - United States, 1998-2008. *MMWR Morb Mortal Wkly Rep.* 2009 Jul 24;58(28):769-73.

Centers for Disease Control and Prevention (CDC). Vital signs: nonsmokers' exposure to secondhand smoke - United States, 1999-2008. *MMWR Morb Mortal Wkly Rep.* 2010 Sep 10;59(35):1141-6.

Centre for Molecular, Environmental, Genetic and Analytic Epidemiology, School of Population Health, The UniverGumowski P, Lech B, Chaves I, Girard JP. Chronic asthma and rhinitis due to Candida albicans, epidermophyton, and trichophyton. *Ann Allergy.* 1987 Jul;59(1):48-51.

Cereijido M, Contreras RG, Flores-Benítez D, Flores-Maldonado C, Larre I, Ruiz A, Shoshani L. New diseases derived or associated with the tight junction. *Arch Med Res.* 2007 Jul;38(5):465-78.

Chafen JJ, Newberry SJ, Riedl MA, Bravata DM, Maglione M, Suttorp MJ, Sundaram V, Paige NM, Towfigh A, Hulley BJ, Shekelle PG. Diagnosing and managing common food allergies: a systematic review. *JAMA.* 2010 May 12;303(18):1848-56.

Chahine BG, Bahna SL. The role of the gut mucosal immunity in the development of tolerance versus development of allergy to food. *Curr Opin Allergy Clin Immunol.* 2010 Aug;10(4):394-9.

Chaitow L, Trenev N. *Probiotics: The revolutionary, 'friendly bacteria way to vital health and well-being.* New York: Thorsons, 1990.

Chaitow L. *Conquer Pain the Natural Way.* San Francisco: Chronicle Books, 2002.

Chakŭrski I, Matev M, Koĭchev A, Angelova I, Stefanov G. Treatment of chronic colitis with an herbal combination of Taraxacum officinale, Hipericum perforatum, Melissa officinaliss, Calendula officinalis and Foeniculum vulgare. *Vutr Boles.* 1981;20(6):51-4.

395

Chan CK, Kuo ML, Shen JJ, See LC, Chang HH, Huang JL. Ding Chuan Tang, a Chinese herb decoction, could improve airway hyper-responsiveness in stabilized asthmatic children: a randomized, double-blind clinical trial. *Pediatr Allergy Immunol.* 2006;17:316-22.

Chan YS, Xia L, Ng TB. White kidney bean lectin exerts anti-proliferative and apoptotic effects on cancer cells. Int J Biol Macromol. 2016 Apr;85:335-45. doi: 10.1016/j.ijbiomac.2015.12.094.

Chandra RK. Prospective studies of the effect of breast feeding on incidence of infection and allergy. *Acta Paediatr Scand.* 1979 Sep;68(5):691-4.

Chaney M, Ross M. *Nutrition.* New York: Houghton Mifflin, 1971.

Chang HT, Tseng LJ, Hung TJ, Kao BT, Lin WY, Fan TC, Chang MD, Pai TW. Inhibition of the interactions between eosinophil cationic protein and airway epithelial cells by traditional Chinese herbs. *BMC Syst Biol.* 2010 Sep 13;4 Suppl 2:S8.

Chang TT, Huang CC, Hsu CH. Clinical evaluation of the Chinese herbal medicine formula STA-1 in the treatment of allergic asthma. *Phytother Res.* 2006;20:342-7.

Chang TT, Huang CC, Hsu CH. Inhibition of mite-induced immunoglobulin E synthesis, airway inflammation, and hyperreactivity by herbal medicine STA-1. *Immunopharmacol Immunotoxicol.* 2006;28:683-95.

Chao A, Thun MJ, Connell CJ, McCullough ML, Jacobs EJ, Flanders WD, Rodriguez C, Sinha R, Calle EE. Meat consumption and risk of colorectal cancer. *JAMA.* 2005 Jan 12;293(2):172-82.

Chapat L, Chemin K, Dubois B, Bourdet-Sicard R, Kaiserlian D. Lactobacillus casei reduces CD8+ T cell-mediated skin inflammation. *Eur J Immunol.* 2004 Sep;34(9):2520-8.

Chapidze G, Kapanadze S, Dolidze N, Bachutashvili Z, Latsabidze N. Prevention of coronary atherosclerosis by the use of combination therapy with antioxidant coenzyme q10 and statins. *Georgian Med News.* 2005 Jan;(1):20-5.

Characterization and quantitation of Antioxidant Constituents of Sweet Pepper (Capsicum annuum - Cayenne). *J Agric Food Chem.* 2004 Jun 16;52(12):3861-9.

Chatzi L, Apostolaki G, Bibakis I, Skypala I, Bibaki-Liakou V, Tzanakis N, Kogevinas M, Cullinan P. Protective effect of fruits, vegetables and the Mediterranean diet on asthma and allergies among children in Crete. *Thorax.* 2007 Aug;62(8):677-83.

Chatzi L, Torrent M, Romieu I, Garcia-Esteban R, Ferrer C, Vioque J, Kogevinas M, Sunyer J. Mediterranean diet in pregnancy is protective for wheeze and atopy in childhood. *Thorax.* 2008 Jun;63(6):507-13.

Chaves TC, de Andrade e Silva TS, Monteiro SA, Watanabe PC, Oliveira AS, Grossi DB. Craniocervical posture and hyoid bone position in children with mild and moderate asthma and mouth breathing. *Int J Pediatr Otorhinolaryngol.* 2010 Sep;74(9):1021-7.

Chawes BL, Bønnelykke K, Kreiner-Møller E, Bisgaard H. Children with allergic and nonallergic rhinitis have a similar risk of asthma. *J Allergy Clin Immunol.* 2010 Sep;126(3):567-73.e1-8.

Chawes BL, Kreiner-Møller E, Bisgaard H. Objective assessments of allergic and nonallergic rhinitis in young children. *Allergy.* 2009 Oct;64(10):1547-53.

Chay WY, Tham CK, Toh HC, Lim HY, Tan CK, Lim C, Wang WW, Choo SP. Coriolus versicolor (Yunzhi) Use as Therapy in Advanced Hepatocellular Carcinoma Patients with Poor Liver Function or Who Are Unfit for Standard Therapy. J Altern Complement Med. 2017 Aug;23(8):648-652. doi: 10.1089/acm.2016.0136.

Chehade M, Aceves SS. Food allergy and eosinophilic esophagitis. *Curr Opin Allergy Clin Immunol.* 2010 Jun;10(3):231-7.

Chellini E, Talassi F, Corbo G, Berti G, De Sario M, Rusconi F, Piffer S, Caranci N, Petronio MG, Sestini P, Dell'Orco V, Bonci E, Armenio L, La Grutta S; Gruppo Collaborativo SIDRIA-2. Environmental, social and demographic characteristics of children and adolescents, resident in different Italian areas. *Epidemiol Prev.* 2005 Mar-Apr;29(2 Suppl):14-23.

Chen HJ, Shih CK, Hsu HY, Chiang W. Mast cell-dependent allergic responses are inhibited by ethanolic extract of adlay (Coix lachryma-jobi L. var. ma-yuen Stapf) testa. *J Agric Food Chem.* 2010 Feb 24;58(4):2596-601.

Chen JT, Tominaga K, Sato Y, Anzai H, Matsuoka R. Maitake mushroom (Grifola frondosa) extract induces ovulation in patients with polycystic ovary syndrome: a possible monotherapy and a combination therapy after failure with first-line clomiphene citrate. J Altern Complement Med. 2010 Dec;16(12):1295-9. doi: 10.1089/acm.2009.0696.

Chen JX, Ji B, Lu ZL, Hu LS. Effects of chai hu (radix burpleuri) containing formulation on plasma beta-endorphin, epinephrine and dopamine on patients. *Am J Chin Med.* 2005;33(5):737-45.

Chen M, Deng J, Su C, Li J, Wang M, Abuaku BK, Hu S, Tan H, Wen SW. Impact of passive smoking, cooking with solid fuel exposure, and MBL/MASP-2 gene polymorphism upon susceptibility to tuberculosis. Int J Infect Dis. 2014 Oct 10. pii: S1201-9712(14)01626-9. doi: 10.1016/j.ijid.2014.08.010.

Chen TQ, Wu JG, Kan YJ, Yang C, Wu YB, Wu JZ. Antioxidant and Hepatoprotective Activities of Reishi, Ganoderma lucidum Crude Polysaccharide Extracts, by Ultrasonic-Circulating Extraction. Int J Med Mushrooms. 2018;20(6):581-593. doi:10.1615/IntJMedMushrooms.2018026536.

Chen Y, Blaser MJ. Helicobacter pylori colonization is inversely associated with childhood asthma. *J Infect Dis.* 2008 Aug 15;198(4):553-60.

Chen Y, Blaser MJ. Inverse associations of Helicobacter pylori with asthma and allergy. *Arch Intern Med.* 2007 Apr 23;167(8):821-7.

Cheney G, Waxler SH, Miller IJ. Vitamin U therapy of peptic ulcer; experience at San Quentin Prison. *Calif Med.* 1956 Jan;84(1):39-42.

Chevallier A. *Encyclopedia of Medicinal Plants.* New York, NY: DK Publishing; 1996.

Chevrier MR, Ryan AE, Lee DY, Zhongze M, Wu-Yan Z, Via CS. Boswellia carterii extract inhibits TH1 cytokines and promotes TH2 cytokines in vitro. *Clin Diagn Lab Immunol.* 2005 May;12(5):575-80.

Chiang BL, Sheih YH, Wang LH, Liao CK, Gill HS. Enhancing immunity by dietary consumption of a probiotic lactic acid bacterium (*Bifidobacterium lactis* HN019): optimization and definition of cellular immune responses. *Eur J Clin Nutr.* 2000 Nov;54(11):849-55.

Chilton F, Tucker L. *Win the War Within.* New York: Rodale, 2006.

Chilton FH, Rudel LL, Parks JS, Arm JP, Seeds MC. Mechanisms by which botanical lipids affect inflammatory disorders. *Am J Clin Nutr.* 2008 Feb;87(2):498S-503S.

Chilton FH, Tucker L. *Win the War Within.* New York: Rodale, 2006.

Chin A Paw MJ, de Jong N, Pallast EG, Kloek GC, Schouten EG, Kok FJ. Immunity in frail elderly: a randomized controlled trial of exercise and enriched foods. *Med Sci Sports Exerc.* 2000 Dec;32(12):2005-11.

Choi YH, Park HS. Apoptosis in leukemia cells from garlic through generation of reactive oxygen species. J Biomed Sci. 2012 May 11;19(1):50.

Chong Neto HJ, Rosário NA; Grupo EISL Curitiba (Estudio Internacional de Sibilancias en Lactantes). Risk factors for wheezing in the first year of life. *J Pediatr.* 2008 Nov-Dec;84(6):495-502.

Chopra RN, Nayar SL, Chopra IC, eds. *Glossary of Indian Medicinal plants.* New Delhi: CSIR, 1956.

Choudhry S, Seibold MA, Borrell LN, Tang H, Serebrisky D, Chapela R, Rodriguez-Santana JR, Avila PC, Ziv E, Rodriguez-Cintron W, Risch NJ, Burchard EG. Dissecting complex diseases in complex populations: asthma in latino americans. *Proc Am Thorac Soc.* 2007 Jul;4(3):226-33.

Chouraqui JP, Grathwohl D, Labaune JM, Hascoet JM, de Montgollier I, Leclaire M, Giarre M, Steenhout P. Assessment of the safety, tolerance, and protective effect against diarrhea of infant formulas containing mixtures of probiotics or probiotics and prebiotics in a randomized controlled trial. *Am J Clin Nutr.* 2008 May;87(5):1365-73.

Christopher JR. *School of Natural Healing.* Springville UT: Christopher Publ, 1976.

Chu YF, Liu RH. Cranberries inhibit LDL oxidation and induce LDL receptor expression in hepatocytes. *Life Sci.* 2005;77(15):1892-1901. 27.

Chu YF, Liu RH. Cranberries inhibit LDL oxidation and induce LDL receptor expression in hepatocytes. *Life Sci.* 2005;77(15):1892-1901.

Chung SY, Butts CL, Maleki SJ, Champagne ET Linking peanut allergenicity to the processes of maturation, curing, and roasting. *J Agric Food Chem.* 2003;51: 4273-4277.

Chwirot WB, Popp F. White-light-induced luminescence and mitotic activity of yeast cells. *Folia Histochemica et Cytobiologica.* 1991;29(4):155.

Cianci A, Giordano R, Delia A, Grasso E, Amodeo A, De Leo V, Caccamo F. Efficacy of *Lactobacillus rhamnosus* GR-1 and of *Lactobacillus reuteri* RC-14 in the treatment and prevention of vaginoses and bacterial vaginitis relapses. *Minerva Ginecol.* 2008 Oct;60(5):369-76.

Cibella F, Cuttitta G. Nocturnal asthma and gastroesophageal reflux. *Am J Med.* 2001 Dec 3;111 Suppl 8A:31S-36S.

Cinatl J, Morgenstern B, Bauer G, Chandra P, Rabenau H, Doerr HW. Glycyrrhizin, an active component of liquorice roots, and replication of SARS-associated coronavirus. Lancet. 2003 Jun 14;361(9374):2045-6. doi: 10.1016/S0140-6736(03)13615-X

Cingi C, Demirbas D, Songu M. Allergic rhinitis caused by food allergies. *Eur Arch Otorhinolaryngol.* 2010 Sep;267(9):1327-35.

Ciprandi G, De Amici M, Negrini S, Marseglia G, Tosca MA. TGF-beta and IL-17 serum levels and specific immunotherapy. *Int Immunopharmacol.* 2009 Sep;9(10):1247-9.

Cisneros C, García-Río F, Romera D, Villasante C, Girón R, Ancochea J. Bronchial reactivity indices are determinants of health-related quality of life in patients with stable asthma. *Thorax.* 2010 Sep;65(9):795-800.

Clark S, Bock SA, Gaeta TJ, Brenner BE, Cydulka RK, Camargo CA; Multicenter Airway Research Collaboration-8 Investigators. Multicenter study of emergency department visits for food allergies. *J Allergy Clin Immunol.* 2004 Feb;113(2):347-52.

REFERENCES AND BIBLIOGRAPHY

Clayton EM, Todd M, Dowd JB, Aiello AE. The impact of bisphenol A and triclosan on immune parameters in the U.S. population, NHANES 2003-2006. Environ Health Perspect. 2011 Mar;119(3):390-6.

Clement YN, Williams AF, Aranda D, Chase R, Watson N, Mohammed R, Stubbs O, Williamson D. Medicinal herb use among asthmatic patients attending a specialty care facility in Trinidad. BMC Complement Altern Med. 2005 Feb 15;5:3.

Clerici M, Balotta C, Meroni L, Ferrario E, Riva C, Trabattoni D, Ridolfo A,Villa M, Shearer GM, Moroni M, Galli M. Type 1 cytokine production and low prevalence of viral isolation correlate with long-term nonprogression in HIV infection. AIDS Res Hum Retroviruses. 1996 Jul 20;12(11):1053-61.

Cobo Sanz JM, Mateos JA, Muñoz Conejo A. Effect of Lactobacillus casei on the incidence of infectious conditions in children. Nutr Hosp. 2006 Jul-Aug;21(4):547-51.

Codispoti CD, Levin L, LeMasters GK, Ryan P, Reponen T, Villareal M, Burkle J, Stanforth S, Lockey JE, Khurana Hershey GK, Bernstein DI. Breast-feeding, aeroallergen sensitization, and environmental exposures during infancy are determinants of childhood allergic rhinitis. J Allergy Clin Immunol. 2010 May;125(5):1054-1060.e1.

Cohen RT, Raby BA, Van Steen K, Fuhlbrigge AL, Celedón JC, Rosner BA, Strunk RC, Zeiger RS, Weiss ST; Childhood Asthma Management Program Research Group. In utero smoke exposure and impaired response to inhaled corticosteroids in children with asthma. J Allergy Clin Immunol. 2010 Sep;126(3):491-7. 2010 Jul 31. ; .

Cohen S, Popp F. Biophoton emission of the human body. J Photochem & Photobio. 1997;B 40:187-189.

Colecchia A, Vestito A, La Rocca A, Pasqui F, Nikiforaki A, Festi D; Symbiotic Study Group. Effect of a symbiotic preparation on the clinical manifestations of irritable bowel syndrome, constipation-variant. Results of an open, uncontrolled multicenter study. Minerva Gastroenterol Dietol. 2006 Dec;52(4):349-58.

Collipp PJ, Goldzier S 3rd, Weiss N, Soleymani Y, Snyder R. Pyridoxine treatment of childhood bronchial asthma. Ann Allergy. 1975 Aug;35(2):93-7.

Colodner R, Edelstein H, Chazan B, Raz R. Vaginal colonization by orally administered Lactobacillus rhamnosus GG. Isr Med Assoc J. 2003 Nov;5(11):767-9.

Conquer JA, Holub BJ. Dietary docosahexaenoic acid as a source of eicosapentaenoic acid in vegetarians and omnivores. Lipids. 1997 Mar;32(3):341-5.

Consumer Reports. Probiotics: Are enough in your diet? Cons Rpts Mag. 2005:34-35.

Conway PL, Gorbach SL, Goldin BR. Survival of lactic acid bacteria in the human stomach and adhesion to intestinal cells. J Dairy Sci. 1987 Jan;70(1):1-12.

Cooper GS, Miller FW, Germolec DR: Occupational exposures and autoimmune diseases. Int Immunopharm 2002, 2:303-313.

Cooper K. The Aerobics Program for Total Well-Being. New York: Evans, 1980.

Corbe C, Boissin JP, Siou A. Light vision and chorioretinal circulation. Study of the effect of procyanidolic oligomers (Endotelon). J Fr Ophtalmol. 1988;11(5):453-60.

Corbe C, Boissin JP, Siou A. Light vision and chorioretinal circulation. Study of the effect of procyanidolic oligomers (Endotelon). J Fr Ophtalmol. 1988;11(5):453-60.

Corbo GM, Forastiere F, De Sario M, Brunetti L, Bonci E, Bugiani M, Chellini E, La Grutta S, Migliore E, Pistelli R, Rusconi F, Russo A, Simoni M, Talassi F, Galassi C; Sidria-2 Collaborative Group. Wheeze and asthma in children: associations with body mass index, sports, television viewing, and diet. Epidemiology. 2008 Sep;19(5):747-55.

Corrêa NB, Péret Filho LA, Penna FJ, Lima FM, Nicoli JR. A randomized formula controlled trial of Bifidobacterium lactis and Streptococcus thermophilus for prevention of antibiotic-associated diarrhea in infants. J Clin Gastroenterol. 2005 May-Jun;39(5):385-9.

Cory S, Ussery-Hall A, Griffin-Blake S, Easton A, Vigeant J, Balluz L, Garvin W, Greenlund K; Centers for Disease Control and Prevention (CDC). Prevalence of selected risk behaviors and chronic diseases and conditions-steps communities, United States, 2006-2007. MMWR Surveill Summ. 2010 Sep 24;59(8):1-37.

Courtney R, Cohen M. Investigating the claims of Konstantin Buteyko, M.D., Ph.D.: the relationship of breath holding time to end tidal CO_2 and other proposed measures of dysfunctional breathing. J Altern Complement Med. 2008 Mar;14(2):115-23.

Couto E, Boffetta P, Lagiou P, Ferrari P, Buckland G, Overvad K, Dahm CC, Tjønneland A, Olsen A, Clavel-Chapelon F, Boutron-Ruault MC, Cottet V, Trichopoulos D, Naska A, Benetou V, Kaaks R, Rohrmann S, Boeing H, von Ruesten A, Panico S, Pala V, Vineis P, Palli D, Tumino R, May A, Peeters PH, Bueno-de-Mesquita HB, Büchner FL, Lund E, Skeie G, Engeset D, Gonzalez CA, Navarro C, Rodríguez L, Sánchez MJ, Amiano P, Barricarte A, Hallmans G, Johansson I, Manjer J, Wirfärt E, Allen NE, Crowe F, Khaw KT, Wareham N, Moskal A, Slimani N, Jenab M, Romaguera D, Mouw T, Norat T, Riboli E, Trichopoulou A. Mediterranean dietary pattern and cancer risk in the EPIC cohort. Br J Cancer. 2011 Apr 26;104(9):1493-9.

Couzy F, Kastenmayer P, Vigo M, Clough J, Munoz-Box R, Barclay DV. Calcium bioavailability from a calcium- and sulfate-rich mineral water, compared with milk, in young adult women. *Am J Clin Nutr.* 1995 Dec;62(6):1239-44.

Covar R, Gleason M, Macomber B, Stewart L, Szefler P, Engelhardt K, Murphy J, Liu A, Wood S, DeMichele S, Gelfand EW, Szefler SJ. Impact of a novel nutritional formula on asthma control and biomarkers of allergic airway inflammation in children. *Clin Exp Allergy.* 2010 Aug;40(8):1163-74. 2010 Jun 7.

Crane J, Ellis I, Siebers R, Grimmet D, Lewis S, Fitzharris P. A pilot study of the effect of mechanical ventilation and heat exchange on house-dust mites and Der p 1 in New Zealand homes. *Allergy.* 1998 Aug;53(8):755-62.

Crescente M, Jessen G, Momi S, Höltje HD, Gresele P, Cerletti C, de Gaetano G. Interactions of gallic acid, resveratrol, quercetin and aspirin at the platelet cyclooxygenase-1 level. Functional and modelling studies. *Thromb Haemost.* 2009 Aug;102(2):336-46.

Crews D, Gillette R, Scarpino SV, Manikkam M, Savenkova MI, Skinner MK. Epigenetic transgenerational inheritance of altered stress responses. Proc Natl Acad Sci U S A. 2012 May 21.

Crinnion WJ. Toxic effects of the easily avoidable phthalates and parabens. *Altern Med Rev.* 2010 Sep;15(3):190-6.

Crinnion WJ. Toxic effects of the easily avoidable phthalates and parabens. Altern Med Rev. 2010 Sep;15(3):190-6.

Cserhati E. Current view on the etiology of childhood bronchial asthma. *Orv Hetil.* 2000;141:759-760.

Cuesta-Herranz J, Barber D, Blanco C, Cistero-Bahíma A, Crespo JF, Fernández-Rivas M, Fernández-Sánchez J, Florido JF, Ibáñez MD, Rodríguez R, Salcedo G, Garcia BE, Lombardero M, Quiralte J, Rodriguez J, Sánchez-Monge R, Vereda A, Villalba M, Alonso Díaz de Durana MD, Basagaña M, Carrillo T, Fernández-Nieto M, Tabar AI. Differences among Pollen-Allergic Patients with and without Plant Food Allergy. *Int Arch Allergy Immunol.* 2010 Apr 23;153(2):182-192.

Cummings M. *Human Heredity: Principles and Issues.* St. Paul, MN: West, 1988.

Custovic A, Simpson BM, Simpson A, Kissen P, Woodcock A; NAC Manchester Asthma and Allergy Study Group. Effect of environmental manipulation in pregnancy and early life on respiratory symptoms and atopy during first year of life: a randomised trial. *Lancet.* 2001 Jul 21;358(9277):188-93.

D'Anneo RW, Bruno ME, Falagiani P. Sublingual allergoid immunotherapy: a new 4-day induction phase in patients allergic to house dust mites. *Int J Immunopathol Pharmacol.* 2010 Apr-Jun;23(2):553-60.

D'Auria E, Sala M, Lodi F, Radaelli G, Riva E, Giovannini M. Nutritional value of a rice-hydrolysate formula in infants with cows' milk protein allergy: a randomized pilot study. *J Int Med Res.* 2003 May-Jun;31(3):215-22.

D'Orazio N, Ficoneri C, Riccioni G, Conti P, Theoharides TC, Bollea MR. Conjugated linoleic acid: a functional food? *Int J Immunopathol Pharmacol.* 2003 Sep-Dec;16(3):215-20.

D'Urbano LE, Pellegrino K, Artesani MC, Donnanno S, Luciano R, Riccardi C, Tozzi AE, Ravà L, De Benedetti F, Cavagni G. Performance of a component-based allergen-microarray in the diagnosis of cow's milk and hen's egg allergy. *Clin Exp Allergy.* 2010 Jul 13.

Dalaly BK, Eitenmiller RR, Friend BA, Shahani KM. Human milk ribonuclease. *Biochim Biophys Acta.* 1980 Oct;615(2):381-91.

Dalaly BK, Eitenmiller RR, Vakil JR, Shahani KM. Simultaneous isolation of human milk ribonuclease and lysozyme. Anal Biochem. 1970 Sep;37(1):208-11.

Dalla Pellegrina C, Perbellini O, Scupoli MT, Tomelleri C, Zanetti C, Zoccatelli G, Fusi M, Peruffo A, Rizzi C, Chignola R. Effects of wheat germ agglutinin on human gastrointestinal epithelium: insights from an experimental model of immune/epithelial cell interaction. Toxicol Appl Pharmacol. 2009 Jun 1;237(2):146-53. doi: 10.1016/j.taap.2009.03.012.

Dallinga JW, Robroeks CM, van Berkel JJ, Moonen EJ, Godschalk RW, Jöbsis Q, Dompeling E, Wouters EF, van Schooten FJ. Volatile organic compounds in exhaled breath as a diagnostic tool for asthma in children. Clin Exp Allergy. 2010 Jan;40(1):68-76.

Davidson T. *Rhinology: The Collected Writings of Maurice H. Cottle, M.D.* San Diego, CA: American Rhinologic Society, 1987.

Davies G. *Timetables of Medicine.* New York: Black Dog & Leventhal, 2000.

Davin JC, Forget P, Mahieu PR. Increased intestinal permeability to (51 Cr) EDTA is correlated with IgA immune complex-plasma levels in children with IgA-associated nephropathies. *Acta Paediatr Scand.* 1988 Jan;77(1):118-24.

de Boissieu D, Dupont C, Badoual J. Allergy to nondairy proteins in mother's milk as assessed by intestinal permeability tests. *Allergy.* 1994 Dec;49(10):882-4.

De Lucca AJ, Bland JM, Vigo CB, Cushion M, Selitrennikoff CP, Peter J, Walsh TJ. CAY-I, a fungicidal saponin from Capsicum sp. fruit. *Med Mycol.* 2002 Apr;40(2):131-7.

De Preter V, Raemen H, Cloetens L, Houben E, Rutgeerts P, Verbeke K. Effect of dietary intervention with different pre- and probiotics on intestinal bacterial enzyme activities. *Eur J Clin Nutr.* 2008 Feb;62(2):225-31.

De Simone C, Ciardi A, Grassi A, Lambert Gardini S, Tzantzoglou S, Trinchieri V, Moretti S, Jirillo E. Effect of *Bifidobacterium bifidum* and *Lactobacillus acidophilus* on gut mucosa and peripheral blood B lymphocytes. *Immunopharmacol Immunotoxicol.* 1992;14(1-2):331-40.

De Smet PA. Herbal remedies. *N Engl J Med.* 2002;347:2046-2056.

de Souza TB, Raimundo PO, Andrade SF, Hipólito TM, Silva NC, Dias AL, Ikegaki M, Rocha RP, Coelho LF, Veloso MP, Carvalho DT, Dias DF. Synthesis and antimicrobial activity of 6-triazolo-6-deoxy eugenol glucosides. Carbohydr Res. 2015 Jun 17;410:1-8. doi: 10.1016/j.carres.2015.04.002.

de Vrese M, Rautenberg P, Laue C, Koopmans M, Herremans T, Schrezenmeir J. Probiotic bacteria stimulate virus-specific neutralizing antibodies following a booster polio vaccination. *Eur J Nutr.* 2005 Oct;44(7):406-13.

de Vrese M, Winkler P, Rautenberg P, Harder T, Noah C, Laue C, Ott S, Hampe J, Schreiber S, Heller K, Schrezenmeir J. Effect of *Lactobacillus gasseri* PA 16/8, *Bifidobacterium longum* SP 07/3, *B. bifidum* MF 20/5 on common cold episodes: a double blind, randomized, controlled trial. *Clin Nutr.* 2005 Aug;24(4):481-91.

Dean C. *Death by Modern Medicine.* Belleville, ON: Matrix Verite-Media, 2005.

Debley JS, Carter ER, Redding GJ. Prevalence and impact of gastroesophageal reflux in adolescents with asthma: a population-based study. *Pediatr Pulmonol.* 2006 May;41(5):475-81.

Dehlink E, Yen E, Leichtner AM, Hait EJ, Fiebiger E. First evidence of a possible association between gastric acid suppression during pregnancy and childhood asthma: a population-based register study. *Clin Exp Allergy.* 2009 Feb;39(2):246-53. 2008 Dec 9.

del Giudice MM, Leonardi S, Maiello N, Brunese FP. Food allergy and probiotics in childhood. *J Clin Gastroenterol.* 2010 Sep;44 Suppl 1:S22-5.

Delacourt C. Bronchial changes in untreated asthma. *Arch Pediatr.* 2004 Jun;11 Suppl 2:71s-73s.

Delia A, Morgante G, Rago G, Musacchio MC, Petraglia F, De Leo V. Effectiveness of oral administration of Lactobacillus paracasei subsp. paracasei F19 in association with vaginal suppositories of Lactobacillus acidofilus in the treatment of vaginosis and in the prevention of recurrent vaginitis. *Minerva Ginecol.* 2006 Jun;58(3):227-31.

Del-Rio-Navarro B, Berber A, Blandón-Vijil V, Ramírez-Aguilar M, Romieu I, Ramírez-Chanona N, Heras-Acevedo S, Serrano-Sierra A, Barraza-Villareal A, Baeza-Bacab M, Sienra-Monge JJ. Identification of asthma risk factors in Mexico City in an International Study of Asthma and Allergy in Childhood survey. *Allergy Asthma Proc.* 2006 Jul-Aug;27(4):325-33.

DeMan, JC, Rogosa M, Sharpe ME. A medium for the cultivation of lactobacilli. *J Bacteriol.* 1960:23;130.

Deng G, Lin H, Seidman A, Fornier M, D'Andrea G, Wesa K, Yeung S, Cunningham-Rundles S, Vickers AJ, Cassileth B. A phase I/II trial of a polysaccharide extract from Grifola frondosa (Maitake mushroom) in breast cancer patients: immunological effects. J Cancer Res Clin Oncol. 2009 Sep;135(9):1215-21. doi: 10.1007/s00432-009-0562-z.

Dengate S, Ruben A. Controlled trial of cumulative behavioural effects of a common bread preservative. *J Paediatr Child Health.* 2002 Aug;38(4):373-6.

Dente FL, Bacci E, Bartoli ML, Cianchetti S, Costa F, Di Franco A, Malagrinò L, Vagaggini B, Paggiaro P. Effects of oral prednisone on sputum eosinophils and cytokines in patients with severe refractory asthma. *Ann Allergy Asthma Immunol.* 2010 Jun;104(6):464-70.

Denys GA, Koch KM, Dowzicky MJ. Distribution of resistant gram-positive organisms across the census regions of the United States and in vitro activity of tigecycline, a new glycylcycline antimicrobial. *Am J Infect Control.* 2007 Oct;35(8):521-6.

Depeint F, Tzortzis G, Vulevic J, I'anson K, Gibson GR. Prebiotic evaluation of a novel galactooligosaccharide mixture produced by the enzymatic activity of *Bifidobacterium bifidum* NCIMB 41171, in healthy humans: a randomized, double-blind, crossover, placebo-controlled intervention study. *Am J Clin Nutr.* 2008 Mar;87(3):785-91.

Derebery MJ, Berliner KI. Allergy and its relation to Meniere's disease. *Otolaryngol Clin North Am.* 2010 Oct;43(5):1047-58.

Desbonnet L, Garrett L, Clarke G, Bienenstock J, Dinan TG. The probiotic Bifidobacteria infantis: An assessment of potential antidepressant properties in the rat. *J Psychiatr Res.* 2008 Dec;43(2):164-74.

Desjeux JF, Heyman M. Milk proteins, cytokines and intestinal epithelial functions in children. *Acta Paediatr Jpn.* 1994 Oct;36(5):592-6.

DesRoches A, Infante-Rivard C, Paradis L, Paradis J, Haddad E. Peanut allergy: is maternal transmission of antigens during pregnancy and breastfeeding a risk factor? *J Investig Allergol Clin Immunol.* 2010;20(4):289-94.

Deutsche Gesellschaft für Ernährung. Drink distilled water? *Med. Mo. Pharm.* 1993;16:146.

Devaraj TL. *Speaking of Ayurvedic Remedies for Common Diseases.* New Delhi: Sterling, 1985.

Devirgiliis C, Zalewski PD, Perozzi G, Murgia C. Zinc fluxes and zinc transporter genes in chronic diseases. *Mutat Res.* 2007 Sep 1;622(1-2):84-93. 2007 Feb 17.

DeWitt RC, Kudsk KA. The gut's role in metabolism, mucosal barrier function, and gut immunology. *Infect Dis Clin North Am.* 1999 Jun;13(2):465-81.

Dharmage SC, Erbas B, Jarvis D, Wjst M, Raherison C, Norbäck D, Heinrich J, Sunyer J, Svanes C. Do childhood respiratory infections continue to influence adult respiratory morbidity? *Eur Respir J.* 2009 Feb;33(2):237-44.

Di Gioacchino M, Cavallucci E, Di Stefano F, Paolini F, Ramondo S, Di Sciascio MB, Ciuffreda S, Riccioni G, Della Vecchia R, Romano A, Boscolo P. Effect of natural allergen exposure on non-specific bronchial reactivity in asthmatic farmers. *Sci Total Environ.* 2001 Apr 10;270(1-3):43-8.

Di Gioacchino M, Cavallucci E, Di Stefano F, Verna N, Ramondo S, Ciuffreda S, Riccioni G, Boscolo P. Influence of total IgE and seasonal increase of eosinophil cationic protein on bronchial hyperreactivity in asthmatic grass-sensitized farmers. *Allergy.* 2000 Nov;55(11):1030-4.

Di Marzio L, Centi C, Cinque B, Masci S, Giuliani M, Arcieri A, Zicari L, De Simone C, Cifone MG. Effect of the lactic acid bacterium *Streptococcus thermophilus* on stratum corneum ceramide levels and signs and symptoms of atopic dermatitis patients. *Exp Dermatol.* 2003 Oct;12(5):615-20.

Dias Rde O, Machado Ldos S, Migliolo L, Franco OL. Insights into animal and plant lectins with antimicrobial activities. Molecules. 2015 Jan 5;20(1):519-41. doi: 10.3390/molecules20010519.

Dierksen KP, Moore CJ, Inglis M, Wescombe PA, Tagg JR. The effect of ingestion of milk supplemented with salivaricin A-producing Streptococcus salivarius on the bacteriocin-like inhibitory activity of streptococcal populations on the tongue. *FEMS Microbiol Ecol.* 2007 Mar;59(3):584-91.

Diğrak M, Ilçim A, Hakki Alma M. Antimicrobial activities of several parts of Pinus brutia, Juniperus oxycedrus, Abies cilicia, Cedrus libani and Pinus nigra. *Phytother Res.* 1999 Nov;13(7):584-7.

DiMango E, Holbrook JT, Simpson E, Reibman J, Richter J, Narula S, Prusakowski N, Mastronarde JG, Wise RA; American Lung Association Asthma Clinical Research Centers. Effects of asymptomatic proximal and distal gastroesophageal reflux on asthma severity. *Am J Respir Crit Care Med.* 2009 Nov 1;180(9):809-16. 2009 Aug 6.

Dimitonova SP, Danova ST, Serkedjieva JP, Bakalov BV. Antimicrobial activity and protective properties of vaginal lactobacilli from healthy Bulgarian women. *Anaerobe.* 2007 Oct-Dec;13(5-6):178-84.

Din FV, Theodoratou E, Farrington SM, Tenesa A, Barnetson RA, Cetnarskyj R, Stark L, Porteous ME, Campbell H, Dunlop MG. Effect of aspirin and NSAIDs on risk and survival from colorectal cancer. *Gut.* 2010 Dec;59(12):1670-9.

Ding X, Yang Q, Kong X, Haffty BG, Gao S, Moran MS. Radiosensitization effect of Huaier on breast cancer cells. Oncol Rep. 2016 May;35(5):2843-50. doi: 10.3892/or.2016.4630.

Ding Y, Seow SV, Huang CH, Liew LM, Lim YC, Kuo IC, Chua KY. Coadministration of Golden needle mushroom Flammulina velutipes and HPV tumors Immunology. 2009 Sep;128(1 Suppl):e881-94. doi: 10.1111/j.1365-2567.2009.03099.x.

Dinleyici EC, Eren M, Yargic ZA, Dogan N, Vandenplas Y. Clinical efficacy of *Saccharomyces boulardii* and metronidazole compared to metronidazole alone in children with acute bloody diarrhea caused by amebiasis: a prospective, randomized, open label study. *Am J Trop Med Hyg.* 2009 Jun;80(6):953-5.

Diop L, Guillou S, Durand H. Probiotic food supplement reduces stress-induced gastrointestinal symptoms in volunteers: a double-blind, placebo-controlled, randomized trial. *Nutr Res.* 2008 Jan;28(1):1-5.

Dixon AE, Kaminsky DA, Holbrook JT, Wise RA, Shade DM, Irvin CG. Allergic rhinitis and sinusitis in asthma: differential effects on symptoms and pulmonary function. *Chest.* 2006 Aug;130(2):429-35.

Dona A, Arvanitoyannis IS. Health risks of genetically modified foods. *Crit Rev Food Sci Nutr.* 2009 Feb;49(2):164-75.

Donatini B. Control of Oral Human Papillomavirus (HPV) by Medicinal Mushrooms, Trametes versicolor and Ganoderma lucidum: A PreliminaryClinical Trial. Int J Med Mushrooms. 2014;16(5):497-8.

Donato F, Monarca S, Premi S., and Gelatti, U. Drinking water hardness and chronic degenerative diseases. Part III. Tumors, urolithiasis, fetal malformations, deterioration of the cognitive function in the aged and atopic eczema. *Ann. Ig.* 2003;15:57-70.

Dooley, M.A. and Hogan S.L. Environmental epidemiology and risk factors for autoimmune disease. *Curr Opin Rheum.* 2003;15(2):99-103.

dos Santos LH, Ribeiro IO, Sánchez PG, Hetzel JL, Felicetti JC, Cardoso PF. Evaluation of pantoprazol treatment response of patients with asthma and gastroesophageal reflux: a randomized prospective double-blind placebo-controlled study. *J Bras Pneumol.* 2007 Apr;33(2):119-27.

Dotolo Institute. *The Study of Colon Hydrotherapy.* Pinellas Park, FL: Dotolo, 2003.

Dove MS, Dockery DW, Connolly GN. Smoke-free air laws and asthma prevalence, symptoms, and severity among nonsmoking youth. *Pediatrics.* 2011 Jan;127(1):102-9. 2010 Dec 13.

Dowd JB, Zajacova A, Aiello A. Early origins of health disparities: burden of infection, health, and socioeconomic status in U.S. children. *Soc Sci Med.* 2009 Feb;68(4):699-707. 2009 Jan 17.

REFERENCES AND BIBLIOGRAPHY

Drago L, De Vecchi E, Nicola L, Zucchetti E, Gismondo MR, Vicariotto F. Activity of a *Lactobacillus acidophilus*-based douche for the treatment of bacterial vaginosis. *J Altern Complement Med.* 2007 May;13(4):435-8.

Drouault-Holowacz S, Bieuvelet S, Burckel A, Cazaubiel M, Dray X, Marteau P. A double blind randomized controlled trial of a probiotic combination in 100 patients with irritable bowel syndrome. *Gastroenterol Clin Biol.* 2008 Feb;32(2):147-52.

Drubaix I, Maraval M, Robert L, Robert AM. Hyaluronic acid (hyaluronan) levels in pathological human saphenous veins. Effects of procyanidol oligomers, *Pathol Biol.* 1997 Jan;45(1):86-91.

Drubaix I, Robert L, Maraval M, Robert AM. Synthesis of glycoconjugates by human diseased veins: modulation by procyanidolic oligomers. *Int J Exp Pathol.* 1997 Apr;78(2):117-21.

Ducrotté P. Irritable bowel syndrome: from the gut to the brain-gut. *Gastroenterol Clin Biol.* 2009 Aug-Sep;33(8-9):703-12.

Duke J. *CRC Handbook of Medicinal Herbs.* Boca Raton: CRC; 1989.

Duke J. *The Green Pharmacy.* New York: St. Martins, 1997.

Dunstan JA, Roper J, Mitoulas L, Hartmann PE, Simmer K, Prescott SL. The effect of supplementation with fish oil during pregnancy on breast milk immunoglobulin A, soluble CD14, cytokine levels and fatty acid composition. *Clin Exp Allergy.* 2004 Aug;34(8):1237-42.

Duong M, Subbarao P, Adelroth E, Obminski G, Strinich T, Inman M, Pedersen S, O'Byrne PM. Sputum eosinophils and the response of exercise-induced bronchoconstriction to corticosteroid in asthma. *Chest.* 2008 Feb;133(2):404-11. 2007 Dec 10.

Dupont C, Barau E, Molkhou P, Raynaud F, Barbet JP, Dehennin L. Food-induced alterations of intestinal permeability in children with cow's milk-sensitive enteropathy and atopic dermatitis. *J Pediatr Gastroenterol Nutr.* 1989 May;8(4):459-65.

Dupont C, Barau E, Molkhou P. Intestinal permeability disorders in children. *Allerg Immunol.* 1991 Mar;23(3):95-103.

Dupont C, Soulaines P, Lapillonne A, Donne N, Kalach N, Benhamou P. Atopy patch test for early diagnosis of cow's milk allergy in preterm infants. *J Pediatr Gastroenterol Nutr.* 2010 Apr;50(4):463-4.

Dupuy P, Cassé M, André F, Dhivert-Donnadieu H, Pinton J, Hernandez-Pion C. Low-salt water reduces intestinal permeability in atopic patients. *Dermatology.* 1999;198(2):153-5.

Duran-Tauleria E, Vignati G, Guedan MJ, Petersson CJ. The utility of specific immunoglobulin E measurements in primary care. *Allergy.* 2004 Aug;59 Suppl 78:35-41.

Duwiejua M, Zeitlin IJ, Waterman PG, Chapman J, Mhango GJ, Provan GJ. Anti-inflammatory activity of resins from some species of the plant family Burseraceae. *Planta Med.* 1993 Feb;59(1):12-6.

Dykewicz MS, Lemmon JK, Keaney DL. Comparison of the Multi-Test II and Skintestor Omni allergy skin test devices. *Ann Allergy Asthma Immunol.* 2007 Jun;98(6):559-62.

Eastham EJ, Walker WA. Effect of cow's milk on the gastrointestinal tract: a persistent dilemma for the pediatrician. *Pediatrics.* 1977 Oct;60(4):477-81.

Eaton KK, Howard M, Howard JM. Gut permeability measured by polyethylene glycol absorption in abnormal gut fermentation as compared with food intolerance. *J R Soc Med.* 1995 Feb;88(2):63-6.

Ebers GC, Kukay K, Bulman DE, Sadovnick AD, Rice G, Anderson C, Armstrong H, Cousin K, Bell RB, Hader W, Paty DW, Hashimoto S, Oger J, Duquette P, Warren S, Gray T, O'Connor P, Nath A, Auty A, Metz L, Francis G, Paulseth JE, Murray TJ, Pryse-Phillips W, Nelson R, Freedman M, Brunet D, Bouchard JP, Hinds D, Risch N. A full genome search in multiple sclerosis. *Nat Genet.* 1996 Aug;13(4):472-6.

Eccles R. Menthol and related cooling compounds. *J Pharm Pharmacol.* 1994 Aug;46(8):618-30.

ECRHS (2002) The European Community Respiratory Health Survey II. *Eur Respir J.* 20: 1071-1079.

Edgecombe K, Latter S, Peters S, Roberts G. Health experiences of adolescents with uncontrolled severe asthma. *Arch Dis Child.* 2010 Dec;95(12):985-91. 2010 Jul 30.

Edgell PG. The psychology of asthma. *Can Med Assoc J.* 1952 Aug;67(2):121-5.

Egashira Y, Nagano H. A multicenter clinical trial of TJ-96 in patients with steroid-dependent bronchial asthma. A comparison of groups allocated by the envelope method. *Ann N Y Acad Sci.* 1993 Jun 23;685:580-3.

Ege MJ, Frei R, Bieli C, Schram-Bijkerk D, Waser M, Benz MR, Weiss G, Nyberg F, van Hage M, Pershagen G, Brunekreef B, Riedler J, Lauener R, Braun-Fahrländer C, von Mutius E; PARSIFAL Study team. Not all farming environments protect against the development of asthma and wheeze in children. *J Allergy Clin Immunol.* 2007 May;119(5):1140-7.

Ege MJ, Herzum I, Büchele G, Krauss-Etschmann S, Lauener RP, Roponen M, Hyvärinen A, Vuitton DA, Riedler J, Brunekreef B, Dalphin JC, Braun-Fahrländer C, Pekkanen J, Renz H, von Mutius E; Protection Against Allergy Study in Rural Environments (PASTURE) Study group. Prenatal exposure to a farm environment modifies atopic sensitization at birth. *J Allergy Clin Immunol.* 2008 Aug;122(2):407-12, 412.e1-4.

Eggermont E. Cow's milk protein allergy. *Tijdschr Kindergeneeskd.* 1981 Feb;49(1):16-20.

Eguchi N, Fujino K, Thanasut K, Taharaguchi M, Motoi M, Motoi A, Oonaka K, Taharaguchi S. In vitro Anti-Influenza Virus Activity of Agaricus brasiliensis KA21. Biocontrol Sci. 2017;22(3):171-174. doi: 10.4265/bio.22.171.

Eguchi N, Fujino K, Thanasut K, Taharaguchi M, Motoi M, Motoi A, Oonaka K, Taharaguchi S. In vitro Anti-Influenza Virus Activity of Agaricus brasiliensis KA21. Biocontrol Sci. 2017;22(3):171-174. doi: 10.4265/bio.22.171.

Ehling S, Hengel M, and Shibamoto T. Formation of acrylamide from lipids. *Adv Exp Med Biol* 2005, 561:223-233.

Ehnert B, Lau-Schadendorf S, Weber A, Buettner P, Schou C, Wahn U. Reducing domestic exposure to dust mite allergen reduces bronchial hyperreactivity in sensitive children with asthma. *J Allergy Clin Immunol.* 1992 Jul;90(1):135-8.

Ehren J, Morón B, Martin E, Bethune MT, Gray GM, Khosla C. A food-grade enzyme preparation with modest gluten detoxification properties. *PLoS One.* 2009 Jul 21;4(7):e6313.

Eijkemans M, Mommers M, de Vries SI, van Buuren S, Stafleu A, Bakker I, Thijs C. Asthmatic symptoms, physical activity, and overweight in young children: a cohort study. *Pediatrics.* 2008 Mar;121(3):e666-72.

Eldridge MW, Peden DB. Allergen provocation augments endotoxin-induced nasal inflammation in subjects with atopic asthma. *J Allergy Clin Immunol.* 2000 Mar;105(3):475-81.

el-Ghazaly M, Khayyal MT, Okpanyi SN, Arens-Corell M. Study of the anti-inflammatory activity of Populus tremula, Solidago virgaurea and Fraxinus excelsior. *Arzneimittelforschung.* 1992 Mar;42(3):333-6.

Ellingwood F. *American Materia Medica, Therapeutics and Pharmacognosy.* Portland: Eclectic Medical Publ., 1983.

Elliott RB, Harris DP, Hill JP, Bibby NJ, Wasmuth HE. Type I (insulin-dependent) diabetes mellitus and cow milk: casein variant consumption. *Diabetologia.* 1999 Mar;42(3):292-6.

Elmer GW, McFarland LV, Surawicz CM, Danko L, Greenberg RN. Behaviour of *Saccharomyces boulardii* in recurrent *Clostridium difficile* disease patients. *Aliment Pharmacol Ther.* 1999 Dec;13(12):1663-8.

Elwood PC. Epidemiology and trace elements. *Clin Endocrinol Metab.* 1985 Aug;14(3):617-28.

Emberlin JC, Lewis RA. Pollen challenge study of a phototherapy device for reducing the symptoms of hay fever. *Curr Med Res Opin.* 2009 Jul;25(7):1635-44.

Emmanouil E, Manios Y, Grammatikaki E, Kondaki K, Oikonomou E, Papadopoulos N, Vassilopoulou E. Association of nutrient intake and wheeze or asthma in a Greek pre-school population. *Pediatr Allergy Immunol.* 2010 Feb;21(1 Pt 1):90-5. 2009 Sep 9.

Engler RJ. Alternative and complementary medicine: a source of improved therapies for asthma? A challenge for redefining the specialty? *J Allergy Clin Immunol.* 2000;106:627-9.

Environmental Working Group. *Human Toxome Project.* 2007. http://www.ewg.org/sites/humantoxome/. Accessed: 2007 Sep.

EPA. *A Brief Guide to Mold, Moisture and Your Home.* Environmental Protection Agency, Office of Air and Radiation/Indoor Environments Division. EPA 2002;402-K-02-003.

Epstein GN, Halper JP, Barrett EA, Birdsall C, McGee M, Baron KP, Lowenstein S. A pilot study of mind-body changes in adults with asthma who practice mental imagery. *Altern Ther Health Med.* 2004 Jul-Aug;10(4):66-71.

Erkkola M, Kaila M, Nwaru BI, Kronberg-Kippilä C, Ahonen S, Nevalainen J, Veijola R, Pekkanen J, Ilonen J, Simell O, Knip M, Virtanen SM. Maternal vitamin D intake during pregnancy is inversely associated with asthma and allergic rhinitis in 5-year-old children. *Clin Exp Allergy.* 2009 Jun;39(6):875-82.

Ernst E. Frankincense: systematic review. *BMJ.* 2008 Dec 17;337:a2813.

Erwin EA, James HR, Gutekunst HM, Russo JM, Kelleher KJ, Platts-Mills TA. Serum IgE measurement and detection of food allergy in pediatric patients with eosinophilic esophagitis. *Ann Allergy Asthma Immunol.* 2010 Jun;104(6):496-502.

EuroPrevall. *WP 1.1 Birth Cohort Update.* 1st Quarter 2006. Berlin, Germany: Charité University Medical Centre.

Evans P, Forte D, Jacobs C, Fredhoi C, Aitchison E, Hucklebridge F, Clow A. Cortisol secretory activity in older people in relation to positive and negative well-being. *Psychoneuroendocrinology.* 2007 Aug 7

Everhart JE. *Digestive Diseases in the United States.* Darby, PA: Diane Pub, 1994.

FAAN. *Public Comment on 2005 Food Safety Survey: Docket No. 2004N-0516 (2005 FSS).* Fairfax, VA: Food Allergy & Anaphylaxis Network.

Fabian E, Elmadfa I. Influence of daily consumption of probiotic and conventional yoghurt on the plasma lipid profile in young healthy women. *Ann Nutr Metab.* 2006;50(4):387-93.

Fabian E, Majchrzak D, Dieminger B, Meyer E, Elmadfa I. Influence of probiotic and conventional yoghurt on the status of vitamins B1, B2 and B6 in young healthy women. *Ann Nutr Metab.* 2008;52(1):29-36.

Fairchild SS, Shannon K, Kwan E, Mishell RI. T cell-derived glucosteroid response-modifying factor (GRMFT): a unique lymphokine made by normal T lymphocytes and a T cell hybridoma. *J Immunol.* 1984 Feb;132(2):821-7.

Fälth-Magnusson K, Kjellman NI, Magnusson KE, Sundqvist T. Intestinal permeability in healthy and allergic children before and after sodium-cromoglycate treatment assessed with different-sized polyethyleneglycols (PEG 400 and PEG 1000). *Clin Allergy*. 1984 May;14(3):277-86.

Fälth-Magnusson K, Kjellman NI, Odelram H, Sundqvist T, Magnusson KE. Gastrointestinal permeability in children with cow's milk allergy: effect of milk challenge and sodium cromoglycate as assessed with polyethyleneglycols (PEG 400 and PEG 1000). *Clin Allergy*. 1986 Nov;16(6):543-51.

Falzarano D, de Wit E, Rasmussen AL, Feldmann F, Okumura A, Scott DP, Brining D, Bushmaker T, Martellaro C, Baseler L, Benecke AG, Katze MG, Munster VJ, Feldmann H. Treatment with interferon-α2b and ribavirin improves outcome in MERS-CoV-infected rhesus macaques. Nat Med. 2013 Oct;19(10):1313-7. doi: 10.1038/nm.3362.

Fan AY, Lao L, Zhang RX, Zhou AN, Wang LB, Moudgil KD, Lee DY, Ma ZZ, Zhang WY, Berman BM. Effects of an acetone extract of Boswellia carterii Birdw. (Burseraceae) gum resin on adjuvant-induced arthritis in lewis rats. *J Ethnopharmacol*. 2005 Oct 3;101(1-3):104-9.

Fanaro S, Marten B, Bagna R, Vigi V, Fabris C, Peña-Quintana, Argüelles F, Scholz-Ahrens KE, Sawatzki G, Zelenka R, Schrezenmeir J, de Vrese M and Bertino E. Galacto-oligosaccharides are bifidogenic and safe at weaning: A double-blind Randomized Multicenter study. *J Pediatr Gastroent Nutr*. 2009 48; 82-88

Fang H, Elina T, Heikki A, Seppo S. Modulation of humoral immune response through probiotic intake. *FEMS Immunol Med Microbiol*. 2000 Sep;29(1):47-52.

Fang SP, Tanaka T, Tago F, Okamoto T, Kojima S. Immunomodulatory effects of gyokuheifusan on INF-gamma/IL-4 (Th1/Th2) balance in ovalbumin (OVA)-induced asthma model mice. *Biol Pharm Bull*. 2005;28:829-33.

Fang T, Liu DD, Ning HM, Dan Liu, Sun JY, Huang XJ, Dong Y, Geng MY, Yun SF, Yan J, Huang RM. Modified citrus pectin inhibited bladder tumor growth through downregulation of galectin-3. Acta Pharmacol Sin. 2018 May 16. doi:10.1038/s41401-018-0004-z.

Fanigliulo L, Comparato G, Aragona G, Cavallaro L, Iori V, Maino M, Cavestro GM, Soliani P, Sianesi M, Franzè A, Di Mario F. Role of gut microflora and probiotic effects in the irritable bowel syndrome. *Acta Biomed*. 2006 Aug;77(2):85-9.

FAO/WHO Expert Committee. *Fats and Oils in Human Nutrition*. Food and Nutrition Paper. 1994;(57).

Farber JE, Ross J, Stephens G. Antibiotic anaphylaxis. *Calif Med*. 1954 Jul;81(1):9-11.

Farber JE, Ross J. Antibiotic anaphylaxis; a note on the treatment and prevention of severe reactions to penicillin, streptomycin and dihydrostreptomycin. *Med Times*. 1952 Jan;80(1):28-30.

Fasano A, Shea-Donohue T. Mechanisms of disease: the role of intestinal barrier function in the pathogenesis of gastrointestinal autoimmune diseases. *Nat Clin Pract Gastroenterol Hepatol*. 2005 Sep;2(9):416-22.

Fawell J, Nieuwenhuijsen MJ. Contaminants in drinking water. *Br Med Bull*. 2003;68:199-208.

Fecka I. Qualitative and quantitative determination of hydrolysable tannins and other polyphenols in herbal products from meadowsweet and dog rose. *Phytochem Anal*. 2009 May;20(3):177-90.

Felley CP, Corthésy-Theulaz I, Rivero JL, Sipponen P, Kaufmann M, Bauerfeind P, Wiesel PH, Brassart D, Pfeifer A, Blum AL, Michetti P. Favourable effect of an acidified milk (LC-1) on *Helicobacter pylori* gastritis in man. *Eur J Gastroenterol Hepatol*. 2001 Jan;13(1):25-9.

Feng Yeh C, Wang KC, Chiang LC, Shieh DE, Yen MH, San Chang J. Water extract of licorice had anti-viral activity against human respiratory syncytial virus in human respiratory tract cell lines. J Ethnopharmacol. 2013 Jul 9;148(2):466-73. doi: 10.1016/j.jep.2013.04.040.

Ferencík M, Ebringer L, Mikes Z, Jahnová E, Ciznár I. Successful modification of human intestinal microflora with oral administration of lactic acid bacteria. *Bratisl Lek Listy*. 1999 May;100(5):238-45.

Ferguson BJ. Categorization of eosinophilic chronic rhinosinusitis. *Curr Opin Otolaryngol Head Neck Surg*. 2004 Jun;12(3):237-42.

Ferrari M, Benini L, Brotto E, Locatelli F, De Iorio F, Bonella F, Tacchella N, Corradini G, Lo Cascio V, Vantini I. Omeprazole reduces the response to capsaicin but not to methacholine in asthmatic patients with proximal reflux. *Scand J Gastroenterol*. 2007 Mar;42(3):299-307.

Ferrier L, Berard F, Debrauwer L, Chabo C, Langella P, Bueno L, Fioramonti J. Impairment of the intestinal barrier by ethanol involves enteric microflora and mast cell activation in rodents. *Am J Pathol*. 2006 Apr;168(4):1148-54.

Ferrier L, Berard F, Debrauwer L, Chabo C, Langella P, Bueno L, Fioramonti J. Impairment of the intestinal barrier by ethanol involves enteric microflora and mast cell activation in rodents. *Am J Pathol*. 2006 Apr;168(4):1148-54.

Feske S, Wulff H, Skolnik EY. Ion channels in innate and adaptive immunity. Annu Rev Immunol. 2015;33:291-353. doi: 10.1146/annurev-immunol-032414-112212.

Field RW, Krewski D, Lubin JH, Zielinski JM, Alavanja M, Catalan VS, Klotz JB, Létourneau EG, Lynch CF, Lyon JL, Sandler DP, Schoenberg JB, Steck DJ, Stolwijk JA, Weinberg C, Wilcox HB. An overview of the North American residential radon and lung cancer case-control studies. *J Toxicol Environ Health A*. 2006 Apr;69(7):599-631.

Field T, Henteleff T, Hernandez-Reif M, Martinez E, Mavunda K, Kuhn C, Schanberg S. Children with asthma have improved pulmonary functions after massage therapy. *J Pediatr.* 1998 May;132(5):854-8.

Finkelman FD, Boyce JA, Vercelli D, Rothenberg ME. Key advances in mechanisms of asthma, allergy, and immunology in 2009. *J Allergy Clin Immunol.* 2010 Feb;125(2):312-8.

Fiocchi, A; Restani, P; Riva, E; Qualizza, R; Bruni, P; Restelli, AR; Galli, CL. Meat allergy: I. Specific IgE to BSA and OSA in atopic, beef sensitive children. *J Am Coll Nutr.* 1995 14: 239-244.

Fiore C, Eisenhut M, Krausse R, Ragazzi E, Pellati D, Armanini D, Bielenberg J. Antiviral effects of Glycyrrhiza species. Phytother Res. 2008 Feb;22(2):141-8. http://dx.doi.org/10.1002/ptr.2295

Firenzuoli, F.; Gori, L.; Lombardo, G. The medicinal mushrooms Agaricus blazeiMurrill: Review of literature and pharmaco-toxicological problems. Evid. Based Complement. Alternat. Med. 2008, 5, 3–15.

Firmesse O, Alvaro E, Mogenet A, Bresson JL, Lemée R, Le Ruyet P, Bonhomme C, Lambert D, Andrieux C, Doré J, Corthier G, Furet JP, Rigottier-Gois L. Fate and effects of Camembert cheese micro-organisms in the human colonic microbiota of healthy volunteers after regular Camembert consumption. *Int J Food Microbiol.* 2008 Jul 15;125(2):176-81.

Fjeld T, Veiersted B, Sandvik L, Riise G, Levy F. The Effect of Indoor Foliage Plants on Health and Discomfort Symptoms among Office Workers. *Ind Built Environ.* 1998 July;7(4): 204-209.

Flandrin, J, Montanari M. (eds.). *Food: A Culinary History from Antiquity to the Present.* New York: Penguin Books, 1999.

Fleischer DM, Conover-Walker MK, Christie L, Burks AW, Wood RA. Peanut allergy: recurrence and its management. *J Allergy Clin Immunol.* 2004 Nov;114(5):1195-201.

Flinterman AE, van Hoffen E, den Hartog Jager CF, Koppelman S, Pasmans SG, Hoekstra MO, Bruijnzeel-Koomen CA, Knulst AC, Knol EF. Children with peanut allergy recognize predominantly Ara h2 and Ara h6, which remains stable over time. *Clin Exp Allergy.* 2007 Aug;37(8):1221-8.

Foliaki S, Annesi-Maesano I, Tuuau-Potoi N, Waqatakirewa L, Cheng S, Douwes J, Pearce N. Risk factors for symptoms of childhood asthma, allergic rhinoconjunctivitis and eczema in the Pacific: an ISAAC Phase III study. *Int J Tuberc Lung Dis.* 2008 Jul;12(7):799-806.

Forbes EE, Groschwitz K, Abonia JP, Brandt EB, Cohen E, Blanchard C, Ahrens R, Seidu L, McKenzie A, Strait R, Finkelman FD, Foster PS, Matthaei KI, Rothenberg ME, Hogan SP. IL-9- and mast cell-mediated intestinal permeability predisposes to oral antigen hypersensitivity. *J Exp Med.* 2008 Apr 14;205(4):897-913.

Forestier C, Guelon D, Cluytens V, Gillart T, Sirot J, De Champs C. Oral probiotic and prevention of Pseudomonas aeruginosa infections: a randomized, double-blind, placebo-controlled pilot study in intensive care unit patients. *Crit Care.* 2008;12(3):R69.

Forestier C, Guelon D, Cluytens V, Gillart T, Sirot J, De Champs C. Oral probiotic and prevention of Pseudomonas aeruginosa infections: a randomized, double-blind, placebo-controlled pilot study in intensive care unit patients. *Crit Care.* 2008;12(3):R69.

Forget-Dubois N, Boivin M, Dionne G, Pierce T, Tremblay RE, Pérusse D. A longitudinal twin study of the genetic and environmental etiology of maternal hostile-reactive behavior during infancy and toddlerhood. *Infant Behav Dev.* 2007

Foster S, Hobbs C. *Medicinal Plants and Herbs.* Boston: Houghton Mifflin, 2002.

Fox RD, *Algoculture.* Doctorate Disseration, 1983 Jul.

Francavilla R, Lionetti E, Castellaneta SP, Magistà AM, Maurogiovanni G, Bucci N, De Canio A, Indrio F, Cavallo L, Ierardi E, Miniello VL. Inhibition of Helicobacter pylori infection in humans by Lactobacillus reuteri ATCC 55730 and effect on eradication therapy: a pilot study. *Helicobacter.* 2008 Apr;13(2):127-34.

Francavilla R, Lionetti E, Castellaneta SP, Magistà AM, Maurogiovanni G, Bucci N, De Canio A, Indrio F, Cavallo L, Ierardi E, Miniello VL. Inhibition of *Helicobacter pylori* infection in humans by *Lactobacillus reuteri* ATCC 55730 and effect on eradication therapy: a pilot study. *Helicobacter.* 2008 Apr;13(2):127-34.

Francis H, Fletcher G, Anthony C, Pickering C, Oldham L, Hadley E, Custovic A, Niven R. Clinical effects of air filters in homes of asthmatic adults sensitized and exposed to pet allergens. *Clin Exp Allergy.* 2003 Jan;33(1):101-5.

Frank PI, Morris JA, Hazell ML, Linehan MF, Frank TL. Long term prognosis in preschool children with wheeze: longitudinal postal questionnaire study 1993-2004. *BMJ.* 2008 Jun 21;336(7658):1423-6. 2008 Jun 16.

Frawley D, Lad V. *The Yoga of Herbs.* Sante Fe: Lotus Press, 1986.

Fredriksen L, Mathiesen G, Moen A, Bron PA, Kleerebezem M, Eijsink VG, Egge-Jacobsen W. The major autolysin Acm2 from Lactobacillus plantarum undergoes cytoplasmic O-glycosylation. J Bacteriol. 2012 Jan;194(2):325-33. doi: 10.1128/JB.06314-11.

Freedman BJ. A dietary free from additives in the management of allergic disease. *Clin Allergy.* 1977 Sep;7(5):417-21.

Fremont S, Moneret-Vautrin DA, Franck P, Morisset M, Croizier A, Codreanu F, Kanny G. Prospective study of sensitization and food allergy to flaxseed in 1317 subjects. *Eur Ann Allergy Clin Immunol.* 2010 Jun;42(3):103-11.

Frias J, Song YS, Martínez-Villaluenga C, González de Mejia E, Vidal-Valverde C. Immunoreactivity and amino acid content of fermented soybean products. *J Agric Food Chem.* 2008 Jan 9;56(1):99-105.

Friedman LS, Harvard Health Publ. Ed. *Controlling GERD and Chronic Heartburn.* Boston: Harvard Health, 2008.

Friend BA, Shahani KM, Long CA, Vaughn LA. The effect of processing and storage on key enzymes, B vitamins, and lipids of mature human milk. Evaluation of fresh samples and effects of freezing and frozen storage. *Pediatr Res.* 1983 Jan;17(1):61-4.

Friend BA, Shahani KM. Characterization and evaluation of Aspergillus oryzae lactase coupled to a regenerable support. *Biotechnol Bioeng.* 1982 Feb;24(2):329-45.

Frumkin H. Beyond toxicity: human health and the natural environment. *Am J Prev Med.* 2001;20(3):234-40.

Fu G, Zhong Y, Li C, Li Y, Lin X, Liao B, Tsang EW, Wu K, Huang S. Epigenetic regulation of peanut allergen gene Ara h 3 in developing embryos. *Planta.* 2010 Apr;231(5):1049-60.

Fu JX. Measurement of MEFV in 66 cases of asthma in the convalescent stage and after treatment with Chinese herbs. *Zhong Xi Yi Jie He Za Zhi.* 1989 Nov;9(11):658-9, 644.

Fu LL, Zhou CC, Yao S, Yu JY, Liu B, Bao JK. Plant lectins: targeting programmed cell death pathways as antitumor agents. Int J Biochem Cell Biol. 2011 Oct;43(10):1442-9. doi: 10.1016/j.biocel.2011.07.004.

Fuiano N, Fusilli S, Passalacqua G, Incorvaia C. Allergen-specific immunoglobulin E in the skin and nasal mucosa of symptomatic and asymptomatic children sensitized to aeroallergens. *J Investig Allergol Clin Immunol.* 2010;20(5):425-30.

Fujii T, Ohtsuka Y, Lee T, Kudo T, Shoji H, Sato H, Nagata S, Shimizu T, Yamashiro Y. Bifidobacterium breve enhances transforming growth factor beta1 signaling by regulating Smad7 expression in preterm in-fants. *J Pediatr Gastroenterol Nutr.* 2006 Jul;43(1):83-8.

Fujii T, Ohtsuka Y, Lee T, Kudo T, Shoji H, Sato H, Nagata S, Shimizu T, Yamashiro Y. *Bifidobacterium breve* enhances transforming growth factor beta1 signaling by regulating Smad7 expression in preterm infants. *J Pediatr Gastroenterol Nutr.* 2006 Jul;43(1):83-8.

Fujimori S, Gudis K, Mitsui K, Seo T, Yonezawa M, Tanaka S, Tatsuguchi A, Sakamoto C. A randomized controlled trial on the efficacy of synbiotic versus probiotic or prebiotic treatment to improve the quality of life in patients with ulcerative colitis. *Nutrition.* 2009 May;25(5):520-5.

Fujita Y, Tsuno H, Nakayama J. Fermented Papaya Preparation Restores Age-Related Reductions in Peripheral Blood Mononuclear Cell Cytolytic Activity in Tube-Fed Patients. PLoS One. 2017 Jan 6;12(1):e0169240. doi: 10.1371/journal.pone.0169240.

Fulgoni VL 3rd. Current protein intake in America: analysis of the National Health and Nutrition Examination Survey, 2003-2004. *Am J Clin Nutr.* 2008 May;87(5):1554S-1557S.

Furrie E, Macfarlane S, Kennedy A, Cummings JH, Walsh SV, O'neil DA, Macfarlane GT. Synbiotic therapy (*Bifidobacterium longum*/Synergy 1) initiates resolution of inflammation in patients with active ulcerative colitis: a randomised controlled pilot trial. *Gut.* 2005 Feb;54(2):242-9.

Furrie E. Probiotics and allergy. *Proc Nutr Soc.* 2005 Nov;64(4):465-9.

Furuhjelm C, Warstedt K, Larsson J, Fredriksson M, Böttcher MF, Fälth-Magnusson K, Duchén K. Fish oil supplementation in pregnancy and lactation may decrease the risk of infant allergy. *Acta Paediatr.* 2009 Sep;98(9):1461-7.

Gabory A, Attig L, Junien C. Sexual dimorphism in environmental epigenetic programming. *Mol Cell Endocrinol.* 2009 May 25;304(1-2):8-18. 2009 Mar 9.

Gamboa PM, Cáceres O, Antepara I, Sánchez-Monge R, Ahrazem O, Salcedo G, Barber D, Lombardero M, Sanz ML. Two different profiles of peach allergy in the north of Spain. *Allergy.* 2007 Apr;62(4):408-14.

Gandhi TK, Weingart SN, Borus J, Seger AC, Peterson J, Burdick E, Seger DL, Shu K, Federico F, Leape LL, Bates DW. Adverse drug events in ambulatory care. N Engl J Med. 2003 Apr 17;348(16):1556-64.

Giampietro PG, Kjellman NI, Oldaeus G, Wouters-Wesseling W, Businco L. Hypoallergenicity of an extensively hydrolyzed whey formula. *Pediatr Allergy Immunol.* 2001 Apr;12(2):83-6.

Gao DN, Zhang Y, Ren YB, Kang J, Jiang L, Feng Z, Qu YN, Qi QH, Meng X. Relationship of Serum Mannose-Binding Lectin Levels with the Development of Sepsis: a Meta-analysis. Inflammation. 2014 Oct 17.

Gao X, Wang W, Wei S, Li W. Review of pharmacological effects of Glycyrrhiza radix and its bioactive compounds. *Zhongguo Zhong Yao Za Zhi.* 2009 Nov;34(21):2695-700.

Gaón D, Doweck Y, Gómez Zavaglia A, Ruiz Holgado A, Oliver G. Lactose digestion by milk fermented with *Lactobacillus acidophilus* and *Lactobacillus casei* of human origin. *Medicina (B Aires).* 1995;55(3):237-42.

Gaón D, García H, Winter L, Rodríguez N, Quintás R, González SN, Oliver G. Effect of Lactobacillus strains and *Saccharomyces boulardii* on persistent diarrhea in children. *Medicina (B Aires).* 2003;63(4):293-8.

Gaón D, Garmendia C, Murrielo NO, de Cucco Games A, Cerchio A, Quintas R, González SN, Oliver G. Effect of Lactobacillus strains (*L. casei* and *L. Acidophilus* Strains cerela) on bacterial overgrowth-related chronic diarrhea. *Medicina.* 2002;62(2):159-63.

Garaczi E, Boros-Gyevi M, Bella Z, Csoma Z, Kemény L, Koreck A. Intranasal phototherapy is more effective than fexofenadine hydrochloride in the treatment of seasonal allergic rhinitis: results of a pilot study. *Photochem Photobiol.* 2011 Mar-Apr;87(2):474-7.

Garavello W, Somigliana E, Acaia B, Gaini L, Pignataro L, Gaini RM. Nasal lavage in pregnant women with seasonal allergic rhinitis: a randomized study. *Int Arch Allergy Immunol.* 2010;151(2):137-41. 2009 Sep 15. 19752567.

Garcia Gomez LJ, Sanchez-Muniz FJ. Review: cardiovascular effect of garlic (Allium sativum). *Arch Latinoam Nutr.* 2000 Sep;50(3):219-29.

Garcia Vilela E, De Lourdes De Abreu Ferrari M, Oswaldo Da Gama Torres H, Guerra Pinto A, Carolina Carneiro Aguirre A, Paiva Martins F, Marcos Andrade Goulart E, Sales Da Cunha A. Influence of *Saccharomyces boulardii* on the intestinal permeability of patients with Crohn's disease in remission. *Scand J Gastroenterol.* 2008;43(7):842-8.

García-Compeán D, González MV, Galindo G, Mar DA, Treviño JL, Martínez R, Bosques F, Maldonado H. Prevalence of gastroesophageal reflux disease in patients with extraesophageal symptoms referred from otolaryngology, allergy, and cardiology practices: a prospective study. *Dig Dis.* 2000;18(3):178-82.

Garcia-Marcos L, Canflanca IM, Garrido JB, Varela AL, Garcia-Hernandez G, Guillen Grima F, Gonzalez-Diaz C, Carvajal-Urueña I, Arnedo-Pena A, Busquets-Monge RM, Morales Suarez-Varela M, Blanco-Quiros A. Relationship of asthma and rhinoconjunctivitis with obesity, exercise and Mediterranean diet in Spanish schoolchildren. *Thorax.* 2007 Jun;62(6):503-8.

Gardner CD, Fortmann SP, Krauss RM. Association of small low-density lipoprotein particles with the incidence of coronary artery disease in men and women. *JAMA.* 1996 Sep 18;276(11):875-81.

Gardner ML. Gastrointestinal absorption of intact proteins. *Annu Rev Nutr.* 1988;8:329-50.

Gary WK, Fanny WS, David SC. Factors associated with difference in prevalence of asthma in children from three cities in China: multicentre epidemiological survey. *BMJ.* 2004;329:1-4.

Garzi A, Messina M, Frati F, Carfagna L, Zagordo L, Belcastro M, Parmiani S, Sensi L, Marcucci F. An extensively hydrolysed cow's milk formula improves clinical symptoms of gastroesophageal reflux and reduces the gastric emptying time in infants. *Allergol Immunopathol (Madr).* 2002 Jan-Feb;30(1):36-41.

Gawrońska A, Dziechciarz P, Horvath A, Szajewska H. A randomized double-blind placebo-controlled trial of Lactobacillus GG for abdominal pain disorders in children. *Aliment Pharmacol Ther.* 2007 Jan 15;25(2):177-84.

Gazdik F, Horvathova M, Gazdikova K, Jahnova E. The influence of selenium supplementation on the immunity of corticoid-dependent asthmatics. *Bratisl Lek Listy.* 2002;103(1):17-21.

Gazdik F, Kadrabova J, Gazdikova K. Decreased consumption of corticosteroids after selenium supplementation in corticoid-dependent asthmatics. *Bratisl Lek Listy.* 2002;103(1):22-5.

Geha RS, Beiser A, Ren C, Patterson R, Greenberger PA, Grammer LC, Ditto AM, Harris KE, Shaughnessy MA, Yarnold PR, Corren J, Saxon A. Multicenter, double-blind, placebo-controlled, multiple-challenge evaluation of reported reactions to monosodium glutamate. *J Allergy Clin Immunol.* 2000 Nov;106(5):973-80.

Gerez IF, Shek LP, Chng HH, Lee BW. Diagnostic tests for food allergy. *Singapore* Med J. 2010 Jan;51(1):4-9.

Gergen PJ, Arbes SJ Jr, Calatroni A, Mitchell HE, Zeldin DC. Total IgE levels and asthma prevalence in the US population: results from the National Health and Nutrition Examination Survey 2005-2006. *J Allergy Clin Immunol.* 2009 Sep;124(3):447-53. 2009 Aug 3.

Ghadioungui P. (transl.) The Ebers Papyrus. Academy of Scientific Research. Cairo, 1987.

Gibbons E. *Stalking the Healthful Herbs.* New York: David McKay, 1966.

Gibson RA. Docosa-hexaenoic acid (DHA) accumulation is regulated by the polyunsaturated fat content of the diet: Is it synthesis or is it incorporation? *Asia Pac J Clin Nutr.* 2004;13(Suppl):S78.

Gilbert CR, Arum SM, Smith CM. Vitamin D deficiency and chronic lung disease. *Can Respir J.* 2009 May-Jun;16(3):75-80.

Gill HS, Rutherfurd KJ, Cross ML, Gopal PK. Enhancement of immunity in the elderly by dietary supplementation with the probiotic Bifidobacterium lactis HN019. *Am J Clin Nutr.* 2001 Dec;74(6):833-9.

Gill HS, Rutherfurd KJ, Cross ML. Dietary probiotic supplementation enhances natural killer cell activity in the elderly: an investigation of age-related immunological changes. *J Clin Immunol.* 2001 Jul;21(4):264-71.

Gillman A, Douglass JA. What do asthmatics have to fear from food and additive allergy? *Clin Exp Allergy.* 2010 Sep;40(9):1295-302.

Ginde AA, Mansbach JM, Camargo CA Jr. Association between serum 25-hydroxyvitamin D level and upper respiratory tract infection in the Third National Health and Nutrition Examination Survey. *Arch Intern Med.* 2009 Feb 23;169(4):384-90.

Gionchetti P, Rizzello F, Venturi A, Brigidi P, Matteuzzi D, Bazzocchi G, Poggioli G, Miglioli M, Campieri M. Oral bacteriotherapy as maintenance treatment in patients with chronic pouchitis: a double-blind, placebo-controlled trial. *Gastroenterology.* 2000 Aug;119(2):305-9.

Gittleman AL. *Guess What Came to Dinner.* New York: Avery, 2001.

Glavas-Dodov M, Steffansen B, Crcarevska MS, Geskovski N, Dimchevska S, Kuzmanovska S, Goracinova K. Wheat germ agglutinin-functionalised crosslinked polyelectrolyte microparticles for local colon delivery of 5-FU: in vitro efficacy and in vivo gastrointestinal distribution. J Microencapsul. 2013;30(7):643-56. doi: 10.3109/02652048.2013.770099.

Glinsky VV, Raz A. Modified citrus pectin anti-metastatic properties: one bullet, multiple targets. Carbohydr Res. 2009 Sep 28;344(14):1788-91. doi:10.1016/j.carres.2008.08.038.

Glück U, Gebbers J. Ingested probiotics reduce nasal colonization with pathogenic bacteria (Staphylococcus aureus, Streptococcus pneumoniae, and b-hemolytic streptococci. *Am J. Clin. Nutr.* 2003;77:517-520.

Glück U, Gebbers J. Ingested probiotics reduce nasal colonization with pathogenic bacteria (*Staphylococcus aureus, Streptococcus pneumoniae,* and b-hemolytic streptococci. *Am J. Clin. Nutr.* 2003;77:517-520.

Goedsche K, Förster M, Kroegel C, Uhlemann C. Repeated cold water stimulations (hydrotherapy according to Kneipp) in patients with COPD. *Forsch Komplementmed.* 2007 Jun;14(3):158-66.

Goel V, Dolan RJ. The functional anatomy of humor: segregating cognitive and affective components. *Nat Neurosci.* 2001;4:237-8.

Gohil K, Packer L. Bioflavonoid-Rich Botanical Extracts Show Antioxidant and Gene Regulatory Activity. *Ann N Y Acad Sci.* 2002:957:70-7.

Goldin BR, Adlercreutz H, Dwyer JT, Swenson L, Warram JH, Gorbach SL. Effect of diet on excretion of estrogens in pre- and postmenopausal women. *Cancer Res.* 1981 Sep;41(9 Pt 2):3771-3.

Goldin BR, Adlercreutz H, Gorbach SL, Warram JH, Dwyer JT, Swenson L, Woods MN. Estrogen excretion patterns and plasma levels in vegetarian and omnivorous women. *N Engl J Med.* 1982 Dec 16;307(25):1542-7.

Goldin BR, Adlercreutz H, Gorbach SL, Warram JH, Dwyer JT, Swenson L, Woods MN. Estrogen excretion patterns and plasma levels in vegetarian and omnivorous women. *N Engl J Med.* 1982 Dec 16;307(25):1542-7.

Goldin BR, Swenson L, Dwyer J, Sexton M, Gorbach SL. Effect of diet and Lactobacillus acidophilus supplements on human fecal bacterial enzymes. *J Natl Cancer Inst.* 1980 Feb;64(2):255-61.

Goldin BR, Swenson L, Dwyer J, Sexton M, Gorbach SL. Effect of diet and *Lactobacillus acidophilus* supplements on human fecal bacterial enzymes. *J Natl Cancer Inst.* 1980 Feb;64(2):255-61.

Goldstein JL, Aisenberg J, Zakko SF, Berger MF, Dodge WE. Endoscopic ulcer rates in healthy subjects associated with use of aspirin (81 mg q.d.) alone or coadministered with celecoxib or naproxen: a randomized, 1-week trial. *Dig Dis Sci.* 2008 Mar;53(3):647-56.

Golub E. *The Limits of Medicine.* New York: Times Books, 1994.

Gonzales M, Malcoe LH, Myers OB, Espinoza J. Risk factors for asthma and cough among Hispanic children in the southwestern United States of America, 2003-2004. *Rev Panam Salud Publica.* 2007 May;21(5):274-81.

González Alvarez R, Arruzazabala ML. Current views of the mechanism of action of prophylactic antiallergic drugs. *Allergol Immunopathol (Madr).* 1981 Nov-Dec;9(6):501-8.

González J, Fernández M, García Fragoso L. Exclusive breastfeeding reduces asthma in a group of children from the Caguas municipality of Puerto Rico. *Bol Asoc Med P R.* 2010 Jan-Mar;102(1):10-2.

González Morales JE, Leal de Hernández L, González Spencer D. Asthma associated with gastroesophageal reflux. *Rev Alerg Mex.* 1998 Jan-Feb;45(1):16-21.

González-Pérez A, Aponte Z, Vidaurre CF, Rodríguez LA. Anaphylaxis epidemiology in patients with and patients without asthma: a United Kingdom database review. *J Allergy Clin Immunol.* 2010 May;125(5):1098-1104.e1.

González-Sánchez R, Trujillo X, Trujillo-Hernández B, Vásquez C, Huerta M, Elizalde A. Forskolin versus sodium cromoglycate for prevention of asthma attacks: a single-blinded clinical trial. *J Int Med Res.* 2006 Mar-Apr;34(2):200-7.

Goossens D, Jonkers D, Russel M, Stobberingh E, Van Den Bogaard A, StockbrUgger R. The effect of *Lactobacillus plantarum* 299v on the bacterial composition and metabolic activity in faeces of healthy volunteers: a placebo-controlled study on the onset and duration of effects. *Aliment Pharmacol Ther.* 2003 Sep 1;18(5):495-505.

Goossens DA, Jonkers DM, Russel MG, Stobberingh EE, Stockbrügger RW. The effect of a probiotic drink with *Lactobacillus plantarum* 299v on the bacterial composition in faeces and mucosal biopsies of rectum and ascending colon. *Aliment Pharmacol Ther.* 2006 Jan 15;23(2):255-63.

Gordon BR. Patch testing for allergies. *Curr Opin Otolaryngol Head Neck Surg.* 2010 Jun;18(3):191-4.

Gore KV, Rao AK, Guruswamy MN. Physiological studies with Tylophora asthmatica in bronchial asthma. *Indian J Med Res.* 1980 Jan;71:144-8.

Goren AI, Hellmann S. Changes prevalence of asthma among schoolchildren in Israel. *Eur Respir J.* 1997;10:2279-2284.

Gotteland M, Poliak L, Cruchet S, Brunser O. Effect of regular ingestion of Saccharomyces boulardii plus inulin or Lactobacillus acidophilus LB in children colonized by Helicobacter pylori. *Acta Paediatr.* 2005 Dec;94(12):1747-51.

Gotteland M, Poliak L, Cruchet S, Brunser O. Effect of regular ingestion of *Saccharomyces boulardii* plus inulin or *Lactobacillus acidophilus* LB in children colonized by *Helicobacter pylori. Acta Paediatr.* 2005 Dec;94(12):1747-51.

Govindan S, Viswanathan S, Vijayasekaran V, Alagappan R. A pilot study on the clinical efficacy of Solanum xanthocarpum and Solanum trilobatum in bronchial asthma. *J Ethnopharmacol.* 1999 Aug;66(2):205-10.

Govindan S, Viswanathan S, Vijayasekaran V, Alagappan R. Further studies on the clinical efficacy of Solanum xanthocarpum and Solanum trilobatum in bronchial asthma. *Phytother Res.* 2004 Oct;18(10):805-9.

Grant WB, Holick MF. Benefits and requirements of vitamin D for optimal health: a review. *Altern Med Rev.* 2005 Jun;10(2):94-111.

Grant WB. Hypothesis—ultraviolet-B irradiance and vitamin D reduce the risk of viral infections and thus their sequelae, including autoimmune diseases and some cancers. *Photochem Photobiol.* 2008 Mar-Apr;84(2):356-65. 2008 Jan 7.

Grasso F, Grillo C, Musumeci F, Triglia A, Rodolico G, Cammisuli F, Rinzivillo C, Fragati G, Santuccio A, Rodolico M. Photon emission from normal and tumour human tissues. *Experientia.* 1992;48:10-13.

Gravina LP, Crespo C, Giugno H, Sen L, Chertkoff L, Mangano A, Castaños C. Mannose-binding lectin gene modifier of cystic fibrosis phenotype in Argentinean pediatric patients. J Cyst Fibros. 2014 Aug 29. pii: S1569-1993(14)00173-8. doi: 10.1016/j.jcf.2014.07.012

Gray H. *Anatomy, Descriptive and Surgical.* 15th Edition. New York: Random House, 1977.

Gray-Davison F. *Ayurvedic Healing.* New York: Keats, 2002.

Greskevitch M, Kullman G, Bang KM, Mazurek JM. Respiratory disease in agricultural workers: mortality and morbidity statistics. J Agromedicine. 2007;12(3):5-10.

Griffith HW. *Healing Herbs: The Essential Guide.* Tucson: Fisher Books, 2000.

Grimm T, Chovanová Z, Muchová J, Sumegová K, Liptáková A, Duracková Z, Högger P. Inhibition of NF-kappaB activation and MMP-9 secretion by plasma of human volunteers after ingestion of maritime pine bark extract (Pycnogenol). J Inflamm (Lond). 2006 Jan 27;3:1.

Grimm T, Schäfer A, Högger P. Antioxidant activity and inhibition of matrix metalloproteinases by metabolites of maritime pine bark extract (pycnogenol). *Free Radic Biol Med.* 2004 Mar 15;36(6):811-22.

Grimm T, Skrabala R, Chovanová Z, Muchová J, Sumegová K, Liptáková A, Duracková Z, Högger P. Single and multiple dose pharmacokinetics of maritime pine bark extract (pycnogenol) after oral administration to healthy volunteers. *BMC Clin Pharmacol.* 2006 Aug 3;6:4.

Grönlund MM, Gueimonde M, Laitinen K, Kociubinski G, Grönroos T, Salminen S, Isolauri E. Maternal breast-milk and intestinal bifidobacteria guide the compositional development of the *Bifidobacterium* microbiota in infants at risk of allergic disease. *Clin Exp Allergy.* 2007 Dec;37(12):1764-72.

Gropper SS, Smith JL, Groff JL. *Advanced nutrition and human metabolism.* Belmonth, CA: Wadsworth Publ, 2008.

Groppo FC, Ramacciato JC, Simões RP, Flório FM, Sartoratto A. Antimicrobial activity of garlic, tea tree oil, and chlorhexidine against oral microorganisms. *Int Dent J.* 2002 Dec;52(6):433-7.

Groschwitz KR, Ahrens R, Osterfeld H, Gurish MF, Han X, Abrink M, Finkelman FD, Pejler G, Hogan SP. Mast cells regulate homeostatic intestinal epithelial migration and barrier function by a chymase/Mcpt4-dependent mechanism. *Proc Natl Acad Sci U S A.* 2009 Dec 29;106(52):22381-6.

Grosser BI, Monti-Bloch L, Jennings-White C, Berliner DL. Behavioral and electrophysiological effects of androstadienone, a human pheromone. *Psychoneuroendocrinology.* 2000 Apr;25(3):289-99.

Grzanna R, Lindmark L, Frondoza CG. Ginger—an herbal medicinal product with broad anti-inflammatory actions. *J Med Food.* 2005 Summer;8(2):125-32.

Guajardo-Flores D, Serna-Saldívar SO, Gutiérrez-Uribe JA. Evaluation of the antioxidant and antiproliferative activities of extracted saponins and flavonols from germinated black beans (Phaseolus vulgaris L.). Food Chem. 2013 Nov 15;141(2):1497-503.

Guandalini S. The influence of gluten: weaning recommendations for healthy children and children at risk for celiac disease. *Nestle Nutr Workshop Ser Pediatr Program.* 2007;60:139-51; discussion 151-5.

Guarino A, Canani RB, Spagnuolo MI, Albano F, Di Benedetto L. Oral bacterial therapy reduces the duration of symptoms and of viral excretion in children with mild diarrhea. *J Pediatr Gastroenterol Nutr.* 1997 Nov;25(5):516-9.

Guerin M, Huntley ME, Olaizola M. Haematococcus astaxanthin: applications for human health and nutrition. *Trends Biotechnol.* 2003 May;21(5):210-6.

REFERENCES AND BIBLIOGRAPHY

Guerin-Danan C, Chabanet C, Pedone C, Popot F, Vaissade P, Bouley C, Szylit O, Andrieux C. Milk fermented with yogurt cultures and *Lactobacillus casei* compared with yogurt and gelled milk: influence on intestinal microflora in healthy infants. *Am J Clin Nutr.* 1998 Jan;67(1):111-7.

Guerrero-Bosagna C, Skinner MK. Environmentally induced epigenetic transgenerational inheritance of phenotype and disease. Mol Cell Endocrinol. 2012 May 6;354(1-2):3-8.

Guinot P, Brambilla C, Duchier J, Braquet P, Bonvoisin B, Cournot A. Effect of BN 52063, a specific PAF-acether antagonist, on bronchial provocation test to allergens in asthmatic patients. A preliminary study. *Prostaglandins.* 1987 Nov;34(5):723-31.

Gundermann KJ, Müller J. Phytodolor—effects and efficacy of a herbal medicine. *Wien Med Wochenschr.* 2007;157(13-14):343-7.

Gupta I, Gupta V, Parihar A, Gupta S, Lüdtke R, Safayhi H, Ammon HP. Effects of Boswellia serrata gum resin in patients with bronchial asthma: results of a double-blind, placebo-controlled, 6-week clinical study. *Eur J Med Res.* 1998 Nov 17;3(11):511-4.

Guslandi M, Giollo P, Testoni PA. A pilot trial of *Saccharomyces boulardii* in ulcerative colitis. *Eur J Gastroenterol Hepatol.* 2003 Jun;15(6):697-8.

Guslandi M, Mezzi G, Sorghi M, Testoni PA. *Saccharomyces boulardii* in maintenance treatment of Crohn's disease. *Dig Dis Sci.* 2000 Jul;45(7):1462-4.

Gutmanis J. *Hawaiian Herbal Medicine.* Waipahu, HI: Island Heritage, 2001.

Guyonnet D, Woodcock A, Stefani B, Trevisan C, Hall C. Fermented milk containing Bifidobacterium lactis DN-173 010 improved self-reported digestive comfort amongst a general population of adults. A randomized, open-label, controlled, pilot study. *J Dig Dis.* 2009 Feb;10(1):61-70.

Haarman M, Knol J. Quantitative real-time PCR assays to identify and quantify fecal *Bifidobacterium* species in infants receiving a prebiotic infant formula. Appl Environ Microbiol. 2005 May;71(5):2318-24.

Haggag EG, Abou-Moustafa MA, Boucher W, Theoharides TC. The effect of a herbal water-extract on histamine release from mast cells and on allergic asthma. *J Herb Pharmacother.* 2003;3(4):41-54.

Haines JL, Ter-Minassian M, Bazyk A, Gusella JF, Kim DJ, Terwedow H, Pericak-Vance MA, Rimmler JB, Haynes CS, Roses AD, Lee A, Shaner B, Menold M, Seboun E, Fitoussi RP, Gartioux C, Reyes C, Ribierre F, Gyapay G, Weissenbach J, Hauser SL, Goodkin DE, Lincoln R, Usuku K, Oksenberg JR, *et al.* A complete genomic screen for multiple sclerosis underscores a role for the major histocompatability complex. The Multiple Sclerosis Genetics Group. *Nat Genet.* 1996 Aug;13(4):469-71..

Halász A, Cserháti E. The prognosis of bronchial asthma in childhood in Hungary: a long-term follow-up. *J Asthma.* 2002 Dec;39(8):693-9.

Halken S, Hansen KS, Jacobsen HP, Estmann A, Faelling AE, Hansen LG, Kier SR, Lassen K, Lintrup M, Mortensen S, Ibsen KK, Osterballe O, Høst A. Comparison of a partially hydrolyzed infant formula with two extensively hydrolyzed formulas for allergy prevention: a prospective, randomized, study. *Pediatr Allergy Immunol.* 2000 Aug;11(3):149-61.

Hallén A, Jarstrand C, Påhlson C. Treatment of bacterial vaginosis with lactobacilli. Sex Transm Dis. 1992 May-Jun;19(3):146-8.

Halpern GM, Miller AH. *Medicinal Mushrooms: Ancient Remedies for Modern Ailments.* New York: M. Evans, 2002.

Hamasaki Y, Kobayashi I, Hayasaki R, Zaitu M, Muro E, Yamamoto S, Ichimaru T, Miyazaki S. The Chinese herbal medicine, shinpi-to, inhibits IgE-mediated leukotriene synthesis in rat basophilic leukemia-2H3 cells. *J Ethnopharmacol.* 1997 Apr;56(2):123-31.

Hamelmann E, Beyer K, Gruber C, Lau S, Matricardi PM, Nickel R, Niggemann B, Wahn U. Primary prevention of allergy: avoiding risk or providing protection? *Clin Exp Allergy.* 2008 Feb;38(2):233-45.

Hamilton RG. Clinical laboratory assessment of immediate-type hypersensitivity. *J Allergy Clin Immunol.* 2010 Feb;125(2 Suppl 2):S284-96.

Hammond BG, Mayhew DA, Kier LD, Mast RW, Sander WJ. Safety assessment of DHA-rich microalgae from Schizochytrium sp. *Regul Toxicol Pharmacol.* 2002 Apr;35(2 Pt 1):255-65.

Han ER, Choi IS, Kim HK, Kang YW, Park JG, Lim JR, Seo JH, Choi JH. Inhaled corticosteroid-related tooth problems in asthmatics. *J Asthma.* 2009 Mar;46(2):160-4.

Han SN, Leka LS, Lichtenstein AH, Ausman LM, Meydani SN. Effect of a therapeutic lifestyle change diet on immune functions of moderately hypercholesterolemic humans. *J Lipid Res.* 2003 Dec;44(12):2304-10.

Hansen KS, Ballmer-Weber BK, Lüttkopf D, Skov PS, Wüthrich B, Bindslev-Jensen C, Vieths S, Poulsen LK. Roasted hazelnuts—allergenic activity evaluated by double-blind, placebo-controlled food challenge. *Allergy.* 2003 Feb;58(2):132-8.

Hansen KS, Ballmer-Weber BK, Sastre J, Lidholm J, Andersson K, Oberhofer H, Lluch-Bernal M, Ostling J, Mattsson L, Schocker F, Vieths S, Poulsen LK. Component-resolved in vitro diagnosis of hazelnut allergy in Europe. *J Allergy Clin Immunol.* 2009 May;123(5):1134-41, 1141.e1-3.

Hansen KS, Khinchi MS, Skov PS, Bindslev-Jensen C, Poulsen LK, Malling HJ. Food allergy to apple and specific immunotherapy with birch pollen. *Mol Nutr Food Res.* 2004 Nov;48(6):441-8.

Haranath PS, Shyamalakumari S. Experimental study on mode of action of Tylophora asthmatica in bronchial asthma. *Indian J Med Res.* 1975 May;63(5):661-70.

Harrington JJ, Lee-Chiong T Jr. Sleep and older patients. *Clin Chest Med.* 2007 Dec;28(4):673-84, v.

Harris LA, Chang L. Irritable bowel syndrome: new and emerging therapies. *Curr Opin Gastroenterol.* 2006 Mar;22(2):128-35.

Hartz C, Lauer I, Del Mar San Miguel Moncin M, Cistero-Bahima A, Foetisch K, Lidholm J, Vieths S, Scheurer S. Comparison of IgE-Binding Capacity, Cross-Reactivity and Biological Potency of Allergenic Non-Specific Lipid Transfer Proteins from Peach, Cherry and Hazelnut. *Int Arch Allergy Immunol.* 2010 Jun 17;153(4):335-346.

Harvald B, Hauge M: Hereditary factors elucidated by twin studies. *In Genetics and the Epidemiology of Chronic Disease.* Edited by Neel JV, Shaw MV, Schull WJ. Washington, DC: Dept Health, Education and Welfare, 1965:64-76.

Harvey HP, Solomon HJ. Acute anaphylactic shock due to para-aminosalicylic acid. *Am Rev Tuberc.* 1958 Mar;77(3):492-5.

Hassan AM. Selenium status in patients with aspirin-induced asthma. *Ann Clin Biochem.* 2008 Sep;45(Pt 5):508-12.

Hasselmark L, Malmgren R, Zetterström O, Unge G. Selenium supplementation in intrinsic asthma. *Allergy.* 1993 Jan;48(1):30-6.

Hata K, Ishikawa K, Hori K, Konishi T. Differentiation-inducing activity of lupeol, a lupane-type triterpene from Chinese dandelion root (Hokouei-kon), on a mouse melanoma cell line. *Biol Pharm Bull.* 2000 Aug;23(8):962-7.

Hata Y, Yamamoto M, Ohni M, Nakajima K, Nakamura Y, Takano T. A placebo-controlled study of the effect of sour milk on blood pressure in hypertensive subjects. *Am J Clin Nutr.* 1996 Nov;64(5):767-71.

Hatakka K, Holma R, El-Nezami H, Suomalainen T, Kuisma M, Saxelin M, Poussa T, Mykkänen H, Korpela R. The influence of *Lactobacillus rhamnosus* LC705 together with Propionibacterium freudenreichii ssp. shermanii JS on potentially carcinogenic bacterial activity in human colon. *Int J Food Microbiol.* 2008 Dec 10;128(2):406-10.

Hattori K, Sasai M, Yamamoto A, Taniuchi S, Kojima T, Kobayashi Y, Iwamoto H, Yaeshima T, Hayasawa H. Intestinal flora of infants with cow milk hypersensitivity fed on casein-hydrolyzed formula supplemented raffinose. *Arerugi.* 2000 Dec;49(12):1146-55.

Hattori K, Yamamoto A, Sasai M, Taniuchi S, Kojima T, Kobayashi Y, Iwamoto H, Namba K, Yaeshima T. Effects of administration of bifidobacteria on fecal microflora and clinical symptoms in infants with atopic dermatitis. *Arerugi.* 2003 Jan;52(1):20-30.

He M, Antoine JM, Yang Y, Yang J, Han H. Influence of live flora on lactose digestion in male adult lactose-malabsorbers after dairy products intake. *Wei Sheng Yan Jiu.* 2004 Sep;33(5):603-5.

He T, Priebe MG, Zhong Y, Huang C, Harmsen HJ, Raangs GC, Antoine JM, Welling GW, Vonk RJ. Effects of yogurt and bifidobacteria supplementation on the colonic microbiota in lactose-intolerant subjects. *J Appl Microbiol.* 2008 Feb;104(2):595-604.

Heaney LG, Brightling CE, Menzies-Gow A, Stevenson M, Niven RM; British Thoracic Society Difficult Asthma Network. Refractory asthma in the UK: cross-sectional findings from a UK multicentre registry. *Thorax.* 2010 Sep;65(9):787-94.

Heaney RP, Dowell MS. Absorbability of the calcium in a high-calcium mineral water. *Osteoporos Int.* 1994 Nov;4(6):323-4.

Heap GA, van Heel DA. Genetics and pathogenesis of coeliac disease. *Semin Immunol.* May 13 2009.

Heine RG, Nethercote M, Rosenbaum J, Allen KJ. Emerging management concepts for eosinophilic esophagitis in children. *J Gastroenterol Hepatol.* 2011 May 4.

Hemilä H, Chalker E. Vitamin C for preventing and treating the common cold. *Cochrane Database Syst Rev.* 2013 Jan 31;1:CD000980. doi: 10.1002/14651858.CD000980.pub4.

Hemmer W, Focke M, Marzban G, Swoboda I, Jarisch R, Laimer M. Identification of Bet v 1-related allergens in fig and other Moraceae fruits. *Clin Exp Allergy.* 2010 Apr;40(4):679-87.

Hendel B, Ferreira P. *Water & Salt: The Essence of Life.* Gaithersburg: Natural Resources, 2003.

Herbert V. Vitamin B12: Plant sources, requirements, and assay. *Am J Clin Nutr.* 1988;48:852-858.

Herman PM, Drost LM. Evaluating the clinical relevance of food sensitivity tests: a single subject experiment. *Altern Med Rev.* 2004 Jun;9(2):198-207.

Hernández-Márquez E, Lagunas-Martínez A, Bermudez-Morales VH, Burgete-García I, León-Rivera I, Montiel-Arcos E, García-Villa E, Gariglio P, Madrid-Marina VV, Ondarza-Vidaurreta RN. Inhibitory activity of Lingzhi or Reishi medicinal mushroom, Ganodermalucidum (higher Basidiomycetes) on transformed cells by human papillomavirus. Int J Med Mushrooms. 2014;16(2):179-87.

Herrera-Ramos E, López-Rodríguez M, Ruíz-Hernández JJ, Horcajada JP, Borderías L, Lerma E, Blanquer J, Pérez-González MC, García-Laorden MI, Florido Y, Mas-Bosch V, Montero M, Ferrer JM, Sorlí L,

Vilaplana C, Rajas O, Briones M, Aspa J, López-Granados E, Solé-Violán J, de Castro FR, Rodríguez-Gallego C. Surfactant protein A genetic variants associate with severe respiratory insufficiency in pandemic influenza A virus infection. *Crit Care.* 2014 Jun 20;18(3):R127. doi: 10.1186/cc13934.

Herzog AM, Black KA, Fountaine DJ, Knotts TR. Reflection and attentional recovery as two distinctive benefits of restorative environments. *J Environ Psychol.* 1997;17:165-70.

Hess-Kosa K. *Indoor Air Quality: Sampling Methodologies.* Boca Rataon: CRC Press, 2002.

Heyman M, Grasset E, Ducroc R, Desjeux JF. Antigen absorption by the jejunal epithelium of children with cow's milk allergy. *Pediatr Res.* 1988 Aug;24(2):197-202.

Hickson M, D'Souza AL, Muthu N, Rogers TR, Want S, Rajkumar C, Bulpitt CJ. Use of probiotic Lactobacillus preparation to prevent diarrhoea associated with antibiotics: randomised double blind placebo controlled trial. *BMJ.* 2007 Jul 14;335(7610):80.

Hide DW, Matthews S, Tariq S, Arshad SH. Allergen avoidance in infancy and allergy at 4 years of age. *Allergy.* 1996 Feb;51(2):89-93.

Hijazi Z, Molla AM, Al-Habashi H, Muawad WM, Molla AM, Sharma PN. Intestinal permeability is increased in bronchial asthma. *Arch Dis Child.* 2004 Mar;89(3):227-9.

Hill J, Micklewright A, Lewis S, Britton J. Investigation of the effect of short-term change in dietary magnesium intake in asthma. *Eur Respir J.* 1997 Oct;10(10):2225-9.

Hilton E, Isenberg HD, Alperstein P, France K, Borenstein MT. Ingestion of yogurt containing *Lactobacillus acidophilus* as prophylaxis for *Candida* vaginitis. *Ann Intern Med.* 1992 Mar 1;116(5):353-7.

Hirose Y, Murosaki S, Yamamoto Y, Yoshikai Y, Tsuru T. Daily intake of heat-killed *Lactobacillus plantarum* L-137 augments acquired immunity in healthy adults. *J Nutr.* 2006 Dec;136(12):3069-73.

Hlivak P, Jahnova E, Odraska J, Ferencik M, Ebringer L, Mikes Z. Long-term (56-week) oral administration of probiotic *Enterococcus faecium* M-74 decreases the expression of sICAM-1 and monocyte CD54, and increases that of lymphocyte CD49d in humans. *Bratisl Lek Listy.* 2005;106(4-5):175-81.

Hlivak P, Odraska J, Ferencik M, Ebringer L, Jahnova E, Mikes Z. One-year application of probiotic strain *Enterococcus faecium* M-74 decreases serum cholesterol levels. *Bratisl Lek Listy.* 2005;106(2):67-72.

Hobbs C. *Kombucha Manchurian Tea Mushroom: The Essential Guide.* Santa Cruz, CA: Botanica Press, 1995.

Hobbs C. *Medicinal Mushrooms.* Summertown, TN: Botanica Press, 2003.

Hobbs C. *Stress & Natural Healing.* Loveland, CO: Interweave Press, 1997.

Hoff S, Seiler H, Heinrich J, Kompauer I, Nieters A, Becker N, Nagel G, Gedrich K, Karg G, Wolfram G, Linseisen J. Allergic sensitisation and allergic rhinitis are associated with n-3 polyunsaturated fatty acids in the diet and in red blood cell membranes. *Eur J Clin Nutr.* 2005 Sep;59(9):1071-80.

Hoffmann D. *Holistic Herbal.* London: Thorsons, 2002.

Hofmann D, Hecker M, Völp A. Efficacy of dry extract of ivy leaves in children with bronchial asthma-a review of randomized controlled trials. *Phytomedicine.* 2003 Mar;10(2-3):213-20.

Höiby AS, Strand V, Robinson DS, Sager A, Rak S. Efficacy, safety, and immunological effects of a 2-year immunotherapy with Depigoid birch pollen extract: a randomized, double-blind, placebo-controlled study. *Clin Exp Allergy.* 2010 Jul;40(7):1062-70.

Holick MF. Sunlight and vitamin D for bone health and prevention of autoimmune diseases, cancers, and cardiovascular disease. *Am J Clin Nutr.* 2004 Dec;80(6 Suppl):1678S-88S.

Holick MF. The vitamin D deficiency pandemic and consequences for nonskeletal health: mechanisms of action. *Mol Aspects Med.* 2008 Dec;29(6):361-8

Holick MF. Vitamin D status: measurement, interpretation, and clinical application. *Ann Epidemiol.* 2009 Feb;19(2):73-8.

Holladay, S.D. Prenatal Immunotoxicant Exposure and Postnatal Autoimmune Disease. *Environ Health Perspect.* 1999; 107(suppl 5):687-691.

Holt GA. Food & Drug Interactions. Chicago: Precept Press, 1998, 83.

Homma M, Oka K, Niitsuma T, Itoh H. A novel 11 beta-hydroxysteroid dehydrogenase inhibitor contained in saiboku-to, a herbal remedy for steroid-dependent bronchial asthma. *J Pharm Pharmacol.* 1994 Apr;46(4):305-9.

Hönscheid A, Rink L, Haase H. T-lymphocytes: a target for stimulatory and inhibitory effects of zinc ions. *Endocr Metab Immune Disord Drug Targets.* 2009 Jun;9(2):132-44.

Hooper R, Calvert J, Thompson RL, Deetlefs ME, Burney P. Urban/rural differences in diet and atopy in South Africa. *Allergy.* 2008 Apr;63(4):425-31.

Hope BE, Massey DG, Fournier-Massey G. Hawaiian materia medica for asthma. *Hawaii Med J.* 1993 Jun;52(6):160-6.

Horak E, Morass B, Ulmer H. Association between environmental tobacco smoke exposure and wheezing disorders in Austrian preschool children. *Swiss Med Wkly.* 2007 Nov 3;137(43-44):608-13.

Hornum M, Bay JT, Clausen P, Melchior Hansen J, Mathiesen ER, Feldt-Rasmussen B, Garred P. High levels of mannose-binding lectin are associated with lower pulse wave velocity in uraemic patients. BMC Nephrol. 2014 Oct 4;15(1):162. doi: 10.1186/1471-2369-15-162.

Horrobin DF. Effects of evening primrose oil in rheumatoid arthritis. *Ann Rheum Dis.* 1989 Nov;48(11):965-6.

Hospers IC, de Vries-Vrolijk K, Brand PL. Double-blind, placebo-controlled cow's milk challenge in children with alleged cow's milk allergies, performed in a general hospital: diagnosis rejected in two-thirds of the children. *Ned Tijdschr Geneeskd.* 2006 Jun 10;150(23):1292-7.

Hosseini S, Pishnamazi S, Sadrzadeh SM, Farid F, Farid R, Watson RR. Pycnogenol((R)) in the Management of Asthma. *J Med Food.* 2001 Winter;4(4):201-209.

Hota B, Ellenbogen C, Hayden MK, Aroutcheva A, Rice TW, Weinstein RA. Community-associated methicillin-resistant *Staphylococcus aureus* skin and soft tissue infections at a public hospital: do public housing and incarceration amplify transmission? *Arch Intern Med.* 2007 May 28;167(10):1026-33.

Hougee S, Vriesema AJ, Wijering SC, Knippels LM, Folkerts G, Nijkamp FP, Knol J, Garssen J. Oral treatment with probiotics reduces allergic symptoms in ovalbumin-sensitized mice: a bacterial strain comparative study. *Int Arch Allergy Immunol.* 2010;151(2):107-17. 2009 Sep 15.

Houle CR, Leo HL, Clark NM. A developmental, community, and psychosocial approach to food allergies in children. *Curr Allergy Asthma Rep.* 2010 Sep;10(5):381-6.

Houssen ME, Ragab A, Mesbah A, El-Samanoudy AZ, Othman G, Moustafa AF, Badria FA. Natural anti-inflammatory products and leukotriene inhibitors as complementary therapy for bronchial asthma. *Clin Biochem.* 2010 Jul;43(10-11):887-90.

Hoyme UB, Saling E. Efficient prematurity prevention is possible by pH-self measurement and immediate therapy of threatening ascending infection. *Eur J Obstet Gynecol Reprod Biol.* 2004 Aug 10;115(2):148-53.

Hoyos AB. Reduced incidence of necrotizing enterocolitis associated with enteral administration of *Lactobacillus acidophilus* and *Bifidobacterium infantis* to neonates in an intensive care unit. *Int J Infect Dis.* 1999 Summer;3(4):197-202.

Hsieh KH. Evaluation of efficacy of traditional Chinese medicines in the treatment of childhood bronchial asthma: clinical trial, immunological tests and animal study. Taiwan Asthma Study Group. *Pediatr Allergy Immunol.* 1996 Aug;7(3):130-40.

Hsu CH, Lu CM, Chang TT. Efficacy and safety of modified Mai-Men-Dong-Tang for treatment of allergic asthma. *Pediatr Allergy Immunol.* 2005;16:76-81.

Hu C, Kitts DD. Antioxidant, prooxidant, and cytotoxic activities of solvent-fractionated dandelion (Taraxacum officinale) flower extracts in vitro. *J Agric Food Chem.* 2003 Jan 1;51(1):301-10.

Hu C, Kitts DD. Dandelion (Taraxacum officinale) flower extract suppresses both reactive oxygen species and nitric oxide and prevents lipid oxidation in vitro. *Phytomedicine.* 2005 Aug;12(8):588-97.

Hu C, Kitts DD. Luteolin and luteolin-7-O-glucoside from dandelion flower suppress iNOS and COX-2 in RAW264.7 cells. *Mol Cell Biochem.* 2004 Oct;265(1-2):107-13.

Hu FB, Willett WC. Optimal diets for prevention of coronary heart disease. *JAMA.* 2002 Nov 27;288(20):2569-78.

Hu Z, Yang A, Fan H, Wang Y, Zhao Y, Zha X, Zhang H, Tu P. Huaier aqueous extract sensitizes cells to rapamycin and cisplatin through activating mTOR signaling. J Ethnopharmacol. 2016 Jun 20;186:143-150. doi: 10.1016/j.jep.2016.03.069.

Hu Z, Yang A, Su G, Zhao Y, Wang Y, Chai X, Tu P. Huaier restrains proliferative and invasive potential of human hepatoma SKHEP-1 cells partially through decreased Lamin B1 and elevated NOV. Sci Rep. 2016 Aug 9;6:31298. doi: 10.1038/srep31298.

Huang D, Ou B, Prior RL. The chemistry behind antioxidant capacity assays. *J Agric Food Chem.* 2005 Mar 23;53(6):1841-56.

Huang M, Wang W, Wei S. Investigation on medicinal plant resources of Glycyrrhiza uralensis in China and chemical assessment of its underground part. *Zhongguo Zhong Yao Za Zhi.* 2010 Apr;35(8):947-52.

Hun L. Bacillus coagulans significantly improved abdominal pain and bloating in patients with IBS. *Postgrad Med.* 2009 Mar;121(2):119-24.

Huntley A, Ernst E: Herbal medicines for asthma: a systematic review. *Thorax.* 2000, 55:925-929.

Hur YM, Rushton JP. Genetic and environmental contributions to prosocial behaviour in 2- to 9-year-old South Korean twins. *Biol Lett.* 2007 Dec 22;3(6):664-6.

Husby S. Dietary antigens: uptake and humoral immunity in man. *APMIS Suppl.* 1988;1:1-40.

Hyndman SJ, Vickers LM, Htut T, Maunder JW, Peock A, Higenbottam TW. A randomized trial of dehumidification in the control of house dust mite. Clin Exp Allergy. 2000 Aug;30(8):1172-80.

Ibernon M, Moreso F, O'Valle F, Grinyo JM, Moral RG, Seron D. Low serum mannose-binding lectin levels are associated with inflammation and apoptosis in early surveillance allograft biopsies. Transpl Immunol. 2014 Sep;31(3):152-6. doi: 10.1016/j.trim.2014.07.001.

Ibero M, Boné J, Martín B, Martínez J. Evaluation of an extensively hydrolysed casein formula (Damira 2000) in children with allergy to cow's milk proteins. *Allergol Immunopathol (Madr).* 2010 Mar-Apr;38(2):60-8.

413

Ibrahim AR, Kawamoto S, Nishimura M, Pak S, Aki T, Diaz-Perales A, Salcedo G, Asturias JA, Hayashi T, Ono K. A new lipid transfer protein homolog identified as an IgE-binding antigen from Japanese cedar pollen. *Biosci Biotechnol Biochem.* 2010;74(3):504-9.

Ichinohe T, Ainai A, Nakamura T, Akiyama Y, Maeyama J, Odagiri T, Tashiro M, Takahashi H, Sawa H, Tamura S, Chiba J, Kurata T, Sata T, Hasegawa H. Induction of cross-protective immunity against influenza A virus H5N1 by an intranasal vaccine with extracts of mushroom mycelia. J Med Virol. 2010 Jan;82(1):128-37.

Ichinohe T, Ainai A, Nakamura T, Akiyama Y, Maeyama J, Odagiri T, Tashiro M, Takahashi H, Sawa H, Tamura S, Chiba J, Kurata T, Sata T, Hasegawa H. Induction of cross-protective immunity against influenza A virus H5N1 by an intranasal vaccine with extracts of mushroom mycelia. J Med Virol. 2010 Jan;82(1):128-37.

Imase K, Tanaka A, Tokunaga K, Sugano H, Ishida H, Takahashi S. *Lactobacillus reuteri* tablets suppress *Helicobacter pylori* infection—a double-blind randomised placebo-controlled cross-over clinical study. *Kansenshogaku Zasshi.* 2007 Jul;81(4):387-93.

Inbar O, Dotan R, Dlin RA, Neuman I, Bar-Or O. Breathing dry or humid air and exercise-induced asthma during swimming. *Eur J Appl Physiol Occup Physiol.* 1980;44(1):43-50.

Indrio F, Ladisa G, Mautone A, Montagna O. Effect of a fermented formula on thymus size and stool pH in healthy term infants. *Pediatr Res.* 2007 Jul;62(1):98-100.

Indrio F, Riezzo G, Raimondi F, Bisceglia M, Cavallo L, Francavilla R. The effects of probiotics on feeding tolerance, bowel habits, and gastrointestinal motility in preterm newborns. *J Pediatr.* 2008 Jun;152(6):801-6.

Ingale AG, Hivrale AU. Plant as a plenteous reserve of lectin. Plant Signal Behav. 2013;8(12):e26595. doi: 10.4161/psb.26595.

Innis SM, Hansen JW. Plasma fatty acid responses, metabolic effects, and safety of microalgal and fungal oils rich in arachidonic and docosahexaenoic acids in adults. *Am J Clin Nutr.* 1996 Aug;64(2):159-67.

Innis SM, Hansen JW. Plasma fatty acid responses, metabolic effects, and safety of microalgal and fungal oils rich in arachidonic and docosahexaenoic acids in healthy adults. *Am J Clin Nutr.* 1996 Aug;64(2):159-67.

Ionescu JG. New insights in the pathogenesis of atopic disease. *J Med Life.* 2009 Apr-Jun;2(2):146-54.

Iovieno A, Lambiase A, Sacchetti M, Stampachiacchiere B, Micera A, Bonini S. Preliminary evidence of the efficacy of probiotic eye-drop treatment in patients with vernal keratoconjunctivitis. *Graefes Arch Clin Exp Ophthalmol.* 2008 Mar;246(3):435-41.

Iribarren C, Tolstykh IV, Miller MK, Eisner MD. Asthma and the prospective risk of anaphylactic shock and other allergy diagnoses in a large integrated health care delivery system. *Ann Allergy Asthma Immunol.* 2010 May;104(5):371-7.

ISAAC. The International Study of Asthma and Allergies in Childhood (ISAAC) Steering Committee. Worldwide variation in prevalence of symptoms of asthma, allergic rhinoconjunctivitis, and atopic eczema: ISAAC. *Lancet.* 1998;351:1225-1232.

Ishida Y, Nakamura F, Kanzato H, Sawada D, Hirata H, Nishimura A, Kajimoto O, Fujiwara S. Clinical effects of *Lactobacillus acidophilus* strain L-92 on perennial allergic rhinitis: a double-blind, placebo-controlled study. *J Dairy Sci.* 2005 Feb;88(2):527-33.

Ishida Y, Nakamura F, Kanzato H, Sawada D, Hirata H, Nishimura A, Kajimoto O, Fujiwara S. Clinical effects of *Lactobacillus acidophilus* strain L-92 on perennial allergic rhinitis: a double-blind, placebo-controlled study. *J Dairy Sci.* 2005 Feb;88(2):527-33.

Ishida Y, Nakamura F, Kanzato H, Sawada D, Yamamoto N, Kagata H, Oh-Ida M, Takeuchi H, Fujiwara S. Effect of milk fermented with *Lactobacillus acidophilus* strain L-92 on symptoms of Japanese cedar pollen allergy: a randomized placebo-controlled trial. *Biosci Biotechnol Biochem.* 2005 Sep;69(9):1652-60.

Ishikawa H, Akedo I, Otani T, Suzuki T, Nakamura T, Takeyama I, Ishiguro S, Miyaoka E, Sobue T, Kakizoe T. Randomized trial of dietary fiber and *Lactobacillus casei* administration for prevention of colorectal tumors. *Int J Cancer.* 2005 Sep 20;116(5):762-7.

Ishtiaq M, Hanif W, Khan MA, Ashraf M, Butt AM. An ethnomedicinal survey and documentation of important medicinal folklore food phytonims of flora of Samahni valley, (Azad Kashmir) Pakistan. *Pak J Biol Sci.* 2007 Jul 1;10(13):2241-56.

Isolauri E, Joensuu J, Suomalainen H, Luomala M, Vesikari T. Improved immunogenicity of oral D x RRV reassortant rotavirus vaccine by *Lactobacillus casei* GG. *Vaccine.* 1995 Feb;13(3):310-2.

Isolauri E, Juntunen M, Rautanen T, Sillanaukee P, Koivula T. A human Lactobacillus strain (*Lactobacillus casei* sp strain GG) promotes recovery from acute diarrhea in children. *Pediatrics.* 1991 Jul;88(1):90-7.

Isolauri E, Kaila M, Mykkänen H, Ling WH, Salminen S. Oral bacteriotherapy for viral gastroenteritis. *Dig Dis Sci.* 1994 Dec;39(12):2595-600.

Itokawa Y. Magnesium intake and cardiovascular disease. *Clin Calcium.* 2005 Feb;15(2):154-9.

Ivory K, Chambers SJ, Pin C, Prieto E, Arqués JL, Nicoletti C. Oral delivery of *Lactobacillus casei* Shirota modifies allergen-induced immune responses in allergic rhinitis. *Clin Exp Allergy.* 2008 Aug;38(8):1282-9.

Izbicki G, Chavko R, Banauch GI, Weiden MD, Berger KI, Aldrich TK, Hall C, Kelly KJ, Prezant DJ. World trade center "sarcoid-like" granulomatous pulmonary disease in New York City fire department rescue workers. *Chest.* 2007 May;131(5):1414-23.

Izquierdo JL, Martín A, de Lucas P, Rodríguez-González-Moro JM, Almonacid C, Paravisini A. Misdiagnosis of patients receiving inhaled therapies in primary care. *Int J Chron Obstruct Pulmon Dis.* 2010 Aug 9;5:241-9.

Izumi K, Aihara M, Ikezawa Z. Effects of non steroidal antiinflammatory drugs (NSAIDs) on immediate-type food allergy analysis of Japanese cases from 1998 to 2009. *Arerugi.* 2009 Dec;58(12):1629-39.

J.A. Smith *et al.* Evaluation of active hexose correlated compound (AHCC) for the eradication of HPV infections in women with HPV positive Pap smears. International Conference of the Society for Integrative Oncology, Houston, October 28, 2014.

Jaber R. Respiratory and allergic diseases: from upper respiratory tract infections to asthma. *Prim Care.* 2002 Jun;29(2):231-61.

Jackson DJ, Lemanske RF Jr. The role of respiratory virus infections in childhood asthma inception. *Immunol Allergy Clin North Am.* 2010 Nov;30(4):513-22, vi.

Jacobs DE, Wilson J, Dixon SL, Smith J, Evens A. The relationship of housing and population health: a 30-year retrospective analysis. *Environ Health Perspect.* 2009 Apr;117(4):597-604. 2008 Dec 16.

Jacobsen CN, Rosenfeldt Nielsen V, Hayford AE, Møller PL, Michaelsen KF, Paerregaard A, Sandström B, Tvede M, Jakobsen M. Screening of probiotic activities of forty-seven strains of Lactobacillus spp. by in vitro techniques and evaluation of the colonization ability of five selected strains in humans. *Appl Environ Microbiol.* 1999 Nov;65(11):4949-56.

Jagetia GC, Aggarwal BB. "Spicing up" of the immune system by curcumin. *J Clin Immunol.* 2007 Jan;27(1):19-35.

Jagetia GC, Nayak V, Vidyasagar MS. Evaluation of the antineoplastic activity of guduchi (Tinospora cordifolia) in cultured HeLa cells. *Cancer Lett.* 1998 May 15;127(1-2):71-82.

Jagetia GC, Rao SK. Evaluation of Cytotoxic Effects of Dichloromethane Extract of Guduchi (Tinospora cordifolia Miers ex Hook F & THOMS) on Cultured HeLa Cells. *Evid Based Complement Alternat Med.* 2006 Jun;3(2):267-72.

Jahnova E, Horvathova M, Gazdik F, Weissova S. Effects of selenium supplementation on expression of adhesion molecules in corticoid-dependent asthmatics. *Bratisl Lek Listy.* 2002;103(1):12-6.

Jain PK, McNaught CE, Anderson AD, MacFie J, Mitchell CJ. Influence of synbiotic containing *Lactobacillus acidophilus* La5, *Bifidobacterium lactis* Bb 12, *Streptococcus thermophilus*, *Lactobacillus bulgaricus* and oligofructose on gut barrier function and sepsis in critically ill patients: a randomised controlled trial. *Clin Nutr.* 2004 Aug;23(4):467-75.

Jaiswal M, Prajapati PK, Patgiri BJ Ravishankar B. A Comparative Pharmaco - Clinical Study on Anti-Asthmatic Effect of Shirisharishta Prepared by Bark, Sapwood and Heartwood of Albizia Lebbeck. *J Res Ayurv.* 2006;27(3):67-74.

Jaiswal M, Prajapati PK, Patgiri BJ, Ravishankar B. Clinical Study on Anti-Asthmatic Effect of Shirisharishta Prepared by Bark, Sapwood and Heartwood of Albizia Lebbeck. *Pharmaco.* 2006 27(3): 67-74

Janelle KC, Barr SI. Nutrient intakes and eating behavior scores of vegetarian and nonvegetarian women. *J Am Diet Assoc.* 1995 Feb;95(2):180-6, 189, quiz 187-8.

Janson C, Anto J, Burney P, Chinn S, de Marco R, Heinrich J, Jarvis D, Kuenzli N, Leynaert B, Luczynska C, Neukirch F, Svanes C, Sunyer J, Wjst M; European Community Respiratory Health Survey II. The European Community Respiratory Health Survey: what are the main results so far? European Community Respiratory Health Survey II. *Eur Respir J.* 2001 Sep;18(3):598-611.

Jarocka-Cyrta E, Baniukiewicz A, Wasilewska J, Pawlak J, Kaczmarski M. Focal villous atrophy of the duodenum in children who have outgrown cow's milk allergy. Chromoendoscopy and magnification endoscopy evaluation. *Med Wieku Rozwoj.* 2007 Apr-Jun;11(2 Pt 1):123-7.

Jauhiainen T, Vapaatalo H, Poussa T, Kyrönpalo S, Rasmussen M, Korpela R. *Lactobacillus helveticus* fermented milk lowers blood pressure in hypertensive subjects in 24-h ambulatory blood pressure measurement. *Am J Hypertens.* 2005 Dec;18(12 Pt 1):1600-5.

Jawad M, Schoop R, Suter A, Klein P, Eccles R. Safety and Efficacy Profile of Echinacea purpurea to Prevent Common Cold Episodes: A Randomized, Double-Blind, Placebo-Controlled Trial. *Evid Based Complement Alternat Med.* 2012;2012:841315.

Jayakumar, T.; Ramesh, E.; Geraldine, P. Antioxidant activity of the oyster mushroom, Pleurotus ostreatus, on CCL4-induced liver injury in rats. *Food Chem. Toxicol.* 2006, 44, 1989–1996.

Jayaprakasam B, Doddaga S, Wang R, Holmes D, Goldfarb J, Li XM. Licorice flavonoids inhibit eotaxin-1 secretion by human fetal lung fibroblasts in vitro. *J Agric Food Chem.* 2009 Feb 11;57(3):820-5.

REFERENCES AND BIBLIOGRAPHY

Jennings S, Prescott SL. Early dietary exposures and feeding practices: role in pathogenesis and prevention of allergic disease? *Postgrad Med J.* 2010 Feb;86(1012):94-9.

Jensen B. *Foods that Heal.* Garden City Park, NY: Avery Publ, 1988, 1993.

Jensen B. *Nature Has a Remedy.* Los Angeles: Keats, 2001.

Jensen HK. The molecular genetic basis and diagnosis of familial hypercholesterolemia in Denmark. *Dan Med Bull.* 2002 Nov;49(4):318-45.

Jeon HJ, Kang HJ, Jung HJ, Kang YS, Lim CJ, Kim YM, Park EH. Anti-inflammatory activity of Taraxacum officinale. J *Ethnopharmacol.* 2008 Jan 4;115(1):82-8.

Jernelöv S, Höglund CO, Axelsson J, Axén J, Grönneberg R, Grunewald J, Stierna P, Lekander M. Effects of examination stress on psychological responses, sleep and allergic symptoms in atopic and non-atopic students. *Int J Behav Med.* 2009;16(4):305-10.

Ji X, Pan C, Li X, Gao Y, Xia L, Quan X, Lv J, Wang R. Trametes robiniophila may induce apoptosis and inhibit MMPs expression in the human gastric carcinoma cell line MKN-45. Oncol Lett. 2017 Feb;13(2):841-846. doi: 10.3892/ol.2016.5517.

Jiang T, Mustapha A, Savaiano DA. Improvement of lactose digestion in humans by ingestion of unfermented milk containing *Bifidobacterium longum.* J *Dairy Sci.* 1996 May;79(5):750-7.

Jiménez E, Fernández L, Maldonado A, Martín R, Olivares M, Xaus J, Rodríguez JM. Oral administration of Lactobacillus strains isolated from breast milk as an alternative for the treatment of infectious mastitis during lactation. *Appl Environ Microbiol.* 2008 Aug;74(15):4650-5.

Joghatai M, Barari L, Mousavie Anijdan SH, Elmi MM. The Evaluation of Radio-sensitivity of Mung Bean Proteins Aqueous Extract on MCF-7, Hela and Fibroblast Cell Line. Int J Radiat Biol. 2018 Feb 26:1-29. doi: 10.1080/09553002.2018.1446226.

Johansson G, Holmén A, Persson L, Högstedt B, Wassén C, Ottova L, Gustafsson JA. Long-term effects of a change from a mixed diet to a lacto-vegetarian diet on human urinary and faecal mutagenic activity. *Mutagenesis.* 1998 Mar;13(2):167-71.

Johansson G, Holmén A, Persson L, Högstedt B, Wassén C, Ottova L, Gustafsson JA. Dietary influence on some proposed risk factors for colon cancer: fecal and urinary mutagenic activity and the activity of some intestinal bacterial enzymes. *Cancer Detect Prev.* 1997;21(3):258-66.

Johansson G, Holmén A, Persson L, Högstedt R, Wassén C, Ottova L, Gustafsson JA. The effect of a shift from a mixed diet to a lacto-vegetarian diet on human urinary and fecal mutagenic activity. *Carcinogenesis.* 1992 Feb;13(2):153-7.

Johansson G, Ravald N. Comparison of some salivary variables between vegetarians and omnivores. *Eur J Oral Sci.* 1995 Apr;103(2 (Pt 1)):95-8.

Johansson GK, Ottova L, Gustafsson JA. Shift from a mixed diet to a lactovegetarian diet: influence on some cancer-associated intestinal bacterial enzyme activities. *Nutr Cancer.* 1990;14(3-4):239-46. PubMed PMID: 2128119.

Johansson ML, Nobaek S, Berggren A, Nyman M, Björck I, Ahrné S, Jeppsson B, Molin G. Survival of Lactobacillus plantarum DSM 9843 (299v), and effect on the short-chain fatty acid content of faeces after ingestion of a rose-hip drink with fermented oats. *Int J Food Microbiol.* 1998 Jun 30;42(1-2):29-38.

Johari H. *Ayurvedic Massage: Traditional Indian Techniques for Balancing Body and Mind.* Rochester, VT: Healing Arts, 1996.

Johnson LM. Gitksan medicinal plants—cultural choice and efficacy. J *Ethnobiol Ethnomed.* 2006 Jun 21;2:29.

Jones MA, Silman AJ, Whiting S, *et al.* Occurrence of rheumatoid arthritis is not increased in the first degree relatives of a population based inception cohort of inflammatory polyarthritis. *Ann Rheum Dis.* 1996;55(2): 89-93.

Jones SE, Versalovic J. Probiotic Lactobacillus reuteri biofilms produce antimicrobial and anti-inflammatory factors. *BMC Microbiol.* 2009 Feb 11;9:35.

José RJ, Roberts J, Bakerly ND. The effectiveness of a social marketing model on case-finding for COPD in a deprived inner city population. *Prim Care Respir J.* 2010 Jun;19(2):104-8.

Joseph SP, Borrell LN, Shapiro A. Self-reported lifetime asthma and nativity status in U.S. children and adolescents: results from the National Health and Nutrition Examination Survey 1999-2004. J *Health Care Poor Underserved.* 2010 May;21(2 Suppl):125-39.

Juergens UR, Dethlefsen U, Steinkamp G, Gillissen A, Repges R, Vetter H. Anti-inflammatory activity of 1.8-cineol (eucalyptol) in bronchial asthma: a double-blind placebo-controlled trial. *Respir Med.* 2003 Mar;97(3):250-6.

Julkunen-Tiitto R. A chemotaxonomic survey of phenolics in leaves of northern Salicaceae species. Phytochemistry. 1986;25(3):663-667.

Jung HA, Yokozawa T, Kim BW, Jung JH, Choi JS. Selective inhibition of prenylated flavonoids from Sophora flavescens against BACE1 and cholinesterases. *Am J Chin Med.* 2010;38(2):415-29.

Jurenka JS. Anti-inflammatory properties of curcumin, a major constituent of Curcuma longa: a review of preclinical and clinical research. *Altern Med Rev.* 2009 Feb;14(2):141-153.

416

Justice JM, Sleasman JW, Lanza DC. Recalcitrant Rhinosinusitis, Innate Immunity, and Mannose-Binding Lectin. Ann Otol Rhinol Laryngol. 2014 Jul 25. pii: 0003489414543680.

Juszkiewicz A, Basta P, Petriczko E, Machaliński B, Trzeciak J, Łuczkowska K, Skarpańska-Stejnborn A. An attempt to induce an immunomodulatory effect in rowers with spirulina extract. J Int Soc Sports Nutr. 2018 Feb 20;15:9. doi:10.1186/s12970-018-0213-3.

Juvonen R, Bloigu A, Peitso A, Silvennoinen-Kassinen S, Saikku P, Leinonen M, Hassi J, Harju T. Training improves physical fitness and decreases CRP also in asthmatic conscripts. J Asthma. 2008 Apr;45(3):237-42.

Kähkönen MP, Hopia AI, Vuorela HJ, Rauha JP, Pihlaja K, Kujala TS, Heinonen M. Antioxidant activity of plant extracts containing phenolic compounds. J Agric Food Chem. 1999 Oct;47(10):3954-62.

Kaila M, Isolauri E, Saxelin M, Arvilommi H, Vesikari T. Viable versus inactivated lactobacillus strain GG in acute rotavirus diarrhoea. Arch Dis Child. 1995 Jan;72(1):51-3.

Kaila M, Vanto T, Valovirta E, Koivikko A, Juntunen-Backman K. Diagnosis of food allergy in Finland: survey of pediatric practices. Pediatr Allergy Immunol. 2000 Nov;11(4):246-9.

Kajander K, Hatakka K, Poussa T, Färkkilä M, Korpela R. A probiotic mixture alleviates symptoms in irritable bowel syndrome patients: a controlled 6-month intervention. Aliment Pharmacol Ther. 2005 Sep 1;22(5):387-94.

Kajander K, Korpela R. Clinical studies on alleviating the symptoms of irritable bowel syndrome. Asia Pac J Clin Nutr. 2006;15(4):576-80.

Kajander K, Krogius-Kurikka L, Rinttilä T, Karjalainen H, Palva A, Korpela R. Effects of multispecies probiotic supplementation on intestinal microbiota in irritable bowel syndrome. Aliment Pharmacol Ther. 2007 Aug 1;26(3):463-73.

Kajander K, Myllyluoma E, Rajilić-Stojanović M, Kyrönpalo S, Rasmussen M, Järvenpää S, Zoetendal EG, de Vos WM, Vapaatalo H, Korpela R. Clinical trial: multispecies probiotic supplementation alleviates the symptoms of irritable bowel syndrome and stabilizes intestinal microbiota. Aliment Pharmacol Ther. 2008 Jan 1;27(1):48-57.

Kalach N, Benhamou PH, Campeotto F, Dupont Ch. Anemia impairs small intestinal absorption measured by intestinal permeability in children. Eur Ann Allergy Clin Immunol. 2007 Jan;39(1):20-2.

Kaliner M, Shelhamer JH, Borson B, Nadel J, Patow C, Marom Z. Human respiratory mucus. Am Rev Respir Dis. 1986 Sep;134(3):612-21.

Kalliomäki M, Salminen S, Arvilommi H, Kero P, Koskinen P, Isolauri E. Probiotics in primary prevention of atopic disease: a randomised placebo-controlled trial. Lancet. 2001 Apr 7;357(9262):1076-9.

Kalliomäki M, Salminen S, Poussa T, Arvilommi H, Isolauri E. Probiotics and prevention of atopic disease: 4-year follow-up of a randomised placebo-controlled trial. Lancet. 2003 May 31;361(9372):1869-71.

Kalliomäki M, Salminen S, Poussa T, Isolauri E. Probiotics during the first 7 years of life: a cumulative risk reduction of eczema in a randomized, placebo-controlled trial. J Allergy Clin Immunol. 2007 Apr;119(4):1019-21.

Kanazawa H, Nagino M, Kamiya S, Komatsu S, Mayumi T, Takagi K, Asahara T, Nomoto K, Tanaka R, Nimura Y. Synbiotics reduce postoperative infectious complications: a randomized controlled trial in biliary cancer patients undergoing hepatectomy. Langenbecks Arch Surg. 2005 Apr;390(2):104-13.

Kang SK, Kim JK, Ahn SH, Oh JE, Kim JH, Lim DH, Son BK. Relationship between silent gastroesophageal reflux and food sensitization in infants and young children with recurrent wheezing. J Korean Med Sci. 2010 Mar;25(3):425-8.

Kankaanpää PE, Yang B, Kallio HP, Isolauri E, Salminen SJ. Influence of probiotic supplemented infant formula on composition of plasma lipids in atopic infants. J Nutr Biochem. 2002 Jun;13(6):364-369.

Kanny G, Grignon G, Dauca M, Guedenet JC, Moneret-Vautrin DA. Ultrastructural changes in the duodenal mucosa induced by ingested histamine in patients with chronic urticaria. Allergy. 1996 Dec;51(12):935-9.

Kano H, Mogami O, Uchida M. Oral administration of milk fermented with Lactobacillus delbrueckii ssp. bulgaricus OLL1073R-1 to DBA/1 mice inhibits secretion of proinflammatory cytokines. Cytotechnology. 2002 Nov;40(1-3):67-73.

Kapil A, Sharma S. Immunopotentiating compounds from Tinospora cordifolia. J Ethnopharmacol. 1997 Oct;58(2):89-95.

Kaplan C. Indoor air pollution from unprocessed solid fuels in developing countries. Rev Environ Health. 2010 Jul-Sep;25(3):221-42.

Kaplan M, Mutlu EA, Benson M, Fields JZ, Banan A, Keshavarzian A. Use of herbal preparations in the treatment of oxidant-mediated inflammatory disorders. Complement Ther Med. 2007 Sep;15(3):207-16. 2006 Aug 21.

Kaplan R. The nature of the view from home: psychological benefits. Environ Behav. 2001;33(4):507-42.

Kaplan R. Wilderness perception and psychological benefits: an analysis of a continuing program. Leisure Sci. 1984;6(3):271-90.

REFERENCES AND BIBLIOGRAPHY

Karkoulias K, Patouchas D, Alahiotis S, Tsiamita M, Vrodakis K, Spiropoulos K. Specific sensitization in wheat flour and contributing factors in traditional bakers. *Eur Rev Med Pharmacol Sci.* 2007 May-Jun;11(3):141-8.

Karpińska J, Mikołuć B, Motkowski R, Piotrowska-Jastrzebska J. HPLC method for simultaneous determination of retinol, alpha-tocopherol and coenzyme Q10 in human plasma. *J Pharm Biomed Anal.* 2006 Sep 18;42(2):232-6.

Kashiwada Y, Takanaka K, Tsukada H, Miwa Y, Taga T, Tanaka S, Ikeshiro Y. Sesquiterpene glucosides from anti-leukotriene B4 release fraction of Taraxacum officinale. *J Asian Nat Prod Res.* 2001;3(3):191-7.

Katial RK, Strand M, Prasertsuntarasai T, Leung R, Zheng W, Alam R. The effect of aspirin desensitization on novel biomarkers in aspirin-exacerbated respiratory diseases. *J Allergy Clin Immunol.* 2010 Oct;126(4):738-44. 2010 Aug 21.

Kattan JD, Srivastava KD, Sampson HA, Li XM. Pharmacologic and Immunologic Effects of Individual Herbs of Food Allergy Herbal Formula 2 in a Murine Model of Peanut Allergy. *J Allergy Clin Immunol.* 2006;117(2):S34.

Kattan JD, Srivastava KD, Zou ZM, Goldfarb J, Sampson HA, Li XM. Pharmacological and immunological effects of individual herbs in the Food Allergy Herbal Formula-2 (FAHF-2) on peanut allergy. *Phytother Res.* 2008 May;22(5):651-9.

Katz DL, Cushman D, Reynolds J, Njike V, Treu JA, Walker J, Smith E, Katz C. Putting physical activity where it fits in the school day: preliminary results of the ABC (Activity Bursts in the Classroom) for fitness program. *Prev Chronic Dis.* 2010 Jul;7(4):A82. 2010 Jun 15.

Katz Y, Rajuan N, Goldberg MR, Eisenberg E, Heyman E, Cohen A, Leshno M. Early exposure to cow's milk protein is protective against IgE-mediated cow's milk protein allergy. *J Allergy Clin Immunol.* 2010 Jul;126(1):77-82.e1.

Kawase M, Hashimoto H, Hosoda M, Morita H, Hosono A. Effect of administration of fermented milk containing whey protein concentrate to rats and healthy men on serum lipids and blood pressure. *J Dairy Sci.* 2000 Feb;83(2):255-63.

Kazaks AG, Uriu-Adams JY, Albertson TE, Shenoy SF, Stern JS. Effect of oral magnesium supplementation on measures of airway resistance and subjective assessment of asthma control and quality of life in men and women with mild to moderate asthma: a randomized placebo controlled trial. *J Asthma.* 2010 Feb;47(1):83-92.

Kazansky DB. MHC restriction and allogeneic immune responses. *J Immunotoxicol.* 2008 Oct;5(4):369-84.

Kazłowska K, Hsu T, Hou CC, Yang WC, Tsai GJ. Anti-inflammatory properties of phenolic compounds and crude extract from Porphyra dentata. *J Ethnopharmacol.* 2010 Mar 2;128(1):123-30.

Ke X, Qian D, Zhu L, Hong S. [Analysis on quality of life and personality characteristics of allergic rhinitis]. *Lin Chung Er Bi Yan Hou Tou Jing Wai Ke Za Zhi.* 2010 Mar;24(5):200-2.

Kecskés G, Belágyi T, Oláh A. Early jejunal nutrition with combined pre- and probiotics in acute pancreatitis—prospective, randomized, double-blind investigations. *Magy Seb.* 2003 Feb;56(1):3-8.

Keita AV, Söderholm JD. The intestinal barrier and its regulation by neuroimmune factors. *Neurogastroenterol Motil.* 2010 Jul;22(7):718-33.

Kekkonen RA, Lummela N, Karjalainen H, Latvala S, Tynkkynen S, Jarvenpaa S, Kautiainen H, Julkunen I, Vapaatalo H, Korpela R. Probiotic intervention has strain-specific anti-inflammatory effects in healthy adults. *World J Gastroenterol.* 2008 Apr 7;14(13):2029-36.

Kekkonen RA, Sysi-Aho M, Seppanen-Laakso T, Julkunen I, Vapaatalo H, Oresic M, Korpela R. Effect of probiotic *Lactobacillus rhamnosus* GG intervention on global serum lipidomic profiles in healthy adults. *World J Gastroenterol.* 2008 May 28;14(20):3188-94.

Kekkonen RA, Vasankari TJ, Vuorimaa T, Haahtela T, Julkunen I, Korpela R. The effect of probiotics on respiratory infections and gastrointestinal symptoms during training in marathon runners. *Int J Sport Nutr Exerc Metab.* 2007 Aug;17(4):352-63.

Kekkonen RA, Vasankari TJ, Vuorimaa T, Haahtela T, Julkunen I, Korpela R. The effect of probiotics on respiratory infections and gastrointestinal symptoms during training in marathon runners. *Int J Sport Nutr Exerc Metab.* 2007 Aug;17(4):352-63.

Kelder P. *Ancient Secret of the Fountain of Youth.* New York: Doubleday, 1998.

Kelly HW, Van Natta ML, Covar RA, Tonascia J, Green RP, Strunk RC; CAMP Research Group. Effect of long-term corticosteroid use on bone mineral density in children: a prospective longitudinal assessment in the childhood Asthma Management Program (CAMP) study. *Pediatrics.* 2008 Jul;122(1):e53-61.

Kelly-Pieper K, Patil SP, Busse P, Yang N, Sampson H, Li XM, Wisnivesky JP, Kattan M. Safety and tolerability of an antiasthma herbal Formula (ASHMI) in adult subjects with asthma: a randomized, double-blinded, placebo-controlled, dose-escalation phase I study. *J Altern Complement Med.* 2009 Jul;15(7):735-43.

Kenia P, Houghton T, Beardsmore C. Does inhaling menthol affect nasal patency or cough? *Pediatr Pulmonol.* 2008 Jun;43(6):532-7.

Keogh JB, Grieger JA, Noakes M, Clifton PM. Flow-Mediated Dilatation Is Impaired by a High-Saturated Fat Diet but Not by a High-Carbohydrate Diet. *Arterioscler Thromb Vasc Biol.* 2005 Mar 17

Keogh JB, Grieger JA, Noakes M, Clifton PM. Flow-Mediated Dilatation Is Impaired by a High-Saturated Fat Diet but Not by a High-Carbohydrate Diet. *Arterioscler Thromb Vasc Biol.* 2005 Mar:17

Kerckhoffs DA, Brouns F, Hornstra G, Mensink RP. Effects on the human serum lipoprotein profile of beta-glucan, soy protein and isoflavones, plant sterols and stanols, garlic and tocotrienols. *J Nutr.* 2002 Sep;132(9):2494-505.

Kerckhoffs DA, Brouns F, Hornstra G, Mensink RP. Effects on the human serum lipoprotein profile of beta-glucan, soy protein and isoflavones, plant sterols and stanols, garlic and tocotrienols. *J Nutr.* 2002 Sep;132(9):2494-505.

Kerkhof M, Postma DS, Brunekreef B, Reijmerink NE, Wijga AH, de Jongste JC, Gehring U, Koppelman GH. Toll-like receptor 2 and 4 genes influence susceptibility to adverse effects of traffic-related air pollution on childhood asthma. *Thorax.* 2010 Aug;65(8):690-7.

Key T, Appleby P, Davey G, Allen N, Spencer E, Travis R. Mortality in British vegetarians: review and preliminary results from EPIC-Oxford. *Amer. Jour. Clin. Nutr. Suppl.* 2003;78(3): 533S-538S.

Keyaerts E, Vijgen L, Pannecouque C, Van Damme E, Peumans W, Egberink H, Balzarini J, Van Ranst M. Plant lectins are potent inhibitors of coronaviruses by interfering with two targets in the viral replication cycle. Antiviral Res. 2007 Sep;75(3):179-87.

Keyaerts E, Vijgen L, Pannecouque C, Van Damme E, Peumans W, Egberink H, Balzarini J, Van Ranst M. Plant lectins are potent inhibitors of coronaviruses by interfering with two targets in the viral replication cycle. Antiviral Res. 2007 Sep;75(3):179-87.

Kiecolt-Glaser JK, Heffner KL, Glaser R, Malarkey WB, Porter K, Atkinson C, Laskowski B, Lemeshow S, Marshall GD. How stress and anxiety can alter immediate and late phase skin test responses in allergic rhinitis. *Psychoneuroendocrinology.* 2009 Jun;34(5):670-80.

Kiefte-de Jong JC, Escher JC, Arends LR, Jaddoe VW, Hofman A, Raat H, Moll HA. Infant nutritional factors and functional constipation in childhood: the Generation R study. *Am J Gastroenterol.* 2010 Apr;105(4):940-5.

Kiessling G, Schneider J, Jahreis G. Long-term consumption of fermented dairy products over 6 months increases HDL cholesterol. *Eur J Clin Nutr.* 2002 Sep;56(9):843-9.

Kilara A, Shahani KM. The use of immobilized enzymes in the food industry: a review. *CRC Crit Rev Food Sci Nutr.* 1979 Dec;12(2):161-98.

Kilpatrick DC. Animal lectins: a historical introduction and overview. Biochim Biophys Acta. 2002 Sep 19;1572(2-3):187-97.

Kim HM, Shin HY, Lim KH, Ryu ST, Shin TY, Chae HJ, Kim HR, Lyu YS, An NH, Lim KS. Taraxacum officinale inhibits tumor necrosis factor-alpha production from rat astrocytes. *Immunopharmacol Immunotoxicol.* 2000 Aug;22(3):519-30.

Kim JH, An S, Kim JE, Choi GS, Ye YM, Park HS. Beef-induced anaphylaxis confirmed by the basophil activation test. *Allergy Asthma Immunol Res.* 2010 Jul;2(3):206-8.

Kim JH, Ellwood PE, Asher MI. Diet and asthma: looking back, moving forward. *Respir Res.* 2009 Jun 12;10:49.

Kim JH, Kim JE, Choi GS, Hwang EK, An S, Ye YM, Park HS. A case of occupational rhinitis caused by rice powder in the grain industry. *Allergy Asthma Immunol Res.* 2010 Apr;2(2):141-3.

Kim JH, Lee SY, Kim HB, Jin HS, Yu JH, Kim BJ, Kim BS, Kang MJ, Jang SO, Hong SJ. TBXA2R gene polymorphism and responsiveness to leukotriene receptor antagonist in children with asthma. *Clin Exp Allergy.* 2008 Jan;38(1):51-9.

Kim JI, Lee MS, Jung SY, Choi JY, Lee S, Ko JM, Zhao H, Zhao J, Kim AR, Shin MS, Kang KW, Jung HJ, Kim TH, Liu B, Choi SM. Acupuncture for persistent allergic rhinitis: a multi-centre, randomised, controlled trial protocol. Trials. 2009 Jul 14;10:54.

Kim JY, Kim DY, Lee YS, Lee BK, Lee KH, Ro JY. DA-9601, Artemisia asiatica herbal extract, ameliorates airway inflammation of allergic asthma in mice. *Mol Cells.* 2006;22:104-12.

Kim LS, Waters RF, Burkholder PM. Immunological activity of larch arabinogalactan and Echinacea: a preliminary, randomized, double-blind, placebo-controlled trial. *Altern Med Rev.* 2002 Apr;7(2):138-49.

Kim MN, Kim N, Lee SH, Park YS, Hwang JH, Kim JW, Jeong SH, Lee DH, Kim JS, Jung HC, Song IS. The effects of probiotics on PPI-triple therapy for *Helicobacter pylori* eradication. *Helicobacter.* 2008 Aug;13(4):261-8.

Kim NI, Jo Y, Ahn SB, Son BK, Kim SH, Park YS, Kim SH, Ju JE. A case of eosinophilic esophagitis with food hypersensitivity. *J Neurogastroenterol Motil.* 2010 Jul;16(3):315-8.

Kim SJ, Jung JY, Kim HW, Park T. Anti-obesity effects of Juniperus chinensis extract are associated with increased AMP-activated protein kinase expression and phosphorylation in the visceral adipose tissue of rats. *Biol Pharm Bull.* 2008 Jul;31(7):1415-21.

Kim TE, Park SW, Noh G, Lee S. Comparison of skin prick test results between crude allergen extracts from foods and commercial allergen extracts in atopic dermatitis by double-blind placebo-controlled food challenge for milk, egg, and soybean. *Yonsei Med J.* 2002 Oct;43(5):613-20.

Kim YG, Moon JT, Lee KM, Chon NR, Park H. The effects of probiotics on symptoms of irritable bowel syndrome. *Korean J Gastroenterol.* 2006 Jun;47(6):413-9.

Kim YH, Kim KS, Han CS, Yang HC, Park SH, Ko KI, Lee SH, Kim KH, Lee NH, Kim JM, Son K. Inhibitory effects of natural plants of Jeju Island on elastase and MMP-1 expression. *Int J Cosmet Sci.* 2007 Dec;29(6):487-8.

Kimata H. Differential effects of laughter on allergen-specific immunoglobulin and neurotrophin levels in tears. *Percept Mot Skills.* 2004 Jun;98(3 Pt 1):901-8.

Kimata H. Effect of viewing a humorous vs. nonhumorous film on bronchial responsiveness in patients with bronchial asthma. *Physiol Behav.* 2004 Jun;81(4):681-4.

Kimata H. Emotion with tears decreases allergic responses to latex in atopic eczema patients with latex allergy. *J Psychosom Res.* 2006 Jul;61(1):67-9.

Kimata H. Increase in dermcidin-derived peptides in sweat of patients with atopic eczema caused by a humorous video. *J Psychosom Res.* 2007 Jan;62(1):57-9.

Kimata H. Laughter counteracts enhancement of plasma neurotrophin levels and allergic skin wheal responses by mobile phone-mediated stress. *Behav Med.* 2004 Winter;29(4):149-52.

Kimata H. Modulation of fecal polyamines by viewing humorous films in patients with atopic dermatitis. *Eur J Gastroenterol Hepatol.* 2010 Jun;22(6):724-8.

Kimata H. Reduction of allergic responses in atopic infants by mother's laughter. *Eur J Clin Invest.* 2004 Sep;34(9):645-6.

Kimata H. Viewing a humorous film decreases IgE production by seminal B cells from patients with atopic eczema. *J Psychosom Res.* 2009 Feb;66(2):173-5.

Kimata H. Viewing humorous film improves nighttime wakening in children with atopic dermatitis. *Indian Pediatr.* 2007 Apr;44(4):281-5.

Kimata M, Inagaki N, Nagai H. Effects of luteolin and other flavonoids on IgE-mediated allergic reactions. *Planta Med.* 2000 Feb;66(1):25-9.

Kimata M, Shichijo M, Miura T, Serizawa I, Inagaki N, Nagai H. Effects of luteolin, quercetin and baicalein on immunoglobulin E-mediated mediator release from human cultured mast cells. *Clin Exp Allergy.* 2000 Apr;30(4):501-8.

Kimmatkar N, Thawani V, Hingorani L, Khiyani R. Efficacy and tolerability of Boswellia serrata extract in treatment of osteoarthritis of knee—a randomized double blind placebo controlled trial. *Phytomedicine.* 2003 Jan;10(1):3-7.

Kinaciyan T, Jahn-Schmid B, Radakovics A, Zwölfer B, Schreiber C, Francis JN, Ebner C, Bohle B. Successful sublingual immunotherapy with birch pollen has limited effects on concomitant food allergy to apple and the immune response to the Bet v 1 homolog Mal d 1. *J Allergy Clin Immunol.* 2007 Apr;119(4):937-43.

Kinross JM, von Roon AC, Holmes E, Darzi A, Nicholson JK. The human gut microbiome: implications for future health care. *Curr Gastroenterol Rep.* 2008 Aug;10(4):396-403.

Kippelen P, Larsson J, Anderson SD, Brannan JD, Dahlén B, Dahlén SE. Effect of sodium cromoglycate on mast cell mediators during hyperpnea in athletes. *Med Sci Sports Exerc.* 2010 Oct;42(10):1853-60.

Kirjavainen PV, Arvola T, Salminen SJ, Isolauri E. Aberrant composition of gut microbiota of allergic infants: a target of bifidobacterial therapy at weaning? *Gut.* 2002 Jul;51(1):51-5.

Kirjavainen PV, Salminen SJ, Isolauri E. Probiotic bacteria in the management of atopic disease: underscoring the importance of viability. *J Pediatr Gastroenterol Nutr.* 2003 Feb;36(2):223-7.

Kirpich IA, Solovieva NV, Leikhter SN, Shidakova NA, Lebedeva OV, Sidorov PI, Bazhukova TA, Soloviev AG, Barve SS, McClain CJ, Cave M. Probiotics restore bowel flora and improve liver enzymes in human alcohol-induced liver injury: a pilot study. *Alcohol.* 2008 Dec;42(8):675-82.

Kisiel W, Barszcz B. Further sesquiterpenoids and phenolics from Taraxacum officinale. *Fitoterapia.* 2000 Jun;71(3):269-73.

Kisiel W, Michalska K. Sesquiterpenoids and phenolics from Taraxacum hondoense. *Fitoterapia.* 2005 Sep;76(6):520-4.

Kitajima H, Sumida Y, Tanaka R, Yuki N, Takayama H, Fujimura M. Early administration of *Bifidobacterium breve* to preterm infants: randomised controlled trial. *Arch Dis Child Fetal Neonatal Ed.* 1997 Mar;76(2):F101-7.

Klarin B, Johansson ML, Molin G, Larsson A, Jeppsson B. Adhesion of the probiotic bacterium *Lactobacillus plantarum* 299v onto the gut mucosa in critically ill patients: a randomised open trial. *Crit Care.* 2005 Jun;9(3):R285-93.

Klarin B, Molin G, Jeppsson B, Larsson A. Use of the probiotic *Lactobacillus plantarum* 299 to reduce pathogenic bacteria in the oropharynx of intubated patients: a randomised controlled open pilot study. *Crit Care.* 2008;12(6):R136.

Klein A, Friedrich U, Vogelsang H, Jahreis G. *Lactobacillus acidophilus* 74-2 and *Bifidobacterium animalis* subsp *lactis* DGCC 420 modulate unspecific cellular immune response in healthy adults. *Eur J Clin Nutr.* 2008 May;62(5):584-93.

Klein E, Smith D, Laxminarayan R. Trends in Hospitalizations and Deaths in the United States Associated with Infections Caused by Staphylococcus aureus and MRSA, 1999-2004. *Emerging Infectious Diseases. University of Florida Rel.* 2007 Dec 3.

Klein R, Landau MG. *Healing: The Body Betrayed.* Minneapolis: DCI:Chronimed, 1992.

Klein U, Kanellis MJ, Drake D. Effects of four anticaries agents on lesion depth progression in an in vitro caries model. *Pediatr Dent.* 1999 May-Jun;21(3):176-80.

Klein-Galczinsky C. Pharmacological and clinical effectiveness of a fixed phytogenic combination trembling poplar (Populus tremula), true goldenrod (Solidago virgaurea) and ash (Fraxinus excelsior) in mild to moderate rheumatic complaints. *Wien Med Wochenschr.* 1999;149(8-10):248-53.

Klemola T, Vanto T, Juntunen-Backman K, Kalimo K, Korpela R, Varjonen E. Allergy to soy formula and to extensively hydrolyzed whey formula in infants with cow's milk allergy: a prospective, randomized study with a follow-up to the age of 2 years. *J Pediatr.* 2002 Feb;140(2):219-24.

Klima H, Haas O, Roschger P. Photon emission from blood cells and its possible role in immune system regulation. In: Jezowska-Trzebiatowska B. (ed.): *Photon Emission from Biological Systems. Singapore: World Sci.* 1987:153-169.

Klingberg TD, Budde BB. The survival and persistence in the human gastrointestinal tract of five potential probiotic lactobacilli consumed as freeze-dried cultures or as probiotic sausage. *Int J Food Microbiol.* 2006 May 25;109(1-2):157-9.

Kloss J. *Back to Eden.* Twin Oaks, WI: Lotus Press, 1939-1999.

Knutson TW, Bengtsson U, Dannaeus A, Ahlstedt S, Knutson L. Effects of luminal antigen on intestinal albumin and hyaluronan permeability and ion transport in atopic patients. *J Allergy Clin Immunol.* 1996 Jun;97(6):1225-32.

Ko J, Busse PJ, Shek L, Noone SA, Sampson HA, Li XM. Effect of Chinese Herbal Formulas on T Cell Responses in Patients with Peanut Allergy or Asthma. *J Allergy Clin Immunol.*2005;115:S34.

Ko J, Lee JI, Munoz-Furlong A, Li XM, Sicherer SH. Use of complementary and alternative medicine by food-allergic patients. *Ann Allergy Asthma Immunol.* 2006;97:365-9.

Kobayashi I, Hamasaki Y, Sato R, Zaitu M, Muro E, Yamamoto S, Ichimaru T, Miyazaki S. Saiboku-To, a herbal extract mixture, selectively inhibits 5-lipoxygenase activity in leukotriene synthesis in rat basophilic leukemia-1 cells. *J Ethnopharmacol.* 1995 Aug 11;48(1):33-41.

Kohlhammer Y, Döring A, Schäfer T, Wichmann HE, Heinrich J; KORA Study Group. Swimming pool attendance and hay fever rates later in life. *Allergy.* 2006 Nov;61(11):1305-9. PubMed PMID: 17002706.

Kohlhammer Y, Zutavern A, Rzehak P, Woelke G, Heinrich J. Influence of physical inactivity on the prevalence of hay fever. *Allergy.* 2006 Nov;61(11):1310-5.

Kojima M, Kimura N, Miura R. Regulation of primary metabolic pathways in oyster mushroom mycelia induced by blue light stimulation: accumulation of shikimic acid. Sci Rep. 2015 Feb 27;5:8630. doi: 10.1038/srep08630.

Kojima M, Kimura N, Miura R. Regulation of primary metabolic pathways in oyster mushroom mycelia induced by blue light stimulation: accumulation of shikimic acid. Sci Rep. 2015 Feb 27;5:8630. doi: 10.1038/srep08630.

Kokwaro JO. *Medicinal Plants of East Africa.* Nairobi: Univ of Neirobi Press, 2009.

Kollaritsch H, Holst H, Grobara P, Wiedermann G. Prevention of traveler's diarrhea with *Saccharomyces boulardii.* Results of a placebo controlled double-blind study. *Fortschr Med.* 1993 Mar 30;111(9):152-6.

Kong LF, Guo LH, Zheng XY. Effect of yiqi bushen huoxue herbs in treating children asthma and on levels of nitric oxide, endothelin-1 and serum endothelial cells. *Zhongguo Zhong Xi Yi Jie He Za Zhi.* 2001 Sep;21(9):667-9.

Koo HN, Hong SH, Song BK, Kim CH, Yoo YH, Kim HM. Taraxacum officinale induces cytotoxicity through TNF-alpha and IL-1alpha secretion in Hep G2 cells. *Life Sci.* 2004 Jan 16;74(9):1149-57.

Koop H, Bachem MG. Serum iron, ferritin, and vitamin B12 during prolonged omeprazole therapy. *J Clin Gastroenterol.* 1992;14:288-92.

Kootstra HS, Vlieg-Boerstra BJ, Dubois AE. Assessment of the reduced allergenic properties of the Santana apple. *Ann Allergy Asthma Immunol.* 2007 Dec;99(6):522-5.

Korschunov VM, Smeianov VV, Efimov BA, Tarabrina NP, Ivanov AA, Baranov AE. Therapeutic use of an antibiotic-resistant *Bifidobacterium* preparation in men exposed to high-dose gamma-irradiation. *J Med Microbiol.* 1996 Jan;44(1):70-4.

Kositz C, Schroecksnadel K, Grander G, Schennach H, Kofler H, Fuchs D. High serum tryptophan concentration in pollinosis patients is associated with unresponsiveness to pollen extract therapy. *Int Arch Allergy Immunol.* 2008;147(1):35-40.

Kotowska M, Albrecht P, Szajewska H. *Saccharomyces boulardii* in the prevention of antibiotic-associated diarrhoea in children: a randomized double-blind placebo-controlled trial. *Aliment Pharmacol Ther.* 2005 Mar 1;21(5):583-90.

Kotzampassi K, Giamarellos-Bourboulis EJ, Voudouris A, Kazamias P, Eleftheriadis E. Benefits of a synbiotic formula (Synbiotic 2000Forte) in critically Ill trauma patients: early results of a randomized controlled trial. *World J Surg.* 2006 Oct;30(10):1848-55.

Kotzampassi K, Giamarellos-Bourboulis EJ, Voudouris A, Kazamias P, Eleftheriadis E. Benefits of a synbiotic formula (Synbiotic 2000Forte) in critically Ill trauma patients: early results of a randomized controlled trial. *World J Surg.* 2006 Oct;30(10):1848-55.

Kovács T, Mette H, Per B, Kun L, Schmelczer M, Barta J, Jean-Claude D, Nagy J. Relationship between intestinal permeability and antibodies against food antigens in IgA nephropathy. *Orv Hetil.* 1996 Jan 14;137(2):65-9.

Kowalchik C, Hylton W (eds). *Rodale's Illustrated Encyclopedia of Herbs.* Emmaus, PA: 1987.

Kowalczyk E, Krzesiński P, Kura M, Niedworok J, Kowalski J, Błaszczyk J. Pharmacological effects of flavonoids from Scutellaria baicalensis. *Przegl Lek.* 2006;63(2):95-6.

Kozlowski LT, Mehta NY, Sweeney CT, Schwartz SS, Vogler GP, Jarvis MJ, West RJ. Filter ventilation and nicotine content of tobacco in cigarettes from Canada, the United Kingdom, and the United States. *Tob Control.* 1998 Winter;7(4):369-75.

Krasse P, Carlsson B, Dahl C, Paulsson A, Nilsson A, Sinkiewicz G. Decreased gum bleeding and reduced gingivitis by the probiotic *Lactobacillus reuteri*. *Swed Dent J.* 2006;30(2):55-60.

Kreig M. *Black Market Medicine.* New York: Bantam, 1968.

Kremmyda LS, Vlachava M, Noakes PS, Diaper ND, Miles EA, Calder PC. Atopy Risk in Infants and Children in Relation to Early Exposure to Fish, Oily Fish, or Long-Chain Omega-3 Fatty Acids: A Systematic Review. *Clin Rev Allergy Immunol.* 2009 Dec 9.

Krogulska A, Dynowski J, Wasowska-Królikowska K. Bronchial reactivity in schoolchildren allergic to food. *Ann Allergy Asthma Immunol.* 2010 Jul;105(1):31-8.

Krogulska A, Wasowska-Królikowska K, Dynowski J. Evaluation of bronchial hyperreactivity in children with asthma undergoing food challenges. *Pol Merkur Lekarski.* 2007 Jul;23(133):30-5.

Krogulska A, Wasowska-Królikowska K, Polakowska E, Chrul S. Cytokine profile in children with asthma undergoing food challenges. *J Investig Allergol Clin Immunol.* 2009;19(1):43-8.

Krogulska A, Wasowska-Królikowska K, Polakowska E, Chrul S. Evaluation of receptor expression on immune system cells in the peripheral blood of asthmatic children undergoing food challenges. *Int Arch Allergy Immunol.* 2009;150(4):377-88. 2009 Jul 1.

Krogulska A, Wasowska-Królikowska K, Trzeźwińska B. Food challenges in children with asthma. *Pol Merkur Lekarski.* 2007 Jul;23(133):22-9.

Kroidl RF, Schwichtenberg U, Frank E. Bronchial asthma due to storage mite allergy. Pneumologie. 2007 Aug;61(8):525-30.

Krueger AP, Reed EJ. Biological impact of small air ions. Science. 1976 Sep 24;193(4259):1209-13.

Kruger K, Kamilli I, Schattenkirchner M. Blastocystis hominis as a rare arthritogenic pathogen. *Z Rheumatol.* 1994 Mar-Apr;53(2):83-5.

Krüger P, Kanzer J, Hummel J, Fricker G, Schubert-Zsilavecz M, Abdel-Tawab M. Permeation of Boswellia extract in the Caco-2 model and possible interactions of its constituents KBA and AKBA with OATP1B3 and MRP2. *Eur J Pharm Sci.* 2009 Feb 15;36(2-3):275-84.

Kubota A, He F, Kawase M, Harata G, Hiramatsu M, Iino H. Diversity of intestinal bifidobacteria in patients with Japanese cedar pollinosis and possible influence of probiotic intervention. *Curr Microbiol.* 2011 Jan;62(1):71-7.

Kubota A, He F, Kawase M, Harata G, Hiramatsu M, Salminen S, Iino H. Lactobacillus strains stabilize intestinal microbiota in Japanese cedar pollinosis patients. *Microbiol Immunol.* 2009 Apr;53(4):198-205.

Kuitunen M, Kukkonen K, Juntunen-Backman K, Korpela R, Poussa T, Tuure T, Haahtela T, Savilahti E. Probiotics prevent IgE-associated allergy until age 5 years in Cesarean-delivered children but not in the total cohort. *J Allergy Clin Immunol.* 2009 Feb;123(2):335-41.

Kuitunen M, Savilahti E, Sarnesto A. Human alpha-lactalbumin and bovine beta-lactoglobulin absorption in infants. *Allergy.* 1994 May;49(5):354-60.

Kuitunen M, Savilahti E. Mucosal IgA, mucosal cow's milk antibodies, serum cow's milk antibodies and gastrointestinal permeability in infants. *Pediatr Allergy Immunol.* 1995 Feb;6(1):30-5.

Kukkonen K, Kuitunen M, Haahtela T, Korpela R, Poussa T, Savilahti E. High intestinal IgA associates with reduced risk of IgE-associated allergic diseases. *Pediatr Allergy Immunol.* 2010 Feb;21(1 Pt 1):67-73.

Kukkonen K, Nieminen T, Poussa T, Savilahti E, Kuitunen M. Effect of probiotics on vaccine antibody responses in infancy—a randomized placebo-controlled double-blind trial. *Pediatr Allergy Immunol.* 2006 Sep;17(6):416-21.

Kukkonen K, Savilahti E, Haahtela T, Juntunen-Backman K, Korpela R, Poussa T, Tuure T, Kuitunen M. Probiotics and prebiotic galacto-oligosaccharides in the prevention of allergic diseases: a randomized, double-blind, placebo-controlled trial. *J Allergy Clin Immunol.* 2007 Jan;119(1):192-8.

Kukkonen K, Savilahti E, Haahtela T, Juntunen-Backman K, Korpela R, Poussa T, Tuure T, Kuitunen M. Long-term safety and impact on infection rates of postnatal probiotic and prebiotic (synbiotic) treatment: randomized, double-blind, placebo-controlled trial. *Pediatrics.* 2008 Jul;122(1):8-12.

Kukkonen K, Savilahti E, Haahtela T, Juntunen-Backman K, Korpela R, Poussa T, Tuure T, Kuitunen M. Probiotics and prebiotic galacto-oligosaccharides in the prevention of allergic diseases: a randomized, double-blind, placebo-controlled trial. *J Allergy Clin Immunol.* 2007 Jan;119(1):192-8.

Kulka M. The potential of natural products as effective treatments for allergic inflammation: implications for allergic rhinitis. *Curr Top Med Chem.* 2009;9(17):1611-24.

Kull I, Bergström A, Lilja G, Pershagen G, Wickman M. Fish consumption during the first year of life and development of allergic diseases during childhood. *Allergy.* 2006 Aug;61(8):1009-15.

Kull I, Melen E, Alm J, Hallberg J, Svartengren M, van Hage M, Pershagen G, Wickman M, Bergström A. Breast-feeding in relation to asthma, lung function, and sensitization in young schoolchildren. *J Allergy Clin Immunol.* 2010 May;125(5):1013-9.

Kullo IJ, Ballantyne CM. Conditional risk factors for atherosclerosis. *Mayo Clin Proc.* 2005 Feb;80(2):219-30.

Kumar A, Panghal S, Mallapur SS, Kumar M, Ram V, Singh BK. Antiinflammatory Activity of Piper longum Fruit Oil. *Indian J Pharm Sci.* 2009 Jul;71(4):454-6.

Kumar A, Saluja AK, Shah UD, Mayavanshi AV. Pharmacological potential of Albizzia lebbeck: A Review. *Pharmacog.* 2007 Jan-May; 1(1) 171-174.

Kumar R, Singh BP, Srivastava P, Sridhara S, Arora N, Gaur SN. Relevance of serum IgE estimation in allergic bronchial asthma with special reference to food allergy. *Asian Pac J Allergy Immunol.* 2006 Dec;24(4):191-9.

Kummeling I, Mills EN, Clausen M, Dubakiene R, Pérez CF, Fernández-Rivas M, Knulst AC, Kowalski ML, Lidholm J, Le TM, Metzler C, Mustakov T, Popov T, Potts J, van Ree R, Sakellariou A, Töndury B, Tzannis K, Burney P. The EuroPrevall surveys on the prevalence of food allergies in children and adults: background and study methodology. *Allergy.* 2009 Oct;64(10):1493-7.

Kung HC, Hoyert DL, Xu J, Murphy SL. Deaths: Final Data for 2005. *National Vital Statistics Reports.* 2008;56(10). http://www.cdc.gov/nchs/data/ nvsr/nvsr56/nvsr56_10.pdf. Accessed: 2008 Jun.

Kunisawa J, Kiyono H. Aberrant interaction of the gut immune system with environmental factors in the development of food allergies. *Curr Allergy Asthma Rep.* 2010 May;10(3):215-21.

Kurth T, Barr RG, Gaziano JM, Buring JE. Randomised aspirin assignment and risk of adult-onset asthma in the Women's Health Study. *Thorax.* 2008 Jun;63(6):514-8. 2008 Mar 13.

Kurugöl Z, Koturoğlu G. Effects of *Saccharomyces boulardii* in children with acute diarrhoea. *Acta Paediatr.* 2005 Jan;94(1):44-7.

Kusunoki T, Morimoto T, Nishikomori R, Yasumi T, Heike T, Mukaida K, Fujii T, Nakahata T. Breastfeeding and the prevalence of allergic diseases in schoolchildren: Does reverse causation matter? *Pediatr Allergy Immunol.* 2010 Feb;21(1 Pt 1):60-6.

Kuvaeva IB. Permeability of the gastronintestinal tract for macromolecules in health and disease. *Hum Physiol.* 1979 Mar-Apr;4(2):272-83.

Kuz'mina IaS, Vavilova NN. Kinesitherapy of patients with bronchial asthma and excessive body weight at the early stage of rehabilitation treatment. *Vopr Kurortol Fizioter Lech Fiz Kult.* 2009 Sep-Oct;(5):17-20.

Kuznetsov VF, Iushchuk ND, Iurko LP, Nabokova NIu. Intestinal dysbacteriosis in yersiniosis patients and the possibility of its correction with biopreparations. *Ter Arkh.* 1994;66(11):17-8.

Kuznetsova TA, Shevchenko NM, Zviagintseva TN, Besednova NN. Biological activity of fucoidans from brown algae and the prospects of their use in medicine]. *Antibiot Khimioter.* 2004;49(5):24-30.

Kvamme JM, Wilsgaard T, Florholmen J, Jacobsen BK. Body mass index and disease burden in elderly men and women: the Tromsø Study. *Eur J Epidemiol.* 2010 Mar;25(3):183-93. 2010 Jan 20.

Lad V. *Ayurveda: The Science of Self-Healing.* Twin Lakes, WI: Lotus Press.

Laitinen K, Isolauri E. Management of food allergy: vitamins, fatty acids or probiotics? *Eur J Gastroenterol Hepatol.* 2005 Dec;17(12):1305-11.

Laitinen K, Poussa T, Isolauri E; Nutrition, Allergy, Mucosal Immunology and Intestinal Microbiota Group. Probiotics and dietary counselling contribute to glucose regulation during and after pregnancy: a randomised controlled trial. *Br J Nutr.* 2009 Jun;101(11):1679-87.

Lam SK, Ng TB. Lectins: production and practical applications. *Appl Microbiol Biotechnol.* 2011 Jan;89(1):45-55. doi: 10.1007/s00253-010-2892-9.

Lamaison JL, Carnat A, Petitjean-Freytet C. Tannin content and inhibiting activity of elastase in Rosaceae. *Ann Pharm Fr.* 1990;48(6):335-40.

Landmark K, Reikvam A. Do vitamins C and E protect against the development of carotid stenosis and cardiovascular disease? *Tidsskr Nor Laegeforen.* 2005 Jan 20;125(2):159-62.

Laney AS, Cragin LA, Blevins LZ, Sumner AD, Cox-Ganser JM, Kreiss K, Moffatt SG, Lohff CJ. Sarcoidosis, asthma, and asthma-like symptoms among occupants of a historically water-damaged office building. *Indoor Air.* 2009 Feb;19(1):83-90.

Lang CJ, Hansen M, Roscioli E, Jones J, Murgia C, Leigh Ackland M, Zalewski P, Anderson G, Ruffin R. Dietary zinc mediates inflammation and protects against wasting and metabolic derangement caused by sustained cigarette smoke exposure in mice. *Biometals.* 2011 Feb;24(1):23-39. 2010 Aug 29.

Lange NE, Rifas-Shiman SL, Camargo CA Jr, Gold DR, Gillman MW, Litonjua AA. Maternal dietary pattern during pregnancy is not associated with recurrent wheeze in children. *J Allergy Clin Immunol.* 2010 Aug;126(2):250-5, 255.e1-4.

Langhendries JP, Detry J, Van Hees J, Lamboray JM, Darimont J, Mozin MJ, Secretin MC, Senterre J. Effect of a fermented infant formula containing viable bifidobacteria on the fecal flora composition and pH of healthy full-term infants. *J Pediatr Gastroenterol Nutr.* 1995 Aug;21(2):177-81.

Lappe FM. *Diet for a Small Planet.* New York: Ballantine, 1971.

Lara-Villoslada F, Sierra S, Boza J, Xaus J, Olivares M. Beneficial effects of consumption of a dairy product containing two probiotic strains, Lactobacillus CECT5711 and *Lactobacillus gasseri* CECT5714 in healthy children. *Nutr Hosp.* 2007 Jul-Aug;22(4):496-502.

Larenas-Linnemann D, Matta JJ, Shah-Hosseini K, Michels A, Mösges R. Skin prick test evaluation of Dermatophagoides pteronyssinus diagnostic extracts from Europe, Mexico, and the United States. *Ann Allergy Asthma Immunol.* 2010 May;104(5):420-5.

Lau BH, Riesen SK, Truong KP, Lau EW, Rohdewald P, Barreta RA. Pycnogenol as an adjunct in the management of childhood asthma. *J Asthma.* 2004;41(8):825-32.

Laubereau B, Filipiak-Pittroff B, von Berg A, Grübl A, Reinhardt D, Wichmann HE, Koletzko S; GINI Study Group. Caesarean section and gastrointestinal symptoms, atopic dermatitis, and sensitisation during the first year of life. *Arch Dis Child.* 2004 Nov;89(11):993-7.

Laurière M, Pecquet C, Bouchez-Mahiout I, Snégaroff J, Bayrou O, Raison-Peyron N, Vigan M. Hydrolysed wheat proteins present in cosmetics can induce immediate hypersensitivities. *Contact Dermatitis.* 2006 May;54(5):283-9.

LaValle JB. *The Cox-2 Connection.* Rochester, VT: Healing Arts, 2001.

Lazarou J, Pomeranz BH, Corey PN. Incidence of adverse drug reactions in hospitalized patients: a meta-analysis of prospective studies. *JAMA.* 1998 Apr.

Leal AL, Eslava-Schmalbach J, Alvarez C, Buitrago G, Méndez M; Grupo para el Control de la Resistencia Bacteriana en Bogotá. Endemic tendencies and bacterial resistance markers in third-level hospitals in Bogotá, Colombia. Rev Salud Publica (Bogota). 2006 May;8 Suppl 1:59-70.

Lean G. US study links more than 200 diseases to pollution. *London Independent.* 2004 Nov 14.

Leander M, Cronqvist A, Janson C, Uddenfeldt M, Rask-Andersen A. Health-related quality of life predicts onset of asthma in a longitudinal population study. *Respir Med.* 2009 Feb;103(2):194-200.

Lecheler J, Pfannebecker B, Nguyen DT, Petzold U, Munzel U, Kremer HJ, Maus J. Prevention of exercise-induced asthma by a fixed combination of disodium cromoglycate plus reproterol compared with montelukast in young patients. *Arzneimittelforschung.* 2008;58(6):303-9.

Lee E, Haa K, Yook JM, Jin MH, Seo CS, Son KH, Kim HP, Bae KH, Kang SS, Son JK, Chang HW. Anti-asthmatic activity of an ethanol extract from Saururus chinensis. *Biol Pharm Bull.* 2006 Feb;29(2):211-5.

Lee JH, Noh J, Noh G, Kim HS, Mun SH, Choi WS, Cho S, Lee S. Allergen-specific B cell subset responses in cow's milk allergy of late eczematous reactions in atopic dermatitis. *Cell Immunol.* 2010;262(1):44-51.

Lee JY, Kim CJ. Determination of allergenic egg proteins in food by protein-, mass spectrometry-, and DNA-based methods. *J AOAC Int.* 2010 Mar-Apr;93(2):462-77.

Lee KH, Yeh MH, Kao ST, Hung CM, Chen BC, Liu CJ, Yeh CC. Xia-bai-san inhibits lipopolysaccharide-induced activation of intercellular adhesion molecule-1 and nuclear factor-kappa B in human lung cells. *J Ethnopharmacol.* 2009 Jul 30;124(3):530-8.

Lee MC, Lin LH, Hung KL, Wu HY. Oral bacterial therapy promotes recovery from acute diarrhea in children. *Acta Paediatr Taiwan.* 2001 Sep-Oct;42(5):301-5.

Lee SJ, Cho SJ, Park EA. Effects of probiotics on enteric flora and feeding tolerance in preterm infants. *Neonatology.* 2007;91(3):174-9.

Lee SJ, Shim YH, Cho SJ, Lee JW. Probiotics prophylaxis in children with persistent primary vesicoureteral reflux. *Pediatr Nephrol.* 2007 Sep;22(9):1315-20.

Lee TH, Hsueh PR, Yeh WC, Wang HP, Wang TH, Lin JT. Low frequency of bacteremia after endoscopic mucosal resection. *Gastrointest Endosc.* 2000 Aug;52(2):223-5.

Lee YS, Kim SH, Jung SH, Kim JK, Pan CH, Lim SS. Aldose reductase inhibitory compounds from Glycyrrhiza uralensis. *Biol Pharm Bull.* 2010;33(5):917-21.

Léger D, Annesi-Maesano I, Carat F, Rugina M, Chanal I, Pribil C, El Hasnaoui A, Bousquet J. Allergic rhinitis and its consequences on quality of sleep: An unexplored area. *Arch Intern Med.* 2006 Sep 18;166(16):1744-8.

Lehmann B. The vitamin D3 pathway in human skin and its role for regulation of biological processes. *Photochem Photobiol.* 2005 Nov-Dec;81(6):1246-51.

Lehto M, Airaksinen L, Puustinen A, Tillander S, Hannula S, Nyman T, Toskala E, Alenius H, Lauerma A. Thaumatin-like protein and baker's respiratory allergy. *Ann Allergy Asthma Immunol.* 2010 Feb;104(2):139-46.

Leitzmann C. Vegetarian diets: what are the advantages? *Forum Nutr.* 2005;(57):147-56.

Léonard R, Wopfner N, Pabst M, Stadlmann J, Petersen BO, Duus JØ, Himly M, Radauer C, Gadermaier G, Razzazi-Fazeli E, Ferreira F, Altmann F. A new allergen from ragweed (Ambrosia artemisiifolia) with homology to art v 1 from mugwort. *J Biol Chem.* 2010 Aug 27;285(35):27192-200.

Lerman RH, Minich DM, Darland G, Lamb JJ, Chang JL, Hsi A, Bland JS, Tripp ML. Subjects with elevated LDL cholesterol and metabolic syndrome benefit from supplementation with soy protein, phytosterols, hops rho iso-alpha acids, and Acacia nilotica proanthocyanidins. *J Clin Lipidol.* 2010 Jan-Feb;4(1):59-68.

Leroy EM, Baize S, Volchkov VE, Fisher-Hoch SP, Georges-Courbot MC, Lansoud-Soukate J, Capron M, Debré P, McCormick JB, Georges AJ. Human asymptomatic Ebola infection and strong inflammatory response. *Lancet.* 2000 Jun 24;355(9222):2210-5.

Leu YL, Shi LS, Damu AG. Chemical constituents of Taraxacum formosanum. *Chem Pharm Bull.* 2003 May;51(5):599-601.

Leu YL, Wang YL, Huang SC, Shi LS. Chemical constituents from roots of Taraxacum formosanum. *Chem Pharm Bull.* 2005 Jul;53(7):853-5.

Leung DY, Sampson HA, Yunginger JW, Burks AW Jr, Schneider LC, Wortel CH, Davis FM, Hyun JD, Shanahan WR Jr; Avon Longitudinal Study of Parents and Children Study Team. Effect of anti-IgE therapy in patients with peanut allergy. *N Engl J Med.* 2003 Mar 13;348(11):986-93.

Leung DY, Shanahan WR Jr, Li XM, Sampson HA. New approaches for the treatment of anaphylaxis. *Novartis Found Symp.* 2004;257:248-60; discussion 260-4, 276-85.

Lewerin C, Jacobsson S, Lindstedt G, Nilsson-Ehle H. Serum biomarkers for atrophic gastritis and antibodies against Helicobacter pylori in the elderly: Implications for vitamin B12, folic acid and iron status and response to oral vitamin therapy. *Scand J Gastroenterol.* 2008;43(9):1050-6.

Lewis SA, Grimshaw KE, Warner JO, Hourihane JO. The promiscuity of immunoglobulin E binding to peanut allergens, as determined by Western blotting, correlates with the severity of clinical symptoms. *Clin Exp Allergy.* 2005 Jun;35(6):767-73.

Lewis WH, Elvin-Lewis MPF. *Medical Botany: Plants Affecting Man's Health.* New York: Wiley, 1977.

Lewontin R. *The Genetic Basis of Evolutionary Change.* New York: Columbia Univ Press, 1974.

Leyel CF. *Culpeper's English Physician & Complete Herbal.* Hollywood, CA: Wilshire, 1971.

Leynadier F. Mast cells and basophils in asthma. Ann Biol Clin (Paris). 1989;47(6):351-6.

Li J, Li J, Aipire A, Luo J, Yuan P, Zhang F. The combination of Pleurotus ferulae water extract and CpG-ODN enhances the immune responses and antitumor efficacy of HPV peptides pulsed dendritic cell-based vaccine. Vaccine. 2016 Jun 30;34(31):3568-75. doi: 10.1016/j.vaccine.2016.05.022.

Li J, Sun B, Huang Y, Lin X, Zhao D, Tan G, Wu J, Zhao H, Cao L, Zhong N. A multicentre study assessing the prevalence of sensitizations in patients with asthma and/or rhinitis in China. *Allergy.* 2009;64:1083-1092.

Li MH, Zhang HL, Yang BY. Effects of ginkgo leaf concentrated oral liquor in treating asthma. *Zhongguo Zhong Xi Yi Jie He Za Zhi.* 1997 Apr;17(4):216-8. 5.

Li Q, Li XL, Yang X, Bao JM, Shen XH. Effects of antiallergic herbal agents on cystic fibrosis transmembrane conductance regulator in nasal mucosal epithelia of allergic rhinitis rabbits. *Chin Med J (Engl).* 2009 Dec 20;122(24):3020-4.

Li S, Li W, Wang Y, Asada Y, Koike K. Prenylflavonoids from Glycyrrhiza uralensis and their protein tyrosine phosphatase-1B inhibitory activities. *Bioorg Med Chem Lett.* 2010 Sep 15;20(18):5398-401.

Li XM, Huang CK, Zhang TF, Teper AA, Srivastava K, Schofield BH, Sampson HA. The chinese herbal medicine formula MSSM-002 suppresses allergic airway hyperreactivity and modulates TH1/TH2 responses in a murine model of allergic asthma. *J Allergy Clin Immunol.* 2000;106:660-8.

Li XM, Srivastava K. Traditional Chinese medicine for the therapy of allergic disorders. *Curr Opin Otolaryngol Head Neck Surg.* 2006 Jun;14(3):191-6.

Li XM, Zhang TF, Huang CK, Srivastava K, Teper AA, Zhang L, Schofield BH, Sampson HA. Food Allergy Herbal Formula-1 (FAHF-1) blocks peanut-induced anaphylaxis in a murine model. *J Allergy Clin Immunol.* 2001;108:639-46.

Li XM, Zhang TF, Sampson H, Zou ZM, Beyer K, Wen MC, Schofield B. The potential use of Chinese herbal medicines in treating allergic asthma. *Ann Allergy Asthma Immunol.* 2004;93:S35-S44.

Li XM. Beyond allergen avoidance: update on developing therapies for peanut allergy. *Curr Opin Allergy Clin Immunol.* 2005;5:287-92.

Li YQ, Yuan W, Zhang SL. Clinical and experimental study of xiao er ke cuan ling oral liquid in the treatment of infantile bronchopneumonia. *Zhongguo Zhong Xi Yi Jie He Za Zhi.* 1992 Dec;12(12):719-21, 737, 708.

Lied GA, Lillestøl K, Valeur J, Berstad A. Intestinal B cell-activating factor: an indicator of non-IgE-mediated hypersensitivity reactions to food? *Aliment Pharmacol Ther.* 2010 Jul;32(1):66-73.

Lieske JC, Goldfarb DS, De Simone C, Regnier C. Use of a probiotic to decrease enteric hyperoxaluria. *Kidney Int.* 2005 Sep;68(3):1244-9.

Lillestøl K, Berstad A, Lind R, Florvaag E, Arslan Lied G, Tangen T. Anxiety and depression in patients with self-reported food hypersensitivity. *Gen Hosp Psychiatry.* 2010 Jan-Feb;32(1):42-8.

Lim W, Park S, Bazer FW, Song G. Apigenin Reduces Survival of Choriocarcinoma Cells by Inducing Apoptosis via the PI3K/AKT and ERK1/2 MAPK Pathways. J Cell Physiol. 2016 Dec;231(12):2690-9. doi: 10.1002/jcp.25372.

Lima JA, Fischer GB, Sarria EE, Mattiello R, Solé D. Prevalence of and risk factors for wheezing in the first year of life. *J Bras Pneumol.* 2010 Oct;36(5):525-31. English, Portuguese.

Limb SL, Brown KC, Wood RA, Wise RA, Eggleston PA, Tonascia J, Hamilton RG, Adkinson NF Jr. Adult asthma severity in individuals with a history of childhood asthma. *J Allergy Clin Immunol.* 2005 Jan;115(1):61-6.

Lin HC, Hsu CH, Chen HL, Chung MY, Hsu JF, Lien RI, Tsao LY, Chen CH, Su BH. Oral probiotics prevent necrotizing enterocolitis in very low birth weight preterm infants: a multicenter, randomized, controlled trial. *Pediatrics.* 2008 Oct;122(4):693-700.

Lin HC, Su BH, Chen AC, Lin TW, Tsai CH, Yeh TF, Oh W. Oral probiotics reduce the incidence and severity of necrotizing enterocolitis in very low birth weight infants. *Pediatrics.* 2005 Jan;115(1):1-4.

Lin JS, Chiu YH, Lin NT, Chu CH, Huang KC, Liao KW, Peng KC. Different effects of probiotic species/strains on infections in preschool children: A double-blind, randomized, controlled study. *Vaccine.* 2009 Feb 11;27(7):1073-9.

Lin SY, Ayres JW, Winkler W Jr, Sandine WE. Lactobacillus effects on cholesterol: in vitro and in vivo results. *J Dairy Sci.* 1989 Nov;72(11):2885-99.

Lindahl O, Lindwall L, Spångberg A, Stenram A, Ockerman PA. Vegan regimen with reduced medication in the treatment of bronchial asthma. *J Asthma.* 1985;22(1):45-55.

Ling H, He J, Tan H, Yi L, Liu F, Ji X, Wu Y, Hu H, Zeng X, Ai X, Jiang H, Su Q. Identification of potential targets for differentiation in human leukemia cells induced by diallyl disulfide. Int J Oncol. 2017 Feb;50(2):697-707. doi: 10.3892/ijo.2017.3839.

Ling WH, Hänninen O. Shifting from a conventional diet to an uncooked vegan diet reversibly alters fecal hydrolytic activities in humans. J Nutr. 1992 Apr;122(4):924-30.

Ling WH, Hänninen O. Shifting from a conventional diet to an uncooked vegan diet reversibly alters fecal hydrolytic activities in humans. *J Nutr.* 1992 Apr;122(4):924-30.

Lininger S, Gaby A, Austin S, Brown D, Wright J, Duncan A. *The Natural Pharmacy.* New York: Three Rivers, 1999.

Lininger S, Gaby A, Austin S, Brown D, Wright J, Duncan A. *The Natural Pharmacy.* New York: Three Rivers, 1999.

Linsalata M, Russo F, Berloco P, Caruso ML, Matteo GD, Cifone MG, Simone CD, Ierardi E, Di Leo A. The influence of Lactobacillus brevis on ornithine decarboxylase activity and polyamine profiles in Helicobacter pylori-infected gastric mucosa. Helicobacter. 2004 Apr;9(2):165-72.

Linsalata M, Russo F, Berloco P, Caruso ML, Matteo GD, Cifone MG, Simone CD, Ierardi E, Di Leo A. The influence of *Lactobacillus brevis* on ornithine decarboxylase activity and polyamine profiles in *Helicobacter pylori*-infected gastric mucosa. *Helicobacter.* 2004 Apr;9(2):165-72.

Lipkind M. Registration of spontaneous photon emission from virus-infected cell cultures: development of experimental system. *Indian J Exp Biol.* 2003 May;41(5):457-72.

Lipski E. *Digestive Wellness.* Los Angeles, CA: Keats, 2000.

Lissiman E, Bhasale AL, Cohen M. Garlic for the common cold. Cochrane Database Syst Rev. 2014 Nov 11;11:CD006206.

Liu AH, Jaramillo R, Sicherer SH, Wood RA, Bock SA, Burks AW, Massing M, Cohn RD, Zeldin DC. National prevalence and risk factors for food allergy and relationship to asthma: results from the National Health and Nutrition Examination Survey 2005-2006. *J Allergy Clin Immunol.* 2010 Oct;126(4):798-806.e13.

Liu F, Zhang J, Liu Y, Zhang N, Holtappels G, Lin P, Liu S, Bachert C. Inflammatory profiles in nasal mucosa of patients with persistent vs intermittent allergic rhinitis. *Allergy.* 2010 Sep;65(9):1149-57.

Liu GM, Cao MJ, Huang YY, Cai QF, Weng WY, Su WJ. Comparative study of in vitro digestibility of major allergen tropomyosin and other food proteins of Chinese mitten crab (Eriocheir sinensis). *J Sci Food Agric.* 2010 Aug 15;90(10):1614-20.

Liu HY, Giday Z, Moore BF. Possible pathogenetic mechanisms producing bovine milk protein inducible malabsorption: a hypothesis. *Ann Allergy.* 1977 Jul;39(1):1-7.

Liu J, Zhang J, Shi Y, Grimsgaard S, Alraek T, Fønnebø V. Chinese red yeast rice (Monascus purpureus) for primary hyperlipidemia: a meta-analysis of randomized controlled trials. *Chin Med.* 2006 Nov 23;1:4.

Liu JY, Hu JH, Zhu QG, Li FQ, Wang J, Sun HJ. Effect of matrine on the expression of substance P receptor and inflammatory cytokines production in human skin keratinocytes and fibroblasts. *Int Immunopharmacol.* 2007 Jun;7(6):816-23.

Liu Q, Chen X, Yang G, Min X, Deng M. Apigenin inhibits cell migration through MAPK pathways in human bladder smooth muscle cells. Biocell. 2011 Dec;35(3):71-9.

Liu T, Valdez R, Yoon PW, Crocker D, Moonesinghe R, Khoury MJ. The association between family history of asthma and the prevalence of asthma among US adults: National Health and Nutrition Examination Survey, 1999-2004. *Genet Med.* 2009 May;11(5):323-8.

Liu X, Beaty TH, Deindl P, Huang SK, Lau S, Sommerfeld C, Fallin MD, Kao WH, Wahn U, Nickel R. Associations between specific serum IgE response and 6 variants within the genes IL4, IL13, and IL4RA in German children: the German Multicenter Atopy Study. *J Allergy Clin Immunol.* 2004 Mar;113(3):489-95.

Liu XH, Li Q, Zhang P, Su Y, Zhang XR, Sun Q. Serum mannose-binding lectin and C-reactive protein are potential biomarkers for patients with community-acquired pneumonia. Genet Test Mol Biomarkers. 2014 Sep;18(9):630-5. doi: 10.1089/gtmb.2014.0038.

Liu XJ, Cao MA, Li WH, Shen CS, Yan SQ, Yuan CS. Alkaloids from Sophora flavescens Aition. *Fitoterapia.* 2010 Sep;81(6):524-7.

Liu Y, Jing H, Wang J, Zhang R, Zhang Y, Zhang Y, Xu Q, Yu X, Xue C. Micronutrients decrease incidence of common infections in type 2 diabetic outpatients. Asia Pac J Clin Nutr. 2011;20(3):375-82.

Liu Z, Bhattacharyya S, Ning B, Midoro-Horiuti T, Czerwinski EW, Goldblum RM, Mort A, Kearney CM. Plant-expressed recombinant mountain cedar allergen Jun a 1 is allergenic and has limited pectate lyase activity. *Int Arch Allergy Immunol.* 2010;153(4):347-58.

Liu Z, Luo Y, Zhou TT, Zhang WZ. Could plant lectins become promising anti-tumour drugs for causing autophagic cell death? Cell Prolif. 2013 Oct;46(5):509-15. doi: 10.1111/cpr.12054.

Lloyd JU. *American Materia Medica, Therapeutics and Pharmacognosy.* Portland, OR: Eclectic Medical Publications, 1989-1983.

Lloyd Spencer J. Immunization via the anal mucosa and adjacent skin to protect against respiratory virus infections and allergic rhinitis: a hypothesis. *Med Hypotheses.* 2010 Mar;74(3):542-6.

Lloyd-Still JD, Powers CA, Hoffman DR, Boyd-Trull K, Lester LA, Benisek DC, Arterburn LM. Bioavailability and safety of a high dose of docosahexaenoic acid triacylglycerol of algal origin in cystic fibrosis patients: a randomized, controlled study. *Nutrition.* 2006 Jan;22(1):36-46.

Locke GR 3rd, Talley NJ, Fett SL, Zinsmeister AR, Melton LJ 3rd. Prevalence and clinical spectrum of gastroesophageal reflux: a population-based study in Olmsted County, Minnesota. *Gastroenterology.* 1997 May;112(5):1448-56.

Loguercio C, Abbiati R, Rinaldi M, Romano A, Del Vecchio Blanco C, Coltorti M. Long-term effects of *Enterococcus faecium* SF68 versus lactulose in the treatment of patients with cirrhosis and grade 1-2 hepatic encephalopathy. *J Hepatol.* 1995 Jul;23(1):39-46.

Loguercio C, Del Vecchio Blanco C, Coltorti M. Enterococcus lactic acid bacteria strain SF68 and lactulose in hepatic encephalopathy: a controlled study. *J Int Med Res.* 1987 Nov-Dec;15(6):335-43.

Loizzo MR, Saab AM, Tundis R, Statti GA, Menichini F, Lampronti I, Gambari R, Cinatl J, Doerr HW. Phytochemical analysis and in vitro antiviral activities of the essential oils of seven Lebanon species. *Chem Biodivers.* 2008 Mar;5(3):461-70.

Lomax AR, Calder PC. Probiotics, immune function, infection and inflammation: a review of the evidence from studies conducted in humans. *Curr Pharm Des.* 2009;15(13):1428-518.

Longhi L, Orsini F, De Blasio D, Fumagalli S, Ortolano F, Locatelli M, Stocchetti N, De Simoni MG. Mannose-binding lectin is expressed after clinical and experimental traumatic brain injury and its deletion is protective. Crit Care Med. 2014 Aug;42(8):1910-8. doi: 10.1097/CCM.0000000000000399

Longo G, Barbi E, Berti I, Meneghetti R, Pittalis A, Ronfani L, Ventura A. Specific oral tolerance induction in children with very severe cow's milk-induced reactions. *J Allergy Clin Immunol.* 2008 Feb;121(2):343-7.

Lopes EA, Fanelli-Galvani A, Prisco CC, Gonçalves RC, Jacob CM, Cabral AL, Martins MA, Carvalho CR. Assessment of muscle shortening and static posture in children with persistent asthma. *Eur J Pediatr.* 2007 Jul;166(7):715-21.

López A, El-Naggar T, Dueñas M, Ortega T, Estrella I, Hernández T, Gómez-Serranillos MP, Palomino OM, Carretero ME. Effect of cooking and germination on phenolic composition and biological properties of dark beans (Phaseolus vulgaris L.). Food Chem. 2013 May 1;138(1):547-55.

López N, de Barros-Mazón S, Vilela MM, Silva CM, Ribeiro JD. Genetic and environmental influences on atopic immune response in early life. *J Investig Allergol Clin Immunol.* 1999 Nov-Dec;9(6):392-8.

Lopez-Garcia E, Schulze MB, Meigs JB, Manson JE, Rifai N, Stampfer MJ, Willett WC, Hu FB. Consumption of trans fatty acids is related to plasma biomarkers of inflammation and endothelial dysfunction. *J Nutr.* 2005 Mar;135(3):562-6.

Lorea Baroja M, Kirjavainen PV, Hekmat S, Reid G. Anti-inflammatory effects of probiotic yogurt in inflammatory bowel disease patients. *Clin Exp Immunol.* 2007 Sep;149(3):470-9.

Lu MK, Shih YW, Chang Chien TT, Fang LH, Huang HC, Chen PS. α-Solanine inhibits human melanoma cell migration and invasion by reducing matrix metalloproteinase-2/9 activities. *Biol Pharm Bull.* 2010;33(10):1685-91.

Lucas A, Brooke OG, Cole TJ, Morley R, Bamford MF. Food and drug reactions, wheezing, and eczema in preterm infants. *Arch Dis Child.* 1990 Apr;65(4):411-5. 8; .

Lucendo AJ, Lucendo B. An update on the immunopathogenesis of eosinophilic esophagitis. *Expert Rev Gastroenterol Hepatol.* 2010 Apr;4(2):141-8.

Luna Vital DA, González de Mejía E, Dia VP, Loarca-Piña G. Peptides in common bean fractions inhibit human colorectal cancer cells. Food Chem. 2014 Aug 15;157:347-55. doi: 10.1016/j.foodchem.2014.02.050.

Lunardi AC, Marques da Silva CC, Rodrigues Mendes FA, Marques AP, Stelmach R, Fernandes Carvalho CR. Musculoskeletal dysfunction and pain in adults with asthma. *J Asthma.* 2011 Feb;48(1):105-10.

Luo J, Xu F, Lu GJ, Lin HC, Feng ZC. Low mannose-binding lectin (MBL) levels and MBL genetic polymorphisms associated with the risk of neonatal sepsis: An updated meta-analysis. Early Hum Dev. 2014 Oct;90(10):557-64. doi: 10.1016/j.earlhumdev.2014.07.007.

Lv X, Xi L, Han D, Zhang L. Evaluation of the psychological status in seasonal allergic rhinitis patients. *ORL J Otorhinolaryngol Relat Spec.* 2010;72(2):84-90.

Lykken DT, Tellegen A, DeRubeis R: Volunteer bias in twin research: the rule of two-thirds. *Soc Biol* 1978, 25(1): 1-9. Phillips DI: Twin studies in medical research: can they tell us whether diseases are genetically determined? *Lancet* 1993;341(8851): 1008-1009.

Lythcott GI. Anaphylaxis to viomycin. *Am Rev Tuberc.* 1957 Jan;75(1):135-8.

Ma J, Xiao L, Knowles SB. Obesity, insulin resistance and the prevalence of atopy and asthma in US adults. Allergy. 2010 Nov;65(11):1455-63.

Ma XP, Muzhapaer D. Efficacy of sublingual immunotherapy in children with dust mite allergic asthma. *Zhongguo Dang Dai Er Ke Za Zhi.* 2010 May;12(5):344-7.

Mabey R, ed. *The New Age Herbalist.* New York: Simon & Schuster, 1941.

Macdonald TT, Monteleone G. Immunity, inflammation, and allergy in the gut. *Science.* 2005 Mar 25;307(5717):1920-5.

Maciorkowska E, Kaczmarski M, Andrzej K. Endoscopic evaluation of upper gastrointestinal tract mucosa in children with food hypersensitivity. *Med Wieku Rozwoj.* 2000 Jan-Mar;4(1):37-48.

Mackerras D, Cunningham J, Hunt A, Brent P. Re: "effect of supplemental folic acid in pregnancy on childhood asthma: a prospective birth cohort study". *Am J Epidemiol.* 2010 Mar 15;171(6):746-7; author reply 747. 2010 Feb 9.

MacRedmond R, Singhera G, Attridge S, Bahzad M, Fava C, Lai Y, Hallstrand TS, Dorscheid DR. Conjugated linoleic acid improves airway hyper-reactivity in overweight mild asthmatics. *Clin Exp Allergy.* 2010 Jul;40(7):1071-8.

Macsali F, Real FG, Omenaas ER, Bjorge L, Janson C, Franklin K, Svanes C. Oral contraception, body mass index, and asthma: a cross-sectional Nordic-Baltic population survey. *J Allergy Clin Immunol.* 2009 Feb;123(2):391-7.

Madden JA, Plummer SF, Tang J, Garaiova I, Plummer NT, Herbison M, Hunter JO, Shimada T, Cheng L, Shirakawa T. Effect of probiotics on preventing disruption of the intestinal microflora following antibiotic therapy: a double-blind, placebo-controlled pilot study. *Int Immunopharmacol.* 2005 Jun;5(6):1091-7.

Maeda N, Inomata N, Morita A, Kirino M, Ikezawa Z. Correlation of oral allergy syndrome due to plant-derived foods with pollen sensitization in Japan. *Ann Allergy Asthma Immunol.* 2010 Mar;104(3):205-10.

Maes HH, Silberg JL, Neale MC, Eaves LJ. Genetic and cultural transmission of antisocial behavior: an extended twin parent model. *Twin Res Hum Genet.* 2007 Feb;10(1):136-50.

Mah KW, Chin VI, Wong WS, Lay C, Tannock GW, Shek LP, Aw MM, Chua KY, Wong HB, Panchalingham A, Lee BW. Effect of a milk formula containing probiotics on the fecal microbiota of asian infants at risk of atopic diseases. *Pediatr Res.* 2007 Dec;62(6):674-9.

Mai XM, Kull I, Wickman M, Bergström A. Antibiotic use in early life and development of allergic diseases: respiratory infection as the explanation. *Clin Exp Allergy.* 2010 Aug;40(8):1230-7.

Mainardi T, Kapoor S, Bielory L. Complementary and alternative medicine: herbs, phytochemicals and vitamins and their immunologic effects. *J Allergy Clin Immunol.* 2009 Feb;123(2):283-94; quiz 295-6.

Majamaa H, Isolauri E, Saxelin M, Vesikari T. Lactic acid bacteria in the treatment of acute rotavirus gastroenteritis. *J Pediatr Gastroenterol Nutr.* 1995 Apr;20(3):333-8.

Majamaa H, Isolauri E. Probiotics: a novel approach in the management of food allergy. *J Allergy Clin Immunol.* 1997 Feb;99(2):179-85.

Makrides M, Neumann M, Gibson R. Effect of maternal docosahexaenoic acid (DHA) supplementation on breast milk composition. *Europ Jrnl of Clin Nutr.* 1996;50:352-357.

Maliakal PP, Wanwimolruk S. Effect of herbal teas on hepatic drug metabolizing enzymes in rats. *J Pharm Pharmacol.* 2001 Oct;53(10):1323-9.

Mälkönen T, Alanko K, Jolanki R, Luukkonen R, Aalto-Korte K, Lauerma A, Susitaival P. Long-term follow-up study of occupational hand eczema. Br J Dermatol. 2010 Aug 13.

Mallol J, Solé D, Baeza-Bacab M, Aguirre-Camposano V, Soto-Quiros M, Baena-Cagnani C; Latin American ISAAC Group. Regional variation in asthma symptom prevalence in Latin American children. *J Asthma.* 2010 Aug;47(6):644-50.

Maneechotesuwan K, Supawita S, Kasetsinsombat K, Wongkajornsilp A, Barnes PJ. Sputum indoleamine-2, 3-dioxygenase activity is increased in asthmatic airways by using inhaled corticosteroids. *J Allergy Clin Immunol.* 2008 Jan;121(1):43-50.

Manley KJ, Fraenkel MB, Mayall BC, Power DA. Probiotic treatment of vancomycin-resistant enterococci: a randomised controlled trial. *Med J Aust.* 2007 May 7;186(9):454-7.

Mansfield LE, Posey CR. Daytime sleepiness and cognitive performance improve in seasonal allergic rhinitis treated with intranasal fluticasone propionate. *Allergy Asthma Proc.* 2007 Mar-Apr;28(2):226-9.

Månsson HL. Fatty acids in bovine milk fat. *Food Nutr Res.* 2008;52. doi: 10.3402/fnr.v52i0.1821.

Manz F. Hydration and disease. *J Am Coll Nutr.* 2007 Oct;26(5 Suppl):535S-541S.

Manzoni P, Mostert M, Leonessa ML, Priolo C, Farina D, Monetti C, Latino MA, Gomirato G. Oral supplementation with *Lactobacillus casei* subspecies *rhamnosus* prevents enteric colonization by *Candida* species in preterm neonates: a randomized study. *Clin Infect Dis.* 2006 Jun 15;42(12):1735-42.

Marcel AK, Ekali LG, Eugene S, Arnold OE, Sandrine ED, von der Weid D, Gbaguidi E, Ngogang J, Mbanya JC. The effect of Spirulina platensis versus soybean on insulin resistance in HIV-infected patients: a randomized pilot study. Nutrients. 2011 Jul;3(7):712-24. doi: 10.3390/nu3070712.

Marcos A, Wärnberg J, Nova E, Gómez S, Alvarez A, Alvarez R, Mateos JA, Cobo JM. The effect of milk fermented by yogurt cultures plus *Lactobacillus casei* DN-114001 on the immune response of subjects under academic examination stress. *Eur J Nutr.* 2004 Dec;43(6):381-9.

Marcucci F, Duse M, Frati F, Incorvaia C, Marseglia GL, La Rosa M. The future of sublingual immunotherapy. *Int J Immunopathol Pharmacol.* 2009 Oct-Dec;22(4 Suppl):31-3.

Margioris AN. Fatty acids and postprandial inflammation. *Curr Opin Clin Nutr Metab Care.* 2009 Mar;12(2):129-37.

Maria KW, Behrens T, Brasky TM. Are asthma and allergies in children and adolescents increasing? Results from ISAAC Phase I and Phase II surveys in Munster, Germany. Allergy. 2003;58:572-579.

Marin C, Ramirez R, Delgado-Lista J, Yubero-Serrano EM, Perez-Martinez P, Carracedo J, Garcia-Rios A, Rodriguez F, Gutierrez-Mariscal FM, Gomez P, Perez-Jimenez F, Lopez-Miranda J. Mediterranean diet reduces endothelial damage and improves the regenerative capacity of endothelium. Am J Clin Nutr. 2011 Feb;93(2):267-74.

Marotta F, Naito Y, Jain S, Lorenzetti A, Soresi V, Kumari A, Carrera Bastos P, Tomella C, Yadav H. Is there a potential application of a fermented nutraceutical in acute respiratory illnesses? An in-vivo placebo-controlled, cross-over clinical study in different age groups of healthy subjects. J Biol Regul Homeost Agents. 2012 Apr-Jun;26(2):285-94.

Marteau P, Pochart P, Bouhnik Y, Zidi S, Goderel I, Rambaud JC. Survival of *Lactobacillus acidophilus* and *Bifidobacterium* sp. in the small intestine following ingestion in fermented milk. A rational basis for the use of probiotics in man. *Gastroenterol Clin Biol.* 1992;16(1):25-8.

Marth K, Novatchkova M, Focke-Tejkl M, Jenisch S, Jäger S, Kabelitz D, Valenta R. Tracing antigen signatures in the human IgE repertoire. *Mol Immunol.* 2010 Aug;47(14):2323-9.

Martin IR, Wickens K, Patchett K, Kent R, Fitzharris P, Siebers R, Lewis S, Crane J, Holbrook N, Town GI, Smith S. Cat allergen levels in public places in New Zealand. *N Z Med J.* 1998 Sep 25;111(1074):356-8.

Martinez M. Docosahexaenoic acid therapy in docosahexaenoic acid-deficient patients with disorders of peroxisomal biogenesis. *Versicherungsmedizin.* 1996;31 Suppl:145-152

Martínez-Augustin O, Boza JJ, Del Pino JI, Lucena J, Martínez-Valverde A, Gil A. Dietary nucleotides might influence the humoral immune response against cow's milk proteins in preterm neonates. *Biol Neonate.* 1997;71(4):215-23.

Martin-Venegas R, Roig-Perez S, Ferrer R, Moreno JJ. Arachidonic acid cascade and epithelial barrier function during Caco-2 cell differentiation. J Lipid Res. 2006 Apr;3.

Martin-Venegas R, Roig-Perez S, Ferrer R, Moreno JJ. Arachidonic acid cascade and epithelial barrier function during Caco-2 cell differentiation. *J Lipid Res.* 2006 Apr;3.

Marushko IuV. The development of a treatment method for streptococcal tonsillitis in children. *Lik Sprava.* 2000 Jan-Feb;(1):79-82.

Maslowski KM, Mackay CR. Diet, gut microbiota and immune responses. *Nat Immunol.* 2011 Jan;12(1):5-9.

Masoli M, Fabian D, Holt S, Beasley R. The global burden of asthma: executive summary of the GINA Dissemination Committee Report. *Allergy*. 2004;59:469-478.

Massey DG, Chien YK, Fournier-Massey G. Mamane: scientific therapy for asthma? *Hawaii Med J*. 1994;53:350-1. 363.

Massicot JG, Cohen SG. Epidemiologic and socioeconomic aspects of allergic diseases. *J Allergy Clin Immunol*. 1986 Nov;78(5 Pt 2):954-8.

Masuno T, Kishimoto S, Ogura T, Honma T, Niitani H, Fukuoka M, Ogawa N. A comparative trial of LC9018 plus doxorubicin and doxorubicin alone for the treatment of malignant pleural effusion secondary to lung cancer. *Cancer*. 1991 Oct 1;68(7):1495-500.

Matasar MJ, Neugut AI. Epidemiology of anaphylaxis in the United States. *Curr Allergy Asthma Rep*. 2003;3:30-35.

Mater DD, Bretigny L, Firmesse O, Flores MJ, Mogenet A, Bresson JL, Corthier G. *Streptococcus thermophilus* and *Lactobacillus delbrueckii* subsp. bulgaricus survive gastrointestinal transit of healthy volunteers consuming yogurt. *FEMS Microbiol Lett*. 2005 Sep 15;250(2):185-7.

Matheson MC, Haydn Walters E, Burgess JA, Jenkins MA, Giles GG, Hopper JL, Abramson MJ, Dharmage SC. Childhood immunization and atopic disease into middle-age—a prospective cohort study. *Pediatr Allergy Immunol*. 2010 Mar;21(2 Pt 1):301-6.

Mathur BN, Shahani KM. Use of total whey constituents for human food. *J Dairy Sci*. 1979 Jan;62(1):99-105.

Matricardi PM, Bockelbrink A, Beyer K, Keil T, Niggemann B, Grüber C, Wahn U, Lau S. Primary versus secondary immunoglobulin E sensitization to soy and wheat in the Multi-Centre Allergy Study cohort. *Clin Exp Allergy*. 2008 Mar;38(3):493-500.

Matsui EC, Matsui W. Higher serum folate levels are associated with a lower risk of atopy and wheeze. *J Allergy Clin Immunol*. 2009 Jun;123(6):1253-9.e2. 2009 May 5.

Matsumoto M, Benno Y. Anti-inflammatory metabolite production in the gut from the consumption of probiotic yogurt containing *Bifidobacterium animalis* subsp. *lactis* LKM512. *Biosci Biotechnol Biochem*. 2006 Jun;70(6):1287-92.

Matsumoto M, Benno Y. Consumption of *Bifidobacterium lactis* LKM512 yogurt reduces gut mutagenicity by increasing gut polyamine contents in healthy adult subjects. *Mutat Res*. 2004 Dec 21;568(2):147-53.

Matsumoto Y, Noguchi E, Imoto Y, Nanatsue K, Takeshita K, Shibasaki M, Arinami T, Fujieda S. Upregulation of IL17RB during natural allergen exposure in patients with seasonal allergic rhinitis. *Allergol Int*. 2011 Mar;60(1):87-92.

Matsuzaki T, Saito M, Usuku K, Nose H, Izumo S, Arimura K, Osame M. A prospective uncontrolled trial of fermented milk drink containing viable *Lactobacillus casei* strain Shirota in the treatment of HTLV-1 associated myelopathy/tropical spastic paraparesis. *J Neurol Sci*. 2005 Oct 15;237(1-2):75-81.

Matthews SG, Phillips DI. Transgenerational inheritance of stress pathology. Exp Neurol. 2012 Jan;233(1):95-101.

Mattila P, Renkonen J, Toppila-Salmi S, Parviainen V, Joenväärä S, Alff-Tuomala S, Nicorici D, Renkonen R. Time-series nasal epithelial transcriptomics during natural pollen exposure in healthy subjects and allergic patients. *Allergy*. 2010 Feb;65(2):175-83.

Maurer HR. Bromelain: biochemistry, pharmacology and medical use. *Cell Mol Life Sci*. 2001 Aug;58(9):1234-45.

Mayes MD. Epidemiologic studies of environmental agents and systemic autoimmune diseases. *Environ Health Perspect*. 1999 Oct;107 Suppl 5:743-8.

Maywald M, Rink L. Zinc supplementation induces CD4(+)CD25(+)Foxp3(+) antigen-specific regulatory T cells and suppresses IFN-γ production by upregulation of Foxp3 and KLF-10 and downregulation of IRF-1. Eur J Nutr. 2016 Jun 3.

McAlindon TE. Nutraceuticals: do they work and when should we use them? *Best Pract Res Clin Rheumatol*. 2006 Feb;20(1):99-115.

McCarney RW, Lasserson TJ, Linde K, Brinkhaus B. An overview of two Cochrane systematic reviews of complementary treatments for chronic asthma: acupuncture and homeopathy. *Respir Med*. 2004 Aug;98(8):687-96.

McCarney RW, Linde K, Lasserson TJ. Homeopathy for chronic asthma. *Cochrane Database Syst Rev*. 2004;(1):CD000353.

McConnaughey E. *Sea Vegetables*. Happy Camp, CA: Naturegraph, 1985.

McDougall J, McDougall M. *The McDougal Plan*. Clinton, NJ: New Win, 1983.

McGuire BW, Sia LL, Haynes JD, Kisicki JC, Gutierrez M, Stokstad EL. Absorption kinetics of orally administered leucovorin calcium. *NCI Monogr*. 1987;(5):47-56.

McGuire BW, Sia LL, Leese PT, Gutierrez ML, Stokstad EL. Pharmacokinetics of leucovorin calcium after intravenous, intramuscular, and oral administration. *Clin Pharm*. 1988 Jan;7(1):52-8.

McHugh MK, Symanski E, Pompeii LA, Delclos GL. Prevalence of asthma by industry and occupation in the U.S. working population. *Am J Ind Med*. 2010 May;53(5):463-75.

McHugh MK, Symanski E, Pompeii LA, Delclos GL. Prevalence of asthma among adult females and males in the United States: results from the National Health and Nutrition Examination Survey (NHANES), 2001-2004. *J Asthma*. 2009 Oct;46(8):759-66.

McKeever TM, Lewis SA, Cassano PA, Ocké M, Burney P, Britton J, Smit HA. Patterns of dietary intake and relation to respiratory disease, forced expiratory volume in 1 s, and decline in 5-y forced expiratory volume. *Am J Clin Nutr*. 2010 Aug;92(2):408-15. 2010 Jun 16.

McKenzie H, Main J, Pennington CR, Parratt D. Antibody to selected strains of Saccharomyces cerevisiae (baker's and brewer's yeast) and Candida albicans in Crohn's disease. *Gut*. 1990 May;31(5):536-8.

McLachlan CN. beta-casein A1, ischaemic heart disease mortality, and other illnesses. *Med Hypotheses*. 2001 Feb;56(2):262-72.

McNally ME, Atkinson SA, Cole DE. Contribution of sulfate and sulfoesters to total sulfur intake in infants fed human milk. *J Nutr*. 1991 Aug;121(8):1250-4.

McNaught CE, Woodcock NP, Anderson AD, MacFie J. A prospective randomised trial of probiotics in critically ill patients. *Clin Nutr*. 2005 Apr;24(2):211-9.

McNaught CE, Woodcock NP, MacFie J, Mitchell CJ. A prospective randomised study of the probiotic *Lactobacillus plantarum* 299V on indices of gut barrier function in elective surgical patients. *Gut*. 2002 Dec;51(6):827-31.

Meglio P, Bartone E, Plantamura M, Arabito E, Giampietro PG. A protocol for oral desensitization in children with IgE-mediated cow's milk allergy. *Allergy*. 2004 Sep;59(9):980-7.

Mehra PN, Puri HS. Studies on Gaduchi satwa. *Indian J Pharm*. 1969;31:180-2.

Meier B, Shao Y, Julkunen-Tiitto R, Bettschart A, Sticher O. A chemotaxonomic survey of phenolic compounds in Swiss willow species. Planta Med. 1992;58:A698.

Meier B, Sticher O, Julkunen-Tiitto R. Pharmaceutical aspects of the use of willows in herbal remedies. Planta Med. 1988;54(6):559-560.

Melcion C, Verroust P, Baud L, Ardaillou N, Morel-Maroger L, Ardaillou R. Protective effect of procyanidolic oligomers on the heterologous phase of glomerulonephritis induced by anti-glomerular basement membrane antibodies. *C R Seances Acad Sci III*. 1982 Dec 6;295(12):721-6.

Men, Research, And The History Of Hay Fever. *OldAndSold.com*, 1943; Accessed May 16, 2011

Mentel R, Meinsen D, Pilgrim H, Herrmann B, Lindequist U. In vitro antiviral effect of extracts of Kuehneromyces mutabilis on influenza virus. Pharmazie. 1994 Nov;49(11):859-60.

Merchant RE and Andre CA. 2001. A review of recent clinical trials of the nutritional supplement Chlorella pyrenoidosa in the treatment of fibromyalgia, hypertension, and ulcerative colitis. *Altern Ther Health Med*. May-Jun;7(3):79-91.

Messina M. Insights gained from 20 years of soy research. *J Nutr*. 2010 Dec;140(12):2289S-2295S. 2010 Oct 27.

Metsälä J, Lundqvist A, Kaila M, Gissler M, Klaukka T, Virtanen SM. Maternal and perinatal characteristics and the risk of cow's milk allergy in infants up to 2 years of age: a case-control study nested in the Finnish population. *Am J Epidemiol*. 2010 Jun 15;171(12):1310-6.

Meyer A, Kirsch H, Domergue F, Abbadi A, Sperling P, Bauer J, Cirpus P, Zank TK, Moreau H, Roscoe TJ, Zahringer U, Heinz E. Novel fatty acid elongases and their use for the reconstitution of docosahexaenoic acid biosynthesis. *J Lipid Res*. 2004 Oct;45(10):1899-909.

Meyer AL, Elmadfa I, Herbacek I, Micksche M. Probiotic, as well as conventional yogurt, can enhance the stimulated production of proinflammatory cytokines. *J Hum Nutr Diet*. 2007 Dec;20(6):590-8.

Michaelsen KF. Probiotics, breastfeeding and atopic eczema. *Acta Derm Venereol Suppl (Stockh)*. 2005 Nov;(215):21-4.

Michail S. The role of probiotics in allergic diseases. Allergy Asthma Clin Immunol. 2009 Oct 22;5(1):5.

Michalska K, Kisiel W. Sesquiterpene lactones from Taraxacum obovatum. *Planta Med*. 2003 Feb;69(2):181-3.

Michelow IC, Lear C, Scully C, Prugar LI, Longley CB, Yantosca LM, Ji X, Karpel M, Brudner M, Takahashi K, Spear GT, Ezekowitz RA, Schmidt EV, Olinger GG. High-dose mannose-binding lectin therapy for Ebola virus infection. J Infect Dis. 2011 Jan 15;203(2):175-9. doi: 10.1093/infdis/jiq025.

Michelson PH, Williams LW, Benjamin DK, Barnato AE. Obesity, inflammation, and asthma severity in childhood: data from the National Health and Nutrition Examination Survey 2001-2004. *Ann Allergy Asthma Immunol*. 2009 Nov;103(5):381-5.

Michetti P, Dorta G, Wiesel PH, Brassart D, Verdu E, Herranz M, Felley C, Porta N, Rouvet M, Blum AL, Corthésy-Theulaz I. Effect of whey-based culture supernatant of *Lactobacillus acidophilus* (johnsonii) La1 on *Helicobacter pylori* infection in humans. *Digestion*. 1999;60(3):203-9.

Michielutti F, Bertini M, Presciuttini B, Andreotti G. Clinical assessment of a new oral bacterial treatment for children with acute diarrhea. *Minerva Med*. 1996 Nov;87(11):545-50.

Mickleborough TD, Lindley MR, Ray S. Dietary salt, airway inflammation, and diffusion capacity in exercise-induced asthma. *Med Sci Sports Exerc*. 2005 Jun;37(6):904-14.

REFERENCES AND BIBLIOGRAPHY

Mikoluc B, Motkowski R, Karpinska J, Piotrowska-Jastrzebska J. Plasma levels of vitamins A and E, coenzyme Q10, and anti-ox-LDL antibody titer in children treated with an elimination diet due to food hypersensitivity. *Int J Vitam Nutr Res.* 2009 Sep;79(5-6):328-36.

Milgrom P, Ly KA, Roberts MC, Rothen M, Mueller G, Yamaguchi DK. Mutans streptococci dose response to xylitol chewing gum. *J Dent Res.* 2006 Feb;85(2):177-81.

Miller AL. The etiologies, pathophysiology, and alternative/complementary treatment of asthma. *Altern Med Rev.* 2001 Feb;6(1):20-47.

Miller GT. *Living in the Environment.* Belmont, CA: Wadsworth, 1996.

Miller JD, Morin LP, Schwartz WJ, Moore RY. New insights into the mammalian circadian clock. *Sleep.* 1996 Oct;19(8):641-67.

Miller K. Cholesterol and In-Hospital Mortality in Elderly Patients. *Am Family Phys.* 2004 May.

Mindell E, Hopkins V. *Prescription Alternatives.* New Canaan, CT: Keats, 1998.

Miranda H, Outeiro TF. The sour side of neurodegenerative disorders: the effects of protein glycation. *J Pathol.* 2010 May;221(1):13-25.

Mitchell AE, Hong YJ, Koh E, Barrett DM, Bryant DE, Denison RF, Kaffka S. Ten-year comparison of the influence of organic and conventional crop management practices on the content of flavonoids in tomatoes. *J Agric Food Chem.* 2007 Jul 25;55(15):6154-9.

Mittag D, Akkerdaas J, Ballmer-Weber BK, Vogel L, Wensing M, Becker WM, Koppelman SJ, Knulst AC, Helbling A, Hefle SL, Van Ree R, Vieths S. Ara h 8, a Bet v 1-homologous allergen from peanut, is a major allergen in patients with combined birch pollen and peanut allergy. *J Allergy Clin Immunol.* 2004 Dec;114(6):1410-7.

Mittag D, Vieths S, Vogel L, Becker WM, Rihs HP, Helbling A, Wüthrich B, Ballmer-Weber BK. Soybean allergy in patients allergic to birch pollen: clinical investigation and molecular characterization of allergens. *J Allergy Clin Immunol.* 2004 Jan;113(1):148-54.

Miyakawa T, Hatano K, Miyauchi Y, Suwa Y, Sawano Y, Tanokura M. A secreted protein with plant-specific cysteine-rich motif functions as a mannose-binding lectin that exhibits antifungal activity. *Plant Physiol.* 2014 Oct;166(2):766-78. doi: 10.1104/pp.114.242636.

Miyake Y, Sasaki S, Tanaka K, Hirota Y. Dairy food, calcium and vitamin D intake in pregnancy, and wheeze and eczema in infants. *Eur Respir J.* 2010 Jun;35(6):1228-34. 2009 Oct 19.

Miyazaki K, Mizutani H, Katabuchi H, Fukuma K, Fujisaki S, Okamura H. Activated (HLA-DR+) T-lymphocyte subsets in cervical carcinoma and effects of radiotherapy and immunotherapy with sizofiran on cell-mediated immunity and survival. Gynecol Oncol. 1995 Mar;56(3):412-20.

Miyazawa T, Itahashi K, Imai T. Management of neonatal cow's milk allergy in high-risk neonates. *Pediatr Int.* 2009 Aug;51(4):544-7.

Moattari A, Aleyasin S, Arabpour M, Sadeghi S. Prevalence of Human Metapneumovirus (hMPV) in Children with Wheezing in Shiraz-Iran. *Iran J Allergy Asthma Immunol.* 2010 Dec;9(4):250-4.

Modern Biology. Austin: Harcourt Brace, 1993.

Mohammad MA, Molloy A, Scott J, Hussein L. Plasma cobalamin and folate and their metabolic markers methylmalonic acid and total homocysteine among Egyptian children before and after nutritional supplementation with the probiotic bacteria *Lactobacillus acidophilus* in yoghurt matrix. *Int J Food Sci Nutr.* 2006 Nov-Dec;57(7-8):470-80.

Mohan R, Koebnick C, Schildt J, Mueller M, Radke M, Blaut M. Effects of *Bifidobacterium lactis* Bb12 supplementation on body weight, fecal pH, acetate, lactate, calprotectin, and IgA in preterm infants. *Pediatr Res.* 2008 Oct;64(4):418-22.

Mohan R, Koebnick C, Schildt J, Schmidt S, Mueller M, Possner M, Radke M, Blaut M. Effects of *Bifidobacterium lactis* Bb12 supplementation on intestinal microbiota of preterm infants: a double-blind, placebo-controlled, randomized study. *J Clin Microbiol.* 2006 Nov;44(11):4025-31.

Mokhtar N, Chan SC. Use of complementary medicine amongst asthmatic patients in primary care. *Med J Malaysia.* 2006 Mar;61(1):125-7.

Monarca S. Zerbini I, Simonati C, Gelatti U. Drinking water hardness and chronic degenerative diseases. Part II. Cardiovascular diseases. *Ann. Ig.* 2003;15:41-56.

Mondal S, Varma S, Bamola VD, Naik SN, Mirdha BR, Padhi MM, Mehta N, Mahapatra SC. Double-blinded randomized controlled trial for immunomodulatory effects of Tulsi (Ocimum sanctum Linn.) leaf extract on healthy volunteers. J Ethnopharmacol. 2011 Jul 14;136(3):452-6. doi: 10.1016/j.jep.2011.05.012.

Moneret-Vautrin DA, Kanny G, Thévenin F. Asthma caused by food allergy. *Rev Med Interne.* 1996;17(7):551-7.

Moneret-Vautrin DA, Morisset M. Adult food allergy. *Curr Allergy Asthma Rep.* 2005 Jan;5(1):80-5.

Monks H, Gowland MH, Mackenzie H, Erlewyn-Lajeunesse M, King R, Lucas JS, Roberts G. How do teenagers manage their food allergies? *Clin Exp Allergy.* 2010 Aug 2.

Moorhead KJ, Morgan HC. *Spirulina: Nature's Superfood.* Kailua-Kona, HI: Nutrex, 1995.

Moreira A, Delgado L, Haahtela T, Fonseca J, Moreira P, Lopes C, Mota J, Santos P, Rytilä P, Castel-Branco MG. Physical training does not increase allergic inflammation in asthmatic children. Eur Respir J. 2008 Dec;32(6):1570-5.

Moreira P, Moreira A, Padrão P, Delgado L. The role of economic and educational factors in asthma: evidence from the Portuguese health survey. Public Health. 2008 Apr;122(4):434-9. 2007 Oct 17.

Morel AF, Dias GO, Porto C, Simionatto E, Stuker CZ, Dalcol II. Antimicrobial activity of extractives of Solidago microglossa. Fitoterapia. 2006 Sep;77(6):453-5.

Morgan DK, Whitelaw E. The case for transgenerational epigenetic inheritance in humans. Mamm Genome. 2008 Jun;19(6):394-7.

Mori T, O'Keefe BR, Sowder RC 2nd, Bringans S, Gardella R, Berg S, Cochran P, Turpin JA, Buckheit RW Jr, McMahon JB, Boyd MR. Isolation and characterization of griffithsin, a novel HIV-inactivating protein, from the red alga Griffithsia sp. J Biol Chem. 2005 Mar 11;280(10):9345-53.

Morimoto K, Takeshita T, Nanno M, Tokudome S, Nakayama K. Modulation of natural killer cell activity by supplementation of fermented milk containing Lactobacillus casei in habitual smokers. Prev Med. 2005 May;40(5):589-94.

Morisset M, Moneret-Vautrin DA, Kanny G, Guénard L, Beaudouin E, Flabbée J, Hatahet R. Thresholds of clinical reactivity to milk, egg, peanut and sesame in immunoglobulin E-dependent allergies: evaluation by double-blind or single-blind placebo-controlled oral challenges. Clin Exp Allergy. 2003 Aug;33(8):1046-51.

Moss M. E. Coli Path Shows Flaws in Ground Beef Inspection. NY Times 2009 Oct 3.

Moussaieff A, Shein NA, Tsenter J, Grigoriadis S, Simeonidou C, Alexandrovich AG, Trembovler V, Ben-Neriah Y, Schmitz ML, Fiebich BL, Munoz E, Mechoulam R, Shohami E. Incensole acetate: a novel neuroprotective agent isolated from Boswellia carterii. J Cereb Blood Flow Metab. 2008 Jul;28(7):1341-52.

Moyle A. Nature Cure for Asthma and Hay Fever. Wellingborough, U.K.: Thorsons, 1978.

Mozafar A. Is there vitamin B12 in plants or not? A plant nutritionist's view. Veg Nutr. 1997;1/2:50-52.

Mozaffarian D, Aro A, Willett WC. Health effects of trans-fatty acids: experimental and observational evidence. Eur J Clin Nutr. 2009 May;63 Suppl 2:S5-21.

Muller H, Lindman AS, Blomfeldt A, Seljeflot I, Pedersen JI. A diet rich in coconut oil reduces diurnal postprandial variations in circulating tissue plasminogen activator antigen and fasting lipoprotein (a) compared with a diet rich in unsaturated fat in women. J Nutr. 2003 Nov;133(11):3422-7.

Müller S, Pühl S, Vieth M, Stolte M. Analysis of symptoms and endoscopic findings in 117 patients with histological diagnoses of eosinophilic esophagitis. Endoscopy. 2007 Apr;39(4):339-44.

Mullié C, Yazourh A, Thibault H, Odou MF, Singer E, Kalach N, Kremp O, Romond MB. Increased poliovirus-specific intestinal antibody response coincides with promotion of Bifidobacterium longum-infantis and Bifidobacterium breve in infants: a randomized, double-blind, placebo-controlled trial. Pediatr Res. 2004 Nov;56(5):791-5.

Mulyaningsih S, Sporer F, Reichling J, Wink M. Antibacterial activity of essential oils from Eucalyptus and of selected components against multidrug-resistant bacterial pathogens. Pharm Biol. 2011 Sep;49(9):893-9. doi: 10.3109/13880209.2011.553625.

Muramatsu D, Iwai A, Aoki S, Uchiyama H, Kawata K, Nakayama Y, Nikawa Y, Kusano K, Okabe M, Miyazaki T. β-Glucan derived from Aureobasidium pullulans is effective for the prevention of influenza in mice. PLoS One. 2012;7(7):e41399.

Muramatsu D, Iwai A, Aoki S, Uchiyama H, Kawata K, Nakayama Y, Nikawa Y, Kusano K, Okabe M, Miyazaki T. β-Glucan derived from Aureobasidium pullulans is effective for the prevention of influenza in mice. PLoS One. 2012;7(7):e41399.

Murray M and Pizzorno J. Encyclopedia of Natural Medicine. 2nd Edition. Roseville, CA: Prima Publishing, 1998.

Murray M, Pizzorno J. Encyclopedia of Natural Medicine. 2nd Edition. Roseville, CA: Prima Publishing, 1998.

Mustapha A, Jiang T, Savaiano DA. Improvement of lactose digestion by humans following ingestion of unfermented acidophilus milk: influence of bile sensitivity, lactose transport, and acid tolerance of Lactobacillus acidophilus. J Dairy Sci. 1997 Aug;80(8):1537-45.

Myllyluoma E, Ahonen AM, Korpela R, Vapaatalo H, Kankuri E. Effects of multispecies probiotic combination on helicobacter pylori infection in vitro. Clin Vaccine Immunol. 2008 Sep;15(9):1472-82.

Nadkarni AK, Nadkarni KM. Indian Materia Medica. (Vols 1 and 2). Bombay, India: Popular Pradashan, 1908, 1976.

Nagai T, Arai Y, Emori M, Nunome SY, Yabe T, Takeda T, Yamada H. Anti-allergic activity of a Kampo (Japanese herbal) medicine "Sho-seiryu-to (Xiao-Qing-Long-Tang)" on airway inflammation in a mouse model. Int Immunopharmacol. 2004 Oct;4(10-11):1353-65.

Nagel G, Linseisen J. Dietary intake of fatty acids, antioxidants and selected food groups and asthma in adults. Eur J Clin Nutr. 2005 Jan;59(1):8-15.

REFERENCES AND BIBLIOGRAPHY

Nagel G, Weinmayr G, Kleiner A, Garcia-Marcos L, Strachan DP; ISAAC Phase Two Study Group. Effect of diet on asthma and allergic sensitisation in the International Study on Allergies and Asthma in Childhood (ISAAC) Phase Two. Thorax. 2010 Jun;65(6):516-22.

Naghii MR, Samman S. The role of boron in nutrition and metabolism. Prog Food Nutr Sci. 1993 Oct-Dec;17(4):331-49.

Nair PK, Rodriguez S, Ramachandran R, Alamo A, Melnick SJ, Escalon E, Garcia PI Jr, Wnuk SF, Ramachandran C. Immune stimulating properties of a novel polysaccharide from the medicinal plant Tinospora cordifolia. Int Immunopharmacol. 2004 Dec 15;4(13):1645-59.

Naito S, Koga H, Yamaguchi A, Fujimoto N, Hasui Y, Kuramoto H, Iguchi A, Kinukawa N; Kyushu University Urological Oncology Group. Prevention of recurrence with epirubicin and Lactobacillus casei after transurethral resection of bladder cancer. J Urol. 2008 Feb;179(2):485-90.

Nakano T, Shimojo N, Morita Y, Arima T, Tomiita M, Kohno Y. Sensitization to casein and beta-lactoglobulin (BLG) in children with cow's milk allergy (CMA). Arerugi. 2010 Feb;59(2):117-22.

Nakau M, Imanishi J, Imanishi J, Watanabe S, Imanishi A, Baba T, Hirai K, Ito T, Chiba W, Morimoto Y. Spiritual care of cancer patients by integrated medicine in urban green space: a pilot study. Explore (NY). 2013 Mar-Apr;9(2):87-90. doi: 10.1016/j.explore.2012.12.002.

Nantz MP, Rowe CA, Muller CE, Creasy RA, Stanilka JM, Percival SS. Supplementation with aged garlic extract improves both NK and γδ-T cell function and reduces the severity of cold and flu symptoms: a randomized, double-blind, placebo-controlled nutrition intervention. Clin Nutr. 2012 Jun;31(3):337-44. doi: 10.1016/j.clnu.2011.11.019.

Napoli, J.E., Brand-Miller, J.C., Conway, P. (2003) Bifidogenic effects of feeding infant formula containing galactooligosaccharides in healthy formula-fed infants. Asia Pac J Clin Nutr. 12(Suppl): S60

Nariya M, Shukla V, Jain S, Ravishankar B. Comparison of enteroprotective efficacy of triphala formulations (Indian Herbal Drug) on methotrexate-induced small intestinal damage in rats. Phytother Res. 2009 Aug;23(8):1092-8.

Naruszewicz M, Daniewski M, Nowicka G, Kozlowska-Wojciechowska M. Trans-unsaturated fatty acids and acrylamide in food as potential atherosclerosis progression factors. Based on own studies. Acta Microbiol Pol. 2003;52 Suppl:75-81.

Naruszewicz M, Johansson ML, Zapolska-Downar D, Bukowska H. Effect of Lactobacillus plantarum 299v on cardiovascular disease risk factors in smokers. Am J Clin Nutr. 2002 Dec;76(6):1249-55.

Naruszewicz M, Johansson ML, Zapolska-Downar D, Bukowska H. Effect of Lactobacillus plantarum 299v on cardiovascular disease risk factors in smokers. Am J Clin Nutr. 2002 Dec;76(6):1249-55.

Narva M, Nevala R, Poussa T, Korpela R. The effect of Lactobacillus helveticus fermented milk on acute changes in calcium metabolism in postmenopausal women. Eur J Nutr. 2004 Apr;43(2):61-8.

Näse L, Hatakka K, Savilahti E, Saxelin M, Pönkä A, Poussa T, Korpela R, Meurman JH. Effect of long-term consumption of a probiotic bacterium, Lactobacillus rhamnosus GG, in milk on dental caries and caries risk in children. Caries Res. 2001 Nov-Dec;35(6):412-20.

National Cooperation Group on Childhood Asthma. A nationwide survey in China on prevalence of asthma in urban children. Chin J Pediatr. pp. 123-127.

National Toxicology Program. Final Report on Carcinogens Background Document for Formaldehyde. Rep Carcinog Backgr Doc. 2010 Jan;(10-5981):i-512.

NDL, BHNRC, ARS, USDA. Oxygen Radical Absorbance Capacity (ORAC) of Selected Foods - 2007. Beltsville, MD: USDA-ARS. 2007.

Nedovic B, Posteraro B, Leoncini E, Ruggeri A, Amore R, Sanguinetti M, Ricciardi W, Boccia S. Mannose-binding lectin codon 54 gene polymorphism and vulvovaginal candidiasis: a systematic review and meta-analysis. Biomed Res Int. 2014;2014:738298. doi: 10.1155/2014/738298.

Nentwich I, Michková E, Nevoral J, Urbanek R, Szépfalusi Z. Cow's milk-specific cellular and humoral immune responses and atopy skin symptoms in infants from atopic families fed a partially (pHF) or extensively (eHF) hydrolyzed infant formula. Allergy. 2001 Dec;56(12):1144-56.

Nestel PJ. Adulthood - prevention: Cardiovascular disease. Med J Aust. 2002 Jun 3;176(11 Suppl):S118-9.

Newall CA, Anderson LA, Phillipson JD (eds). Herbal Medicines: A Guide for Health-Care Professionals. London: Pharmaceut Press; 1996.

Newmark T, Schulick P. Beyond Aspirin. Prescott, AZ: Holm, 2000.

Neyestani TR, Shariatzadeh N, Gharavi A, Kalayi A, Khalaji N. Physiological dose of lycopene suppressed oxidative stress and enhanced serum levels of immunoglobulin M in patients with Type 2 diabetes mellitus: a possible role in the prevention of long-term complications. J Endocrinol Invest. 2007 Nov;30(10):833-8.

Ngai SP, Jones AY, Hui-Chan CW, Ko FW, Hui DS. Effect of Acu-TENS on post-exercise expiratory lung volume in subjects with asthma-A randomized controlled trial. Respir Physiol Neurobiol. 2009 Jul 31;167(3):348-53. 2009 Jun 18.

Nicholls SJ, Lundman P, Harmer JA, Cutri B, Griffiths KA, Rye KA, Barter PJ, Celermajer DS. Consumption of saturated fat impairs the anti-inflammatory properties of high-density lipoproteins and endothelial function. *J Am Coll Cardiol.* 2006 Aug 15;48(4):715-20.

Nicolaou N, Poorafshar M, Murray C, Simpson A, Winell H, Kerry G, Härlin A, Woodcock A, Ahlstedt S, Custovic A. Allergy or tolerance in children sensitized to peanut: prevalence and differentiation using component-resolved diagnostics. *J Allergy Clin Immunol.* 2010 Jan;125(1):191-7.e1-13.

Niederau C, Göpfert E. The effect of chelidonium- and turmeric root extract on upper abdominal pain due to functional disorders of the biliary system. Results from a placebo-controlled double-blind study. *Med Klin.* 1999 Aug 15;94(8):425-30.

Niedzielin K, Kordecki H, Birkenfeld B. A controlled, double-blind, randomized study on the efficacy of *Lactobacillus plantarum* 299V in patients with irritable bowel syndrome. *Eur J Gastroenterol Hepatol.* 2001 Oct;13(10):1143-7.

Nielsen OH, Jørgensen S, Pedersen K, Justesen T. Microbiological evaluation of jejunal aspirates and faecal samples after oral administration of bifidobacteria and lactic acid bacteria. *J Appl Bacteriol.* 1994 May;76(5):469-74.

Nielsen RG, Bindslev-Jensen C, Kruse-Andersen S, Husby S. Severe gastroesophageal reflux disease and cow milk hypersensitivity in infants and children: disease association and evaluation of a new challenge procedure. J *Pediatr Gastroenterol Nutr.* 2004 Oct;39(4):383-91.

Nielsen SE, Young JF, Daneshvar B, Lauridsen ST, Knuthsen P, Sandström B, Dragsted LO. Effect of parsley (Petroselinum crispum) intake on urinary apigenin excretion, blood antioxidant enzymes and biomarkers for oxidative stress in human subjects. Br J Nutr. 1999 Jun;81(6):447-55.

Niggemann B, von Berg A, Bollrath C, Berdel D, Schauer U, Rieger C, Haschke-Becher E, Wahn U. Safety and efficacy of a new extensively hydrolyzed formula for infants with cow's milk protein allergy. *Pediatr Allergy Immunol.* 2008 Jun;19(4):348-54.

Nightingale JA, Rogers DF, Hart LA, Kharitonov SA, Chung KF, Barnes PJ. Effect of inhaled endotoxin on induced sputum in normal, atopic, and atopic asthmatic subjects. *Thorax.* 1998 Jul;53(7):563-71.

NIH Clinical Trials. Phase II Evaluation of AHCC for the Eradication of HPV Infections (AHCC4HPV). NIH. May 2018.

Niimi A, Nguyen LT, Usmani O, Mann B, Chung KF. Reduced pH and chloride levels in exhaled breath condensate of patients with chronic cough. *Thorax.* 2004 Jul;59(7):608-12.

Nilson KM, Vakil JR, Shahani KM. B-complex vitamin content of cheddar cheese. *J Nutr.* 1965 Aug;86:362-8.

Ninan TK, Russell G. Respiratory symptoms and atopy in Aberdeen schoolchildren: evidence from two surveys 25 years apart. BMJ. 1992;304:873-875.

Nishida K, Hasegawa A, Nakae S, Oboki K, Saito H, Yamasaki S, Hirano T. Zinc transporter Znt5/Slc30a5 is required for the mast cell-mediated delayed-type allergic reaction but not the immediate-type reaction. J Exp Med. 2009 Jun 8;206(6):1351-64.

Njoroge GN, Bussmann RW. Traditional management of ear, nose and throat (ENT) diseases in Central Kenya. *J Ethnobiol Ethnomed.* 2006 Dec 27;2:54.

Nobaek S, Johansson ML, Molin G, Ahrné S, Jeppsson B. Alteration of intestinal microflora is associated with reduction in abdominal bloating and pain in patients with irritable bowel syndrome. *Am J Gastroenterol.* 2000 May;95(5):1231-8.

Nodake Y, Fukumoto S, Fukasawa M, Sakakibara R, Yamasaki N. Reduction of the immunogenicity of beta-lactoglobulin from cow's milk by conjugation with a dextran derivative. *Biosci Biotechnol Biochem.* 2010;74(4):721-6.

Noh J, Lee JH, Noh G, Bang SY, Kim HS, Choi WS, Cho S, Lee SS. Characterisation of allergen-specific responses of IL-10-producing regulatory B cells (Br1) in Cow Milk Allergy. *Cell Immunol.* 2010;264(2):143-9.

Nonaka M, Imaeda H, Matsumoto S, Yong Ma B, Kawasaki N, Mekata E, Andoh A, Saito Y, Tani T, Fujiyama Y, Kawasaki T. Mannan-binding protein, a C-type serum lectin, recognizes primary colorectal carcinomas through tumor-associated Lewis glycans. J Immunol. 2014 Feb 1;192(3):1294-301. doi: 10.4049/jimmunol.1203023.

Noone EJ, Roche HM, Nugent AP, Gibney MJ. The effect of dietary supplementation using isomeric blends of conjugated linoleic acid on lipid metabolism in healthy human subjects. *Br J Nutr.* 2002 Sep;88(3):243-51.

Noorbakhsh R, Mortazavi SA, Sankian M, Shahidi F, Assarehzadegan MA, Varasteh A. Cloning, expression, characterization, and computational approach for cross-reactivity prediction of manganese superoxide dismutase allergen from pistachio nut. *Allergol Int.* 2010 Sep;59(3):295-304.

Nopchinda S, Varavithya W, Phuapradit P, Sangchai R, Suthutvoravut U, Chantraruksa V, Haschke F. Effect of bifidobacterium Bb12 with or without *Streptococcus thermophilus* supplemented formula on nutritional status. *J Med Assoc Thai.* 2002 Nov;85 Suppl 4:S1225-31.

Norris R. "Flush-free niacin": Dietary supplement may be "benefit-free." *Prev Cardio.* 2006 Winter: 64.

Nova E, Toro O, Varela P, López-Vidriero I, Morandé G, Marcos A. Effects of a nutritional intervention with yogurt on lymphocyte subsets and cytokine production capacity in anorexia nervosa patients. *Eur J Nutr.* 2006 Jun;45(4):225-33.

Novembre E, Dini L, Bernardini R, Resti M, Vierucci A. Unusual reactions to food additives. *Pediatr Med Chir.* 1992 Jan-Feb;14(1):39-42.

Nowak JE, Harmon K, Caldwell CC, Wong HR. Prophylactic zinc supplementation reduces bacterial load and improves survival in a murine model of sepsis. Pediatr Crit Care Med. 2012 Sep;13(5):e323-9. doi: 10.1097/PCC.0b013e31824fbd90.

Nowak-Wegrzyn A, Fiocchi A. Is oral immunotherapy the cure for food allergies? *Curr Opin Allergy Clin Immunol.* 2010 Jun;10(3):214-9.

Nsouli TM. Long-term use of nasal saline irrigation: harmful or helpful? *Amer Acad of Allergy, Asthma and Immunol.* 2009; Abstract O32.

Nurmatov U, Devereux G, Sheikh A. Nutrients and foods for the primary prevention of asthma and allergy: Systematic review and meta-analysis. *J Allergy Clin Immunol.* 2010 Dec 23.

Nusem D, Panasoff J. Beer anaphylaxis. *Isr Med Assoc J.* 2009 Jun;11(6):380-1.

Nwaru BI, Erkkola M, Ahonen S, Kaila M, Haapala AM, Kronberg-Kippilä C, Salmelin R, Veijola R, Ilonen J, Simell O, Knip M, Virtanen SM. Age at the introduction of solid foods during the first year and allergic sensitization at age 5 years. *Pediatrics.* 2010 Jan;125(1):50-9. 2009 Dec 7.

O'Connor J., Bensky D. (ed). *Shanghai College of Traditional Chinese Medicine: Acupuncture: A Comprehensive Text.* Seattle: Eastland Press, 1981.

O'Neil C, Helbling AA, Lehrer SB. Allergic reactions to fish. *Clin Rev Allergy.* 1993;11(2):183-200.

Obi N, Hayashi K, Miyahara T, Shimada Y, Terasawa K, Watanabe M, Takeyama M, Obi R, Ochiai H. Inhibitory Effect of TNF-alpha Produced by Macrophages Stimulated with Grifola frondosa Extract (ME) on the Growth of Influenza A/Aichi/2/68 Virus in MDCK Cells. Am J Chin Med. 2008;36(6):1171-83.

Obi N, Hayashi K, Miyahara T, Shimada Y, Terasawa K, Watanabe M, Takeyama M, Obi R, Ochiai H. Inhibitory Effect of TNF-alpha Produced by Macrophages Stimulated with Grifola frondosa Extract (ME) on the Growth of Influenza A/Aichi/2/68 Virus in MDCK Cells. Am J Chin Med. 2008;36(6):1171-83.

O'Brien SJ, Shannon JE, Gail MH. A molecular approach to the identification and individualization of human and animal cells in culture: isozyme and allozyme genetic signatures. *In Vitro.* 1980 Feb;16(2):119-35.

Odamaki T, Xiao JZ, Iwabuchi N, Sakamoto M, Takahashi N, Kondo S, Miyaji K, Iwatsuki K, Togashi H, Enomoto T, Benno Y. Influence of Bifidobacterium longum BB536 intake on faecal microbiota in individuals with Japanese cedar pollinosis during the pollen season. *J Med Microbiol.* 2007 Oct;56(Pt 10):1301-8.

Odamaki T, Xiao JZ, Iwabuchi N, Sakamoto M, Takahashi N, Kondo S, Iwatsuki K, Kokubo S, Togashi H, Enomoto T, Benno Y. Fluctuation of fecal microbiota in individuals with Japanese cedar pollinosis during the pollen season and influence of probiotic intake. *J Investig Allergol Clin Immunol.* 2007;17(2):92-100.

Oehme FW (ed.). *Toxicity of heavy metals in the environment. Part 1.* New York: M.Dekker, 1979.

Ogawa T, Hashikawa S, Asai Y, Sakamoto H, Yasuda K, Makimura Y. A new synbiotic, Lactobacillus casei subsp. casei together with dextran, reduces murine and human allergic reaction. *FEMS Immunol Med Microbiol.* 2006 Apr;46(3):400-9.

Ogawa T, Hashikawa S, Asai Y, Sakamoto H, Yasuda K, Makimura Y. A new synbiotic, *Lactobacillus casei* subsp. casei together with dextran, reduces murine and human allergic reaction. *FEMS Immunol Med Microbiol.* 2006 Apr;46(3):400-9.

Oh CK, Lücker PW, Wetzelsberger N, Kuhlmann F. The determination of magnesium, calcium, sodium and potassium in assorted foods with special attention to the loss of electrolytes after various forms of food preparations. *Mag.-Bull.* 1986;8:297-302.

Oh SY, Chung J, Kim MK, Kwon SO, Cho BH. Antioxidant nutrient intakes and corresponding biomarkers associated with the risk of atopic dermatitis in young children. *Eur J Clin Nutr.* 2010 Mar;64(3):245-52. 2010 Jan 27.

Ohashi Y, Nakai S, Tsukamoto T, Masumori N, Akaza H, Miyanaga N, Kitamura T, Kawabe K, Kotake T, Kuroda M, Naito S, Koga H, Saito Y, Nomata K, Kitagawa M, Aso Y. Habitual intake of lactic acid bacteria and risk reduction of bladder cancer. *Urol Int.* 2002;68(4):273-80.

Ok IS, Kim SH, Kim BK, Lee JC, Lee YC. Pinellia ternata, Citrus reticulata, and their combinational prescription inhibit eosinophil infiltration and airway hyperresponsiveness by suppressing CCR3+ and Th2 cytokines production in the ovalbumin-induced asthma model. *Mediators Inflamm.* 2009;2009:413270.

Okamura T, Maehara Y, Sugimachi K. Phase II clinical study of LC9018 on carcinomatous peritonitis of gastric cancer. Subgroup for Carcinomatous Peritonitis, Cooperative, Study Group of LC9018. *Gan To Kagaku Ryoho.* 1989 Jun;16(6):2257-62.

Okawa T, Niibe H, Arai T, Sekiba K, Noda K, Takeuchi S, Hashimoto S, Ogawa N. Effect of LC9018 combined with radiation therapy on carcinoma of the uterine cervix. A phase III, multicenter, randomized, controlled study. *Cancer.* 1993 Sep 15;72(6):1949-54.

Oláh A, Belágyi T, Issekutz A, Gamal ME, Bengmark S. Randomized clinical trial of specific lactobacillus and fibre supplement to early enteral nutrition in patients with acute pancreatitis. *Br J Surg.* 2002 Sep;89(9):1103-7.

Ołdak E, Kurzatkowska B, Stasiak-Barmuta A. Natural course of sensitization in children: follow-up study from birth to 6 years of age, I. Evaluation of total serum IgE and specific IgE antibodies with regard to atopic family history. *Rocz Akad Med Bialymst.* 2000;45:87-95.

Oleĭnichenko EV, Mitrokhin SD, Nonikov VE, Minaev VI. Effectiveness of acipole in prevention of enteric dysbacteriosis due to antibacterial therapy. *Antibiot Khimioter.* 1999;44(1):23-5.

Olivares M, Díaz-Ropero MA, Gómez N, Lara-Villoslada F, Sierra S, Maldonado JA, Martín R, López-Huertas E, Rodríguez JM, Xaus J. Oral administration of two probiotic strains, *Lactobacillus gasseri* CECT5714 and Lactobacillus coryniformis CECT5711, enhances the intestinal function of healthy adults. *Int J Food Microbiol.* 2006 Mar 15;107(2):104-11.

Olivares M, Paz Díaz-Ropero M, Gómez N, Sierra S, Lara-Villoslada F, Martín R, Miguel Rodríguez J, Xaus J. Dietary deprivation of fermented foods causes a fall in innate immune response. Lactic acid bacteria can counteract the immunological effect of this deprivation. *J Dairy Res.* 2006 Nov;73(4):492-8.

O'Mahony L, McCarthy J, Kelly P, Hurley G, Luo F, Chen K, O'Sullivan GC, Kiely B, Collins JK, Shanahan F, Quigley EM. Lactobacillus and bifidobacterium in irritable bowel syndrome: symptom responses and relationship to cytokine profiles. *Gastroenterology.* 2005 Mar;128(3):541-51.

Ombra MN, d'Acierno A, Nazzaro F, Riccardi R, Spigno P, Zaccardelli M, Pane C, Maione M, Fratianni F. Phenolic Composition and Antioxidant and Antiproliferative Activities of the Extracts of Twelve Common Bean (Phaseolus vulgaris L.) Endemic Ecotypes of Southern Italy before and after Cooking. Oxid Med Cell Longev. 2016;2016:1398298. doi: 10.1155/2016/1398298.

Onbasi K, Sin AZ, Doganavsargil B, Onder GF, Bor S, Sebik F. Eosinophil infiltration of the oesophageal mucosa in patients with pollen allergy during the season. *Clin Exp Allergy.* 2005 Nov;35(11):1423-31.

Onder G, *et al.* Serum cholesterol levels and in-hospital mortality in the elderly. *Am J Med.* 2003 Sept;115:265-71.

Onwulata CI, Rao DR, Vankineni P. Relative efficiency of yogurt, sweet acidophilus milk, hydrolyzed-lactose milk, and a commercial lactase tablet in alleviating lactose maldigestion. *Am J Clin Nutr.* 1989 Jun;49(6):1233-7.

Ooi, V.E.C. Hepatoprotective effect of some edible mushrooms. Phytotherapy Res. 1996, 10, 536–538.

Oozeer R, Leplingard A, Mater DD, Mogenet A, Michelin R, Seksek I, Marteau P, Doré J, Bresson JL, Corthier G. Survival of *Lactobacillus casei* in the human digestive tract after consumption of fermented milk. *Appl Environ Microbiol.* 2006 Aug;72(8):5615-7.

Oreskovic NM, Sawicki GS, Kinane TB, Winickoff JP, Perrin JM. Travel patterns to school among children with asthma. *Clin Pediatr.* 2009 Jul;48(6):632-40. 2009 May 6.

Orsatti CL, Nahás EA, Nahas-Neto J, Orsatti FL, Linhares IM, Witkin SS. Mannose-binding lectin gene polymorphism and risk factors for cardiovascular disease in postmenopausal women. Mol Immunol. 2014 Sep;61(1):23-7. doi: 10.1016/j.molimm.2014.05.003.

Ortiz-Andrellucchi A, Sánchez-Villegas A, Rodríguez-Gallego C, Lemes A, Molero T, Soria A, Peña-Quintana L, Santana M, Ramírez O, García J, Cabrera F, Cobo J, Serra-Majem L. Immunomodulatory effects of the intake of fermented milk with Lactobacillus casei DN114001 in lactating mothers and their children. *Br J Nutr.* 2008 Oct;100(4):834-45.

Osguthorpe JD. Immunotherapy. *Curr Opin Otolaryngol Head Neck Surg.* 2010 Jun;18(3):206-12.

Otto SJ, van Houwelingen AC, Hornstra G. The effect of supplementation with docosahexaenoic and arachidonic acid derived from single cell oils on plasma and erythrocyte fatty acids of pregnant women in the second trimester. *Prostaglandins Leukot Essent Fatty Acids.* 2000 Nov;63(5):323-8.

Ou CC, Tsao SM, Lin MC, Yin MC. Protective action on human LDL against oxidation and glycation by four organosulfur compounds derived from garlic. *Lipids.* 2003 Mar;38(3):219-24.

Ouwehand AC, Bergsma N, Parhiala R, Lahtinen S, Gueimonde M, Finne-Soveri H, Strandberg T, Pitkälä K, Salminen S. *Bifidobacterium* microbiota and parameters of immune function in elderly subjects. *FEMS Immunol Med Microbiol.* 2008 Jun;53(1):18-25.

Ouwehand AC, Nermes M, Collado MC, Rautonen N, Salminen S, Isolauri E. Specific probiotics alleviate allergic rhinitis during the birch pollen season. *World J Gastroenterol.* 2009 Jul 14;15(26):3261-8.

Ouwehand AC, Tiihonen K, Saarinen M, Putaala H, Rautonen N. Influence of a combination of *Lactobacillus acidophilus* NCFM and lactitol on healthy elderly: intestinal and immune parameters. *Br J Nutr.* 2009 Feb;101(3):367-75.

Ouwehand AC. Antiallergic effects of probiotics. *J Nutr.* 2007 Mar;137(3 Suppl 2):794S-7S.

Ovelgönne JH, Koninkx JF, Pusztai A, Bardocz S, Kok W, Ewen SW, Hendriks HG, van Dijk JE. Decreased levels of heat shock proteins in gut epithelial cells after exposure to plant lectins. Gut. 2000 May;46(5):679-87.

Overbeck S, Uciechowski P, Ackland ML, Ford D, Rink L. Intracellular zinc homeostasis in leukocyte subsets is regulated by different expression of zinc exporters ZnT-1 to ZnT-9. J Leukoc Biol. 2008 Feb;83(2):368-80.

Ozdemir O. Any benefits of probiotics in allergic disorders? *Allergy Asthma Proc.* 2010 Mar;31(2):103-11.

Ozkan TB, Sahin E, Erdemir G, Budak F. Effect of *Saccharomyces boulardii* in children with acute gastroenteritis and its relationship to the immune response. *J Int Med Res.* 2007 Mar-Apr;35(2):201-12.

Paganelli R, Pallone F, Montano S, Le Moli S, Matricardi PM, Fais S, Paoluzi P, D'Amelio R, Aiuti F. Isotypic analysis of antibody response to a food antigen in inflammatory bowel disease. *Int Arch Allergy Appl Immunol.* 1985;78(1):81-5.

Pahud JJ, Schwarz K. Research and development of infant formulae with reduced allergenic properties. *Ann Allergy.* 1984 Dec;53(6 Pt 2):609-14.

Paineau D, Carcano D, Leyer G, Darquy S, Alyanakian MA, Simoneau G, Bergmann JF, Brassart D, Bornet F, Ouwehand AC. Effects of seven potential probiotic strains on specific immune responses in healthy adults: a double-blind, randomized, controlled trial. *FEMS Immunol Med Microbiol.* 2008 Jun;53(1):107-13.

Pakhale S, Doucette S, Vandemheen K, Boulet LP, McIvor RA, Fitzgerald JM, Hernandez P, Lemiere C, Sharma S, Field SK, Alvarez GG, Dales RE, Aaron SD. A comparison of obese and nonobese people with asthma: exploring an asthma-obesity interaction. *Chest.* 2010 Jun;137(6):1316-23. 2010 Feb 12.

Palacin A, Bartra J, Muñoz R, Diaz-Perales A, Valero A, Salcedo G. Anaphylaxis to wheat flour-derived foodstuffs and the lipid transfer protein syndrome: a potential role of wheat lipid transfer protein Tri a 14. *Int Arch Allergy Immunol.* 2010;152(2):178-83.

Palacios R, Sugawara I. Hydrocortisone abrogates proliferation of T cells in autologous mixed lymphocyte reaction by rendering the interleukin-2 Producer T cells unresponsive to interleukin-1 and unable to synthesize the T-cell growth factor. *Scand J Immunol.* 1982 Jan;15(1):25-31. 7.

Palacios R. HLA-DR antigens render interleukin-2-producer T lymphocytes sensitive to interleukin-1. *Scand J Immunol.* 1981 Sep;14(3):321-6.

Palmer DJ, Gold MS, Makrides M. Effect of cooked and raw egg consumption on ovalbumin content of human milk: a randomized, double-blind, cross-over trial. *Clin Exp Allergy.* 2005 Feb;35(2):173-8.

Panghal S, Mallapur SS, Kumar M, Ram V, Singh BK. Antiinflammatory Activity of Piper longum Fruit Oil. *Indian J Pharm Sci.* 2009 Jul;71(4):454-6.

Panigrahi P, Parida S, Pradhan L, Mohapatra SS, Misra PR, Johnson JA, Chaudhry R, Taylor S, Hansen NI, Gewolb IH. Long-term colonization of a *Lactobacillus plantarum* synbiotic preparation in the neonatal gut. *J Pediatr Gastroenterol Nutr.* 2008 Jul;47(1):45-53.

Pant H, Ferguson BJ, Macardle PJ. The role of allergy in rhinosinusitis. *Curr Opin Otolaryngol Head Neck Surg.* 2009 Jun;17(3):232-8.

Pant H, Kette FE, Smith WB, Wormald PJ, Macardle PJ. Fungal-specific humoral response in eosinophilic mucus chronic rhinosinusitis. *Laryngoscope.* 2005 Apr;115(4):601-6.

Panzani R, Ariano R, Mistrello G. Cypress pollen does not cross-react to plant-derived foods. *Eur Ann Allergy Clin Immunol.* 2010 Jun;42(3):125-6.

Papandreou C, Becerra-Tomás N, Bulló M, Martínez-González MÁ, Corella D, Estruch R, Ros E, Arós F, Schroder H, Fitó M, Serra-Majem L, Lapetra J, Fiol M, Ruiz-Canela M, Sorli JV, Salas-Salvadó J. Legume consumption and risk of all-cause, cardiovascular, and cancer mortality in the PREDIMED study. Clin Nutr. 2018 Jan 9. pii: S0261-5614(17)31439-5. doi: 10.1016/j.clnu.2017.12.019.

Pápay ZE, Kósa A, Boldizsár I, Ruszkai A, Balogh E, Klebovich I, Antal I. Pharmaceutical and formulation aspects of Petroselinum crispum extract. Acta Pharm Hung. 2012;82(1):3-14.

Parcell S. Sulfur in human nutrition and applications in medicine. *Altern Med Rev.* 2002 Feb;7(1):22-44.

Park BJ, Tsunetsugu Y, Kasetani T, Kagawa T, Miyazaki Y. The physiological effects of Shinrin-yoku (taking in the forest atmosphere or forest bathing): evidence from field experiments in 24 forests across Japan. *Environ Health Prev Med.* 2010 Jan;15(1):18-26.

Parra D, De Morentin BM, Cobo JM, Mateos A, Martinez JA. Monocyte function in healthy middle-aged people receiving fermented milk containing *Lactobacillus casei*. *J Nutr Health Aging.* 2004;8(4):208-11.

Parra MD, Martínez de Morentin BE, Cobo JM, Mateos A, Martínez JA. Daily ingestion of fermented milk containing *Lactobacillus casei* DN114001 improves innate-defense capacity in healthy middle-aged people. *J Physiol Biochem.* 2004 Jun;60(2):85-91.

Partridge MR, Dockrell M, Smith NM: The use of complementary medicines by those with asthma. Respir Med 2003, 97:436-438.

Passeron T, Lacour JP, Fontas E, Ortonne JP. Prebiotics and synbiotics: two promising approaches for the treatment of atopic dermatitis in children above 2 years. *Allergy.* 2006 Apr;61(4):431-7.

Pastorello EA, Farioli L, Conti A, Pravettoni V, Bonomi S, Iametti S, Fortunato D, Scibilia J, Bindslev-Jensen C, Ballmer-Weber B, Robino AM, Ortolani C. Wheat IgE-mediated food allergy in European patients: alpha-amylase inhibitors, lipid transfer proteins and low-molecular-weight glutenins. Allergenic molecules recognized by double-blind, placebo-controlled food challenge. *Int Arch Allergy Immunol.* 2007;144(1):10-22.

Pastorello EA, Pompei C, Pravettoni V, Farioli L, Calamari AM, Scibilia J, Robino AM, Conti A, Iametti S, Fortunato D, Bonomi S, Ortolani C. Lipid-transfer protein is the major maize allergen maintaining IgE-binding activity after cooking at 100 degrees C, as demonstrated in anaphylactic patients and patients with positive double-blind, placebo-controlled food challenge results. *J Allergy Clin Immunol.* 2003 Oct;112(4):775-83.

Patchett K, Lewis S, Crane J, Fitzharris P. Cat allergen (Fel d 1) levels on school children's clothing and in primary school classrooms in Wellington, New Zealand. *J Allergy Clin Immunol.* 1997 Dec;100(6 Pt 1):755-9.

Patel DS, Rafferty GF, Lee S, Hannam S, Greenough A. Work of breathing and volume targeted ventilation in respiratory distress. *Arch Dis Child Fetal Neonatal Ed.* 2010 Nov;95(6):F443-6.

Patriarca G, Nucera E, Pollastrini E, Roncallo C, De Pasquale T, Lombardo C, Pedone C, Gasbarrini G, Buonomo A, Schiavino D. Oral specific desensitization in food-allergic children. *Dig Dis Sci.* 2007 Jul;52(7):1662-72.

Patriarca G, Nucera E, Roncallo C, Pollastrini E, Bartolozzi F, De Pasquale T, Buonomo A, Gasbarrini G, Di Campli C, Schiavino D. Oral desensitizing treatment in food allergy: clinical and immunological results. *Aliment Pharmacol Ther.* 2003 Feb;17(3):459-65.

Patterson DB. Anaphylactic shock from chloromycetin. Northwest Med. 1950 May;49(5):352-3.Agarwal KN, Bhasin SK. Feasibility studies to control acute diarrhoea in children by feeding fermented milk preparations Actimel and Indian Dahi. *Eur J Clin Nutr.* 2002 Dec;56 Suppl 4:S56-9.

Patwardhan B, Gautam M. Botanical immunodrugs: scope and opportunities. *Drug Discov Today.* 2005 Apr 1;10(7):495-502.

Paul M, Somkuti GA. Hydrolytic breakdown of lactoferricin by lactic acid bacteria. J Ind Microbiol Biotechnol. 2010 Feb;37(2):173-8. Epub 2009 Nov 19.

Payment P, Franco E, Richardson L, Siemiatyck, J. Gastrointestinal health effects associated with the consumption of drinking water produced by point-of-use domestic reverse-osmosis filtration units. *Appl. Environ. Microbiol.* 1991;57:945-948.

Peat JK, van den Berg RH, Green WF, Mellis CM, Leeder SR, Woolcock AJ. Changing prevalence of asthma in Australian children. *BMJ.* 1994;308:1591-1596.

Peat JK. The rising trend in allergic illness: which environmental factors are important? Clin Exp Allergy. 1994 Sep;24(9):797-800.

Pedone CA, Arnaud CC, Postaire ER, Bouley CF, Reinert P. Multicentric study of the effect of milk fermented by *Lactobacillus casei* on the incidence of diarrhoea. *Int J Clin Pract.* 2000 Nov;54(9):568-71.

Pedone CA, Bernabeu AO, Postaire ER, Bouley CF, Reinert P. The effect of supplementation with milk fermented by *Lactobacillus casei* (strain DN-114 001) on acute diarrhoea in children attending day care centres. *Int J Clin Pract.* 1999 Apr-May;53(3):179-84.

Pedrosa MC, Golner BB, Goldin BR, Barakat S, Dallal GE, Russell RM. Survival of yogurt-containing organisms and *Lactobacillus gasseri* (ADH) and their effect on bacterial enzyme activity in the gastrointestinal tract of healthy and hypochlorhydric elderly subjects. *Am J Clin Nutr.* 1995 Feb;61(2):353-9.

Pehowich DJ, Gomes AV, Barnes JA. Fatty acid composition and possible health effects of coconut constituents. *West Indian Med J.* 2000 Jun;49(2):128-33.

Peral MC, Martinez MA, Valdez JC. Bacteriotherapy with *Lactobacillus plantarum* in burns. *Int Wound J.* 2009 Feb;6(1):73-81.

Perez-Galvez A, Martin HD, Sies H, Stahl W. Incorporation of carotenoids from paprika oleoresin into human chylomicrons. *Br J Nutr.* 2003 Jun;89(6):787-93.

Perez-Pena R. Secrets of the Mummy's Medicine Chest. *NY Times.* 2005 Sept 10.

Persson R, Orbaek P, Kecklund G, Akerstedt T. Impact of an 84-hour workweek on biomarkers for stress, metabolic processes and diurnal rhythm. *Scand J Work Environ Health.* 2006 Oct;32(5):349-58.

Pessi T, Sütas Y, Hurme M, Isolauri E. Interleukin-10 generation in atopic children following oral *Lactobacillus rhamnosus* GG. *Clin Exp Allergy.* 2000 Dec;30(12):1804-8.

Peters JI, McKinney JM, Smith B, Wood P, Forkner E, Galbreath AD. Impact of obesity in asthma: evidence from a large prospective disease management study. *Ann Allergy Asthma Immunol.* 2011 Jan;106(1):30-5.

Peterson CG, Hansson T, Skott A, Bengtsson U, Ahlstedt S, Magnussons J. Detection of local mast-cell activity in patients with food hypersensitivity. *J Investig Allergol Clin Immunol.* 2007;17(5):314-20.

Peterson KA, Samuelson WM, Ryujin DT, Young DC, Thomas KL, Hilden K, Fang JC. The role of gastroesophageal reflux in exercise-triggered asthma: a randomized controlled trial. *Dig Dis Sci.* 2009 Mar;54(3):564-71. 2008 Aug 8.

Petlevski R, Hadzija M, Slijepcević M, Juretić D, Petrik J. Glutathione S-transferases and malondialdehyde in the liver of NOD mice on short-term treatment with plant mixture extract P-9801091. *Phytother Res.* 2003 Apr;17(4):311-4.

Petricevic L, Unger FM, Viernstein H, Kiss H. Randomized, double-blind, placebo-controlled study of oral lactobacilli to improve the vaginal flora of postmenopausal women. *Eur J Obstet Gynecol Reprod Biol.* 2008 Nov;141(1):54-7.

Petricevic L, Witt A. The role of *Lactobacillus casei* rhamnosus Lcr35 in restoring the normal vaginal flora after antibiotic treatment of bacterial vaginosis. *BJOG.* 2008 Oct;115(11):1369-74.

Petrunov B, Marinova S, Markova R, Nenkov P, Nikolaeva S, Nikolova M, Taskov H, Cvetanov J. Cellular and humoral systemic and mucosal immune responses stimulated in volunteers by an oral polybacterial immunomodulator "Dentavax". *Int Immunopharmacol.* 2006 Jul;6(7):1181-93.

Petti S, Tarsitani G, D'Arca AS. A randomized clinical trial of the effect of yoghurt on the human salivary microflora. *Arch Oral Biol.* 2001 Aug;46(8):705-12.

Pfefferle PI, Sel S, Ege MJ, Büchele G, Blümer N, Krauss-Etschmann S, Herzum I, Albers CE, Lauener RP, Roponen M, Hirvonen MR, Vuitton DA, Riedler J, Brunekreef B, Dalphin JC, Braun-Fahrländer C, Pekkanen J, von Mutius E, Renz H; PASTURE Study Group. Cord blood allergen-specific IgE is associated with reduced IFN-gamma production by cord blood cells: the Protection against Allergy-Study in Rural Environments (PASTURE) Study. *J Allergy Clin Immunol.* 2008 Oct;122(4):711-6.

Pfundstein B, El Desouky SK, Hull WE, Haubner R, Erben G, Owen RW. Polyphenolic compounds in the fruits of Egyptian medicinal plants (Terminalia bellerica, Terminalia chebula and Terminalia horrida): characterization, quantitation and determination of antioxidant capacities. *Phytochemistry.* 2010 Jul;71(10):1132-48.

Phuapradit P, Varavithya W, Vathanophas K, Sangchai R, Podhipak A, Suthutvoravut U, Nopchinda S, Chantraruksa V, Haschke F. Reduction of rotavirus infection in children receiving bifidobacteria-supplemented formula. *J Med Assoc Thai.* 1999 Nov;82 Suppl 1:S43-8.

Physicians' Desk Reference. Montvale, NJ: Thomson, 2003-2008.

Pierce SK, Klinman NR. Antibody-specific immunoregulation. *J Exp Med.* 1977 Aug 1;146(2):509-19.

Piirainen L, Haahtela S, Helin T, Korpela R, Haahtela T, Vaarala O. Effect of Lactobacillus rhamnosus GG on rBet v1 and rMal d1 specific IgA in the saliva of patients with birch pollen allergy. *Ann Allergy Asthma Immunol.* 2008 Apr;100(4):338-42.

Piirainen L, Haahtela S, Helin T, Korpela R, Haahtela T, Vaarala O. Effect of *Lactobacillus rhamnosus* GG on rBet v1 and rMal d1 specific IgA in the saliva of patients with birch pollen allergy. *Ann Allergy Asthma Immunol.* 2008 Apr;100(4):338-42.

Pike MG, Heddle RJ, Boulton P, Turner MW, Atherton DJ. Increased intestinal permeability in atopic eczema. *J Invest Dermatol.* 1986 Feb;86(2):101-4.

Pines JM, Prabhu A, Hilton JA, Hollander JE, Datner EM. The effect of emergency department crowding on length of stay and medication treatment times in discharged patients with acute asthma. *Acad Emerg Med.* 2010 Aug;17(8):834-9.

Piraino F, Brandt CR. Isolation and partial characterization of an antiviral, RC-183, from the edible mushroom Rozites caperata. *Antiviral Res.* 1999 Sep;43(2):67-78.

Piraino F, Brandt CR. Isolation and partial characterization of an antiviral, RC-183, from the edible mushroom Rozites caperata. *Antiviral Res.* 1999 Sep;43(2):67-78.

Pitkala KH, Strandberg TE, Finne Soveri UH, Ouwehand AC, Poussa T, Salminen S. Fermented cereal with specific bifidobacteria normalizes bowel movements in elderly nursing home residents. A randomized, controlled trial. *J Nutr Health Aging.* 2007 Jul-Aug;11(4):305-11.

Pitten FA, Scholler M, Krüger U, Effendy I, Kramer A. Filamentous fungi and yeasts on mattresses covered with different encasings. Eur J Dermatol. 2001 Nov-Dec;11(6):534-7.

Pitt-Rivers R, Trotter WR. *The Thyroid Gland.* London: Butterworth Publ, 1954.

Plaschke P, Janson C, Norrman E, Björnsson E, Ellbjär S, Järvholm B. Association between atopic sensitization and asthma and bronchial hyperresponsiveness in swedish adults: pets, and not mites, are the most important allergens. *J Allergy Clin Immunol.* 1999 Jul;104(1):58-65.

Plaut M, Valentine MD. Clinical practice. Allergic rhinitis. *N Engl J Med.* 2005 Nov 3;353(18):1934-44.

Plaut TE, Jones TB. *Dr. Tom Plaut's Asthma guide for people of all ages.* Amherst, MA: Pedipress, 1999.

Plaza V, Miguel E, Bellido-Casado J, Lozano MP, Ríos L, Bolíbar I. [Usefulness of the Guidelines of the Spanish Society of Pulmonology and Thoracic Surgery (SEPAR) in identifying the causes of chronic cough]. Arch Bronconeumol. 2006 Feb;42(2):68-73.

Plein K, Hotz J. Therapeutic effects of *Saccharomyces boulardii* on mild residual symptoms in a stable phase of Crohn's disease with special respect to chronic diarrhea—a pilot study. *Z Gastroenterol.* 1993 Feb;31(2):129-34.

Plohmann B, Bader G, Hiller K, Franz G. Immunomodulatory and antitumoral effects of triterpenoid saponins. *Pharmazie*. 1997 Dec;52(12):953-7.

Plummer M, Schiffman M, Castle PE, Maucort-Boulch D, Wheeler, CM, ALTS Group. A 2-year prospective study of human papillomaviruspersistence among women with a cytological diagnosis of atypical squamous cells of undetermined significance or low-grade squamous intraepithelial lesion. J Infect Dis. 2007;195(11):1582-9.

Poblocka-Olech L, Krauze-Baranowska M. SPE-HPTLC of procyanidins from the barks of different species and clones of Salix. *J Pharm Biomed Anal*. 2008 Nov 4;48(3):965-8.

Pohjavuori E, Viljanen M, Korpela R, Kuitunen M, Tiittanen M, Vaarala O, Savilahti E. Lactobacillus GG effect in increasing IFN-gamma production in infants with cow's milk allergy. *J Allergy Clin Immunol*. 2004 Jul;114(1):131-6.

Polito A, Aboab J, Annane D. The hypothalamic pituitary adrenal axis in sepsis. *Novartis Found Symp*. 2007;280:182-203.

Polk S, Sunyer J, Muñoz-Ortiz L, Barnes M, Torrent M, Figueroa C, Harris J, Vall O, Antó JM, Cullinan P. A prospective study of Fel d1 and Der p1 exposure in infancy and childhood wheezing. *Am J Respir Crit Care Med*. 2004 Aug 1;170(3):273-8.

Pollini F, Capristo C, Boner AL. Upper respiratory tract infections and atopy. *Int J Immunopathol Pharmacol*. 2010 Jan-Mar;23(1 Suppl):32-7.

Ponsonby AL, McMichael A, van der Mei I. Ultraviolet radiation and autoimmune disease: insights from epidemiological research. *Toxicology*. 2002 Dec 27;181-182:71-8.

Postlethwait EM. Scavenger receptors clear the air. *J Clin Invest*. 2007 Mar;117(3):601-4.

Postma DS. Gender Differences in Asthma Development and Progression. *Gender Medicine*. 2007;4:S133-146.

Postolache TT, Lapidus M, Sander ER, Langenberg P, Hamilton RG, Soriano JJ, McDonald JS, Furst N, Bai J, Scrandis DA, Cabassa JA, Stiller JW, Balis T, Guzman A, Togias A, Tonelli LH. Changes in allergy symptoms and depression scores are positively correlated in patients with recurrent mood disorders exposed to seasonal peaks in aeroallergens. *ScientificWorldJournal*. 2007 Dec 17;7:1968-77.

Potterton D. (Ed.) *Culpeper's Color Herbal*. New York: Sterling, 1983.

Poulos LM, Waters AM, Correll PK, Loblay RH, Marks GB. Trends in hospitalizations for anaphylaxis, angioedema, and urticaria in Australia, 1993-1994 to 2004-2005. *J Allergy Clin Immunol*. 2007 Oct;120(4):878-84.

Powe DG, Groot Kormelink T, Sisson M, Blokhuis BJ, Kramer MF, Jones NS, Redegeld FA. Evidence for the involvement of free light chain immunoglobulins in allergic and nonallergic rhinitis. *J Allergy Clin Immunol*. 2010 Jan;125(1):139-45.e1-3.

Pregliasco F, Anselmi G, Fonte L, Giussani F, Schieppati S, Soletti L. A new chance of preventing winter diseases by the administration of synbiotic formulations. *J Clin Gastroenterol*. 2008 Sep;42 Suppl 3 Pt 2:S224-33.

Prescott SL, Wickens K, Westcott L, Jung W, Currie H, Black PN, Stanley TV, Mitchell EA, Fitzharris P, Siebers R, Wu L, Crane J; Probiotic Study Group. Supplementation with Lactobacillus rhamnosus or Bifidobacterium lactis probiotics in pregnancy increases cord blood interferon-gamma and breast milk transforming growth factor-beta and immunoglobin A detection. *Clin Exp Allergy*. 2008 Oct;38(10):1606-14.

Prescott SL, Wickens K, Westcott L, Jung W, Currie H, Black PN, Stanley TV, Mitchell EA, Fitzharris P, Siebers R, Wu L, Crane J; Probiotic Study Group. Supplementation with *Lactobacillus rhamnosus* or *Bifidobacterium lactis* probiotics in pregnancy increases cord blood interferon-gamma and breast milk transforming growth factor-beta and immunoglobin A detection. *Clin Exp Allergy*. 2008 Oct;38(10):1606-14.

Priftis KN, Panagiotakos DB, Anthracopoulos MB, Papadimitriou A, Nicolaidou P. Aims, methods and preliminary findings of the Physical Activity, Nutrition and Allergies in Children Examined in Athens (PANACEA) epidemiological study. *BMC Public Health*. 2007 Jul 4;7:140.

Prioult G, Fliss I, Pecquet S. Effect of probiotic bacteria on induction and maintenance of oral tolerance to beta-lactoglobulin in gnotobiotic mice. *Clin Diagn Lab Immunol*. 2003 Sep;10(5):787-92.

Prucksunand C, Indrasukhsri B, Leethochawalit M, Hungspreugs K. Phase II clinical trial on effect of the long turmeric (Curcuma longa Linn) on healing of peptic ulcer. *Southeast Asian J Trop Med Public Health*. 2001 Mar;32(1):208-15.

Pruthi S, Thapa MM. Infectious and inflammatory disorders. *Magn Reson Imaging Clin N Am*. 2009 Aug;17(3):423-38, v.

Pu JY, He L, Wu SY, Zhang P, Huang X. Anti-virus research of triterpenoids in licorice. Bing Du Xue Bao. 2013 Nov;29(6):673-9.

Qin HL, Zheng JJ, Tong DN, Chen WX, Fan XB, Hang XM, Jiang YQ. Effect of Lactobacillus plantarum enteral feeding on the gut permeability and septic complications in the patients with acute pancreatitis. *Eur J Clin Nutr*. 2008 Jul;62(7):923-30.

Qin HL, Zheng JJ, Tong DN, Chen WX, Fan XB, Hang XM, Jiang YQ. Effect of *Lactobacillus plantarum* enteral feeding on the gut permeability and septic complications in the patients with acute pancreatitis. *Eur J Clin Nutr.* 2008 Jul;62(7):923-30.

Qu C, Srivastava K, Ko J, Zhang TF, Sampson HA, Li XM. Induction of tolerance after establishment of peanut allergy by the food allergy herbal formula-2 is associated with up-regulation of interferon-gamma. *Clin Exp Allergy.* 2007 Jun;37(6):846-55.

Radon K, Danuser B, Iversen M, Jörres R, Monso E, Opravil U, Weber C, Donham KJ, Nowak D. Respiratory symptoms in European animal farmers. *Eur Respir J.* 2001 Apr;17(4):747-54.

Rafter J, Bennett M, Caderni G, Clune Y, Hughes R, Karlsson PC, Klinder A, O'Riordan M, O'Sullivan GC, Pool-Zobel B, Rechkemmer G, Roller M, Rowland I, Salvadori M, Thijs H, Van Loo J, Watzl B, Collins JK. Dietary synbiotics reduce cancer risk factors in polypectomized and colon cancer patients. *Am J Clin Nutr.* 2007 Feb;85(2):488-96.

Raherison C, Pénard-Morand C, Moreau D, Caillaud D, Charpin D, Kopferschmitt C, Lavaud F, Taytard A, Maesano IA. Smoking exposure and allergic sensitisation in children according to maternal allergies. *Ann Allergy Asthma Immunol.* 2008 Apr;100(4):351-7.

Rahman MM, Bhattacharya A, Fernandes G. Docosahexaenoic acid is more potent inhibitor of osteoclast differentiation in RAW 264.7 cells than eicosapentaenoic acid. *J Cell Physiol.* 2008 Jan;214(1):201-9.

Raithel M, Weidenhiller M, Abel R, Baenkler HW, Hahn EG. Colorectal mucosal histamine release by mucosa oxygenation in comparison with other established clinical tests in patients with gastrointestinally mediated allergy. *World J Gastroenterol.* 2006 Aug 7;12(29):4699-705.

Raloff J. Ill Winds. *Science News:* 2001;160(14):218.

Ramos Alvarenga RF, Wan B, Inui T, Franzblau SG, Pauli GF, Jaki BU. Airborne antituberculosis activity of Eucalyptus citriodora essential oil. *J Nat Prod.* 2014 Mar 28;77(3):603-10. doi: 10.1021/np400872m.

Rampton DS, Murdoch RD, Sladen GE. Rectal mucosal histamine release in ulcerative colitis. *Clin Sci (Lond).* 1980 Nov;59(5):389-91.

Rancé F, Kanny G, Dutau G, Moneret-Vautrin DA. Food allergens in children. *Arch Pediatr.* 1999;6(Suppl 1):61S-66S.

Randal Bollinger R, Barbas AS, Bush EL, Lin SS, Parker W. Biofilms in the large bowel suggest an apparent function of the human vermiform appendix. *J Theor Biol.* 2007 Dec 21;249(4):826-31.

Rangavajhyala N, Shahani KM, Sridevi G, Srikumaran S. Nonlipopolysaccharide component(s) of Lactobacillus acidophilus stimulate(s) the production of interleukin-1 alpha and tumor necrosis factor-alpha by murine macrophages. *Nutr Cancer.* 1997;28(2):130-4.

Ranilla LG, Genovese MI, Lajolo FM. Polyphenols and antioxidant capacity of seed coat and cotyledon from Brazilian and Peruvian bean cultivars (Phaseolus vulgaris L.). *J Agric Food Chem.* 2007 Jan 10;55(1):90-8.

Ranjbaran Z, Keefer L, Stepanski E, Farhadi A, Keshavarzian A. The relevance of sleep abnormalities to chronic inflammatory conditions. *Inflamm Res.* 2007 Feb;56(2):51-7.

Rankin LC, Groom JR, Chopin M, Herold MJ, Walker JA, Mielke LA, McKenzie AN, Carotta S, Nutt SL, Belz GT. Leafy Greens and Gut: The transcription factor T-bet is essential for the development of NKp46(+) innate lymphocytes via the Notch pathway. Nat Immunol. 2013 Mar 3. doi: 10.1038/ni.2545.

Rao SK, Rao PS, Rao BN. Preliminary investigation of the radiosensitizing activity of guduchi (Tinospora cordifolia) in tumor-bearing mice. *Phytother Res.* 2008 Nov;22(11):1482-9.

Rapin JR, Wiernsperger N. Possible links between intestinal permeablity and food processing: A potential therapeutic niche for glutamine. *Clinics (Sao Paulo).* 2010 Jun;65(6):635-43.

Rappoport J. Both sides of the pharmaceutical death coin. *Townsend Letter for Doctors and Patients.* 2006 Oct.

Rauha JP, Remes S, Heinonen M, Hopia A, Kähkönen M, Kujala T, Pihlaja K, Vuorela H, Vuorela P. Antimicrobial effects of Finnish plant extracts containing flavonoids and other phenolic compounds. *Int J Food Microbiol.* 2000 May 25;56(1):3-12.

Rauma A. Antioxidant status in vegetarians versus omnivores. *Nutrition.* 2003;16(2): 111-119.

Rautava S, Isolauri E. Cow's milk allergy in infants with atopic eczema is associated with aberrant production of interleukin-4 during oral cow's milk challenge. *J Pediatr Gastroenterol Nutr.* 2004 Nov;39(5):529-35.

Rautava S, Salminen S, Isolauri E. Specific probiotics in reducing the risk of acute infections in infancy—a randomised, double-blind, placebo-controlled study. *Br J Nutr.* 2009 Jun;101(11):1722-6.

Rayes N, Seehofer D, Hansen S, Boucsein K, Müller AR, Serke S, Bengmark S, Neuhaus P. Early enteral supply of lactobacillus and fiber versus selective bowel decontamination: a controlled trial in liver transplant recipients. *Transplantation.* 2002 Jul 15;74(1):123-7.

Rayes N, Seehofer D, Müller AR, Hansen S, Bengmark S, Neuhaus P. Influence of probiotics and fibre on the incidence of bacterial infections following major abdominal surgery - results of a prospective trial. *Z Gastroenterol.* 2002 Oct;40(10):869-76.

Raza S, Graham SM, Allen SJ, Sultana S, Cuevas L, Hart CA, Kaila M, Isolauri E, Saxelin M, Arvilommi H, *et al.* Lactobacillus GG in acute diarrhea. *Indian Pediatr.* 1995 Oct;32(10):1140-2.

Raza S, Graham SM, Allen SJ, Sultana S, Cuevas L, Hart CA. Lactobacillus GG promotes recovery from acute nonbloody diarrhea in Pakistan. Pediatr Infect Dis J. 1995 Feb;14(2):107-11.

Rebhun J. Coexisting immune complex diseases in atopy. Ann Allergy. 1980 Dec;45(6):368-71.

Reddy KP, Shahani KM, Kulkarni SM. B-complex vitamins in cultured and acidified yogurt. J Dairy Sci. 1976 Feb;59(2):191-5.

Regente M, Taveira GB, Pinedo M, Elizalde MM, Ticchi AJ, Diz MS, Carvalho AO, de la Canal L, Gomes VM. A sunflower lectin with antifungal properties and putative medical mycology applications. Curr Microbiol. 2014 Jul;69(1):88-95. doi: 10.1007/s00284-014-0558-z.

Reger D, Goode S, Mercer E. Chemistry: Principles & Practice. Fort Worth, TX: Harcourt Brace, 1993.

Regis E. Virus Ground Zero. New York: Pocket, 1996.

Reha CM, Ebru A. Specific immunotherapy is effective in the prevention of new sensitivities. Allergol Immunopathol (Madr). 2007 Mar-Apr;35(2):44-51.

Rehm J, Taylor B, Mohapatra S, Irving H, Baliunas D, Patra J, Roerecke M. Alcohol as a risk factor for liver cirrhosis: a systematic review and meta-analysis. Drug Alcohol Rev. 2010 Jul;29(4):437-45.

Reid G, Beuerman D, Heinemann C, Bruce AW. Probiotic Lactobacillus dose required to restore and maintain a normal vaginal flora. FEMS Immunol Med Microbiol. 2001 Dec;32(1):37-41.

Reid G, Burton J, Hammond JA, Bruce AW. Nucleic acid-based diagnosis of bacterial vaginosis and improved management using probiotic lactobacilli. J Med Food. 2004 Summer;7(2):223-8.

Reid G, Charbonneau D, Erb J, Kochanowski B, Beuerman D, Poehner R, Bruce AW. Oral use of Lactobacillus rhamnosus GR-1 and L. fermentum RC-14 significantly alters vaginal flora: randomized, placebo-controlled trial in 64 healthy women. FEMS Immunol Med Microbiol. 2003 Mar 20;35(2):131-4.

Renkonen R, Renkonen J, Joenväärä S, Mattila P, Parviainen V, Toppila-Salmi S. Allergens are transported through the respiratory epithelium. Expert Rev Clin Immunol. 2010 Jan;6(1):55-9.

Renvert S, Lindahl C, Renvert H, Persson GR. Clinical and microbiological analysis of subjects treated with Brånemark or AstraTech implants: a 7-year follow-up study. Clin Oral Implants Res. 2008 Apr;19(4):342-7.

Reuter A, Lidholm J, Andersson K, Ostling J, Lundberg M, Scheurer S, Enrique E, Cistero-Bahima A, San Miguel-Moncin M, Ballmer-Weber BK, Vieths S. A critical assessment of allergen component-based in vitro diagnosis in cherry allergy across Europe. Clin Exp Allergy. 2006 Jun;36(6):815-23.

Reznik M, Sharif I, Ozuah PO. Rubbing ointments and asthma morbidity in adolescents. J Altern Complement Med. 2004 Dec;10(6):1097-9.

Ribeiro LZ, Tripp RA, Rossi LM, Palma PV, Yokosawa J, Mantese OC, Oliveira TF, Nepomuceno LL, Queiróz DA. Serum mannose-binding lectin levels are linked with respiratory syncytial virus (RSV) disease. J Clin Immunol. 2008 Mar;28(2):166-73.

Riccia DN, Bizzini F, Perilli MG, Polimeni A, Trinchieri V, Amicosante G, Cifone MG. Anti-inflammatory effects of Lactobacillus brevis (CD2) on periodontal disease. Oral Dis. 2007 Jul;13(4):376-85.

Riccioni G, Barbara M, Bucciarelli T, di Ilio C, D'Orazio N. Antioxidant vitamin supplementation in asthma. Ann Clin Lab Sci. 2007 Winter;37(1):96-101.

Riccioni G, Bucciarelli T, Mancini B, Di Ilio C, Della Vecchia R, D'Orazio N. Plasma lycopene and antioxidant vitamins in asthma: the PLAVA study. J Asthma. 2007 Jul-Aug;44(6):429-32.

Riccioni G, D'Orazio N. The role of selenium, zinc and antioxidant vitamin supplementation in the treatment of bronchial asthma: adjuvant therapy or not? Expert Opin Investig Drugs. 2005 Sep;14(9):1145-55.

Riccioni G, Di Stefano F, De Benedictis M, Verna N, Cavallucci E, Paolini F, Di Sciascio MB, Della Vecchia R, Schiavone C, Boscolo P, Conti P, Di Gioacchino M. Seasonal variability of non-specific bronchial responsiveness in asthmatic patients with allergy to house dust mites. Allergy Asthma Proc. 2001 Jan-Feb;22(1):5-9.

Riedler J, Braun-Fahrländer C, Eder W, Schreuer M, Waser M, Maisch S, Carr D, Schierl R, Nowak D, von Mutius E; ALEX Study Team. Exposure to farming in early life and development of asthma and allergy: a cross-sectional survey. Lancet. 2001 Oct 6;358(9288):1129-33.

Rimkiene S, Ragazinskiene O, Savickiene N. The cumulation of Wild pansy (Viola tricolor L.) accessions: the possibility of species preservation and usage in medicine. Medicina (Kaunas). 2003;39(4):411-6.

Rinne M, Kalliomaki M, Arvilommi H, Salminen S, Isolauri E. Effect of probiotics and breastfeeding on the bifidobacterium and lactobacillus/enterococcus microbiota and humoral immune responses. J Pediatr. 2005 Aug;147(2):186-91.

Rinne M, Kalliomaki M, Arvilommi H, Salminen S, Isolauri E. Effect of probiotics and breastfeeding on the bifidobacterium and lactobacillus/enterococcus microbiota and humoral immune responses. J Pediatr. 2005 Aug;147(2):186-91.

Rinne M, Kalliomäki M, Salminen S, Isolauri E. Probiotic intervention in the first months of life: short-term effects on gastrointestinal symptoms and long-term effects on gut microbiota. J Pediatr Gastroenterol Nutr. 2006 Aug;43(2):200-5.

Río ME, Zago Beatriz L, Garcia H, Winter L. The nutritional status change the effectiveness of a dietary supplement of lactic bacteria on the emerging of respiratory tract diseases in children. *Arch Latinoam Nutr.* 2002 Mar;52(1):29-34.

Río ME, Zago LB, Garcia H, Winter L. Influence of nutritional status on the effectiveness of a dietary supplement of live lactobacillus to prevent and cure diarrhoea in children. *Arch Latinoam Nutr.* 2004 Sep;54(3):287-92.

Robert AM, Groult N, Six C, Robert L. The effect of procyanidolic oligomers on mesenchymal cells in culture II—Attachment of elastic fibers to the cells. *Pathol Biol.* 1990 Jun;38(6):601-7.

Robert AM, Robert L, Renard G. Protection of cornea against proteolytic damage. Experimental study of procyanidolic oligomers (PCO) on bovine cornea. *J Fr Ophtalmol.* 2002 Apr;25(4):351-5.

Robert AM, Tixier JM, Robert L, Legeais JM, Renard G. Effect of procyanidolic oligomers on the permeability of the blood-brain barrier. *Pathol Biol.* 2001 May;49(4):298-304.

Roberts G, Lack G. Diagnosing peanut allergy with skin prick and specific IgE testing. *J Allergy Clin Immunol.* 2005 Jun;115(6):1291-6.

Robinson L, Cherewatenko VS, Reeves S. *Epicor: The Key to a Balanced Immune System.* Sherman Oaks, CA: Health Point, 2009.

Rodriguez E, Valbuena MC, Rey M, Porras de Quintana L. Causal agents of photoallergic contact dermatitis diagnosed in the national institute of dermatology of Colombia. *Photodermatol Photoimmunol Photomed.* 2006 Aug;22(4):189-92.

Rodriguez J, Crespo JF, Burks W, Rivas-Plata C, Fernandez-Anaya S, Vives R, Daroca P. Randomized, double-blind, crossover challenge study in 53 subjects reporting adverse reactions to melon (Cucumis melo). *J Allergy Clin Immunol.* 2000 Nov;106(5):968-72.

Rodriguez-Fragoso L, Reyes-Esparza J, Burchiel SW, Herrera-Ruiz D, Torres E. Risks and benefits of commonly used herbal medicines in Mexico. *Toxicol Appl Pharmacol.* 2008 Feb 15;227(1):125-35.

Rodríguez-Ortiz PG, Muñoz-Mendoza D, Arias-Cruz A, González-Díaz SN, Herrera-Castro D, Vidaurri-Ojeda AC. Epidemiological characteristics of patients with food allergy assisted at Regional Center of Allergies and Clinical Immunology of Monterrey. *Rev Alerg Mex.* 2009 Nov-Dec;56(6):185-91.

Roduit C, Scholtens S, de Jongste JC, Wijga AH, Gerritsen J, Postma DS, Brunekreef B, Hoekstra MO, Aalberse R, Smit HA. Asthma at 8 years of age in children born by caesarean section. *Thorax.* 2009 Feb;64(2):107-13.

Roessler A, Friedrich U, Vogelsang H, Bauer A, Kaatz M, Hipler UC, Schmidt I, Jahreis G. The immune system in healthy adults and patients with atopic dermatitis seems to be affected differently by a probiotic intervention. *Clin Exp Allergy.* 2008 Jan;38(1):93-102.

Roger A, Justicia JL, Navarro LÁ, Eseverri JL, Ferrès J, Malet A, Alvà V. Observational study of the safety of an ultra-rush sublingual immunotherapy regimen to treat rhinitis due to house dust mites. *Int Arch Allergy Immunol.* 2011;154(1):69-75. 2010 Jul 27.

Roller M, Clune Y, Collins K, Rechkemmer G, Watzl B. Consumption of prebiotic inulin enriched with oligofructose in combination with the probiotics *Lactobacillus rhamnosus* and *Bifidobacterium lactis* has minor effects on selected immune parameters in polypectomised and colon cancer patients. *Br J Nutr.* 2007 Apr;97(4):676-84.

Romeo J, Wärnberg J, Nova E, Díaz LE, González-Gross M, Marcos A. Changes in the immune system after moderate beer consumption. *Ann Nutr Metab.* 2007;51(4):359-66.

Romieu I, Barraza-Villarreal A, Escamilla-Núñez C, Texcalac-Sangrador JL, Hernandez-Cadena L, Díaz-Sánchez D, De Batlle J, Del Rio-Navarro BE. Dietary intake, lung function and airway inflammation in Mexico City school children exposed to air pollutants. *Respir Res.* 2009 Dec 10;10:122.

Ronteltap A, van Schaik J, Wensing M, Rynja FJ, Knulst AC, de Vries JH. Sensory testing of recipes masking peanut or hazelnut for double-blind placebo-controlled food challenges. Allergy. 2004 Apr;59(4):457-60. Clark S, Bock SA, Gaeta TJ, Brenner BE, Cydulka RK, Camargo CA; Multicenter Airway Research Collaboration-8 Investigators. Multicenter study of emergency department visits for food allergies. *J Allergy Clin Immunol.* 2004 Feb;113(2):347-52.

Rook GA, Hernandez-Pando R. Pathogenetic role, in human and murine tuberculosis, of changes in the peripheral metabolism of glucocorticoids and antiglucocorticoids. *Psychoneuroendocrinology.* 1997;22 Suppl 1:S109-13.

Ros E, Mataix J. Fatty acid composition of nuts—implications for cardiovascular health. *Br J Nutr.* 2006 Nov;96 Suppl 2:S29-35.

Rosander A, Connolly E, Roos S. Removal of antibiotic resistance gene-carrying plasmids from *Lactobacillus reuteri* ATCC 55730 and characterization of the resulting daughter strain, *L. reuteri* DSM 17938. *Appl Environ Microbiol.* 2008 Oct;74(19):6032-40.

Rose NR, Bona C. Defining criteria for autoimmune diseases (Witebsky's postulates revisited). Immunol Today. 1993 Sep;14(9):426-30.

Rosenfeldt V, Benfeldt E, Nielsen SD, Michaelsen KF, Jeppesen DL, Valerius NH, Paerregaard A. Effect of probiotic Lactobacillus strains in children with atopic dermatitis. *J Allergy Clin Immunol.* 2003 Feb;111(2):389-95.

Rosenfeldt V, Benfeldt E, Valerius NH, Paerregaard A, Michaelsen KF. Effect of probiotics on gastrointestinal symptoms and small intestinal permeability in children with atopic dermatitis. *J Pediatr.* 2004 Nov;145(5):612-6.

Rosenfeldt V, Michaelsen KF, Jakobsen M, Larsen CN, Møller PL, Pedersen P, Tvede M, Weyrehter H, Valerius NH, Paerregaard A. Effect of probiotic Lactobacillus strains in young children hospitalized with acute diarrhea. *Pediatr Infect Dis J.* 2002 May;21(5):411-6.

Rosenkranz E, Maywald M, Hilgers RD, Brieger A, Clarner T, Kipp M, Plümäkers B, Meyer S, Schwerdtle T, Rink L. Induction of regulatory T cells in Th1-/Th17-driven experimental autoimmune encephalomyelitis by zinc administration. *J Nutr Biochem.* 2016 Mar;29:116-23. doi: 10.1016/j.jnutbio.2015.11.010.

Rosenkranz SK, Swain KE, Rosenkranz RR, Beckman B, Harms CA. Modifiable lifestyle factors impact airway health in non-asthmatic prepubescent boys but not girls. *Pediatr Pulmonol.* 2010 Dec 30.

Rosenlund H, Bergström A, Alm JS, Swartz J, Scheynius A, van Hage M, Johansen K, Brunekreef B, von Mutius E, Ege MJ, Riedler J, Braun-Fahrländer C, Waser M, Pershagen G; PARSIFAL Study Group. Allergic disease and atopic sensitization in children in relation to measles vaccination and measles infection. *Pediatrics.* 2009 Mar;123(3):771-8.

Rousseaux C, Thuru X, Gelot A, Barnich N, Neut C, Dubuquoy L, Dubuquoy C, Merour E, Geboes K, Chamaillard M, Ouwehand A, Leyer G, Carcano D, Colombel JF, Ardid D, Desreumaux P. Lactobacillus acidophilus modulates intestinal pain and induces opioid and cannabinoid receptors. *Nat Med.* 2007 Jan;13(1):35-7

Royer RJ, Schmidt CL. Evaluation of venotropic drugs by venous gas plethysmography. A study of procyanidolic oligomers *Sem Hop.* 1981 Dec 18-25;57(47-48):2009-13.

Rozycki VR, Baigorria CM, Freyre MR, Bernard CM, Zannier MS, Charpentier M. Nutrient content in vegetable species from the Argentine Chaco. *Arch Latinoam Nutr.* 1997 Sep;47(3):265-70.

Rubin E., Farber JL. *Pathology.* 3rd Ed. Philadelphia: Lippincott-Raven, 1999.

Rudders SA, Espinola JA, Camargo CA Jr. North-south differences in US emergency department visits for acute allergic reactions. *Ann Allergy Asthma Immunol.* 2010 May;104(5):413-6.

Rynard PB, Palij B, Galloway CA, Roughley FR. Resperin inhalation treatment for chronic respiratory diseases. *Can Fam Physician.* 1968 Oct;14(10):70-1.

Saarinen KM, Juntunen-Backman K, Järvenpää AL, Klemetti P, Kuitunen P, Lope L, Renlund M, Siivola M, Vaarala O, Savilahti E. Breast-feeding and the development of cows' milk protein allergy. *Adv Exp Med Biol.* 2000;478:121-30.

Saavedra JM, Abi-Hanna A, Moore N, Yolken RH. Long-term consumption of infant formulas containing live probiotic bacteria: tolerance and safety. *Am J Clin Nutr.* 2004 Feb;79(2):261-7.

Saavedra JM, Bauman NA, Oung I, Perman JA, Yolken RH. Feeding of *Bifidobacterium bifidum* and *Streptococcus thermophilus* to infants in hospital for prevention of diarrhoea and shedding of rotavirus. *Lancet.* 1994 Oct 15;344(8929):1046-9.

Saggioro A. Probiotics in the treatment of irritable bowel syndrome. *J Clin Gastroenterol.* 2004 Jul;38(6 Suppl):S104-6.

Sahagún-Flores JE, López-Peña LS, de la Cruz-Ramírez Jaimes J, García-Bravo MS, Peregrina-Gómez R, de Alba-García JE. Eradication of Helicobacter pylori: triple treatment scheme plus Lactobacillus vs. triple treatment alone. *Cir Cir.* 2007 Sep-Oct;75(5):333-6.

Sahakian NM, White SK, Park JH, Cox-Ganser JM, Kreiss K. Identification of mold and dampness-associated respiratory morbidity in 2 schools: comparison of questionnaire survey responses to national data. *J Sch Health.* 2008 Jan;78(1):32-7.

Sahin-Yilmaz A, Nocon CC, Corey JP. Immunoglobulin E-mediated food allergies among adults with allergic rhinitis. *Otolaryngol Head Neck Surg.* 2010 Sep;143(3):379-85.

Salazar F, Sewell HF, Shakib F, Ghaemmaghami AM. The role of lectins in allergic sensitization and allergic disease. J Allergy Clin Immunol. 2013 Jul;132(1):27-36. doi: 10.1016/j.jaci.2013.02.001.

Salazar-Lindo E, Figueroa-Quintanilla D, Caciano MI, Reto-Valiente V, Chauviere G, Colin P; Lacteol Study Group. Effectiveness and safety of Lactobacillus LB in the treatment of mild acute diarrhea in children. *J Pediatr Gastroenterol Nutr.* 2007 May;44(5):571-6.

Salazar-Lindo E, Miranda-Langschwager P, Campos-Sanchez M, Chea-Woo E, Sack RB. *Lactobacillus casei* strain GG in the treatment of infants with acute watery diarrhea: a randomized, double-blind, placebo controlled clinical trial [ISRCTN67363048]. *BMC Pediatr.* 2004 Sep 2;4:18.

Salem N, Wegher B, Mena P, Uauy R. Arachidonic and docosahexaenoic acids are biosynthesized from their 18-carbon precursors in human infants. *Proc Natl Acad Sci.* 1996;93:49-54.

Salib RJ, Howarth PH. Remodelling of the upper airways in allergic rhinitis: is it a feature of the disease? *Clin Exp Allergy.* 2003 Dec;33(12):1629-33.

Salim AS. Sulfhydryl-containing agents in the treatment of gastric bleeding induced by nonsteroidal anti-inflammatory drugs. *Can J Surg*. 1993 Feb;36(1):53-8.

Salmi H, Kuitunen M, Viljanen M, Lapatto R. Cow's milk allergy is associated with changes in urinary organic acid concentrations. *Pediatr Allergy Immunol*. 2010 Mar;21(2 Pt 2):e401-6.

Salminen E, Elomaa I, Minkkinen J, Vapaatalo H, Salminen S. Preservation of intestinal integrity during radiotherapy using live *Lactobacillus acidophilus* cultures. *Clin Radiol*. 1988 Jul;39(4):435-7.

Salminen S, Isolauri E, Salminen E. Clinical uses of probiotics for stabilizing the gut mucosal barrier: successful strains and future challenges. *Antonie Van Leeuwenhoek*. 1996 Oct;70(2-4):347-58.

Salom IL, Silvis SE, Doscherholmen A. Effect of cimetidine on the absorption of vitamin B12. *Scand J Gastroenterol*. 1982;17:129-31.

Salome CM, Marks GB. Sex, asthma and obesity: an intimate relationship? *Clin Exp Allergy*. 2011 Jan;41(1):6-8.

Salpietro CD, Gangemi S, Briuglia S, Meo A, Merlino MV, Muscolino G, Bisignano G, Trombetta D, Saija A. The almond milk: a new approach to the management of cow-milk allergy/intolerance in infants. *Minerva Pediatr*. 2005 Aug;57(4):173-80.

Salvi SS, Barnes PJ. Chronic obstructive pulmonary disease in non-smokers. *Lancet*. 2009 Aug 29;374(9691):733-43.

Samanta M, Sarkar M, Ghosh P, Ghosh J, Sinha M, Chatterjee S. Prophylactic probiotics for prevention of necrotizing enterocolitis in very low birth weight newborns. *J Trop Pediatr*. 2009 Apr;55(2):128-31.

Sancho AI, Hoffmann-Sommergruber K, Alessandri S, Conti A, Giuffrida MG, Shewry P, Jensen BM, Skov P, Vieths S. Authentication of food allergen quality by physicochemical and immunological methods. *Clin Exp Allergy*. 2010 Jul;40(7):973-86.

Santos A, Dias A, Pinheiro JA. Predictive factors for the persistence of cow's milk allergy. *Pediatr Allergy Immunol*. 2010 Apr 27.

Sanz Ortega J, Martorell Aragonés A, Michavila Gómez A, Nieto García A; Grupo de Trabajo para el Estudio de la Alergia Alimentaria. Incidence of IgE-mediated allergy to cow's milk proteins in the first year of life. *An Esp Pediatr*. 2001 Jun;54(6):536-9.

Saran S, Gopalan S, Krishna TP. Use of fermented foods to combat stunting and failure to thrive. *Nutrition*. 2002 May;18(5):393-6.

Sato Y, Akiyama H, Matsuoka H, Sakata K, Nakamura R, Ishikawa S, Inakuma T, Totsuka M, Sugita-Konishi Y, Ebisawa M, Teshima R. Dietary carotenoids inhibit oral sensitization and the development of food allergy. *J Agric Food Chem*. 2010 Jun 23;58(12):7180-6.

Satyanarayana S, Sushruta K, Sarma GS, Srinivas N, Subba Raju GV. Antioxidant activity of the aqueous extracts of spicy food additives—evaluation and comparison with ascorbic acid in in-vitro systems. *J Herb Pharmacother*. 2004;4(2):1-10.

Savage JH, Kaeding AJ, Matsui EC, Wood RA. The natural history of soy allergy. *J Allergy Clin Immunol*. 2010 Mar;125(3):683-6.

Savilahti EM, Karinen S, Salo HM, Klemetti P, Saarinen KM, Klemola T, Kuitunen M, Hautaniemi S, Savilahti E, Vaarala O. Combined T regulatory cell and Th2 expression profile identifies children with cow's milk allergy. *Clin Immunol*. 2010 Jul;136(1):16-20.

Savilahti EM, Rantanen V, Lin JS, Karinen S, Saarinen KM, Goldis M, Mäkelä MJ, Hautaniemi S, Savilahti E, Sampson HA. Early recovery from cow's milk allergy is associated with decreasing IgE and increasing IgG4 binding to cow's milk epitopes. *J Allergy Clin Immunol*. 2010 Jun;125(6):1315-1321.e9.

Savino F, Pelle E, Palumeri E, Oggero R, Miniero R. *Lactobacillus reuteri* (American Type Culture Collection Strain 55730) versus simethicone in the treatment of infantile colic: a prospective randomized study. Pediatrics. 2007 Jan;119(1):e124-30.

Sazanova NE, Varnacheva LN, Novikova AV, Pletneva NB. Immunological aspects of food intolerance in children during first years of life. *Pediatriia*. 1992;(3):14-8.

Scadding G, Bjarnason I, Brostoff J, Levi AJ, Peters TJ. Intestinal permeability to 51Cr-labelled ethylenediaminetetraacetate in food-intolerant subjects. *Digestion*. 1989;42(2):104-9.

Scalabrin DM, Johnston WH, Hoffman DR, P'Pool VL, Harris CL, Mitmesser SH. Growth and tolerance of healthy term infants receiving hydrolyzed infant formulas supplemented with Lactobacillus rhamnosus GG: randomized, double-blind, controlled trial. *Clin Pediatr (Phila)*. 2009 Sep;48(7):734-44.

Schaafsma G, Meuling WJ, van Dokkum W, Bouley C. Effects of a milk product, fermented by *Lactobacillus acidophilus* and with fructo-oligosaccharides added, on blood lipids in male volunteers. *Eur J Clin Nutr*. 1998 Jun;52(6):436-40.

Schauenberg P, Paris F. *Guide to Medicinal Plants*. New Canaan, CT: Keats Publ, 1977.

Schauss AG, Wu X, Prior RL, Ou B, Huang D, Owens J, Agarwal A, Jensen GS, Hart AN, Shanbrom E. Antioxidant capacity and other bioactivities of the freeze-dried Amazonian palm berry, Euterpe oleraceae mart. (acai). *J Agric Food Chem*. 2006 Nov 1;54(22):8604-10.

Schempp H, Weiser D, Elstner EF. Biochemical model reactions indicative of inflammatory processes. Activities of extracts from Fraxinus excelsior and Populus tremula. *Arzneimittelforschung.* 2000 Apr;50(4):362-72.

Schiffrin EJ, Brassart D, Servin AL, Rochat F, Donnet-Hughes A. Immune modulation of blood leukocytes in humans by lactic acid bacteria: criteria for strain selection. *Am J Clin Nutr.* 1997 Aug;66(2):515S-520S.

Schillaci D, Arizza V, Dayton T, Camarda L, Di Stefano V. In vitro anti-biofilm activity of Boswellia spp. oleogum resin essential oils. *Lett Appl Microbiol.* 2008 Nov;47(5):433-8.

Schlumpf M, Cotton B, Conscience M, Haller V, Steinmann B, Lichtensteiger W. In vitro and in vivo estrogenicity of UV screens. *Environ Health Perspect.* 2001 Mar;109(3):239-44.

Schmid B, Kötter I, Heide L. Pharmacokinetics of salicin after oral administration of a standardised willow bark extract. *Eur J Clin Pharmacol.* 2001 Aug;57(5):387-91.

Schmitt DA, Maleki SJ (2004) Comparing the effects of boiling, frying and roasting on the allergenicity of peanuts. *J Allergy Clin Immunol.* 113: S155.

Schnappinger M, Sausenthaler S, Linseisen J, Hauner H, Heinrich J. Fish consumption, allergic sensitisation and allergic diseases in adults. *Ann Nutr Metab.* 2009;54(1):67-74.

Scholz-Ahrens KE, Ade P, Marten B, Weber P, Timm W, Açil Y, Glüer CC, Schrezenmeir J. Prebiotics, probiotics, and synbiotics affect mineral absorption, bone mineral content, and bone structure. *J Nutr.* 2007 Mar;137(3 Suppl 2):838S-46S.

Schönfeld P. Phytanic Acid toxicity: implications for the permeability of the inner mitochondrial membrane to ions. *Toxicol Mech Methods.* 2004;14(1-2):47-52.

Schottner M, Gansser D, Spiteller G. Lignans from the roots of Urtica dioica and their metabolites bind to human sex hormone binding globulin (SHBG). *Planta Med.* 1997;65:529-532.

Schouten B, van Esch BC, Hofman GA, Boon L, Knippels LM, Willemsen LE, Garssen J. Oligosaccharide-induced whey-specific CD25(+) regulatory T-cells are involved in the suppression of cow milk allergy in mice. *J Nutr.* 2010 Apr;140(4):835-41.

Schröder L, Koch J, Mahner S, Kost BP, Hofmann S, Jeschke U, Haumann J, Schmedt J, Richter DU. The Effects of Petroselinum Crispum on Estrogen Receptor-positive Benign and Malignant Mammary Cells (MCF12A/MCF7). Anticancer Res. 2017 Jan;37(1):95-102.

Schroecksnadel S, Jenny M, Fuchs D. Sensitivity to sulphite additives. *Clin Exp Allergy.* 2010 Apr;40(4):688-9.

Schulick P. *Ginger: Common Spice & Wonder Drug.* Brattleboro, VT: Herbal Free Perss, 1996.

Schulman G. A nexus of progression of chronic kidney disease: charcoal, tryptophan and profibrotic cytokines. *Blood Purif.* 2006;24(1):143-8.

Schulz V, Hansel R, Tyler VE. *Rational Phytotherapy.* Berlin: Springer-Verlag; 1998.

Schumacher P. *Biophysical Therapy Of Allergies.* Stuttgart: Thieme, 2005.

Schütz K, Carle R, Schieber A. Taraxacum—a review on its phytochemical and pharmacological profile. *J Ethnopharmacol.* 2006 Oct 11;107(3):313-23.

Schwab D, Hahn EG, Raithel M. Enhanced histamine metabolism: a comparative analysis of collagenous colitis and food allergy with respect to the role of diet and NSAID use. *Inflamm Res.* 2003 Apr;52(4):142-7.

Schwab D, Müller S, Aigner T, Neureiter D, Kirchner T, Hahn EG, Raithel M. Functional and morphologic characterization of eosinophils in the lower intestinal mucosa of patients with food allergy. *Am J Gastroenterol.* 2003 Jul;98(7):1525-34.

Schwelberger HG. Histamine intolerance: a metabolic disease? *Inflamm Res.* 2010 Mar;59 Suppl 2:S219-21.

Schwellenbach LJ, Olson KL. McConnell KJ, Stolepart RS, Nash JD, Merenich JA. The triglyceride-lowering effects of a modest dose of docosahexaenoic acid alone versus in combination with low dose eicosapentaenoic acid in patients with coronary artery disease and elevated triglycerides. *J Am Coll Nutr.* 2006;25(6):480-485.

Scott-Taylor TH, O'B Hourihane J, Strobel S. Correlation of allergen-specific IgG subclass antibodies and T lymphocyte cytokine responses in children with multiple food allergies. *Pediatr Allergy Immunol.* 2010 Sep;21(6):935-44.

Scurlock AM, Jones SM. An update on immunotherapy for food allergy. *Curr Opin Allergy Clin Immunol.* 2010 Dec;10(6):587-93.

Sealey-Voyksner JA, Khosla C, Voyksner RD, Jorgenson JW. Novel aspects of quantitation of immunogenic wheat gluten peptides by liquid chromatography-mass spectrometry. *J Chromatogr A.* 2010 Jun 18;1217(25):4167-83.

Searing DA, Leung DY. Vitamin D in atopic dermatitis, asthma and allergic diseases. *Immunol Allergy Clin North Am.* 2010 Aug;30(3):397-409.

Sekine K, Toida T, Saito M, Kuboyama M, Kawashima T, Hashimoto Y. A new morphologically characterized cell wall preparation (whole peptidoglycan) from *Bifidobacterium* infantis with a higher efficacy on the regression of an established tumor in mice. *Cancer Res.* 1985 Mar;45(3):1300-7.

REFERENCES AND BIBLIOGRAPHY

Selmi C, Leung PS, Fischer L, German B, Yang CY, Kenny TP, Cysewski GR, Gershwin ME. The effects of Spirulina on anemia and immune function in senior citizens. Cell Mol Immunol. 2011 May;8(3):248-54. doi: 10.1038/cmi.2010.76.

Senior F. Fallout. *New York Magazine*. Fall: 2003.

Senna G, Gani F, Leo G, Schiappoli M. Alternative tests in the diagnosis of food allergies. *Recenti Prog Med*. 2002 May;93(5):327-34.

Seo K, Jung S, Park M, Song Y, Choung S. Effects of leucocyanidines on activities of metabolizing enzymes and antioxidant enzymes. *Biol Pharm Bull*. 2001 May;24(5):592-3.

Seo SW, Koo HN, An HJ, Kwon KB, Lim BC, Seo EA, Ryu DG, Moon G, Kim HY, Kim HM, Hong SH. Taraxacum officinale protects against cholecystokinin-induced acute pancreatitis in rats. *World J Gastroenterol*. 2005 Jan 28;11(4):597-9.

Seppo L, Jauhiainen T, Poussa T, Korpela R. A fermented milk high in bioactive peptides has a blood pressure-lowering effect in hypertensive subjects. *Am J Clin Nutr*. 2003 Feb;77(2):326-30.

Seppo L, Korpela R, Lönnerdal B, Metsäniitty L, Juntunen-Backman K, Klemola T, Paganus A, Vanto T. A follow-up study of nutrient intake, nutritional status, and growth in infants with cow milk allergy fed either a soy formula or an extensively hydrolyzed whey formula. *Am J Clin Nutr*. 2005 Jul;82(1):140-5.

Serra A, Cocuzza S, Poli G, La Mantia I, Messina A, Pavone P. Otologic findings in children with gastroesophageal reflux. *Int J Pediatr Otorhinolaryngol*. 2007 Nov;71(11):1693-7. 2007 Aug 22.

Sevar R. Audit of outcome in 455 consecutive patients treated with homeopathic medicines. *Homeopathy*. 2005 Oct;94(4):215-21.

Shahani KM, Ayebo AD. Role of dietary lactobacilli in gastrointestinal microecology. *Am J Clin Nutr*. 1980 Nov;33(11 Suppl):2448-57.

Shahani KM, Chandan RC. Nutritional and healthful aspects of cultured and culture-containing dairy foods. *J Dairy Sci*. 1979 Oct;62(10):1685-94.

Shahani KM, Friend BA. Properties of and prospects for cultured dairy foods. *Soc Appl Bacteriol Symp Ser*. 1983;11:257-69.

Shahani KM, Herper WJ, Jensen RG, Parry RM Jr, Zittle CA. Enzymes in bovine milk: a review. *J Dairy Sci*. 1973 May;56(5):531-43.

Shahani KM, Kwan AJ, Friend BA. Role and significance of enzymes in human milk. *Am J Clin Nutr*. 1980 Aug;33(8):1861-8.

Shahani KM, Meshbesher BF, Mangalampalli V. *Cultivate Health From Within*. Danbury, CT: Vital Health Publ, 2005.

Shaheen S, Potts J, Gnatiuc L, Makowska J, Kowalski ML, Joos G, van Zele T, van Durme Y, De Rudder I, Wöhrl S, Godnic-Cvar J, Skadhauge L, Thomsen G, Zuberbier T, Bergmann KC, Heinzerling L, Gjomarkaj M, Bruno A, Pace E, Bonini S, Fokkens W, Weersink EJ, Loureiro C, Todo-Bom A, Villanueva CM, Sanjuas C, Zock JP, Janson C, Burney P; Selenium and Asthma Research Integration project; GA2LEN. The relation between paracetamol use and asthma: a GA2LEN European case-control study. *Eur Respir J*. 2008 Nov;32(5):1231-6.

Shaheen SO, Newson RB, Rayman MP, Wong AP, Tumilty MK, Phillips JM, Potts JF, Kelly FJ, White PT, Burney PG. Randomised, double blind, placebo-controlled trial of selenium supplementation in adult asthma. *Thorax*. 2007 Jun;62(6):483-90.

Shakib F, Brown HM, Phelps A, Redhead R. Study of IgG sub-class antibodies in patients with milk intolerance. *Clin Allergy*. 1986 Sep;16(5):451-8.

Shalev E, Battino S, Weiner E, Colodner R, Keness Y. Ingestion of yogurt containing *Lactobacillus acidophilus* compared with pasteurized yogurt as prophylaxis for recurrent *Candida* vaginitis and bacterial vaginosis. *Arch Fam Med*. 1996 Nov-Dec;5(10):593-6.

Shamir R, Makhoul IR, Etzioni A, Shehadeh N. Evaluation of a diet containing probiotics and zinc for the treatment of mild diarrheal illness in children younger than one year of age. *J Am Coll Nutr*. 2005 Oct;24(5):370-5.

Shan L, Li Y, Jiang H, Tao Y, Qian Z, Li L, Cai F, Ma L, Yu Y. Huaier Restrains Migratory Potential of Hepatocellular Carcinoma Cells Partially Through Decreased Yes-Associated Protein 1. J Cancer. 2017 Nov 6;8(19):4087-4097. doi: 10.7150/jca.21018.

Shariata A, FarhangibAM, Zeinalianc R. Spirulina platensis supplementation, macrophage inhibitory cytokine-1 (MIC-1), oxidative stress markers and anthropometric features in obese individuals: A randomized controlled trial. J Herbal Med. 2019 Sept-Dec;17-18.

Sharma P, Sharma BC, Puri V, Sarin SK. An open-label randomized controlled trial of lactulose and probiotics in the treatment of minimal hepatic encephalopathy. *Eur J Gastroent Hepatol*. 2008 Jun;20(6):506-11.

Sharma SC, Sharma S, Gulati OP. Pycnogenol inhibits the release of histamine from mast cells. *Phytother Res*. 2003 Jan;17(1):66-9.

Sharnan J, Kumar L, Singh S. Comparison of results of skin prick tests, enzyme-linked immunosorbent assays and food challenges in children with respiratory allergy. *J Trop Pediatr*. 2001 Dec;47(6):367-8.

Shawcross DL, Wright G, Olde Damink SW, Jalan R. Role of ammonia and inflammation in minimal hepatic encephalopathy. *Metab Brain Dis.* 2007 Mar;22(1):125-38.

Shea KM, Trucker RT, Weber RW, Peden DB. Climate change and allergic disease. *Clin Rev Allergy Immunol.* 2008;6:443-453.

Shea-Donohue T, Stiltz J, Zhao A, Notari L. Mast Cells. *Curr Gastroenterol Rep.* 2010 Aug 14.

Sheih YH, Chiang BL, Wang LH, Liao CK, Gill HS. Systemic immunity-enhancing effects in healthy subjects following dietary consumption of the lactic acid bacterium *Lactobacillus rhamnosus* HN001. *J Am Coll Nutr.* 2001 Apr;20(2 Suppl):149-56.

Shen FY, Lee MS, Jung SK. Effectiveness of pharmacopuncture for asthma: a systematic review and meta-analysis. *Evid Based Complement Alternat Med.* 2011;2011. pii: 678176.

Sheth SS, Waserman S, Kagan R, Alizadehfar R, Primeau MN, Elliot S, St Pierre Y, Wickett R, Joseph L, Harada L, Dufresne C, Allen M, Allen M, Godefroy SB, Clarke AE. Role of food labels in accidental exposures in food-allergic individuals in Canada. *Ann Allergy Asthma Immunol.* 2010 Jan;104(1):60-5.

Shi S, Zhao Y, Zhou H, Zhang Y, Jiang X, Huang K. Identification of antioxidants from Taraxacum mongolicum by high-performance liquid chromatography-diode array detection-radical-scavenging detection-electrospray ionization mass spectrometry and nuclear magnetic resonance experiments. *J Chromatogr A.* 2008 Oct 31;1209(1-2):145-52

Shi S, Zhou H, Zhang Y, Huang K, Liu S. Chemical constituents from Neo-Taraxacum siphonathum. *Zhongguo Zhong Yao Za Zhi.* 2009 Apr;34(8):1002-4.

Shi SY, Zhou CX, Xu Y, Tao QF, Bai H, Lu FS, Lin WY, Chen HY, Zheng W, Wang LW, Wu YH, Zeng S, Huang KX, Zhao Y, Li XK, Qu J. Studies on chemical constituents from herbs of Taraxacum mongolicum. *Zhongguo Zhong Yao Za Zhi.* 2008 May;33(10):1147-57.

Shi YQ, He Q, Zhao YJ, Wang EH, Wu GP. Lectin microarrays differentiate carcinoma cells from reactive mesothelial cells in pleural effusions. Cytotechnology. 2013 May;65(3):355-62. doi: 10.1007/s10616-012-9474-x.

Shibata H, Nabe T, Yamamura H, Kohno S. l-Ephedrine is a major constituent of Mao-Bushi-Saishin-To, one of the formulas of Chinese medicine, which shows immediate inhibition after oral administration of passive cutaneous anaphylaxis in rats. *Inflamm Res.* 2000 Aug;49(8):398-403.

Shichinohe K, Shimizu M, Kurokawa K. Effect of M-711 on experimental asthma in rats. *J Vet Med Sci.* 1996 Jan;58(1):55-9.

Shimauchi H, Mayanagi G, Nakaya S, Minamibuchi M, Ito Y, Yamaki K, Hirata H. Improvement of periodontal condition by probiotics with *Lactobacillus salivarius* WB21: a randomized, double-blind, placebo-controlled study. *J Clin Periodontol.* 2008 Oct;35(10):897-905.

Shimizu K, Ogura H, Goto M, Asahara T, Nomoto K, Morotomi M, Matsushima A, Tasaki O, Fujita K, Hosotsubo H, Kuwagata Y, Tanaka H, Shimazu T, Sugimoto H. Synbiotics decrease the incidence of septic complications in patients with severe SIRS: a preliminary report. *Dig Dis Sci.* 2009 May;54(5):1071-8.

Shimizu Y, Teshima H, Chen JT, Fujimoto I, Hasumi K, Masubuchi K. [Augmentative effect of sizofiran on the immune functions of regional lymph nodes in patients with cervical cancer]. Nihon Sanka Fujinka Gakkai Zasshi. 1991 Jun;43(6):581-8.

Shimoi T, Ushiyama H, Kan K, Saito K, Kamata K, Hirokado M. Survey of glycoalkaloids content in the various potatoes. *Shokuhin Eiseigaku Zasshi.* 2007 Jun;48(3):77-82.

Shishehbor F, Behroo L, Ghafouriyan Broujerdnia M, Namjoyan F, Latifi SM. Quercetin effectively quells peanut-induced anaphylactic reactions in the peanut sensitized rats. *Iran J Allergy Asthma Immunol.* 2010 Mar;9(1):27-34.

Shishodia S, Harikumar KB, Dass S, Ramawat KG, Aggarwal BB. The guggul for chronic diseases: ancient medicine, modern targets. *Anticancer Res.* 2008 Nov-Dec;28(6A):3647-64.

Shivpuri DN, Menon MP, Parkash D. Preliminary studies in Tylophora indica in the treatment of asthma and allergic rhinitis. *J Assoc Physicians India.* 1968 Jan;16(1):9-15.

Shivpuri DN, Menon MP, Prakash D. A crossover double-blind study on Tylophora indica in the treatment of asthma and allergic rhinitis. *J Allergy.* 1969 Mar;43(3):145-50.

Shivpuri DN, Singhal SC, Parkash D. Treatment of asthma with an alcoholic extract of Tylophora indica: a cross-over, double-blind study. *Ann Allergy.* 1972; 30:407-12.

Shoaf K, Mulvey GL, Armstrong GD, Hutkins RW. Prebiotic galactooligosaccharides reduce adherence of enteropathogenic *Escherichia coli* to tissue culture cells. Infect Immun. 2006 Dec;74(12):6920-8.

Shoaf, K., Muvey, G.L., Armstrong, G.D., Hutkins, R.W. (2006) Prebiotic galactooligosaccharides reduce adherence of enteropathogenic Escherichia coli to tissue culture cells. *Infect Immun.* Dec;74(12):6920-8.

Shornikova AV, Casas IA, Isolauri E, Mykkänen H, Vesikari T. *Lactobacillus reuteri* as a therapeutic agent in acute diarrhea in young children. *J Pediatr Gastroenterol Nutr.* 1997 Apr;24(4):399-404.

Shornikova AV, Casas IA, Mykkänen H, Salo E, Vesikari T. Bacteriotherapy with *Lactobacillus reuteri* in rotavirus gastroenteritis. *Pediatr Infect Dis J.* 1997 Dec;16(12):1103-7.

REFERENCES AND BIBLIOGRAPHY

Sicherer SH, Muñoz-Furlong A, Godbold JH, Sampson HA. US prevalence of self-reported peanut, tree nut, and sesame allergy: 11-year follow-up. *J Allergy Clin Immunol.* 2010 Jun;125(6):1322-6.

Sicherer SH, Noone SA, Koerner CB, Christie L, Burks AW, Sampson HA. Hypoallergenicity and efficacy of an amino acid-based formula in children with cow's milk and multiple food hypersensitivities. *J Pediatr.* 2001 May;138(5):688-93.

Sicherer SH, Sampson HA. Food allergy. *J Allergy Clin Immunol.* 2010 Feb;125(2 Suppl 2):S116-25.

Sidoroff V, Hyvärinen M, Piippo-Savolainen E, Korppi M. Lung function and overweight in school aged children after early childhood wheezing. *Pediatr Pulmonol.* 2010 Dec 30.

Sigstedt SC, Hooten CJ, Callewaert MC, Jenkins AR, Romero AE, Pullin MJ, Kornienko A, Lowrey TK, Slambrouck SV, Steelant WF. Evaluation of aqueous extracts of Taraxacum officinale on growth and invasion of breast and prostate cancer cells. *Int J Oncol.* 2008 May;32(5):1085-90.

Sildorf SM, Eising S, Hougaard DM, Mortensen HB, Skogstrand K, Pociot F, Johannesen J, Svensson J. Differences in MBL levels between juvenile patients newly diagnosed with type 1 diabetes and their healthy siblings. *Mol Immunol.* 2014 Nov;62(1):71-6. doi: 10.1016/j.molimm.2014.06.001.

Silman AJ, MacGregor AJ, Thomson W, Holligan S, Carthy D, Farhan A, Ollier WE. Twin concordance rates for rheumatoid arthritis: results from a nationwide study. *Br J Rheumatol.* 1993 Oct;32(10):903-7.

Silva MF, Kamphorst AO, Hayashi EA, Bellio M, Carvalho CR, Faria AM, Sabino KC, Coelho MG, Nobrega A, Tavares D, Silva AC. Innate profiles of cytokines implicated on oral tolerance correlate with low- or high-suppression of humoral response. *Immunology.* 2010 Jul;130(3):447-57.

Silva MR, Dias G, Ferreira CL, Franceschini SC, Costa NM. Growth of preschool children was improved when fed an iron-fortified fermented milk beverage supplemented with *Lactobacillus acidophilus. Nutr Res.* 2008 Apr;28(4):226-32.

Simakachorn N, Pichaipat V, Rithipornpaisarn P, Kongkaew C, Tongpradit P, Varavithya W. Clinical evaluation of the addition of lyophilized, heat-killed *Lactobacillus acidophilus* LB to oral rehydration therapy in the treatment of acute diarrhea in children. *J Pediatr Gastroenterol Nutr.* 2000 Jan;30(1):68-72.

Simenhoff ML, Dunn SR, Zollner GP, Fitzpatrick ME, Emery SM, Sandine WE, Ayres JW. Biomodulation of the toxic and nutritional effects of small bowel bacterial overgrowth in end-stage kidney disease using freeze-dried *Lactobacillus acidophilus. Miner Electrolyte Metab.* 1996;22(1-3):92-6.

Simeone D, Miele E, Boccia G, Marino A, Troncone R, Staiano A. Prevalence of atopy in children with chronic constipation. *Arch Dis Child.* 2008 Dec;93(12):1044-7.

Simões EA, Carbonell-Estrany X, Rieger CH, Mitchell I, Fredrick L, Groothuis JR; Palivizumab Long-Term Respiratory Outcomes Study Group. The effect of respiratory syncytial virus on subsequent recurrent wheezing in atopic and nonatopic children. *J Allergy Clin Immunol.* 2010 Aug;126(2):256-62. 2010 Jul 10.

Simons FER. What's in a name? The allergic rhinitis-asthma connection. *Clin Exp All Rev.* 2003;3:9-17.

Simonte SJ, Ma S, Mofidi S, Sicherer SH. Relevance of casual contact with peanut butter in children with peanut allergy. *J Allergy Clin Immunol.* 2003 Jul;112(1):180-2.

Simopoulos AP. Essential fatty acids in health and chronic disease. *Am J Clin Nutr.* 1999 Sep;70(3 Suppl):560S-569S.

Simpson A, Tan VY, Winn J, Svensén M, Bishop CM, Heckerman DE, Buchan I, Custovic A. Beyond atopy: multiple patterns of sensitization in relation to asthma in a birth cohort study. *Am J Respir Crit Care Med.* 2010 Jun 1;181(11):1200-6.

Simpson AB, Yousef E, Hossain J. Association between peanut allergy and asthma morbidity. *J Pediatr.* 2010 May;156(5):777-81.

Sin A, Terzioğlu E, Kokuludağ A, Sebik F, Kabakçi T. Serum eosinophil cationic protein (ECP) levels in patients with seasonal allergic rhinitis and allergic asthma. *Allergy Asthma Proc.* 1998 Mar-Apr;19(2):69-73.

Singer P, Shapiro H, Theilla M, Anbar R, Singer J, Cohen J. Anti-inflammatory properties of omega-3 fatty acids in critical illness: novel mechanisms and an integrative perspective. *Intensive Care Med.* 2008 Sep;34(9):1580-92.

Singh BB, Khorsan R, Vinjamury SP, Der-Martirosian C, Kizhakkeveettil A, Anderson TM. Herbal treatments of asthma: a systematic review. *J Asthma.* 2007 Nov;44(9):685-98.

Singh M, Das RR. Zinc for the common cold. *Cochrane Database Syst Rev.* 2013 Jun 18;(6):CD001364. doi: 10.1002/14651858.CD001364.pub4.

Singh RS, Thakur SR, Bansal P. Algal lectins as promising biomolecules for biomedical research. *Crit Rev Microbiol.* 2013 Jul 16.

Singh S, Khajuria A, Taneja SC, Johri RK, Singh J, Qazi GN. Boswellic acids: A leukotriene inhibitor also effective through topical application in inflammatory disorders. *Phytomedicine.* 2008 Jun;15(6-7):400-7.

Singh V, Jain NK. Asthma as a cause for, rather than a result of, gastroesophageal reflux. *J Asthma.* 1983;20(4):241-3. 3.

Sinn DH, Song JH, Kim HJ, Lee JH, Son HJ, Chang DK, Kim YH, Kim JJ, Rhee JC, Rhee PL. Therapeutic effect of *Lactobacillus acidophilus*-SDC 2012, 2013 in patients with irritable bowel syndrome. *Dig Dis Sci.* 2008 Oct;53(10):2714-8.

Sirvent S, Palomares O, Vereda A, Villalba M, Cuesta-Herranz J, Rodríguez R. nsLTP and profilin are allergens in mustard seeds: cloning, sequencing and recombinant production of Sin a 3 and Sin a 4. *Clin Exp Allergy.* 2009 Dec;39(12):1929-36.

Sistek D, Kelly R, Wickens K, Stanley T, Fitzharris P, Crane J. Is the effect of probiotics on atopic dermatitis confined to food sensitized children? *Clin Exp Allergy.* 2006 May;36(5):629-33.

Skamstrup Hansen K, Vieths S, Vestergaard H, Skov PS, Bindslev-Jensen C, Poulsen LK. Seasonal variation in food allergy to apple. *J Chromatogr B Biomed Sci Appl.* 2001 May 25;756(1-2):19-32.

Skovbjerg S, Roos K, Holm SE, Grahn Håkansson E, Nowrouzian F, Ivarsson M, Adlerberth I, Wold AE. Spray bacteriotherapy decreases middle ear fluid in children with secretory otitis media. *Arch Dis Child.* 2009 Feb;94(2):92-8.

Skripak JM, Nash SD, Rowley H, Brereton NH, Oh S, Hamilton RG, Matsui EC, Burks AW, Wood RA. A randomized, double-blind, placebo-controlled study of milk oral immunotherapy for cow's milk allergy. *J Allergy Clin Immunol.* 2008 Dec;122(6):1154-60.

Sletten GB, Halvorsen R, Egaas E, Halstensen TS. Changes in humoral responses to beta-lactoglobulin in tolerant patients suggest a particular role for IgG4 in delayed, non-IgE-mediated cow's milk allergy. *Pediatr Allergy Immunol.* 2006 Sep;17(6):435-43.

Smith J. *Genetic Roulette: The Documented Health Risks of Genetically Engineered Foods.* White River Jct, Vermont: Chelsea Green, 2007.

Smith JA, *et al.* In vitro and in vivo evaluation of Active Hexose Correlated Compound (AHCC) for the Eradication of HPV. Gynec Oncology. 2014. June 133;1;189.

Smith K, Warholak T, Armstrong E, Leib M, Rehfeld R, Malone D. Evaluation of risk factors and health outcomes among persons with asthma. *J Asthma.* 2009 Apr;46(3):234-7.

Smith LJ, Holbrook JT, Wise R, Blumenthal M, Dozor AJ, Mastronarde J, Williams L; American Lung Association Asthma Clinical Research Centers. Dietary intake of soy genistein is associated with lung function in patients with asthma. *J Asthma.* 2004;41(8):833-43.

Smith S, Sullivan K. Examining the influence of biological and psychological factors on cognitive performance in chronic fatigue syndrome: a randomized, double-blind, placebo-controlled, crossover study. *Int J Behav Med.* 2003;10(2):162-73.

Soares AA, de Sá-Nakanishi AB, Bracht A, da Costa SM, Koehnlein EA, de Souza CG, Peralta RM. Hepatoprotective effects of mushrooms. Molecules. 2013 Jul 1;18(7):7609-30.

Sofic E, Denisova N, Youdim K, Vatrenjak-Velagic V, De Filippo C, Mehmedagic A, Causevic A, Cao G, Joseph JA, Prior RL. Antioxidant and pro-oxidant capacity of catecholamines and related compounds. Effects of hydrogen peroxide on glutathione and sphingomyelinase activity in pheochromocytoma PC12 cells: potential relevance to age-related diseases. *J Neural Transm.* 2001;108(5):541-57.

Soga K, Teruya F, Tateno H, Hirabayashi J, Yamamoto K. Terminal N -acetylgalactosamine-specific leguminous lectin from Wisteria japonica as a probe for human lung squamous cell carcinoma. PLoS One. 2013 Dec 13;8(12):e83886. doi: 10.1371/journal.pone.0083886.

Soleo L, Colosio C, Alinovi R, Guarneri D, Russo A, Lovreglio P, Vimercati L, Birindelli S, Cortesi I, Flore C, Carta P, Colombi A, Parrinello G, Ambrosi L. Immunologic effects of exposure to low levels of inorganic mercury. *Med Lav.* 2002 May-Jun;93(3):225-32.

Solomons NW, Guerrero AM, Torun B. Effective in vivo hydrolysis of milk lactose by beta-galactosidases in the presence of solid foods. *Am J Clin Nutr.* 1985 Feb;41(2):222-7.

Sompamit K, Kukongviriyapan U, Nakmareong S, Pannangpetch P, Kukongviriyapan V. Curcumin improves vascular function and alleviates oxidative stress in non-lethal lipopolysaccharide-induced endotoxaemia in mice. *Eur J Pharmacol.* 2009 Aug 15;616(1-3):192-9.

Song GG, Bae SC, Seo YH, Kim JH, Choi SJ, Ji JD, Lee YH. Meta-analysis of functional MBL polymorphisms. Associations with rheumatoid arthritis and primary Sjögren's syndrome. Z Rheumatol. 2014 Sep;73(7):657-64. doi: 10.1007/s00393-014-1408-x.

Song X, Li Y, Zhang H, Yang Q. The anticancer effect of Huaier (Review). Oncol Rep. 2015 Jul;34(1):12-21. doi: 10.3892/or.2015.3950.

Sonibare MA, Gbile ZO. Ethnobotanical survey of anti-asthmatic plants in South Western Nigeria. *Afr J Tradit Complement Altern Med.* 2008 Jun 18;5(4):340-5.

Sontag SJ, O'Connell S, Khandelwal S, Greenlee H, Schnell T, Nemchausky B, Chejfec G, Miller T, Seidel J, Sonnenberg A. Asthmatics with gastroesophageal reflux: long term results of a randomized trial of medical and surgical antireflux therapies. *Am J Gastroenterol.* 2003 May;98(5):987-99.

Sosa M, Saavedra P, Valero C, Guañabens N, Nogués X, del Pino-Montes J, Mosquera J, Alegre J, Gómez-Alonso C, Muñoz-Torres M, Quesada M, Pérez-Cano R, Jódar E, Torrijos A, Lozano-Tonkin C, Díaz-Curiel M; GIUMO Study Group. Inhaled steroids do not decrease bone mineral density but increase risk of fractures: data from the GIUMO Study Group. J Clin Densitom. 2006 Apr-Jun;9(2):154-8.

Soyka F, Edmonds A. *The Ion Effect: How Air Electricity Rules your Life and Health.* Bantam, New York: Bantam, 1978.

Spence A. *Basic Human Anatomy.* Menlo Park, CA: Benjamin/Commings, 1986.

Spiller G. *The Super Pyramid.* New York: HRS Press, 1993.

Sporik R, Squillace SP, Ingram JM, Rakes G, Honsinger RW, Platts-Mills TA. Mite, cat, and cockroach exposure, allergen sensitisation, and asthma in children: a case-control study of three schools. *Thorax.* 1999 Aug;54(8):675-80.

Srivastava K, Zou ZM, Sampson HA, Dansky H, Li XM. Direct Modulation of Airway Reactivity by the Chinese Anti-Asthma Herbal Formula ASHMI. *J Allergy Clin Immunol.* 2005;115:S7.

Srivastava KD, Qu C, Zhang T, Goldfarb J, Sampson HA, Li XM. Food Allergy Herbal Formula-2 silences peanut-induced anaphylaxis for a prolonged posttreatment period via IFN-gamma-producing CD8+ T cells. *J Allergy Clin Immunol.* 2009 Feb;123(2):443-51.

Srivastava KD, Zhang TF, Qu C, Sampson HA, Li XM. Silencing Peanut Allergy: A Chinese Herbal Formula, FAHF-2, Completely Blocks Peanut-induced Anaphylaxis for up to 6 Months Following Therapy in a Murine Model Of Peanut Allergy. *J Allergy Clin Immunol.* 2006;117:S328.

Stach A, Emberlin J, Smith M, Adams-Groom B, Myszkowska D. Factors that determine the severity of Betula spp. pollen seasons in Poland (Poznań and Krakow) and the United Kingdom (Worcester and London). *Int J Biometeorol.* 2008 Mar;52(4):311-21.

Stachowska E, Dolegowska B, Chlubek D, Wesolowska T, Ciechanowski K, Gutowski P, Szumilowicz H, Turowski R. Dietary trans fatty acids and composition of human atheromatous plaques. *Eur J Nutr.* 2004 Oct;43(5):313-8.

Staden U, Rolinck-Werninghaus C, Brewe F, Wahn U, Niggemann B, Beyer K. Specific oral tolerance induction in food allergy in children: efficacy and clinical patterns of reaction. *Allergy.* 2007 Nov;62(11):1261-9.

Stadlbauer V, Mookerjee RP, Hodges S, Wright GA, Davies NA, Jalan R. Effect of probiotic treatment on deranged neutrophil function and cytokine responses in patients with compensated alcoholic cirrhosis. *J Hepatol.* 2008 Jun;48(6):945-51.

Stahl SM. Selective histamine H1 antagonism: novel hypnotic and pharmacologic actions challenge classical notions of antihistamines. *CNS Spectr.* 2008 Dec;13(12):1027-38.

State Pharmacopoeia Commission of The People's Republic of China. *Pharmacopoeia of the People's Republic of China.* Beijing: Chemical Industry Press; 2005.

Steinman HA, Le Roux M, Potter PC. Sulphur dioxide sensitivity in South African asthmatic children. *S Afr Med J.* 1993 Jun;83(6):387-90.

Stenberg JA, Hambäck PA, Ericson L. Herbivore-induced "rent rise" in the host plant may drive a diet breadth enlargement in the tenant. *Ecology.* 2008 Jan;89(1):126-33.

Stengler M. *The Natural Physician's Healing Therapies.* Stamford, CT: Bottom Line Books, 2008.

Stensrud T, Carlsen KH. Can one single test protocol for provoking exercise-induced bronchoconstriction also be used for assessing aerobic capacity? *Clin Respir J.* 2008 Jan;2(1):47-53.

Steurer-Stey C, Russi EW, Steurer J: Complementary and alternative medicine in asthma: do they work? *Swiss Med Wkly.* 2002, 132:338-344.

Stillerman A, Nachtsheim C, Li W, Albrecht M, Waldman J. Efficacy of a novel air filtration pillow for avoidance of perennial allergens in symptomatic adults. *Ann Allergy Asthma Immunol.* 2010 May;104(5):440-9.

Stirapongsasuti P, Tanglertsampan C, Aunhachoke K, Sangasapaviliya A. Anaphylactic reaction to phuk-waan-ban in a patient with latex allergy. *J Med Assoc Thai.* 2010 May;93(5):616-9.

Størdal K, Johannesdottir GB, Bentsen BS, Knudsen PK, Carlsen KC, Closs O, Handeland M, Holm HK, Sandvik L. Acid suppression does not change respiratory symptoms in children with asthma and gastro-oesophageal reflux disease. *Arch Dis Child.* 2005 Sep;90(9):956-60.

Stoye D, Schubert C, Goihl A, Guttek K, Reinhold A, Brocke S, Grüngreiff K, Reinhold D. Zinc aspartate suppresses T cell activation in vitro and relapsing experimental autoimmune encephalomyelitis. *Biometals.* 2012 Jun;25(3):529-39. doi: 10.1007/s10534-012-9532-z.

Stratiki Z, Costalos C, Sevastiadou S, Kastanidou O, Skouroliakou M, Giakoumatou A, Petrohilou V. The effect of a bifidobacter supplemented bovine milk on intestinal permeability of preterm infants. *Early Hum Dev.* 2007 Sep;83(9):575-9.

Strinnholm A, Brulin C, Lindh V. Experiences of double-blind, placebo-controlled food challenges (DBPCFC): a qualitative analysis of mothers' experiences. *J Child Health Care.* 2010 Jun;14(2):179-88.

Strozzi GP, Mogna L. Quantification of folic acid in human feces after administration of Bifidobacterium probiotic strains. *J Clin Gastroenterol.* 2008 Sep;42 Suppl 3 Pt 2:S179-84.

Stuck BA, Czajkowski J, Hagner AE, Klimek L, Verse T, Hörmann K, Maurer JT. Changes in daytime sleepiness, quality of life, and objective sleep patterns in seasonal allergic rhinitis: a controlled clinical trial. *J Allergy Clin Immunol.* 2004 Apr;113(4):663-8.

Stull DE, Schaefer M, Crespi S, Sandor DW. Relative strength of relationships of nasal congestion and ocular symptoms with sleep, mood and productivity. *Curr Med Res Opin.* 2009 Jul;25(7):1785-92.

Sturtzel B, Mikulits C, Gisinger C, Elmadfa I. Use of fiber instead of laxative treatment in a geriatric hospital to improve the wellbeing of seniors. *J Nutr Health Aging.* 2009 Feb;13(2):136-9.

Stutius LM, Sheehan WJ, Rangsithienchai P, Bharmanee A, Scott JE, Young MC, Dioun AF, Schneider LC, Phipatanakul W. Characterizing the relationship between sesame, coconut, and nut allergy in children. *Pediatr Allergy Immunol.* 2010 Dec;21(8):1114-8.

Su P, Henriksson A, Tandianus JE, Park JH, Foong F, Dunn NW. Detection and quantification of *Bifidobacterium lactis* LAFTI B94 in human faecal samples from a consumption trial. *FEMS Microbiol Lett.* 2005 Mar 1;244(1):99-103.

Sugawara G, Nagino M, Nishio H, Ebata T, Takagi K, Asahara T, Nomoto K, Nimura Y. Perioperative synbiotic treatment to prevent postoperative infectious complications in biliary cancer surgery: a randomized controlled trial. *Ann Surg.* 2006 Nov;244(5):706-14.

Sugimachi K, Maehara Y, Ogawa M, Kakegawa T, Tomita M. Dose intensity of uracil and tegafur in postoperative chemotherapy for patients with poorly differentiated gastric cancer. Cancer Chemother Pharmacol. 1997;40(3):233-8.

Sugnanam KK, Collins JT, Smith PK, Connor F, Lewindon P, Cleghorn G, Withers G. Dichotomy of food and inhalant allergen sensitization in eosinophilic esophagitis. *Allergy.* 2007 Nov;62(11):1257-60.

Sullivan A, Barkholt L, Nord CE. *Lactobacillus acidophilus, Bifidobacterium lactis* and *Lactobacillus* F19 prevent antibiotic-associated ecological disturbances of Bacteroides fragilis in the intestine. *J Antimicrob Chemother.* 2003 Aug;52(2):308-11.

Sulman FG, Levy D, Lunkan L, Pfeifer Y, Tal E. New methods in the treatment of weather sensitivity. Fortschr Med. 1977 Mar 17;95(11):746-52.

Sulman FG. Migraine and headache due to weather and allied causes and its specific treatment. Ups J Med Sci Suppl. 1980;31:41-4.

Sumantran VN, Kulkarni AA, Harsulkar A, Wele A, Koppikar SJ, Chandwaskar R, Gaire V, Dalvi M, Wagh UV. Hyaluronidase and collagenase inhibitory activities of the herbal formulation Triphala guggulu. *J Biosci.* 2007 Jun;32(4):755-61.

Sumiyoshi M, Sakanaka M, Kimura Y. Effects of Red Ginseng extract on allergic reactions to food in Balb/c mice. *J Ethnopharmacol.* 2010 Aug 14.

Sung JH, Lee JO, Son JK, Park NS, Kim MR, Kim JG, Moon DC. Cytotoxic constituents from Solidago virga-aurea var. gigantea MIQ. *Arch Pharm Res.* 1999 Dec;22(6):633-7.

Suomalainen H, Isolauri E. New concepts of allergy to cow's milk. *Ann Med.* 1994 Aug;26(4):289-96.

Sur S, Camara M, Buchmeier A, Morgan S, Nelson HS. Double-blind trial of pyridoxine (vitamin B6) in the treatment of steroid-dependent asthma. Ann Allergy. 1993 Feb;70(2):147-52.

Sütas Y, Kekki OM, Isolauri E. Late onset reactions to oral food challenge are linked to low serum interleukin-10 concentrations in patients with atopic dermatitis and food allergy. *Clin Exp Allergy.* 2000 Aug;30(8):1121-8.

Suzuki F, Suzuki C, Shimomura E, Maeda H, Fujii T, Ishida N. Antiviral and interferon-inducing activities of a new peptidomannan, KS-2, extracted from culture mycelia of Lentinus edodes. J Antibiot (Tokyo). 1979 Dec;32(12):1336-45.

Suzuki Y, Kondo K, Ichise H, Tsukamoto Y, Urano T, Umemura K. Dietary supplementation with fermented soybeans suppresses intimal thickening. *Nutrition.* 2003 Mar;19(3):261-4.

Svanes C, Heinrich J, Jarvis D, Chinn S, Omenaas E, Gulsvik A, Künzli N, Burney P. Pet-keeping in childhood and adult asthma and hay fever: European community respiratory health survey. *J Allergy Clin Immunol.* 2003 Aug;112(2):289-300.

Svendsen AJ, Holm NV, Kyvik K, *et al.* Relative importance of genetic effects in rheumatoid arthritis: historical cohort study of Danish nationwide twin population. *BMJ* 2002;324(7332): 264-266.

Swale A, Miyajima F, Kolamunnage-Dona R, Roberts P, Little M, Beeching NJ, Beadsworth MB, Liloglou T, Pirmohamed M. Serum Mannose-Binding Lectin Concentration, but Not Genotype, Is Associated With Clostridium difficile Infection Recurrence: A Prospective Cohort Study. Clin Infect Dis. 2014 Nov 15;59(10):1429-36. doi: 10.1093/cid/ciu666.

Sweeney B, Vora M, Ulbricht C, Basch E. Evidence-based systematic review of dandelion (Taraxacum officinale) by natural standard research collaboration. *J Herb Pharmacother.* 2005;5(1):79-93.

Swett. JA. *A Treatise on Disease of the Chest.* New York, 1852.

Swiderska-Kiełbik S, Krakowiak A, Wiszniewska M, Dudek W, Walusiak-Skorupa J, Krawczyk-Szulc P, Michowicz A, Pałczyński C. Health hazards associated with occupational exposure to birds. *Med Pr.* 2010;61(2):213-22.

Swierzko AS, Szala A, Sawicki S, Szemraj J, Sniadecki M, Sokolowska A, Kaluzynski A, Wydra D, Cedzynski M. Mannose-Binding Lectin (MBL) and MBL-associated serine protease-2 (MASP-2) in women with malignant and benign ovarian tumours. Cancer Immunol Immunother. 2014 Nov;63(11):1129-40. doi: 10.1007/s00262-014-1579-y.

Szyf M, McGowan P, Meaney MJ. The social environment and the epigenome. *Environ Mol Mutagen.* 2008 Jan;49(1):46-60.

Szymański H, Chmielarczyk A, Strus M, Pejcz J, Jawień M, Kochan P, Heczko PB. Colonisation of the gastrointestinal tract by probiotic *L. rhamnosus* strains in acute diarrhoea in children. *Dig Liver Dis.* 2006 Dec;38 Suppl 2:S274-6.

Szymański H, Pejcz J, Jawień M, Chmielarczyk A, Strus M, Heczko PB. Treatment of acute infectious diarrhoea in infants and children with a mixture of three *Lactobacillus rhamnosus* strains—a randomized, double-blind, placebo-controlled trial. *Aliment Pharmacol Ther.* 2006 Jan 15;23(2):247-53.

Takada Y, Ichikawa H, Badmaev V, Aggarwal BB. Acetyl-11-keto-beta-boswellic acid potentiates apoptosis, inhibits invasion, and abolishes osteoclastogenesis by suppressing NF-kappa B and NF-kappa B-regulated gene expression. *J Immunol.* 2006 Mar 1;176(5):3127-40.

Takagi A, Ikemura H, Matsuzaki T, Sato M, Nomoto K, Morotomi M, Yokokura T. Relationship between the in vitro response of dendritic cells to *Lactobacillus* and prevention of tumorigenesis in the mouse. *J Gastroenterol.* 2008;43(9):661-9.

Takahashi N, Eisenhuth G, Lee I, Schachtele C, Laible N, Binion S. Nonspecific antibacterial factors in milk from cows immunized with human oral bacterial pathogens. *J Dairy Sci.* 1992 Jul;75(7):1810-20.

Takasaki M, Konoshima T, Tokuda H, Masuda K, Arai Y, Shiojima K, Ageta H. Anti-carcinogenic activity of Taraxacum plant. I. *Biol Pharm Bull.* 1999 Jun;22(6):602-5.

Takebe Y, Saucedo CJ, Lund G, Uenishi R, Hase S, Tsuchiura T, Kneteman N, Ramessar K, Tyrrell DL, Shirakura M, Wakita T, McMahon JB, O'Keefe BR. Antiviral lectins from red and blue-green algae show potent in vitro and in vivo activity against hepatitis C virus. PLoS One. 2013 May 21;8(5):e64449. doi: 10.1371/journal.pone.0064449.

Takeda K, Okumura K. Effects of a fermented milk drink containing *Lactobacillus casei* strain Shirota on the human NK-cell activity. *J Nutr.* 2007 Mar;137(3 Suppl 2):791S-3S.

Takeda K, Suzuki T, Shimada SI, Shida K, Nanno M, Okumura K. Interleukin-12 is involved in the enhancement of human natural killer cell activity by *Lactobacillus casei* Shirota. *Clin Exp Immunol.* 2006 Oct;146(1):109-15.

Tamaoki J, Chiyotani A, Sakai A, Takemura H, Konno K. Effect of menthol vapour on airway hyperresponsiveness in patients with mild asthma. *Respir Med.* 1995 Aug;89(7):503-4.

Tamura M, Shikina T, Morihana T, Hayama M, Kajimoto O, Sakamoto A, Kajimoto Y, Watanabe O, Nonaka C, Shida K, Nanno M. Effects of probiotics on allergic rhinitis induced by Japanese cedar pollen: randomized double-blind, placebo-controlled clinical trial. *Int Arch Allergy Imml.* 2007;143(1):75-82.

Taniguchi C, Homma M, Takano O, Hirano T, Oka K, Aoyagi Y, Niitsuma T, Hayashi T. Pharmacological effects of urinary products obtained after treatment with saiboku-to, a herbal medicine for bronchial asthma, on type IV allergic reaction. *Planta Med.* 2000 Oct;66(7):607-11.

Tapiero H, Ba GN, Couvreur P, Tew KD. Polyunsaturated fatty acids (PUFA) and eicosanoids in human health and pathologies. *Biomed Pharmacother.* 2002 Jul;56(5):215-22.

Tapsell LC, Hemphill I, Cobiac L, Patch CS, Sullivan DR, Fenech M, Roodenrys S, Keogh JB, Clifton PM, Williams PG, Fazio VA, Inge KE. Health benefits of herbs and spices: the past, the present, the future. *Med J Aust.* 2006 Aug 21;185(4 Suppl):S4-24.

Tasli L, Mat C, De Simone C, Yazici H. Lactobacilli lozenges in the management of oral ulcers of Behçet's syndrome. *Clin Exp Rheumatol.* 2006 Sep-Oct;24(5 Suppl 42):S83-6.

Taussig SJ, Batkin S. Bromelain, the enzyme complex of pineapple (Ananas comosus) and its clinical application. An update. *J Ethnopharmacol.* 1988 Feb-Mar;22(2):191-203.

Tavil B, Koksal E, Yalcin SS, Uckan D. Pretransplant nutritional habits and clinical outcome in children undergoing hematopoietic stem cell transplant. Exp Clin Transplant. 2012 Feb;10(1):55-61.

Taylor AL, Dunstan JA, Prescott SL. Probiotic supplementation for the first 6 months of life fails to reduce the risk of atopic dermatitis and increases the risk of allergen sensitization in high-risk children: a randomized controlled trial. *J Allergy Clin Immunol.* 2007 Jan;119(1):184-91.

Taylor AL, Hale J, Wiltschut J, Lehmann H, Dunstan JA, Prescott SL. Effects of probiotic supplementation for the first 6 months of life on allergen- and vaccine-specific immune responses. *Clin Exp Allergy.* 2006 Oct;36(10):1227-35.

Taylor RB, Lindquist N, Kubanek J, Hay ME. Intraspecific variation in palatability and defensive chemistry of brown seaweeds: effects on herbivore fitness. *Oecologia.* 2003 Aug;136(3):412-23.

Teitelbaum J. *From Fatigue to Fantastic.* New York: Avery, 2001.

Teplyakova TV, Psurtseva NV, Kosogova TA, Mazurkova NA, Khanin VA, Vlasenko VA. Antiviral activity of polyporoid mushrooms (higher Basidiomycetes) from Altai Mountains (Russia). Int J Med Mushrooms. 2012;14(1):37-45.

Terheggen-Lagro SW, Khouw IM, Schaafsma A, Wauters EA. Safety of a new extensively hydrolysed formula in children with cow's milk protein allergy: a double blind crossover study. *BMC Pediatr.* 2002 Oct 14;2:10.

Terracciano L, Bouygue GR, Sarratud T, Veglia F, Martelli A, Fiocchi A. Impact of dietary regimen on the duration of cow's milk allergy: a random allocation study. *Clin Exp Allergy.* 2010 Apr;40(4):637-42.

Tesse R, Schieck M, Kabesch M. Asthma and endocrine disorders: Shared mechanisms and genetic pleiotropy. *Mol Cell Endocrinol.* 2010 Dec 4. [ahead of print] .

Tevini M, ed. *UV-B Radiation and Ozone Depletion: Effects on humans, animals, plants, microorganisms and materials.* Boca Raton: Lewis Pub, 1993.

Thakkar K, Boatright RO, Gilger MA, El-Serag HB. Gastroesophageal reflux and asthma in children: a systematic review. *Pediatrics.* 2010 Apr;125(4):e925-30. 2010 Mar 29.

Tham KW, Zuraimi MS, Koh D, Chew FT, Ooi PL. Associations between home dampness and presence of molds with asthma and allergic symptoms among young children in the tropics. *Pediatr Allergy Immunol.* 2007 Aug;18(5):418-24.

Thampithak A, Jaisin Y, Meesarapee B, Chongthammakun S, Piyachaturawat P, Govitrapong P, Supavilai P, Sanvarinda Y. Transcriptional regulation of iNOS and COX-2 by a novel compound from Curcuma comosa in lipopolysaccharide-induced microglial activation. *Neurosci Lett.* 2009 Sep 22;462(2):171-5.

Theler B, Brockow K, Ballmer-Weber BK. Clinical presentation and diagnosis of meat allergy in Switzerland and Southern Germany. *Swiss Med Wkly.* 2009 May 2;139(17-18):264-70.

Theofilopoulos AN, Kono DH: The genes of systemic autoimmunity. *Proc Assoc Am Physicians.* 1999;111(3): 228-240.

Thibault H, Aubert-Jacquin C, Goulet O. Effects of long-term consumption of a fermented infant formula (with *Bifidobacterium breve* c50 and *Streptococcus thermophilus* 065) on acute diarrhea in healthy infants. *J Pediatr Gastroenterol Nutr.* 2004 Aug;39(2):147-52.

Thiruvengadam KV, Haranath K, Sudarsan S, Sekar TS, Rajagopal KR, Zacharian MG, Devarajan TV. Tylophora indica in bronchial asthma (a controlled comparison with a standard anti-asthmatic drug). *J Indian Med Assoc.* 1978 Oct 1;71(7):172-6.

Thomas M. Are breathing exercises an effective strategy for people with asthma? *Nurs Times.* 2009 Mar 17-23;105(10):22-7.

Thomas Y, Schiff M, Belkadi L, Jurgens P, Kahhak L, Benveniste J. Activation of human neutrophils by electronically transmitted phorbol-myristate acetate. *Med Hypoth.* 2000;54: 33-39.

Thomas, R.G., Gebhardt, S.E. 2008. Nutritive value of pomegranate fruit and juice. *Maryland Dietetic Association Annual Meeting, USDA-ARS.* 2008 April 11.

Thompson D. *On Growth and Form.* Cambridge: Cambridge University Press, 1992.

Thompson T, Lee AR, Grace T. Gluten contamination of grains, seeds, and flours in the United States: a pilot study. *J Am Diet Assoc.* 2010 Jun;110(6):937-40.

Tierra L. *The Herbs of Life.* Freedom, CA: Crossing Press, 1992.

Tierra M. *The Way of Herbs.* New York: Pocket Books, 1990.

Tietze H. *Kombucha: The Miracle Fungus.* Gateway Books: Bath, UK, 1995.

Tisserand R. *The Art of Aromatherapy.* New York: Inner Traditions, 1979.

Tiwari M. *Ayurveda: A Life of Balance.* Rochester, VT: Healing Arts, 1995.

Tlaskalová-Hogenová H, Stepánková R, Hudcovic T, Tucková L, Cukrowska B, Lodinová-Zádníková R, Kozáková H, Rossmann P, Bártová J, Sokol D, Funda DP, Borovská D, Reháková Z, Sinkora J, Hofman J, Drastich P, Kokesová A. Commensal bacteria (normal microflora), mucosal immunity and chronic inflammatory and autoimmune diseases. *Immunol Lett.* 2004 May 15;93(2-3):97-108.

Todd GR, Acerini CL, Ross-Russell R, Zahra S, Warner JT, McCance D. Survey of adrenal crisis associated with inhaled corticosteroids in the United Kingdom. *Arch Dis Child.* 2002 Dec;87(6):457-61.

Tonkal AM, Morsy TA. An update review on Commiphora molmol and related species. *J Egypt Soc Parasitol.* 2008 Dec;38(3):763-96.

Topçu G, Erenler R, Cakmak O, Johansson CB, Celik C, Chai HB, Pezzuto JM. Diterpenes from the berries of Juniperus excelsa. *Phytochemistry.* 1999 Apr;50(7):1195-9.

Toppila-Salmi S, Renkonen J, Joenväärä S, Mattila P, Renkonen R. Allergen interactions with epithelium. *Curr Opin Allergy Clin Immunol.* 2011 Feb;11(1):29-32.

Tordesillas L, Pacios LF, Palacín A, Cuesta-Herranz J, Madero M, Díaz-Perales A. Characterization of IgE epitopes of Cuc m 2, the major melon allergen, and their role in cross-reactivity with pollen profilins. *Clin Exp Allergy.* 2010 Jan;40(1):174-81.

Tormo Carnicer R, Infante Piña D, Roselló Mayans E, Bartolomé Comas R. Intake of fermented milk containing *Lactobacillus casei* DN-114 001 and its effect on gut flora. *An Pediatr.* 2006 Nov;65(5):448-53.

Torrent M, Sunyer J, Muñoz L, Cullinan P, Iturriaga MV, Figueroa C, Vall O, Taylor AN, Anto JM. Early-life domestic aeroallergen exposure and IgE sensitization at age 4 years. *J Allergy Clin Immunol.* 2006 Sep;118(3):742-8.

Touhami M, Boudraa G, Mary JY, Soltana R, Desjeux JF. Clinical consequences of replacing milk with yogurt in persistent infantile diarrhea. *Ann Pediatr.* 1992 Feb;39(2):79-86.

Towers GH. FAHF-1 purporting to block peanut-induced anaphylaxis. *J Allergy Clin Immunol.* 2003 May;111(5):1140; author reply 1140-1.

Towle A. *Modern Biology.* Austin: Harcourt Brace, 1993.

Tran HB, Ahern J, Hodge G, Holt P, Dean MM, Reynolds PN, Hodge S. Oxidative stress decreases functional airway mannose binding lectin in COPD. PLoS One. 2014 Jun 5;9(6):e98571. doi: 10.1371/journal.pone.0098571. eCollection 2014.

Trenev N. *Probiotics: Nature's Internal Healers.* New York: Avery, 1998.

Trois L, Cardoso EM, Miura E. Use of probiotics in HIV-infected children: a randomized double-blind controlled study. *J Trop Pediatr.* 2008 Feb;54(1):19-24.

Trojanová I, Rada V, Kokoska L, Vlková E. The bifidogenic effect of Taraxacum officinale root. *Fitoterapia.* 2004 Dec;75(7-8):760-3.

Troncone R, Caputo N, Florio G, Finelli E. Increased intestinal sugar permeability after challenge in children with cow's milk allergy or intolerance. *Allergy.* 1994 Mar;49(3):142-6.

Trout L, King M, Feng W, Inglis SK, Ballard ST. Inhibition of airway liquid secretion and its effect on the physical properties of airway mucus. *Am J Physiol.* 1998 Feb;274(2 Pt 1):L258-63.

Tsai JC, Tsai S, Chang WC. Comparison of two Chinese medical herbs, Huangbai and Qianniuzi, on influence of short circuit current across the rat intestinal epithelia. *J Ethnopharmacol.* 2004 Jul;93(1):21-5.

Tsang KW, Lam CL, Yan C, Mak JC, Ooi GC, Ho JC, Lam B, Man R, Sham JS, Lam WK. Coriolus versicolor polysaccharide peptide slows progression of advanced non-small cell lung cancer. Respir Med. 2003 Jun;97(6):618-24.

Tsang KW, Lam CL, Yan C, Mak JC, Ooi GC, Ho JC, Lam B, Man R, Sham JS, Lam WK. Coriolus versicolor polysaccharide peptide slows progression of advanced non-small cell lung cancer. Respir Med. 2003 Jun;97(6):618-24.

Tsong T. Deciphering the language of cells. *Trends in Biochem Sci.* 1989;14:89-92.

Tsuchiya J, Barreto R, Okura R, Kawakita S, Fesce E, Marotta F. Single-blind follow-up study on the effectiveness of a symbiotic preparation in irritable bowel syndrome. *Chin J Dig Dis.* 2004;5(4):169-74.

Tubelius P, Stan V, Zachrisson A. Increasing work-place healthiness with the probiotic *Lactobacillus reuteri*: a randomised, double-blind placebo-controlled study. *Environ Health.* 2005 Nov 7;4:25.

Tucker KL, Olson B, Bakun P, Dallal GE, Selhub J, Rosenberg IH. Breakfast cereal fortified with folic acid, vitamin B-6, and vitamin B-12 increases vitamin concentrations and reduces homocysteine concentrations: a randomized trial. *Am J Clin Nutr.* 2004 May;79(5):805-11.

Tulk HM, Robinson LE. Modifying the n-6/n-3 polyunsaturated fatty acid ratio of a high-saturated fat challenge does not acutely attenuate postprandial changes in inflammatory markers in men with meta-bolic syndrome. *Metabolism.* 2009 Jul 20.

Tunnicliffe WS, Burge PS, Ayres JG. Effect of domestic concentrations of nitrogen dioxide on airway responses to inhaled allergen in asthmatic patients. *Lancet.* 1994 Dec 24-31;344(8939-8940):1733-6.

Tunnicliffe WS, Fletcher TJ, Hammond K, Roberts K, Custovic A, Simpson A, Woodcock A, Ayres JG. Sensitivity and exposure to indoor allergens in adults with differing asthma severity. *Eur Respir J.* 1999 Mar;13(3):654-9.

Tuomilehto J, Lindström J, Hyyrynen J, Korpela R, Karhunen ML, Mikkola I, Jauhiainen T, Seppo L, Nissinen A. Effect of ingesting sour milk fermented using *Lactobacillus helveticus* bacteria producing tripeptides on blood pressure in subjects with mild hypertension. *J Hum Hypertens.* 2004 Nov;18(11):795-802.

Turchet P, Laurenzano M, Auboiron S, Antoine JM. Effect of fermented milk containing the probiotic *Lactobacillus casei* DN-114001 on winter infections in free-living elderly subjects: a randomised, controlled pilot study. *J Nutr Health Aging.* 2003;7(2):75-7.

Tursi A, Brandimarte G, Giorgetti GM, Elisei W. Mesalazine and/or Lactobacillus casei in maintaining long-term remission of symptomatic uncomplicated diverticular disease of the colon. *Hepatogastroenterology.* 2008 May-Jun;55(84):916-20.

Twetman S, Derawi B, Keller M, Ekstrand K, Yucel-Lindberg T, Stecksen-Blicks C. Short-term effect of chewing gums containing probiotic *Lactobacillus reuteri* on the levels of inflammatory mediators in gingival crevicular fluid. *Acta Odontol Scand.* 2009 Feb;67(1):19-24.

Twum C, Wei Y. The association between urinary concentrations of dichlorophenol pesticides and obesity in children. Rev Environ Health. 2011;26(3):215-9.

U.S. Food and Drug Administration *Guidance for Industry Botanical Drug Products.* CfDEaR. 2000

Uddenfeldt M, Janson C, Lampa E, Leander M, Norbäck D, Larsson L, Rask-Andersen A. High BMI is related to higher incidence of asthma, while a fish and fruit diet is related to a lower- Results from a long-term follow-up study of three age groups in Sweden. *Respir Med.* 2010 Jul;104(7):972-80.

Udupa AL, Udupa SL, Guruswamy MN. The possible site of anti-asthmatic action of Tylophora asthmatica on pituitary-adrenal axis in albino rats. *Planta Med.* 1991 Oct;57(5):409-13.

Ueno H, Yoshioka K, Matsumoto T. Usefulness of the skin index in predicting the outcome of oral challenges in children. *J Investig Allergol Clin Immunol.* 2007;17(4):207-10.

Ueno M, Adachi A, Fukumoto T, Nishitani N, Fujiwara N, Matsuo H, Kohno K, Morita E. Analysis of causative allergen of the patient with baker's asthma and wheat-dependent exercise-induced anaphylaxis (WDEIA). *Arerugi.* 2010 May;59(5):552-7.

Ukabam SO, Mann RJ, Cooper BT. Small intestinal permeability to sugars in patients with atopic eczema. *Br J Dermatol.* 1984 Jun;110(6):649-52.

Ulrich RS, Simons RF, Losito BD, Fiorito E, Miles MA, Zelson M. Stress recovery during exposure to natural and urban environments. J Envir Psychol. 1991;11:201-30.

Une S, Nonaka K, Akiyama J. Lectin Isolated from Japanese Red Sword Beans (Canavalia gladiata) as a Potential Cancer Chemopreventive Agent. J Food Sci. 2018 Feb 13. doi: 10.1111/1750-3841.14057.

Unknown. Proteolytic activity of various lactic acid bacteria. *Japan Jnl Dairy Food Sci.* 1990;39(4).

Unsel M, Sin AZ, Ardeniz O, Erdem N, Ersoy R, Gulbahar O, Mete N, Kokuludağ A. New onset egg allergy in an adult. *J Investig Allergol Clin Immunol.* 2007;17(1):55-8.

Upadhyay AK, Kumar K, Kumar A, Mishra HS. Tinospora cordifolia (Willd.) Hook. f. and Thoms. (Guduchi) - validation of the Ayurvedic pharmacology through experimental and clinical studies. *Int J Ayurveda Res.* 2010 Apr;1(2):112-21.

Urata Y, Yoshida S, Irie Y, Tanigawa T, Amayasu H, Nakabayashi M, Akahori K. Treatment of asthma patients with herbal medicine TJ-96: a randomized controlled trial. *Respir Med.* 2002 Jun;96(6):469-74.

Vakil JR, Shahani KM. Carbohydrate metabolism of lactic acid cultures. V. Lactobionate and gluconate metabolism of *Streptococcus lactis* UN. *J Dairy Sci.* 1969 Dec;52(12):1928-34.

Valeur N, Engel P, Carbajal N, Connolly E, Ladefoged K. Colonization and immunomodulation by *Lactobacillus reuteri* ATCC 55730 in the human gastrointestinal tract. *Appl Environ Microbiol.* 2004 Feb;70(2):1176-81.

Vally H, Thompson PJ, Misso NL. Changes in bronchial hyperresponsiveness following high- and low-sulphite wine challenges in wine-sensitive asthmatic patients. *Clin Exp Allergy.* 2007 Jul;37(7):1062-6.

van Baarlen P, Troost FJ, van Hemert S, van der Meer C, de Vos WM, de Groot PJ, Hooiveld GJ, Brummer RJ, Kleerebezem M. Differential NF-kappaB pathways induction by *Lactobacillus plantarum* in the duodenum of healthy humans correlating with immune tolerance. *Proc Natl Acad Sci U S A.* 2009 Feb 17;106(7):2371-6

van Beelen VA, Roeleveld J, Mooibroek H, Sijtsma L, Bino RJ, Bosch D, Rietjens IM, Alink GM. A comparative study on the effect of algal and fish oil on viability and cell proliferation of Caco-2 cells. *Food Chem Toxicol.* 2007 May;45(5):716-24.

van den Heuvel EG, Schoterman MH, Muijs T. Transgalactooligosaccharides stimulate calcium absorption in postmenopausal women. *J Nutr.* 2000 Dec;130(12):2938-42.

van Elburg RM, Uil JJ, de Monchy JG, Heymans HS. Intestinal permeability in pediatric gastroenterology. *Scand J Gastroenterol Suppl.* 1992;194:19-24.

van Huisstede A, Braunstahl GJ. Obesity and asthma: co-morbidity or causal relationship? *Monaldi Arch Chest Dis.* 2010 Sep;73(3):116-23.

van Kampen V, Merget R, Rabstein S, Sander I, Bruening T, Broding HC, Keller C, Muesken H, Overlack A, Schultze-Werninghaus G, Walusiak J, Raulf-Heimsoth M. Comparison of wheat and rye flour solutions for skin prick testing: a multi-centre study (Stad 1). *Clin Exp Allergy.* 2009 Dec;39(12):1896-902.

van Odijk J, Peterson CG, Ahlstedt S, Bengtsson U, Borres MP, Hulthén L, Magnusson J, Hansson T. Measurements of eosinophil activation before and after food challenges in adults with food hypersensitivity. *Int Arch Allergy Immunol.* 2006;140(4):334-41.

van Zwol A, Moll HA, Fetter WP, van Elburg RM. Glutamine-enriched enteral nutrition in very low birthweight infants and allergic and infectious diseases at 6 years of age. *Paediatr Perinat Epidemiol.* 2011 Jan;25(1):60-6.

Vanderhoof JA. Probiotics in allergy management. J Pediatr Gastroenterol Nutr. 2008 Nov;47 Suppl 2:S38-40.

VanHaitsma TA, Mickleborough T, Stager JM, Koceja DM, Lindley MR, Chapman R. Comparative effects of caffeine and albuterol on the bronchoconstrictor response to exercise in asthmatic athletes. *Int J Sports Med.* 2010 Apr;31(4):231-6.

Vanto T, Helppilä S, Juntunen-Backman K, Kalimo K, Klemola T, Korpela R, Koskinen P. Prediction of the development of tolerance to milk in children with cow's milk hypersensitivity. *J Pediatr.* 2004 Feb;144(2):218-22.

Vargas C, Bustos P, Diaz PV, Amigo H, Rona RJ. Childhood environment and atopic conditions, with emphasis on asthma in a Chilean agricultural area. *J Asthma.* 2008 Jan-Feb;45(1):73-8.

Varonier HS, de Haller J, Schopfer C. Prevalence of allergies in children and adolescents. *Helv Paediatr Acta.* 1984;39:129-136.

Varraso R, Fung TT, Barr RG, Hu FB, Willett W, Camargo CA Jr. Prospective study of dietary patterns and chronic obstructive pulmonary disease among US women. *Am J Clin Nutr.* 2007 Aug;86(2):488-95.

Varraso R, Fung TT, Hu FB, Willett W, Camargo CA. Prospective study of dietary patterns and chronic obstructive pulmonary disease among US men. *Thorax.* 2007 Sep;62(9):786-91. 2007 May 15.

Varraso R, Jiang R, Barr RG, Willett WC, Camargo CA Jr. Prospective study of cured meats consumption and risk of chronic obstructive pulmonary disease in men. *Am J Epidemiol.* 2007 Dec 15;166(12):1438-45. 2007 Sep 4. 17785711; .

Vassallo MF, Banerji A, Rudders SA, Clark S, Mullins RJ, Camargo CA Jr. Season of birth and food allergy in children. *Ann Allergy Asthma Immunol.* 2010 Apr;104(4):307-13.

Vauthier JM, Lluch A, Lecomte E, Artur Y, Herbeth B. Family resemblance in energy and macronutrient intakes: the Stanislas Family Study. *Int J Epidemiol.*1996 Oct;25(5):1030-7.

Vempati R, Bijlani RL, Deepak KK. The efficacy of a comprehensive lifestyle modification programme based on yoga in the management of bronchial asthma: a randomized controlled trial. *BMC Pulm Med.* 2009 Jul 30;9:37.

Vendt N, Grünberg H, Tuure T, Malminiemi O, Wuolijoki E, Tillmann V, Sepp E, Korpela R. Growth during the first 6 months of life in infants using formula enriched with *Lactobacillus rhamnosus* GG: double-blind, randomized trial. *J Hum Nutr Diet.* 2006 Feb;19(1):51-8.

Venkatachalam KV. Human 3'-phosphoadenosine 5'-phosphosulfate (PAPS) synthase: biochemistry, molecular biology and genetic deficiency. *IUBMB Life.* 2003 Jan;55(1):1-11.

Venkatesan N, Punithavathi D, Babu M. Protection from acute and chronic lung diseases by curcumin. *Adv Exp Med Biol.* 2007;595:379-405.

Venter C, Hasan Arshad S, Grundy J, Pereira B, Bernie Clayton C, Voigt K, Higgins B, Dean T. Time trends in the prevalence of peanut allergy: three cohorts of children from the same geographical location in the UK. *Allergy.* 2010 Jan;65(1):103-8.

Venter C, Meyer R. Session 1: Allergic disease: The challenges of managing food hypersensitivity. *Proc Nutr Soc.* 2010 Feb;69(1):11-24.

Ventura MT, Polimeno L, Amoruso AC, Gatti F, Annoscia E, Marinaro M, Di Leo E, Matino MG, Buquicchio R, Bonini S, Tursi A, Francavilla A. Intestinal permeability in patients with adverse reactions to food. *Dig Liver Dis.* 2006 Oct;38(10):732-6.

Venturi A, Gionchetti P, Rizzello F, Johansson R, Zucconi E, Brigidi P, Matteuzzi D, Campieri M. Impact on the composition of the faecal flora by a new probiotic preparation: preliminary data on maintenance treatment of patients with ulcerative colitis. *Aliment Pharmacol Ther.* 1999 Aug;13(8):1103-8.

Verhasselt V. Oral tolerance in neonates: from basics to potential prevention of allergic disease. *Mucosal Immunol.* 2010 Jul;3(4):326-33.

Verstege A, Mehl A, Rolinck-Werninghaus C, Staden U, Nocon M, Beyer K, Niggemann B. The predictive value of the skin prick test weal size for the outcome of oral food challenges. Clin Exp Allergy. 2005 Sep;35(9):1220-6. Rolinck-Werninghaus C, Staden U, Mehl A, Hamelmann E, Beyer K, Niggemann B. Specific oral tolerance induction with food in children: transient or persistent effect on food allergy? *Allergy.* 2005 Oct;60(10):1320-2.

Vidgren HM, Agren JJ, Schwab U, Rissanen T, Hanninen O, Uusitupa MI. Incorporation of n-3 fatty acids into plasma lipid fractions, and erythrocyte membranes and platelets during dietary supplementation with fish, fish oil, and docosahexaenoic acid-rich oil among healthy young men. *Lipids.* 1997 Jul;32(7):697-705.

Viinanen A, Munhbayarlah S, Zevgee T, Narantsetseg L, Naidansuren Ts, Koskenvuo M, Helenius H, Terho EO. Prevalence of asthma, allergic rhinoconjunctivitis and allergic sensitization in Mongolia. *Allergy.* 2005;60:1370-1377.

Vila R, Mundina M, Tomi F, Furlán R, Zacchino S, Casanova J, Cañigueral S. Composition and antifungal activity of the essential oil of Solidago chilensis. *Planta Med.* 2002 Feb;68(2):164-7.

Viljanen M, Kuitunen M, Haahtela T, Juntunen-Backman K, Korpela R, Savilahti E. Probiotic effects on faecal inflammatory markers and on faecal IgA in food allergic atopic eczema/dermatitis syndrome infants. *Pediatr Allergy Immunol.* 2005 Feb;16(1):65-71.

Viljanen M, Savilahti E, Haahtela T, Juntunen-Backman K, Korpela R, Poussa T, Tuure T, Kuitunen M. Probiotics in the treatment of atopic eczema/dermatitis syndrome in infants: a double-blind placebo-controlled trial. *Allergy.* 2005 Apr;60(4):494-500.

Villarruel G, Rubio DM, Lopez F, Cintioni J, Gurevech R, Romero G, Vandenplas Y. *Saccharomyces boulardii* in acute childhood diarrhoea: a randomized, placebo-controlled study. *Acta Paediatr.* 2007 Apr;96(4):538-41.

Vinson JA, Proch J, Bose P. MegaNatural((R)) Gold Grapeseed Extract: In Vitro Antioxidant and In Vivo Human Supplementation Studies. *J Med Food.* 2001 Spring;4(1):17-26.

Visitsunthorn N, Pacharn P, Jirapongsananuruk O, Weeravejsukit S, Sripramong C, Sookrung N, Bunnag C. Comparison between Siriraj mite allergen vaccine and standardized commercial mite vaccine by skin prick testing in normal Thai adults. *Asian Pac J Allergy Immunol.* 2010 Mar;28(1):41-5.

Visness CM, London SJ, Daniels JL, Kaufman JS, Yeatts KB, Siega-Riz AM, Liu AH, Calatroni A, Zeldin DC. Association of obesity with IgE levels and allergy symptoms in children and adolescents: results from the National Health and Nutrition Examination Survey 2005-2006. *J Allergy Clin Immunol.* 2009 May;123(5):1163-9, 1169.e1-4.

Visness CM, London SJ, Daniels JL, Kaufman JS, Yeatts KB, Siega-Riz AM, Calatroni A, Zeldin DC. Association of childhood obesity with atopic and nonatopic asthma: results from the National Health and Nutrition Examination Survey 1999-2006. *J Asthma.* 2010 Sep;47(7):822-9.

Vivatvakin B, Kowitdamrong E. Randomized control trial of live *Lactobacillus acidophilus* plus *Bifidobacterium infantis* in treatment of infantile acute watery diarrhea. *J Med Assoc Thai.* 2006 Sep;89 Suppl 3:S126-33.

Vlieg-Boerstra BJ, Dubois AE, van der Heide S, Bijleveld CM, Wolt-Plompen SA, Oude Elberink JN, Kukler J, Jansen DF, Venter C, Duiverman EJ. Ready-to-use introduction schedules for first exposure to allergenic foods in children at home. *Allergy.* 2008 Jul;63(7):903-9.

Vlieg-Boerstra BJ, van der Heide S, Bijleveld CM, Kukler J, Duiverman EJ, Wolt-Plompen SA, Dubois AE. Dietary assessment in children adhering to a food allergen avoidance diet for allergy prevention. *Eur J Clin Nutr.* 2006 Dec;60(12):1384-90.

Voicekovska JG, Orlikov GA, Karpov IuG, Teibe U, Ivanov AD, Baidekalne I, Voicehovskis NV, Maulins E. External respiration function and quality of life in patients with bronchial asthma in correction of selenium deficiency. *Ter Arkh.* 2007;79(8):38-41.

Voïtsekhovskaia IuG, Skesters A, Orlikov GA, Silova AA, Rusakova NE, Larmane LT, Karpov IuG, Ivanov AD, Maulins E. Assessment of some oxidative stress parameters in bronchial asthma patients beyond add-on selenium supplementation. *Biomed Khim.* 2007 Sep-Oct;53(5):577-84.

Vojdani A. Antibodies as predictors of complex autoimmune diseases. *Int J Immunopathol Pharmacol.* 2008 Apr-Jun;21(2):267-78.

von Berg A, Filipiak-Pittroff B, Krämer U, Link E, Bollrath C, Brockow I, Koletzko S, Grübl A, Heinrich J, Wichmann HE, Bauer CP, Reinhardt D, Berdel D; GINIplus study group. Preventive effect of hydrolyzed infant formulas persists until age 6 years: long-term results from the German Infant Nutritional Intervention Study (GINI). *J Allergy Clin Immunol.* 2008 Jun;121(6):1442-7.

von Berg A, Koletzko S, Grübl A, Filipiak-Pittroff B, Wichmann HE, Bauer CP, Reinhardt D, Berdel D; German Infant Nutritional Intervention Study Group. The effect of hydrolyzed cow's milk formula for allergy prevention in the first year of life: the German Infant Nutritional Intervention Study, a randomized double-blind trial. *J Allergy Clin Immunol.* 2003 Mar;111(3):533-40.

von Kruedener S, Schneider W, Elstner EF. A combination of Populus tremula, Solidago virgaurea and Fraxinus excelsior as an anti-inflammatory and antirheumatic drug. A short review. *Arzneimittelforschung.* 1995 Feb;45(2):169-71.

von Mutius E, Vercelli D. Farm living: effects on childhood asthma and allergy. *Nat Rev Immunol.* 2010 Dec;10(12):861-8. 2010 Nov 9.

Vorup-Jensen T, Sørensen ES, Jensen UB, Schwaeble W, Kawasaki T, Ma Y, Uemura K, Wakamiya N, Suzuki Y, Jensen TG, Takahashi K, Ezekowitz RA, Thiel S, Jensenius JC. Recombinant expression of human mannan-binding lectin. Int Immunopharmacol. 2001 Apr;1(4):677-87.

Vuksan V, Whitham D, Sievenpiper JL, Jenkins AL, Rogovik AL, Bazinet RP, Vidgen E, Hanna A. Supplementation of conventional therapy with the novel grain Salba (Salvia hispanica L.) improves major and emerging cardiovascular risk factors in type 2 diabetes: results of a randomized controlled trial. Diabetes Care. 2007 Nov;30(11):2804-10.

Vulevic J, Drakoularakou A, Yaqoob P, Tzortzis G and Gibson GR; Modulation of the fecal microflora profile and immune function by a novel trans-galactooligosaccharide mixture (B-GOS) in healthy elderly volunteers. *Am J Clin Nutr.* 1988 88;1438-1446.

Waddell L. Food allergies in children: the difference between cow's milk protein allergy and food intolerance. *J Fam Health Care.* 2010;20(3):104.

Wahler D, Gronover CS, Richter C, Foucu F, Twyman RM, Moerschbacher BM, Fischer R, Muth J, Prufer D. Polyphenoloxidase silencing affects latex coagulation in Taraxacum spp. *Plant Physiol.* 2009 Jul 15.

Waite DA, Eyles EF, Tonkin SL, O'Donnell TV. Asthma prevalence in Tokelauan children in two environments. *Clin Allergy.* 1980;10:71-75.

Waked M, Salameh P. Risk factors for asthma and allergic diseases in school children across Lebanon. *J Asthma Allergy.* 2008 Nov 11;2:1-7.

Walders-Abramson N, Wamboldt FS, Curran-Everett D, Zhang L. Encouraging physical activity in pediatric asthma: a case-control study of the wonders of walking (WOW) program. *Pediatr Pulmonol.* 2009 Sep;44(9):909-16.

Walker S, Wing A. Allergies in children. *J Fam Health Care.* 2010;20(1):24-6.

Walker WA. Antigen absorption from the small intestine and gastrointestinal disease. *Pediatr Clin North Am.* 1975 Nov;22(4):731-46.

Walker WA. Antigen handling by the small intestine. *Clin Gastroenterol.* 1986 Jan;15(1):1-20.

Walle UK, Walle T. Transport of the cooked-food mutagen 2-amino-1-methyl-6-phenylimidazo- 4,5-b pyridine (PhIP) across the human intestinal Caco-2 cell monolayer: role of efflux pumps. *Carcinogenesis.* 1999 Nov;20(11):2153-7.

Walsh MG. Toxocara infection and diminished lung function in a nationally representative sample from the United States population. *Int J Parasitol.* 2010 Nov 8.

459

REFERENCES AND BIBLIOGRAPHY

Walsh SJ, Rau LM: Autoimmune diseases: a leading cause of death among young and middle-aged women in the United States. *Am J Public Health* 2000, 90(9): 1463-1466.

Wang G, Liu CT, Wang ZL, Yan CL, Luo FM, Wang L, Li TQ. Effects of Astragalus membranaceus in promoting T-helper cell type 1 polarization and interferon-gamma production by up-regulating T-bet expression in patients with asthma. *Chin J Integr Med.* 2006 Dec;12(4):262-7.

Wang H, Chang B, Wang B. The effect of herbal medicine including astragalus membranaceus (fisch) bge, codonpsis pilosula and glycyrrhiza uralensis fisch on airway responsiveness. *Zhonghua Jie He He Hu Xi Za Zhi.* 1998 May;21(5):287-8.

Wang J, Dong B, Tan Y, Yu S, Bao YX. A study on the immunomodulation of polysaccharopeptide through the TLR4-TIRAP/MAL-MyD88 signaling pathway in PBMCs from breast cancer patients. *Immunopharmacol Immunotoxicol.* 2013 Aug;35(4):497-504. doi: 10.3109/08923973.2013.805764.

Wang J, Lin J, Bardina L, Goldis M, Nowak-Wegrzyn A, Shreffler WG, Sampson HA. Correlation of IgE/IgG4 milk epitopes and affinity of milk-specific IgE antibodies with different phenotypes of clinical milk allergy. *J Allergy Clin Immunol.* 2010 Mar;125(3):695-702, 702.e1-702.e6.

Wang J, Patil SP, Yang N, Ko J, Lee J, Noone S, Sampson HA, Li XM. Safety, tolerability, and immunologic effects of a food allergy herbal formula in food allergic individuals: a randomized, double-blinded, placebo-controlled, dose escalation, phase 1 study. *Ann Allergy Asthma Immunol.* 2010 Jul;105(1):75-84.

Wang J. Management of the patient with multiple food allergies. *Curr Allergy Asthma Rep.* 2010 Jul;10(4):271-7.

Wang JL, Shaw NS, Kao MD. Magnesium deficiency and its lack of association with asthma in Taiwanese elementary school children. *Asia Pac J Clin Nutr.* 2007;16 Suppl 2:579-84.

Wang JS, Hung WP. The effects of a swimming intervention for children with asthma. *Respirology.* 2009 Aug;14(6):838-42.

Wang KY, Li SN, Liu CS, Perng DS, Su YC, Wu DC, Jan CM, Lai CH, Wang TN, Wang WM. Effects of ingesting Lactobacillus- and Bifidobacterium-containing yogurt in subjects with colonized Helicobacter pylori. *Am J Clin Nutr.* 2004 Sep;80(3):737-41.

Wang KY, Li SN, Liu CS, Perng DS, Su YC, Wu DC, Jan CM, Lai CH, Wang TN, Wang WM. Effects of ingesting *Lactobacillus-* and *Bifidobacterium-*containing yogurt in subjects with colonized *Helicobacter pylori.* *Am J Clin Nutr.* 2004 Sep;80(3):737-41.

Wang L, Hou Y. Determination of trace elements in anti-influenza virus mushrooms. Biol Trace Elem Res. 2011 Dec;143(3):1799-807.

Wang YH, Yang CP, Ku MS, Sun HL, Lue KH. Efficacy of nasal irrigation in the treatment of acute sinusitis in children. *Int J Pediatr Otorhinolaryngol.* 2009 Dec;73(12):1696-701. 2009 Sep 27.

Wang YM, Huan GX. *Utilization of Classical Formulas.* Beijing, China: Chinese Medicine and Pharmacology Publishing Co, 1998.

Wangkheirakpam SD, Joshi DD, Leishangthem GD, Biswas D, Deb L. Hepatoprotective Effect of Auricularia delicata mushroom (Agaricomycetes) from India in Rats: Biochemical and Histopathological Studies and Antimicrobial Activity. Int J Med Mushrooms. 2018;20(3):213-225. doi: 10.1615/IntJMedMushrooms.2018025886.

Waring G, Levy D. Challenging adverse reactions in children with food allergies. *Paediatr Nurs.* 2010 Jul;22(6):16-22.

Waser M, Michels KB, Bieli C, Flöistrup H, Pershagen G, von Mutius E, Ege M, Riedler J, Schram-Bijkerk D, Brunekreef B, van Hage M, Lauener R, Braun-Fahrländer C; PARSIFAL Study team. Inverse association of farm milk consumption with asthma and allergy in rural and suburban populations across Europe. *Clin Exp Allergy.* 2007 May;37(5):661-70.

Watkins BA, Hannon K, Ferruzzi M, Li Y. Dietary PUFA and flavonoids as deterrents for environmental pollutants. *J Nutr Biochem.* 2007 Mar;18(3):196-205.

Watson L. *Supernature.* New York: Bantam, 1973.

Watson R. Preedy VR. Botanical Medicine in Clinical Practice. Oxfordshire: CABI, 2008.

Watve MG, Tickoo R, Jog MM, Bhole BD. How many antibiotics are produced by the genus Streptomyces? *Arch Microbiol.* 2001 Nov;176(5):386-90.

Watzl B, Bub A, Blockhaus M, Herbert BM, Lührmann PM, Neuhäuser-Berthold M, Rechkemmer G. Prolonged tomato juice consumption has no effect on cell-mediated immunity of well-nourished elderly men and women. *J Nutr.* 2000 Jul;130(7):1719-23.

Webber CM, England RW. Oral allergy syndrome: a clinical, diagnostic, and therapeutic challenge. *Ann Allergy Asthma Immunol.* 2010 Feb;104(2):101-8; quiz 109-10, 117.

Webster D, Taschereau P, Belland RJ, Sand C, Rennie RP. Antifungal activity of medicinal plant extracts; preliminary screening studies. *J Ethnopharmacol.* 2008 Jan 4;115(1):140-6.

Weekes DJ. Management of Herpes Simplex with Virostatic Bacterial Agent. *EENT Dig.* 1963;25(12).

Weekes DJ. The treatment of aphthous stomatitis with Lactobacillus tablets. *NY State J Med.* 1958 Aug 15;58(16):2672-3.

460

Wegrowski J, Robert AM, Moczar M. The effect of procyanidolic oligomers on the composition of normal and hypercholesterolemic rabbit aortas. *Biochem Pharmacol.* 1984 Nov 1;33(21):3491-7.

Wei A, Shibamoto T. Antioxidant activities and volatile constituents of various essential oils. *J Agric Food Chem.* 2007 Mar 7;55(5):1737-42.

Weiler JM, Layton T, Hunt M. Asthma in United States Olympic athletes who participated in the 1996 Summer Games. J Allergy Clin Immunol. 1998 Nov;102(5):722-6. 7.

Weiner MA. *Secrets of Fijian Medicine.* Berkeley, CA: Univ. of Calif., 1969.

Weisgerber M, Webber K, Meurer J, Danduran M, Berger S, Flores G. Moderate and vigorous exercise programs in children with asthma: safety, parental satisfaction, and asthma outcomes. Pediatr Pulmonol. 2008 Dec;43(12):1175-82.

Weiss RF. *Herbal Medicine.* Gothenburg, Sweden: Beaconsfield, 1988.

Weizman Z, Asli G, Alsheikh A. Effect of a probiotic infant formula on infections in child care centers: comparison of two probiotic agents. *Pediatrics.* 2005 Jan;115(1):5-9.

Wen MC, Huang CK, Srivastava KD, Zhang TF, Schofield B, Sampson HA, Li XM. Ku-Shen (Sophora flavescens Ait), a single Chinese herb, abrogates airway hyperreactivity in a murine model of asthma. *J Allergy Clin Immunol.* 2004;113:218.

Wen MC, Taper A, Srivastava KD, Huang CK, Schofield B, Li XM. Immunology of T cells by the Chinese Herbal Medicine Ling Zhi (Ganoderma lucidum) *J Allergy Clin Immunol.* 2003;111:S320.

Wen MC, Wei CH, Hu ZQ, Srivastava K, Ko J, Xi ST, Mu DZ, Du JB, Li GH, Wallenstein S, Sampson H, Kattan M, Li XM. Efficacy and tolerability of anti-asthma herbal medicine intervention in adult patients with moderate-severe allergic asthma. *J Allergy Clin Immunol.* 2005;116:517-24.

Wenus C, Goll R, Loken EB, Biong AS, Halvorsen DS, Florholmen J. Prevention of antibiotic-associated diarrhoea by a fermented probiotic milk drink. *Eur J Clin Nutr.* 2008 Feb;62(2):299-301.

Werbach M. *Nutritional Influences on Illness.* Tarzana, CA: Third Line Press, 1996.

Wesa KM, Cunningham-Rundles S, Klimek VM, Vertosick E, Coleton MI, Yeung KS, Lin H, Nimer S, Cassileth BR. Maitake mushroom extract in myelodysplastic syndromes (MDS): a phase II study. Cancer Immunol Immunother. 2015 Feb;64(2):237-47. doi: 10.1007/s00262-014-1628-6.

West CE, Hammarström ML, Hernell O. Probiotics during weaning reduce the incidence of eczema. *Pediatr Allergy Immunol.* 2009 Aug;20(5):430-7.

West R. Risk of death in meat and non-meat eaters. *BMJ.* 1994 Oct 8;309(6959):955.

Westerholm-Ormio M, Vaarala O, Tiittanen M, Savilahti E. Infiltration of Foxp3- and Toll-like receptor-4-positive cells in the intestines of children with food allergy. *J Pediatr Gastroenterol Nutr.* 2010 Apr;50(4):367-76.

Wheeler JG, Bogle ML, Shema SJ, Shirrell MA, Stine KC, Pittler AJ, Burks AW, Helm RM. Impact of dietary yogurt on immune function. *Am J Med Sci.* 1997 Feb;313(2):120-3.

Wheeler JG, Shema SJ, Bogle ML, Shirrell MA, Burks AW, Pittler A, Helm RM. Immune and clinical impact of *Lactobacillus acidophilus* on asthma. *Ann Allergy Asthma Immunol.* 1997 Sep;79(3):229-33.

White LB, Foster S. The Herbal Drugstore. Emmaus, PA: Rodale, 2000.

Whitfield KE, Wiggins SA, Belue R, Brandon DT. Genetic and environmental influences on forced expiratory volume in African Americans: the Carolina African-American Twin Study of Aging. *Ethn Dis.* 2004 Spring;14(2):206-11.

WHO. *Guidelines for Drinking-water Quality.* 2nd ed, vol. 2. Geneva: World Health Organization, 1996.

WHO. How trace elements in water contribute to health. *WHO Chronicle.* 1978;32:382-385.

WHO. *INFOSAN Food Allergies. Information Note No. 3.* Geneva, Switzerland: World Health Organization, 2006.

Whorwell PJ, Altringer L, Morel J, Bond Y, Charbonneau D, O'Mahony L, Kiely B, Shanahan F, Quigley EM. Efficacy of an encapsulated probiotic *Bifidobacterium infantis* 35624 in women with irritable bowel syndrome. *Am J Gastroenterol.* 2006 Jul;101(7):1581-90.

Wickens K, Black PN, Stanley TV, Mitchell E, Fitzharris P, Tannock GW, Purdie G, Crane J; Probiotic Study Group. A differential effect of 2 probiotics in the prevention of eczema and atopy: a double-blind, randomized, placebo-controlled trial. *J Allergy Clin Immunol.* 2008 Oct;122(4):788-94.

Widdicombe JG, Ernst E. Clinical cough V: complementary and alternative medicine: therapy of cough. *Handb Exp Pharmacol.* 2009;(187):321-42.

Wildt S, Munck LK, Vinter-Jensen L, Hanse BF, Nordgaard-Lassen I, Christensen S, Avnstroem S, Rasmussen SN, Rumessen JJ. Probiotic treatment of collagenous colitis: a randomized, double-blind, placebo-controlled trial with *Lactobacillus acidophilus* and *Bifidobacterium animalis* subsp. *Lactis. Inflamm Bowel Dis.* 2006 May;12(5):395-401.

Wilkens H, Wilkens JH, Uffmann J, Bövers J, Fröhlich JC, Fabel H. Effect of the platelet-activating factor antagonist BN 52063 on exertional asthma. *Pneumologie.* 1990 Feb;44 Suppl 1:347-8.

Willard T, Jones K. *Reishi Mushroom: Herb of Spiritual Potency and Medical Wonder.* Issaquah, Washington: Sylvan Press, 1990.

Willard T. *Edible and Medicinal Plants of the Rocky Mountains and Neighbouring Territories.* Calgary: 1992.

Willemsen LE, Koetsier MA, Balvers M, Beermann C, Stahl B, van Tol EA. Polyunsaturated fatty acids support epithelial barrier integrity and reduce IL-4 mediated permeability in vitro. *Eur J Nutr.* 2008 Jun;47(4):183-91.

Williams AB, Yu C, Tashima K, Burgess J, Danvers K. Evaluation of two self-care treatments for prevention of vaginal candidiasis in women with HIV. *J Assoc Nurses AIDS Care.* 2001 Jul-Aug;12(4):51-7.

Williams DM. Considerations in the long-term management of asthma in ambulatory patients. *AM J Health Sits Pham.* 2006;63:S14-21.

Wilson D, Evans M, Guthrie N, Sharma P, Baisley J, Schonlau F, Burki C. A randomized, double-blind, placebo-controlled exploratory study to evaluate the potential of pycnogenol for improving allergic rhinitis symptoms. *Phytother Res.* 2010 Aug;24(8):1115-9.

Wilson K, McDowall L, Hodge D, Chetcuti P, Cartledge P. Cow's milk protein allergy. *Community Pract.* 2010 May;83(5):40-1.

Wilson L. *Nutritional Balancing and Hair Mineral Analysis.* Prescott, AZ: LD Wilson, 1998.

Wilson NM, Charette L, Thomson AH, Silverman M. Gastro-oesophageal reflux and childhood asthma: the acid test. *Thorax.* 1985 Aug;40(8):592-7.

Winchester AM. *Biology and its Relation to Mankind.* New York: Van Nostrand Reinhold, 1969.

Winter FS, Emakam F, Kfutwah A, Hermann J, Azabji-Kenfack M, Krawinkel MB. The effect of Arthrospira platensis capsules on CD4 T-cells and antioxidative capacity in a randomized pilot study of adult women infected with human immunodeficiency virus not under HAART in Yaoundé, Cameroon. Nutrients. 2014 Jul 23;6(7):2973-86. doi: 10.3390/nu6072973.

Winther K, Warholm L, Campbell-Tofte J, Marstrand K. Effect of Rosa canina L. (Rose-hip) on cold during winter season in a middle-class population: A randomized, double-blinded, placebo-controlled trial. Journal of Herbal Medicine, Volume 13, September 2018, Pages 34-41.

Wiseman H. Vitamin D is a membrane antioxidant. Ability to inhibit iron-dependent lipid peroxidation in liposomes compared to cholesterol, ergosterol and tamoxifen and relevance to anticancer action. FEBS Lett. 1993 Jul 12;326(1-3):285-8.

Witsell DL, Garrett CG, Yarbrough WG, Dorrestein SP, Drake AF, Weissler MC. Effect of *Lactobacillus acidophilus* on antibiotic-associated gastrointestinal morbidity: a prospective randomized trial. *J Otolaryngol.* 1995 Aug;24(4):230-3.

Wittenberg JS. *The Rebellious Body.* New York: Insight, 1996.

Woessner KM, Simon RA, Stevenson DD. Monosodium glutamate sensitivity in asthma. *J Allergy Clin Immunol.* 1999 Aug;104(2 Pt 1):305-10.

Wöhrl S, Hemmer W, Focke M, Rappersberger K, Jarisch R. Histamine intolerance-like symptoms in healthy volunteers after oral provocation with liquid histamine. *Allergy Asthma Proc.* 2004 Sep-Oct;25(5):305-11.

Wolvers DA, van Herpen-Broekmans WM, Logman MH, van der Wielen RP, Albers R. Effect of a mixture of micronutrients, but not of bovine colostrum concentrate, on immune function parameters in healthy volunteers: a randomized placebo-controlled study. *Nutr J.* 2006 Nov 21;5:28.

Wolverton BC. *How to grow fresh air: 50 houseplants that purify your home or office.* New York: Penguin, 1997.

Wong CK, Bao YX, Wong EL, Leung PC, Fung KP, Lam CW. Immunomodulatory activities of Yunzhi and Danshen in post-treatment breast cancer patients. Am J Chin Med. 2005;33(3):381-95.

Wong GWK, Hui DSC, Chan HH, Fox TF, Leung R, Zhong NS, Chen YZ, Lai CKW. Prevalence of respiratory and atopic disorders in Chinese schoolchildren. *Clinical and Experimental Allergy.* 2001;31:1125-1231.

Wong WM, Lai KC, Lam KF, Hui WM, Hu WH, Lam CL, Xia HH, Huang JQ, Chan CK, Lam SK, Wong BC. Prevalence, clinical spectrum and health care utilization of gastro-oesophageal reflux disease in a Chinese population: a population-based study. *Aliment Pharmacol Ther.* 2003 Sep 15;18(6):595-604.

Wong, W.-L.; Abdulla, M.A.; Chua, K.-H.; Kuppusamy, U.R.; Tan, Y.-S.; Sabaratnam, V. Hepatoprotective effects of Panus giganteus mushroom against thioacetamide (TAA) induced liver injury in rats. Evid. Based Complement. Alternat. Med. 2012, 2012, 170303.

Wood M. *The Book of Herbal Wisdom.* Berkeley, CA: North Atlantic, 1997.

Wood RA, Kraynak J. *Food Allergies for Dummies.* Hoboken, NJ: Wiley Publ, 2007.

Woods RK, Abramson M, Bailey M, Walters EH. International prevalences of reported food allergies and intolerances. Comparisons arising from the European Community Respiratory Health Survey (ECRHS) 1991-1994. *Eur J Clin Nutr* 2001;55:298-304.

Woods RK, Abramson M, Raven JM, Bailey M, Weiner JM, Walters EH. Reported food intolerance and respiratory symptoms in young adults. *Eur Respir J.* 1998;11: 151-155.

Wouters EF, Reynaert NL, Dentener MA, Vernooy JH. Systemic and local inflammation in asthma and chronic obstructive pulmonary disease: is there a connection? *Proc Am Thorac Soc.* 2009 Dec;6(8):638-47.

Wright GR, Howieson S, McSharry C, McMahon AD, Chaudhuri R, Thompson J, Donnelly I, Brooks RG, Lawson A, Jolly L, McAlpine L, King EM, Chapman MD, Wood S, Thomson NC. Effect of improved home ventilation on asthma control and house dust mite allergen levels. *Allergy.* 2009 Nov;64(11):1671-80.

Wright RJ. Epidemiology of stress and asthma: from constricting communities and fragile families to epigenetics. *Immunol Allergy Clin North Am.* 2011 Feb;31(1):19-39.

Wu B, Yu J, Wang Y. Effect of Chinese herbs for tonifying Shen on balance of Th1 /Th2 in children with asthma in remission stage. *Zhongguo Zhong Xi Yi Jie He Za Zhi.* 2007 Feb;27(2):120-2.

Wu Q, Wu K, Ye Y, Dong X, Zhang J. Quorum sensing and its roles in pathogenesis among animal-associated pathogens—a review. *Wei Sheng Wu Xue Bao.* 2009 Jul 4;49(7):853-8.

Xi L, Han DM, Lü XF, Zhang L. Psychological characteristics in patients with allergic rhinitis and its associated factors analysis.. *Zhonghua Er Bi Yan Hou Tou Jing Wai Ke Za Zhi.* 2009 Dec;44(12):982-5.

Xiao JZ, Kondo S, Takahashi N, Miyaji K, Oshida K, Hiramatsu A, Iwatsuki K, Kokubo S, Hosono A. Effects of milk products fermented by *Bifidobacterium longum* on blood lipids in rats and healthy adult male volunteers. *J Dairy Sci.* 2003 Jul;86(7):2452-61.

Xiao JZ, Kondo S, Yanagisawa N, Miyaji K, Enomoto K, Sakoda T, Iwatsuki K, Enomoto T. Clinical efficacy of probiotic *Bifidobacterium longum* for the treatment of symptoms of Japanese cedar pollen allergy in subjects evaluated in an environmental exposure unit. *Allergol Int.* 2007 Mar;56(1):67-75.

Xiao JZ, Kondo S, Yanagisawa N, Takahashi N, Odamaki T, Iwabuchi N, Miyaji K, Iwatsuki K, Togashi H, Enomoto K, Enomoto T. Probiotics in the treatment of Japanese cedar pollinosis: a double-blind placebo-controlled trial. *Clin Exp Allergy.* 2006 Nov;36(11):1425-35.

Xiao JZ, Kondo S, Yanagisawa N, Takahashi N, Odamaki T, Iwabuchi N, Iwatsuki K, Kokubo S, Togashi H, Enomoto K, Enomoto T. Effect of probiotic *Bifidobacterium longum* BB536 in relieving clinical symptoms and modulating plasma cytokine levels of Japanese cedar pollinosis during the pollen season. A randomized double-blind, placebo-controlled trial. *J Investig Allergol Clin Immunol.* 2006;16(2):86-93.

Xiao P, Kubo H, Ohsawa M, Higashiyama K, Nagase H, Yan YN, Li JS, Kamei J, Ohmiya S. kappa-Opioid receptor-mediated antinociceptive effects of stereoisomers and derivatives of (+)-matrine in mice. *Planta Med.* 1999 Apr;65(3):230-3.

Xiao SD, Zhang DZ, Lu H, Jiang SH, Liu HY, Wang GS, Xu GM, Zhang ZB, Lin GJ, Wang GL. Multicenter, randomized, controlled trial of heat-killed *Lactobacillus acidophilus* LB in patients with chronic diarrhea. *Adv Ther.* 2003 Sep-Oct;20(5):253-60.

Xie JY, Dong JC, Gong ZH. Effects on herba epimedii and radix Astragali on tumor necrosis factor-alpha and nuclear factor-kappa B in asthmatic rats. *Zhongguo Zhong Xi Yi Jie He Za Zhi.* 2006 Aug;26(8):723-7.

Xu X, Zhang D, Zhang H, Wolters PJ, Killeen NP, Sullivan BM, Locksley RM, Lowell CA, Caughey GH. Neutrophil histamine contributes to inflammation in mycoplasma pneumonia. *J Exp Med.* 2006 Dec 25;203(13):2907-17.

Xu Y, Na L, Ren Z, Xu J, Sun C, Smith D, Meydani SN, Wu D. Effect of dietary supplementation with white button mushrooms on host resistance to influenza infection and immune function in mice. Br J Nutr. 2012 Jul 11:1-10.

Xu Z, Zheng G, Wang Y, Zhang C, Yu J, Teng F, Lv H, Cheng X. Aqueous Huaier Extract Suppresses Gastric Cancer Metastasis and Epithelial to Mesenchymal Transition by Targeting Twist. J Cancer. 2017 Oct 19;8(18):3876-3886. doi: 10.7150/jca.20380.

Yadav H, Jain S, Sinha PR. Antidiabetic effect of probiotic dahl containing *Lactobacillus acidophilus* and *Lactobacillus casei* in high fructose fed rats. *Nutrition.* 2007 Jan;23(1):62-8.

Yadav N, Chandra H. Suppression of inflammatory and infection responses in lung macrophages by eucalyptus oil and its constituent 1,8-cineole: Role of pattern recognition receptors TREM-1 and NLRP3, the MAP kinase regulator MKP-1, and NFκB. PLoS One. 2017 Nov 15;12(11):e0188232. doi:10.1371/journal.pone.0188232.

Yadav RK, Ray RB, Vempati R, Bijlani RL. Effect of a comprehensive yoga-based lifestyle modification program on lipid peroxidation. *Indian J Physiol Pharmacol.* 2005 Jul-Sep;49(3):358-62.

Yadav VS, Mishra KP, Singh DP, Mehrotra S, Singh VK. Immunomodulatory effects of curcumin. *Immunopharmacol Immunotoxicol.* 2005;27(3):485-97.

Yadzir ZH, Misnan R, Abdullah N, Bakhtiar F, Arip M, Murad S. Identification of Ige-binding proteins of raw and cooked extracts of Loligo edulis (white squid). *Southeast Asian J Trop Med Public Health.* 2010 May;41(3):653-9.

Yamamura S, Morishima H, Kumano-go T, Suganuma N, Matsumoto H, Adachi H, Sigedo Y, Mikami A, Kai T, Masuyama A, Takano T, Sugita Y, Takeda M. The effect of *Lactobacillus helveticus* fermented milk on sleep and health perception in elderly subjects. *Eur J Clin Nutr.* 2009 Jan;63(1):100-5.

Yang A, Zhao Y, Wang Y, Zha X, Zhao Y, Tu P, Hu Z. Huaier suppresses proliferative potential of prostate cancer PC3 cells via downregulation of Lamin B1 and induction of autophagy. Oncol Rep. 2018 Apr 5. doi: 10.3892/or.2018.6358.

Yang AL, Hu ZD, Tu PF. Research progress on anti-tumor effect of Huaier. Zhongguo Zhong Yao Za Zhi. 2015 Dec;40(24):4805-10.

Yang D, Li S, Wang H, Li X, Liu S, Han W, Hao J, Zhang H. Prevention of postoperative recurrence of bladder cancer: a clinical study. Zhonghua Wai Ke Za Zhi. 1999 Aug;37(8):464-5.

Yang DA, Li SQ, Li XT. [Prophylactic effects of zhuling and BCG on postoperative recurrence of bladder cancer]. Zhonghua Wai Ke Za Zhi. 1994 Jul;32(7):433-4.

Yang Z. Are peanut allergies a concern for using peanut-based formulated foods in developing countries? Food Nutr Bull. 2010 Jun;31(2 Suppl):S147-53.

Yasuda T, Takeyama Y, Ueda T, Shinzeki M, Sawa H, Nakajima T, Kuroda Y. Breakdown of Intestinal Mucosa Via Accelerated Apoptosis Increases Intestinal Permeability in Experimental Severe Acute Pancreatitis. J Surg Res. 2006 Apr 4.

Ye X, Zhou X, Wong LY, Calafat AM. Concentrations of Bisphenol A and Seven Other Phenols in Pooled Sera from 3-11 Year Old Children: 2001-2002 National Health and Nutrition Examination Survey. Environ Sci Technol. 2012 Oct 26.

Yeager S. The Doctor's Book of Food Remedies. Emmaus, PA: Rodale Press, 1998.

Yeager S. The Doctor's Book of Food Remedies. Emmaus, PA: Rodale Press, 1998.

Yeh CC, Lin CC, Wang SD, Chen YS, Su BH, Kao ST. Protective and anti-inflammatory effect of a traditional Chinese medicine, Xia-Bai-San, by modulating lung local cytokine in a murine model of acute lung injury. Int Immunopharmacol. 2006 Sep;6(9):1506-14.

Yin B, Liu W, Yu P, Liu C, Chen Y, Duan X, Liao Z, Chen Y, Wang X, Pan X, Tao Z. Association between human papillomavirus and prostate cancer: A meta-analysis. Oncol Lett. 2017 Aug;14(2):1855-1865. doi: 10.3892/ol.2017.6367.

Yonekura S, Okamoto Y, Okawa T, Hisamitsu M, Chazono H, Kobayashi K, Sakurai D, Horiguchi S, Hanazawa T. Effects of daily intake of Lactobacillus paracasei strain KW3110 on Japanese cedar pollinosis. Allergy Asthma Proc. 2009 Jul-Aug;30(4):397-405.

Yu K, Li B, Zhang T. Direct rapid analysis of multiple PPCPs in municipal wastewater using ultrahigh performance liquid chromatography-tandem mass spectrometry without SPE pre-concentration. Anal Chim Acta. 2012 Aug 13;738:59-68. doi: 10.1016/j.aca.2012.05.057.

Yu L, Zhang Y, Chen C, Cui HF, Yan XK. Meta-analysis on randomized controlled clinical trials of acupuncture for asthma. Zhongguo Zhen Jiu. 2010 Sep;30(9):787-92.

Yu LC. The epithelial gatekeeper against food allergy. Pediatr Neonatol. 2009 Dec;50(6):247-54.

Yusoff NA, Hampton SM, Dickerson JW, Morgan JB. The effects of exclusion of dietary egg and milk in the management of asthmatic children: a pilot study. J R Soc Promot Health. 2004 Mar;124(2):74-80.

Zambrano E. [The transgenerational mechanisms in developmental programming of metabolic diseases]. Rev Invest Clin. 2009 Jan-Feb;61(1):41-52.

Zanjanian MH. The intestine in allergic diseases. Ann Allergy. 1976 Sep;37(3):208-18.

Zarate G, Gonzalez S, Chaia AP. Assessing survival of dairy propionibacteria in gastrointestinal conditions and adherence to intestinal epithelia. Centro de Referencia para Lactobacilos-CONICET. Tucuman, Argentina: Humana Press. 2004.

Zarkadas M, Scott FW, Salminen J, Ham Pong A. Common Allergenic Foods and Their Labelling in Canada. Can J Allergy Clin Immun. 1999; 4:118-141.

Zeiger RS, Heller S. The development and prediction of atopy in high-risk children: follow-up at age seven years in a prospective randomized study of combined maternal and infant food allergen avoidance. J Allergy Clin Immunol. 1995 Jun;95(6):1179-90.

Zeng J, Li YQ, Zuo XL, Zhen YB, Yang J, Liu CH. Clinical trial: effect of active lactic acid bacteria on mucosal barrier function in patients with diarrhoea-predominant irritable bowel syndrome. Aliment Pharmacol Ther. 2008 Oct 15;28(8):994-1002.

Zhang CS, Yang AW, Zhang AL, Fu WB, Thien FU, Lewith G, Xue CC. Ear-acupressure for allergic rhinitis: a systematic review. Clin Otolaryngol. 2010 Feb;35(1):6-12.

Zhang M, Cheung PC, Ooi VE, Zhang L. Evaluation of sulfated fungal beta-glucans from the sclerotium of Pleurotus tuber-regium as a potential water-soluble anti-viral agent. Carbohydr Res. 2004 Sep 13;339(13):2297-301.

Zhang T, Srivastava K, Wen MC, Yang N, Cao J, Busse P, Birmingham N, Goldfarb J, Li XM. Pharmacology and immunological actions of a herbal medicine ASHMI on allergic asthma. Phytother Res. 2010 Jul;24(7):1047-55.

Zhang Z, Lai HJ, Roberg KA, Gangnon RE, Evans MD, Anderson EL, Pappas TE, Dasilva DF, Tisler CJ, Salazar LP, Gern JE, Lemanske RF Jr. Early childhood weight status in relation to asthma development in high-risk children. J Allergy Clin Immunol. 2010 Dec;126(6):1157-62. 2010 Nov 4.

Zhao FD, Dong JC, Xie JY. Effects of Chinese herbs for replenishing shen and strengthening qi on some indexes of neuro-endocrino-immune network in asthmatic rats. Zhongguo Zhong Xi Yi Jie He Za Zhi. 2007 Aug;27(8):715-9.

Zhao HY, Wang HJ, Lu Z, Xu SZ. Intestinal microflora in patients with liver cirrhosis. Chin J Dig Dis. 2004;5(2):64-7.

Zhao J, Bai J, Shen K, Xiang L, Huang S, Chen A, Huang Y, Wang J, Ye R. Self-reported prevalence of childhood allergic diseases in three cities of China: a multicenter study. *BMC Public Health*. 2010 Sep 13;10:551.

Zheng M. Experimental study of 472 herbs with antiviral action against the herpes simplex virus. *Zhong Xi Yi Jie He Za Zhi*. 1990 Jan;10(1):39-41, 6.

Zhong K, Tong L, Liu L, Zhou X, Liu X, Zhang Q, Zhou S. Immunoregulatory and antitumor activity of schizophyllan under ultrasonic treatment. Int J Biol Macromol. 2015 Sep;80:302-8. doi: 10.1016/j.ijbiomac.2015.06.052.

Zhou Q, Zhang B, Verne GN. Intestinal membrane permeability and hypersensitivity in the irritable bowel syndrome. *Pain*. 2009 Nov;146(1-2):41-6.

Zhu DD, Zhu XW, Jiang XD, Dong Z. Thymic stromal lymphopoietin expression is increased in nasal epithelial cells of patients with mugwort pollen sensitive-seasonal allergic rhinitis. *Chin Med J (Engl)*. 2009 Oct 5;122(19):2303-7.

Zhu HH, Chen YP, Yu JE, Wu M, Li Z. Therapeutic effect of Xincang Decoction on chronic airway inflammation in children with bronchial asthma in remission stage. *Zhong Xi Yi Jie He Xue Bao*. 2005 Jan;3(1):23-7.

Ziaei Kajbaf T, Asar S, Alipoor MR. Relationship between obesity and asthma symptoms among children in Ahvaz, Iran:A cross sectional study. *Ital J Pediatr*. 2011 Jan 6;37(1):1.

Zielen S, Kardos P, Madonini E. Steroid-sparing effects with allergen-specific immunotherapy in children with asthma: a randomized controlled trial. *J Allergy Clin Immunol*. 2010 Nov;126(5):942-9. 2010 Jul 10.

Ziemniak W. Efficacy of *Helicobacter pylori* eradication taking into account its resistance to antibiotics. *J Physiol Pharmacol*. 2006 Sep;57 Suppl 3:123-41.

Ziment I, Tashkin DP. Alternative medicine for allergy and asthma. *J Allergy Clin Immunol*. 2000 Oct;106(4):603-14.

Ziment I. Alternative therapies for asthma. *Curr Opin Pulm Med*. 1997 Jan;3(1):61-71.

Zizza, C. The nutrient content of the Italian food supply 1961-1992. *Euro J Clin Nutr*. 1997;51: 259-265.

Zoccatelli G, Pokoj S, Foetisch K, Bartra J, Valero A, Del Mar San Miguel-Moncin M, Vieths S, Scheurer S. Identification and characterization of the major allergen of green bean (Phaseolus vulgaris) as a non-specific lipid transfer protein (Pha v 3). *Mol Immunol*. 2010 Apr;47(7-8):1561-8.

Zwolińska-Wcisło M, Brzozowski T, Mach T, Budak A, Trojanowska D, Konturek PC, Pajdo R, Drozdowicz D, Kwiecień S. Are probiotics effective in the treatment of fungal colonization of the gastrointestinal tract? Experimental and clinical studies. *J Physiol Pharmacol*. 2006 Nov;57 Suppl 9:35-49.

Index

www.ingramcontent.com/pod-product-compliance
Lightning Source LLC
Chambersburg PA
CBHW071532200326
41519CB00021BB/6452

* 9 7 8 1 9 3 6 2 5 1 4 4 5 *